BASIC MECHANISMS
IN HEARING

ACADEMIC PRESS RAPID MANUSCRIPT REPRODUCTION

*Proceedings of the
First Royal Swedish Academy of Sciences Symposium
Held October 30 - November 1, 1972
at the Academy, Stockholm, Sweden*

BASIC MECHANISMS IN HEARING

EDITED BY

AAGE R. MØLLER

Division of Physiological Acoustics
Department of Physiology
Karolinska Institute
Stockholm, Sweden

ASSISTANT EDITOR

PAMELA BOSTON

Department of Environmental Hygiene
Karolinska Institute
Stockholm, Sweden

ACADEMIC PRESS, INC. New York and London 1973

A Subsidiary of Harcourt Brace Jovanovich, Publishers

COPYRIGHT © 1973, BY ACADEMIC PRESS, INC.
ALL RIGHTS RESERVED.
NO PART OF THIS PUBLICATION MAY BE REPRODUCED OR
TRANSMITTED IN ANY FORM OR BY ANY MEANS, ELECTRONIC
OR MECHANICAL, INCLUDING PHOTOCOPY, RECORDING, OR ANY
INFORMATION STORAGE AND RETRIEVAL SYSTEM, WITHOUT
PERMISSION IN WRITING FROM THE PUBLISHER.

ACADEMIC PRESS, INC.
111 Fifth Avenue, New York, New York 10003

United Kingdom Edition published by
ACADEMIC PRESS, INC. (LONDON) LTD.
24/28 Oval Road, London NW1

Library of Congress Cataloging in Publication Data
Main entry under title:

Basic mechanisms in hearing.

  Proceedings of the 1st Royal Swedish Academy of Sciences symposium, held Oct. 30–Nov. 1, 1972, at the Academy, Stockholm.
  1. Hearing–Congresses. 2. Cochlea–Congresses.
3. Neurophysiology–Congresses.   I. Møller, Aage R., Date ed. II. Boston, Pamela, ed. III. Svenska vetenskapsakademien, Stockholm.
QP460.B37   612'.85   73-14701
ISBN 0–12–504250–7

PRINTED IN THE UNITED STATES OF AMERICA

CONTENTS

CONTRIBUTORS ix
PREFACE xi

Introduction: v. Békésy 1
    H. Davis

I. COCHLEAR MECHANICS

Cochlear Nonlinearities 11
    Juergen Tonndorf

An Investigation of Post-Mortem
Cochlear Mechanics Using the Mössbauer Effect 49
    William S. Rhode

A Possibility for Sub-Tectorial Membrane Fluid Motion . . 69
    C. R. Steele

Observations of the Mechanical Disturbances
along the Basilar Membrane with Laser Illumination . . . 95
    L. U. E. Kohllöffel

Concluding Remarks 119
    Jozef J. Zwislocki

II. COCHLEAR MORPHOLOGY

The Normal Organ of Corti 125
    C. Angelborg and H. Engström

The Innervation of the Cochlear Receptor 185
    H. Spoendlin

Problems and Pitfalls in Studies of Cochlear Hair Cell Pathology 235
    Jan Wersäll

III. COCHLEAR PHYSIOLOGY

The Cocktail Hour before the Serious Banquet 259
    H. Davis

The Physiology of Individual Hair Cells and Their Synapses 273
  Åke Flock, Mørup Jørgensen, and Ian Russell

The Ionic Receptive Mechanism in the Acoustico-Lateralis System 307
  Yasuji Katsuki

Cochlear Potentials and Cochlear Mechanics 335
  Peter J. Dallos

Neuropharmacology and Potentials of the Inner Ear 377
  Jörgen Fex

Inner Ear Potentials in
Lower Vertebrates: Dependence on Metabolism. 423
  J. Schwartzkopff

IV. NEURAL CODING AT LOWER LEVELS

Stimulus Coding at Caudal Levels of the Cat's Auditory
Nervous System: I. Response Characteristics of Single Units 455
  N. Y. S. Kiang, D. K. Morest, D. A. Godfrey, J. J. Guinan, Jr.,
  and E. C. Kane

Stimulus Coding at Caudal Levels of the Cat's
Auditory Nervous System: II. Patterns of Synaptic Organization 479
  D. K. Morest, N. Y. S. Kiang, E. C. Kane, J. J. Guinan, Jr., and
  D. A. Godfrey

Studies of Phase-Locked Cochlear Output in Cells
of the Anteroventral Nucleus in the Cochlear Complex of the Cat 511
  J. E. Rose, M. M. Gibson, L. M. Kitzes, and J. E. Hind

The Frequency Selectivity of the Cochlea 519
  E. F. Evans and J. P. Wilson

Considerations of Nonlinear Response
Properties of Single Cochlear Nerve Fibers 555
  Russell R. Pfeiffer and Duck On Kim

Coding of Amplitude Modulated
Sounds in the Cochlear Nucleus of the Rat 593
  Aage R. Møller

V. NEURAL CODING AT HIGHER LEVELS

Time Dependent Features of Adequate Sound Stimuli
and the Functional Organization of Central Auditory Neurons 623
  G. V. Gersuni and I. A. Vartanian

Feature Extraction in the Auditory System of Bats 675
  Nobuo Suga

Patterns of Activity of Single Neurons of the Auditory Cortex in Monkey   745
  John F. Brugge and Michael M. Merzenich

Efferent Crossed Inhibition in the Ventral Cochlear Nuclei 773
  R. Pfalz

VI. PSYCHOACOUSTICS

In Search of Physiological Correlates of Psychoacoustic Characteristics   787
  Jozef J. Zwislocki

Temporal Effects in Psychoacoustical Excitation 809
  E. Zwicker

Minimum Integration Time 829
  David M. Green

VII. SPECIALIZED HEARING IN ANIMALS

Echolocation 849
  Donald R. Griffin

Function of the Swimbladder in Fish Hearing 893
  Olav Sand and Per Stockfelth Enger

The Mechanics of the Locust Ear: An Invertebrate Frequency Analyzer .   911
  Axel Michelsen

SUBJECT INDEX 935

CONTRIBUTORS

John F. Brugge, Laboratory of Neurophysiology, 283 Medical Sciences Building, The University of Wisconsin, Madison, Wisconsin 53706

Peter J. Dallos, Auditory Research Laboratory, Speech Annex Building, Northwestern University, Evanston, Illinois 60201

H. Davis, Central Institute for the Deaf, 818 South Euclid, St. Louis, Missouri 63110

Per Stockfelth Enger, Zoofysiologisk Institutt, Universitetet i Oslo, Postboks 1051, Blindern, Oslo 3, Norway

H. Engström, Oronkliniken, Akademiska Sjukhuset, Fack, 750 14 Uppsala 14, Sweden

E. F. Evans, Department of Communication, Unversity of Keele, Keele, Staffordshire ST5 5BG, England

Jörgen Fex, Center of Neural Sciences, Indiana University, Bloomington, Indiana 47401

Åke Flock, Gustaf 5:s Forskningsinstitut, Karolinska Sjukhuset, 104 01 Stockholm 60, Sweden

G. V. Gersuni, Sechenov Institute of Evolutionary Physiology and Biochemistry of the Academy of Sciences of the USSR, Avenue Torez 52, Leningrad K 223, USSR

David M. Green, Department of Psychology, University of California at San Diego, P. O. Box 109, La Jolla, California 92037

Donald R. Griffin, Rockefeller University, York Avenue and 66th Street, New York, New York 10021

Yasuji Katsuki, Department of Physiology, Tsurumi Women's University, School of Dental Medicine, 84 Tsurumi, Tsurumi-Ku, Yokahama, 230, Japan

N. Y. S. Kiang, Massachusetts Eye and Ear Infirmary, 243 Charles Street, Boston, Massachusetts 02114

CONTRIBUTORS

L. U. E. Kohllöffel, Massachusetts Eye and Ear Infirmary, 243 Charles Street, Boston, Massachusetts 02114

Axel Michelsen, Department of Biology, Odense University, Odense, Denmark

Aage R. Møller, Division of Physiological Acoustics, Fysiologiska Institutionen II, Karolinska Institutet, 104 01 Stockholm 60, Sweden

Habil R. Pfalz, Universität ULM, Abt. für HNO-Heilkunde, D-79 ULM, West Germany

Russell R. Pfeiffer, School of Engineering and Applied Sciences, Washington University, St. Louis, Missouri 63130

William S. Rhode, Laboratory of Neurophysiology, Medical School, 283 Medical Sciences Building, The University of Wisconsin, Madison, Wisconsin 53706

J. E. Rose, Laboratory of Neurophysiology, 283 Medical Sciences Building, The University of Wisconsin, Madison, Wisconsin 53706

J. Schwartzkopff, Lehrstuhl für Allgemeine Zoologie, Ruhr-Universität Bochum, Postfach 2148, 463 Bochum-Querenburg, West Germany

H. Spoendlin, ORL Klinik, Kantonsspital, Rämistrasse 100, 8000 Zürich, Switzerland

C. R. Steele, Department of Aeronautics on Astronautics, Stanford University, Stanford, California 94305

Nobuo Suga, Department of Biology, Washington University, St. Louis, Missouri 63130

Juergen Tonndorf, Department of Otolaryngology, College of Physicians and Surgeons, Columbia University, 630 West 168th Street, New York, New York 10032

Jan Wersäll, Gustaf 5:s Forskningsinstitut, Karolinska Sjukhuset, 104 01 Stockholm 60, Sweden

E. Zwicker, Institutes für Elektroakustik der Techn. Hochschule, Franz-Joseph-Strasse 38, 8000 München, West Germany

Jozef J. Zwislocki, Laboratory of Sensory Communication, Syracuse University, New York 13210

PREFACE

The study of the function of the auditory system has advanced rapidly during the past decade or so. New techniques have made it possible to probe the vibration of the basilar membrane in anesthetized animals at physiological sound levels, and recording with microelectrodes from single nerve cells has come into common practice. Recent developments in computer techniques allow elaborate statistical analysis of the recorded discharge pattern of single elements in the nervous system. The intimate correlation of physiology with anatomy and experimental psychology during the past decade has been a great step forward; we have today a much better knowledge about the function of the periphery of the auditory system than we had only a few years ago.

The multidisciplinary nature of auditory research is subject to the problem that researchers in these diverging fields seldom meet at congresses and symposia. The objective of the symposium BASIC MECHANISMS IN HEARING was therefore to create a form under which a multidisciplinary representation could be realized. Those invited were asked to present their new results. Perhaps more importantly, they could analyze each others' results in an unusually broad perspective and examine hypotheses pertaining to the various complex functions in the auditory system.

The present volume comprises the papers presented at the symposium and the edited discussions following the oral presentations. The result is a broad analysis of the present knowledge of the function of the auditory system covering ultrastructure, physiology and experimental psychology.

Many people have contributed to the preparation of this volume. Lisbeth Magnusson performed the major part of the exacting task of typing to suit the camera-ready method. I am also indebted to Annikki Ahlqvist, Carina Erickson, Ingrid Møller, and Karin Stenbäck for their contributions.

I am pleased to express my gratitude to the participants of the symposium for their excellent cooperation and for their submitting of the manuscripts so promptly.

The symposium as well as the preparation of this volume was sponsored by the Swedish Medical Research Council (Grant 51S-3935), the Natural Science Research Council and by the Royal Swedish Academy of Sciences.

Aage R. Møller

BASIC MECHANISMS IN HEARING

INTRODUCTION: v. BÉKÉSY

Prof. H. Davis

Central Institute for the Deaf
St. Louis, Missouri
USA

In the original plan of this symposium on Basic Mechanisms in Hearing it was intended that an introductory lecture be given by the Nobel laureate in hearing (1961), Georg von Békésy. However, as you all know, Prof. v. Békésy died on 13 June 1972. It is appropriate that we do him honor here today, because of his profound influence on the development of auditory biophysics, physiology and psychoacoustics during the last forty years.

Georg von Békésy was a solitary genius. He never married and he had few intimate friends. It is amazing how great an influence he exerted through the sheer force of his experimental skill and his insight, without students and without collaborators, and rarely appearing in public even to lecture. He made his measurements and his observations over and over again and then wrote out what he did and what he saw and gave us a few samples of representative data and curves. No statistics whatever, but meticulous measurements and brilliant stimulating ideas.

v. Békésy was originally and primarily a physicist. As an investigator he was imaginative, ingenious, precise, immensely patient, and single-minded. He was a master of the art of devising new and special tools such as drills and micro-manipulators for special tasks. He became a legend in his own lifetime. Foremost among his many contributions to otology, to auditory physiology and to psycho-physics are his epoch-making descriptions, based on physical measurements and visual observation, of the traveling-wave pattern of vibration of the basilar membrane and the relation of the location and extent of this pattern to the acoustic frequency. The basis of the pattern he elucidated in terms of physical concepts such as sound pressures, transfer functions, phase differences, and the acoustic damping and the graded stiffness of the basilar membrane. In this way he set the style of auditory biophysics and auditory theory for a generation.

With his Spartan way of life and his intense devotion to his laboratory only a few of his friends were aware of v. Békésy's intense appreciation of art, particularly music and the visual arts. His remarkable memory made him an authority in several curious specialties such as mediaeval time-pieces. It is rumored that when he was invited to address a scientific symposium or congress his first consideration for acceptance was the presence in the host city of a first rate art museum that he had not yet visited to his heart's content.

Archeological art was the special hobby which both refreshed and stimulated his mind when he was not actively engaged in laboratory experiments. He decorated the walls of his laboratory with choice specimens of exotic oriental art, and over the years he gathered a very fine personal collection. Fortunately he was persuaded to exhibit some of the items and expound some of his ideas about them in a motion-picture lecture entitled "Concerning originality and success in science and in art". The film was made less than a year before v. Békésy's death, under the auspices of the Los Angeles Otologic Foundation. It is v. Békésy himself who is the narrator, and it is a beautiful and impressive record of his face, his voice, his style, his art treasures and his philosophy. It is his final development of ideas that he introduced in his Nobel oration here in Stockholm.

I knew v. Békésy personally but not intimately, and I am sure that he would prefer that I say no more about him but speak about his work and his influence. This I shall do, but in a very personal way by emphasizing the influence that v. Békésy had on me and my own thinking, including some errors in evaluation on my part which I wish to correct in retrospect.

Remember that v. Békésy began his scientific career in hearing as a physicist in the Post-Office department of Hungary. This is an implausible beginning,

but remember that the Post-Office department included
the national telephone and telegraph systems, and v.
Békésy had the rocponsibility of improving the telephones. He was the counterpart of Harvoy Fletcher and
all the rest of the Bell Telephone Laboratories in
the U.S.A. I have heard him say that the reason he
started to study the ear was to be sure that it would
be worth the time and money to improve telephones. If
the ear were no better as an acoustic instrument than
a telephone (of 1925) it would be wasteful to try to
make the telephone still better. He soon satisfied
himself that the ear was far superior; so good in
fact that he was fascinated to try to discover just
how nature did such an amazing job of acoustical
engineering.

He attacked the problem in two ways. One was to open
the cochlea and observe directly the movements of the
cochlear partition; the other was to construct and
study models of the cochlea partition and the columns
of fluid above and below it. Both methods yielded the
famous traveling-wave pattern, first described in
1928. Closely following this was a study of auditory
localization, done in order to determine the "group
velocity" of waves traveling along the cochlea in response to a click.

Then came the era of his study of transfer functions
in the ear, of establishing equivalence of air and
bone conduction, further experiments in psychoacoustics, on cochlear hydrodynamics, and on room acoustics.

A simple experiment of this period was one that v.
Békésy regarded with particular pride. This was his
demonstration that the basilar membrane at rest is
not under tension, as had been assumed since the days
of Helmholtz. The necessary equipment was a drill to
open the cochlea, a microscope, a tiny knife and a
set of fine glass fibers (or human hairs). When a
slit was cut in the basilar membrane, either longitudinally or transversely, the edges did not retract.
When gentle local pressure was exerted with one of
the fibers the depression was broad and circular. The
conclusion was the same: symmetry and no tension. The
next steps in the development were to replace the
hypothesis of transverse tension with the concept of
graded volume elasticity: and to measure it.

v. Békésy's publications were in German, many of them in an obscure acoustical journal. I believe we all of us owe a great debt to my colleague S. Smith Stevens of Harvard who came upon these papers, recognized their quality and importance, visited v. Békésy in Budapest in 1937, incorporated many of his data and ideas in our book, <u>Hearing</u> (1939), and later arranged for v. Békésy to settle permanently at Harvard (1947) after a memorable interlude here in Stockholm.

v. Békésy did his work on middle ear and cochlear mechanics without high-speed movies, computers, lasers or Mössbauer effects. These restrictions forced him to emphasize high sound intensities and low frequencies. We shall hear this morning of some of the superstructure that has been built on Békésy's foundations and of certain corrections and important additions. At the time I accepted v. Békésy's data as the best available and built my own thinking around the traveling wave on the basilar membrane, eddies in the perilymph and endolymph, and the crude but fundamental frequency analysis of the basilar membrane. I was concerned about the sharper frequency analysis revealed by psychoacoustics (recognized from the start by v. Békésy) and by our own first response-areas of single auditory neurons (Galambos and Davis, 1942). I took comfort, however, in v. Békésy's vague analogy to Mach's law of contrast and what we now call "lateral inhibition". I thought that his reliance on a "nerve network like that in the skin" was much too optimistic, and I still do. The problem of "sharpening" is still with us, and I believe the innervation and interactions in the ear are much more complex than those in the skin. About all this we shall hear much more this afternoon.

To return to cochlear mechanics; neither v. Békésy nor any of the rest of us recognized the great importance of nonlinearity in the ear. I assumed that the eddies were important at low intensities until Juergen Tonndorf taught me better; and I accepted the details of v. Békésy's description of the complex movements of the organ of Corti, until I realized that my generalizations were in conflict with the principle of directional sensitivity in relation to the orientation of the pattern of cilia on the hair cells, - as established by Drs. Engström, Wersäll, Flock and other good friends.

v. Békésy made some startling calculations, on the basis of his acoustic and microscopic measurements, and he extrapolated an estimate of the amplitude of movement of the basilar membrane at the most sensitive human threshold level. The result was "less than one percent of the diameter of the hydrogen atom". I have often shown Békésy's graph to students and have republished it in books, but I always kept my tongue in cheek and omitted v. Békésy's words "one percent of". I think that because of nonlinearities his extrapolations are in error by two or three orders of magnitude: but even so the amplitude of movement is uncomfortably small for anyone who attempts to make a model of how bending the cilia initiates a chemical reaction or modifies the permeability of a membrane to ions. v. Békésy was not concerned with such models: he "hewed to his line and let the chips fall where they might".

I wonder now to what extent nonlinearity of the ear and lack of spatial resolution of our tools of observation may have concealed a less damped resonance and a sharper response pattern than the classical Békésy envelope of displacement of the cochlear partition. This we shall learn more about in a few moments. It will be a great intellectual relief if we can finally say that the sharpness of neural tuning is physically determined in the organ of Corti. But, beware, I say, of wishful thinking!

Let me jump here to the final chapter of v. Békésy's work, the subject of Sensory Inhibition. This work is psycho-physics, done with v. Békésy's well known ingenuity of experimentation and directness of argument and exposition. His ideas will appear implicitly in the presentations tomorrow concerning the central nervous system. The principle of suppression of some sensory information to obtain better contrast, discrimination or localization seems to apply to all sensory systems. It is worth recalling how v. Békésy turned to this idea very early in order to reconcile his observations of the movements of the basilar membrane with the data of psycho-acoustics, and for him auditory theory meant practically the theory of frequency discrimination.

Now a brief salute to v. Békésy's immortal contribution to otology and psycho-acoustics, the patient-controlled recording audiometer, developed here in Stockholm. One of my medical professors once told our class that the easiest way to achieve immortality in medicine is to contrive a new position in which to place the patient for physical examination. In audiology and psycho-acoustics it is to invent a new test and the instrument with which to perform it. Békésy's name will remain immortal in the Békésy audiometer, (but in U.S.A. it will be spelled without accents). His audiometer is now a standard and very useful instrument in the clinic and an indispensable tool in psycho-acoustics for the study of changing auditory sensitivity as in fatigue or temporary threshold shift.

v. Békésy came closest to biology in his morphological and electrical studies of the cochlea. For me the live dissection of the tectorial membrane, the description of its physical properties and the attachment to it of cilia of the hair cells were particularly important. He also discovered the positive dc polarization of the scala media. This curious phenomenon brings us to the area of metabolism, chemistry, and the physiological response of sensory cells. v. Békésy by-passed the problem of excitation, but he was aware of it. v. Békésy also showed that the electrical response to displacement of the tectorial membrane was related to amplitude, not to the velocity, of the displacement and to its direction, and that the electrical energy released in the ear could be greater than the energy applied in the stimulus. These are three very fundamental propositions for the theory of mechano-electrical or mechano-chemical neural transductions, - although I shudder when I think of the nonlinear distortions involved in some of the experiments with his vibrating electrode.

v. Békésy's influence lives on, as evidenced by the acknowledgement in a paper dealing with the increase in mechano-excitability in free neuromasts and pit organs of various fish and amphibia caused by high potassium concentration in the medium. I hope that Dr. Katsuki will tell us about this phenomenon this afternoon; but his acknowledgement (JASA, Aug. 1972) reads: "The authors express their thanks to Dr. G. von Békésy for invaluable advice". How many ideas Georg von Békésy has suggested indirectly to all the rest of us! We honor him as the posthumous patron of this symposium.

Acknowledgement

The preparation of this manuscript was supported by Grant NS 03856 from the National Institute of Neurological Diseases and Stroke.

I
COCHLEAR MECHANICS

COCHLEAR NONLINEARITIES

Juergen Tonndorf

Columbia University
New York, N.Y.
U.S.A.

Implicit in Békésy's description of the cochlear traveling waves (1928) was the notion that they represent an <u>interface</u> phenomenon between two non-mixing bodies of fluid that are separated by an elastic partition. Interface waves are closely related to surface waves, and the latter are known for their pronounced nonlinearities. This point was first made by Zwislocki (1948) with respect to the problem of cochlear mechanics. The most obvious nonlinearity is given by Békésy's eddies which, being rectified events, are nonlinear phenomena by definition. When I began (1957) studying cochlear hydrodynamics in physical models, nonlinear phenomena were bound to turn up sooner or later. The first such observations were reported in 1958.

It seems strange today that cochlear nonlinearities did not receive more attention until such a late date. One reason may lie in the fact that Helmholtz's concept of localized mechanical resonances in the cochlea did not really leave room for nonlinearities. The cochlea was considered a linear transducer, and this long-standing opinion was not immediately affected by Békésy's discovery. Another reason for the general reluctance to abandon the concept of cochlear linearity might have been associated with the difficulties involved in the mathematical analysis of non-linear phenomena. They had to be solved by linear approximations. Thus, there was neither much awareness nor interest in nonlinearities. Today, of course, it is realized that there are very few, if any, events in which nonlinearities do not play an important role.

From time to time, some evidence has actually been presented that was not compatible with the assumption of cochlear linearity. One may recall the well-known controversy between Stumpf and Helmholtz concerning the origin of complex aural beats ("mistuned consonances"). Helmholtz (1863) refuted Stumpf's argument by claiming that the primary signals were probably distorted, and that such distortion could account for the observed beat rate. Ultimately, i.e., after Helmholtz's death, Stumpf (1910) was able to show that his signals were free of distortion; yet, his subjects clearly perceived complex beats. As an alternative, Helmholtz had considered the possibility that the nonlinearities might arise in the middle ear. Lewis and Reger (1933) showed that subjects that were deprived of their middle ears were able to perceive beats and combination tones as well as persons with intact middle ears - that is, provided one took their hearing losses into account. Thus, the distortion could not arise in the middle ear either. In fact, as was shown more recently (Guinan and Peake, 1967), the middle ear has a remarkably wide dynamic range. Apparently, the only type of nonlinearity that occurs here at physiological levels is the generation of subharmonics (Dallos and Linnell, 1966).

Nonlinearities also appear in the electrical cochlear responses. As far as I am aware of, the first record of a nonlinear cochlear microphonic response was presented by Wever and Bray (1938), the waveform of a beat that was clearly asymmetrical. This finding suggests once more a cochlear origin. By now, there is a voluminous literature on the subject, and the cochlear microphonic generators have been considered a primary source of the observed nonlinearities (e.g., Engebretson and Eldredge, 1968, Dallos and Sweetman, 1969). This notion was aided by the observation made on vestibular hair cells by Lowenstein and Wersäll (1959), i.e., that the degree of electrical depolarization caused by displacements of the sensory hairs toward the kinocilium (the basal body of the cochlear hair cells) is larger than that of the hyperpolarization caused by displacements of equal magnitude but of opposite sign.

The effects of nonlinearities that occur somewhere at lower stations manifest themselves in phenomena observable in the first order neuron (Goblick and

Pfeiffer, 1969, Goldstein and Kiang, 1968). Since the middle ear can be safely excluded as a source, they point once more to a cochlear origin.

The present paper will assess cochlear nonlinearities of _hydrodynamic_ origin. However, this does not imply that _all_ cochlear nonlinearities are of this kind. The evidence concerning the cochlear microphonic generators has just been mentioned.

At the time these studies were originally undertaken (1958-1962), _physical_ models appeared to be the only ones suited for such investigations. They are least abstract so that even phenomena whose parameters are not well understood beforehand may be approached with some chance of success. Today, this type of reasoning may no longer be valid. First of all, much progress has been made in recent years in the mathematical approach to problems involving nonlinear phenomena. Secondly, the data obtained in the earlier studies on physical models make it now possible to set up more general mathematical models.

Physical models have the advantage of displaying complex dynamic events _in toto_, alleviating the necessity of _post-hoc_, piecemeal reconstruction. They can be modified systematically, although not as easily as mathematical models. Their weak point is scaling. However, this must not be considered a major drawback when one is interested in principles of operation, and dimensional analysis may be applied in such cases (Tonndorf, 1960).

At this point, some hydrodynamic principles must be introduced that are essential for the discussion at hand. More extensive treatments may be found in Kinsman (1965) and Batchelor (1967). Lamb (1879) is still a valuable source book in spite of its age, and a brief account by von Kármán (1954) should also be mentioned.

As was already stated, interface waves occur along elastic boundaries between two bodies of fluid. If one fluid is replaced by a gas, one speaks of surface waves. Although, in first approximation, these gases behave very much like fluids, the densities on the two sides of the boundary often differ by several orders of magnitude so that the presence of the gas may be altogether disregarded.

The present discussion will be limited to surface waves, since they have been more extensively studied. There are a number of different types, the two most common ones being: (A) (longer) _gravity_ waves, in which gravity represents the surface-restoring force, and (B) (shorter) _capillary_ waves, in which this role is played by surface tension. The two types are often referred to as Gerstner-Rankine waves or Rayleigh waves respectively. In a given situation, the dividing line is a matter of wavelength; in the case of an air/water boundary, the critical wavelength is $\lambda = 1.73$ cm, a point that is well-defined by different characteristics of the two types of waves. For example, in capillary waves, the speed of propagation decreases with wavelength; in gravity waves, it increases again. At the critical wavelength, the speed is minimal.

With distance of travel, short waves are dissipated faster than long waves. The water surface acts as a spatially-distributed low-pass filter system.

However, this is not the only reason why short waves vanish with time and distance of travel. In contrast to other propagating waves, such as sound waves, for example, the speed of surface waves traveling on open water increases with distance - and so does the wavelength - while the wave height decreases. Consequently, tidal waves, so called "tsunamis", which are caused by submarine earthquakes, for example, may reach very high speeds, while their diminishing heights make them hard to spot. This latter change has nothing to do with energy dissipation. It represents a mere exchange between potential and kinetic energy - wave height and travel speed respectively. Witness tsunamis when they encounter shallow water. The process reverses itself; they are slowed down, i.e., the wavelength becomes shorter, and their height increases once more. However, when waves become steeper, they become increasingly unstable, the limit being a height-to-length ratio of 1:7. As soon as this limit is exceeded, waves begin to break. The entire phenomenon is known as _surf_. It should be noted that, superimposed upon the ac wave motion, there is a closed-loop, dc stream, moving forward along the surface and returning along the bottom,

the well-known undertow. It is this movement that
contributes to the breaking of waves.

The surface of open water is considered a dispersive
medium for reasons of the two properties just described: (a) the dependence of travel speed on wavelength
and (b) the increase of travel speed (and wavelength)

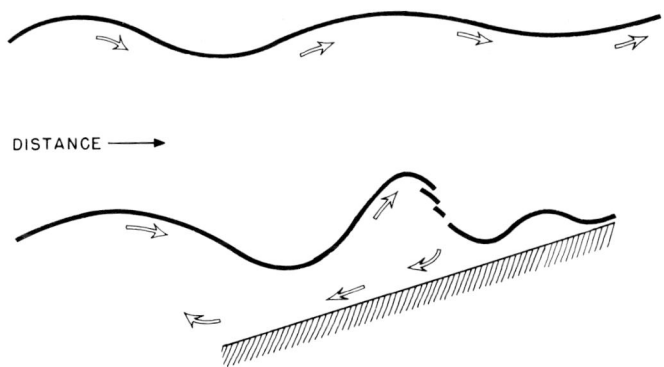

Fig. 1   Progression of surface waves (highly schematic). In open water (top portion), wavelength
and propagation velocity increase with distance of travel, while wave height decreases.
(The rate of exchange is grossly overstated
here for the sake of illustration.) --

Against a sloping bottom (lower portion),
velocity is slowed down cumulatively, and
wavelength decreases in a like manner, while
wave height increases. Waves become unstable,
i.e., they break, when a certain height-to-
length ratio (1:7) is exceeded. Breaking is
aided by the action of an eddy current (arrows), going inward with the crests along the
surface and outward along the bottom. Expressed differently, the sloping bottom represents a delay line; i.e., as soon as the
point is reached at which the diminishing
pass band does no longer contain the frequency of the waves in question, they become attenuated. -- Note that in both drawings waveforms are assumed to be sinusoidal (for
their correct shape cf. Fig. 2).

with distance of travel. By definition then, wave motion in surf is non-dispersive. Fig. 1 compares the wave motion in open water and in surf. The similarities between surf and the cochlear event were described earlier (Tonndorf, 1956).

With respect to the present discussion, fluids must be regarded as being incompressible. Therefore, surface waves entail a peculiar type of particle motion that does not require changes in density. It is made possible by a characteristic property of fluids, i.e., by the fact that their particles can slide past one another. In other words, there is a shearing motion. The mode of particle motion of surface waves is known as trochoidal, i.e., "rolling" (Fig. 2a). As long as no dc motion is superimposed, particles travel along closed orbits which represent a combination of longitudinal and transversal displacements, with the transversal component leading the other one by a phase angle of 90° (insert Fig. 2a). These orbits represent Lissajous figures and can be reconstructed as such. A given particle completes one orbit with each passing wave, moving forward with its crest and returning in its trough.

Because of the incompressibility of fluids, the trochoidal particle motion cannot be limited to the surface layer. In deep open water, the magnitude of the orbits, which are then circular in shape, decreases exponentially with depth, indicating a gradual dissipation of energy (Fig. 2a).

When the water is shallow, specifically when the depth <1/2 λ (Fig. 2b), the energy cannot be fully dissipated over such a limited range, but there can be no vertical components immediately close to the bottom. Thus, along the bottom, only the horizontal components exist. However, even along the surface, the effects of the bottom make themselves felt in that the orbits are elliptical in shape. With depth, only the vertical components decrease in size.

Although the displacements of particles along their individual orbits may be perfectly sinusoidal, the spatial waveform is not so (Fig. 2). Crests are sharper and troughs wider. This is especially so in shallow-water waves. (Theoretically, the crests should be cusp-like. However, in most cases, band-

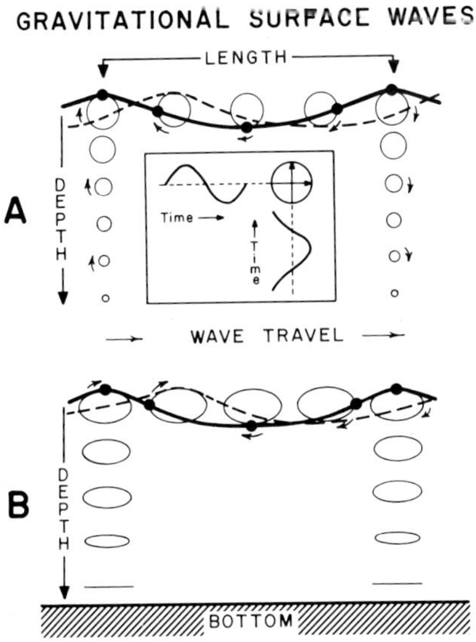

GRAVITATIONAL SURFACE WAVES

Fig. 2 Lagrangian presentation of surface waves which includes pathways of particle motion: (a) in deep water; (b) in shallow water of constant depth. (This is contrasted by the Eulerain presentation which demonstrates the flow field.) Waves propagate from left to right, i.e., the solid outline precedes the dashed one by 1/2 π. Note the waveform asymmetry in both top and bottom figures. This distortion is due to the mode of fluid particle motion. The latter is a resultant of the two displacement vectors that are $90°$ apart in phase (cf. insert), with the transversal vector leading the longitudinal one. Particles revolve along closed orbits as indicated by small arrows, and this mode of motion is known as <u>trochoidal</u>. In deep water, particle orbits decrease exponentially with depth (top figure), whereas in shallow water, the decline is limited to that of the transversal vectors (bottom figure) (from Tonndorf, 1970).

width limitations give them the rounded-off appearance of Fig. 2). This latter nonlinearity is a direct corollary of the trochoidal fluid motion. That is, it is the position of particles at both zero-crossings that makes the crests sharper and the troughs wider. This type of nonlinearity was already recognized by Strutt, Lord Rayleigh (1877) and by Lamb (1879) in their formulations of the classical equations describing surface waves.

Particle motion in capillary waves is essentially the same as that in gravity waves. Nevertheless, when channel dimensions become small, another boundary effect -- in addition to surface tension -- makes itself felt, i.e., that of the so called <u>boundary layer</u>. As with surface tension, its origin is due to molecular forces. Above surfaces, particle density is so small that the molecules of the top fluid layer attract each other, forming a tension in the place of the surface. In contrast, the molecules of the first fluid layer along a wall are in strong mutual attraction with those across the interface. Thus, when a stream of fluid goes by, these particles remain "glued" to their respective sites and cannot participate in the streaming motion. Fluid particles were said to be capable of slipping past one another. Such slippage is opposed by the inherent friction of the fluid, i.e., by its <u>viscosity</u>. Starting at the wall where motion was said to be zero, there is a certain amount of slippage between each sublayer and the next one so that a <u>gradient</u> of <u>velocity</u> is formed that ranges from zero along the wall ("no-slip" condition) to that of the "free" fluid stream where motion is uniform. The thickness of this boundary layer, and thus the steepness of the velocity gradient, varies with inverse viscosity. In a laminar dc flow, then, viscosity is effective only in the boundary layer but not in the free system. The slippage between particles forms a shearing stress that is highest directly at the wall and diminishes gradually with distance.

An ac fluid motion, such as the trochoidal motion of capillary surface waves, is also affected by the shearing stresses within the boundary layer. However, as the trochoidal motion is not limited to the boundary layer proper, this effect extends well beyond it. This point will presently be illustrated by cochlear model findings.

The events in cochlear models will be discussed in two sections: (1) those observed at amplitudes below the onset of Békésy's eddies and (2) those associated with the eddy motion. The eddy is, of course, the equivalent of the undertow found in surf. It is doubtful that surf can develop without an undertow. In the cochlea, however, where viscous damping plays a much bigger role, the onset of eddy motion is a well-marked event, and, at lower magnitudes, there are traveling waves without eddies.

Although the present models were five times the size of a human cochlea, and consequently, the wavelengths in response to low-frequency signals were quite long, the traveling waves were found to be independent of gravity (Tonndorf, 1960). Thus, by definition, they are capillary waves, or expressed differently, the restoring force is entirely determined by the elastic properties of the partition.

Wave propagation was of the non-dispersive kind for the following three reasons: (a) As is typically seen in Békésy-type waves, wavelength and speed of progression decrease monotonically with distance along the partition; (b) in response to complex signals, all component-frequencies travel with the same speed, although their relative magnitude changes with distance on account of the low-pass filter action along the cochlear partition; and (c) the particle orbits within the cochlear fluids are of the kind found in shallow water (Fig. 3).

With distance along the partition, the transversal components of particle motion showed precisely the same amplitude changes as the traveling wave, i.e., their envelopes were identical (Fig. 3). The longitudinal components decreased monotonically in amplitude, once more over the range of the traveling-wave envelope.

As is the case with all traveling waves (cf. Fig. 2), the cumulative phase shift of the cochlear traveling wave with distance along the partition (Békésy, 1947) affected both components of particle motion in the same manner. That is to say, the phase difference between the two components remained at a value of approximately $90°$ all along the partition, except for some small deviations around the places of maximal

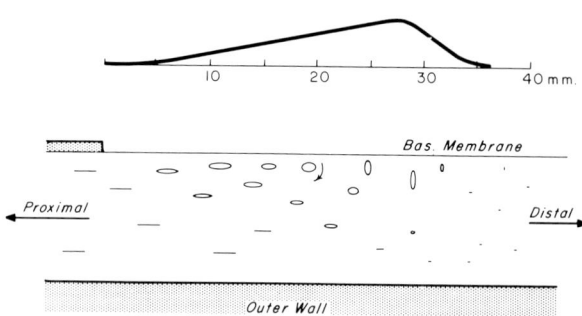

Fig. 3 Trochoidal fluid particle motion in one scala of a cochlear model in response to a sinusoidal input (schematic). Particles revolve along their orbits in the manner of surface (or interface) waves (see arrow in midsection). The longitudinal vectors decrease monotonically with distance. The decrement of the transversal vectors with depth is indicative of shallow-water waves. The build-up and subsequent decline of the transversal vectors with distance duplicates the envelope over the traveling waves: see figure on top in which amplitude is grossly overstated. The displacement of the partition is omitted from the lower graph (from Tonndorf, 1970).

displacement. These will be described later (cf. Fig. 11 below).

The phase relation between particles facing each other across the partition was 180° at every instant of time (Fig. 4). This finding is consistent with the general notion that fluid motions in the perilymphatics scalae are in phase opposition. The situations labelled 0° and 180° in Fig. 4 require some special comments. At both of these instances, displacements of the partition are zero, but the particles on either side are in their positions of maximal horizontal displacement which happen to be opposite to each other. The comparable situation in surface waves (cf. Fig. 2) has led to a nonlinear distortion of the spatial waveform. In the cochlear interface waves, however, the effects of the fluid particles on either side of the partition should cancel each other on account of their opposite posi-

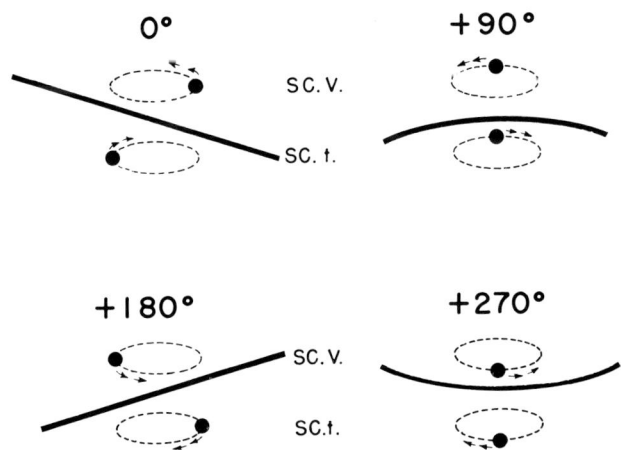

Fig. 4 Particle displacements along their respective orbits on both sides of the cochlear partition at four separate instances of time: sinusoidal input signal; direction of particle movement given by arrows; windows on the left; the displacement of the partition at each instance is schematically indicated. To realize the full waveform, Fig. 2 should be consulted (adapted from Tonndorf, 1959b).

tions. Indeed, at first glance the waveform of the traveling waves in response to sinusoidal inputs appeared to be quasi-sinusoidal, i.e., if one disregarded the characteristic changes Békésy-waves undergo with distance of travel. Nevertheless, it is suggested by Fig. 4 that, at the instant the partition passes through its resting position, considerable shearing stresses should be brought about between the partition and the adjacent fluids of the boundary layers on either side.

Decisions on linearity should not be left to mere inspection. A check for intermodulation distortion constitutes a more reliable test. Significantly, electrical cochlear analogs, the Peterson-Bogert model (1959), for example, are known to react linearly in such situations. That is to say, a delay line, that consists of linear elements, is essentially a linear device, in spite of the waveform changes with distance of travel.

In physical cochlear models, intermodulation distortion was seen to occur. Nevertheless, some of the findings could be fully explained on the basis of linear superposition.

Most of the data cited in the following stemmed from experiments involving beat signals. However, other signals, such as tone pips, missing fundamentals, etc., were also employed. Although the others were not studied in the same detail, the overall results were essentially the same in all cases.

In response to beat signal (imperfect unison, best beats), the traveling waves, i.e., their apparent frequency and maximum displacement, correspond to the average of the two primaries, $1/2 (f_1 + f_2)$. Its instantaneous amplitude waxed and waned with the beat rate, $f_1 - f_2$, ranging from zero to twice the amplitude occurring in response to one of the primaries alone. Moreover, when one of the primaries exceeded the other in magnitude, the amplitude fluctuations became smaller, and a synchronous frequency modulation of a small degree was noted that included appropriate shifts in the place of maximal displacement. This frequency modulation followed exactly the rules given by Helmholtz (1863).

All of these events follow from the rules of linear superposition. In fact, they were no different from what can be seen on an oscilloscope screen under comparable conditions. There was one important exception: The amplitude of the traveling wave was asymmetrical, i.e., displacements of the partition toward scala tympani were consistently larger than those toward scala vestibuli.

Since the present models were not quite symmetrically built -- one scala was slightly larger than the other -- it was checked if this structural asymmetry might not be the cause of the asymmetrical displacement observed. This was not the case.

The asymmetry of the cochlear response could best be observed and measured in the fluid particle motion.

The mode of beating of particle orbits is illustrated
in Fig. 5. A given orbit was seen to wax and wane
with the beat rate. However, in doing so, it did not
expand and contract equally in all directions as in
Fig. 5a. Rather, both vectors changed their size in
an asymmetrical fashion, i.e., the apparent centers
of a given orbit at the instant of minimal size and
at that of full expansion did not coincide with each
other. There was a shift both along the longitudinal
and transversal axes (Fig. 5b). Particles facing each
other across the partition displayed this asymmetry
in a push-pull manner. In scala vestibuli, orbital
expansions were invariably larger toward the cochlear
apex and toward the partition than in the opposite
directions, while in scala tympani the signs were
reversed (Fig. 5c).

At a given place of observation, the degree of the
asymmetrical beat response did not vary with the in-

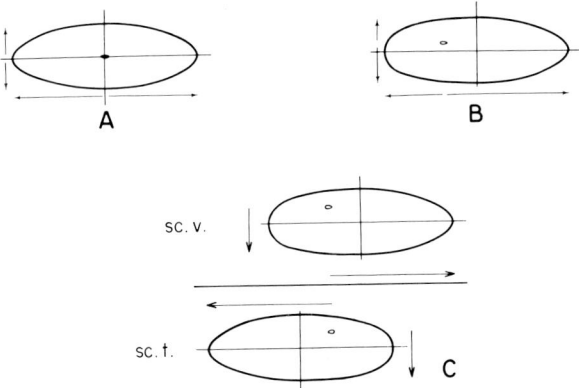

Fig. 5   Particle orbits in response to simple beats.
The larger orbits represent the instant of
the beat maximum and the smaller ones inside
them that of the minimum. (A) Symmetrical
beat motion; (B) asymmetrical beat motion as
actually observed in the model; (C) across
the partition, the asymmetrical beat motion
occurred in a phase opposite manner. In scala
vestibuli, orbital expansions were invariably
larger toward the helicotrema and toward the
partition; in scala tympani, opposite directions prevailed (from Tonndorf, 1959a).

tensity of the applied signal. In other words, it was an amplitude-independent event.

It is realized from the push-pull type of asymmetrical beat responses illustrated in Fig. 5c that the beat rate had manifested itself as a new component that contained energy. Progressing in the direction of the cochlear apex, its amplitude became larger, a finding that was to be expected on account of its small frequency value. When the beat rate was sufficiently high in frequency, it was seen to form a traveling wave of its own.

That this was a true process of demodulation or envelope detection became clear from observations on complex beats. The newly generated low-frequency component always corresponded to the periodicity of the envelope. It should also be mentioned that the visual detectability of the asymmetrical beat motion in the model varied with the complexity of the beating signal in the same manner (although not to exactly the same degree) as had been observed by Helmholtz (1863) with respect to the audible detectability of complex beats.

In an effort to find out if the helicotrema or the cochlear windows had anything to do with the origin of the nonlinear beat response, two different pairs of primaries were employed, although both had the same beat rate (5 Hz). First, a high-frequency pair was used (400 and 405 Hz) such that neither primary by itself could produce a measurable fluid displacement in the helicotrema (Fig. 6, top). The resulting response along the partition was clearly asymmetrical, indicating that the helicotrema did not contribute to its origin. Thereafter, a low-frequency pair was used (30 and 35 Hz) that formed its traveling wave maximum at quite a distance away from the windows (Fig. 6, bottom). In that case, the fluid motion directly adjacent to the windows did not reveal any asymmetry, indicating that the cochlear window had not been responsible for the asymmetrical response either. Significantly, the asymmetry did not make its appearance until the region of the displacement maximum was reached.

When the frequency range between the extremes of Fig. 6 was systematically explored, the degree of asym-

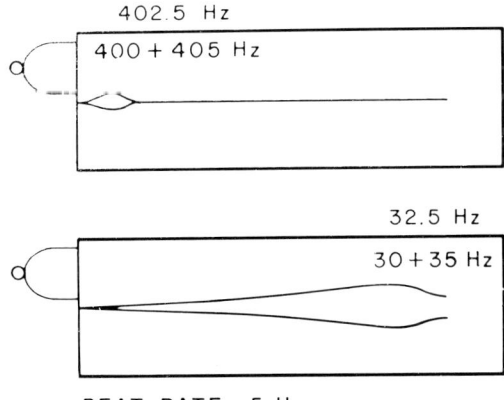

Fig. 6   Traveling-wave envelopes for a pair of high-frequency primaries (top figure) and a pair of low-frequency primaries (bottom figure) at the instant of the beat maximum. Primary frequencies, their averages, and the beat rate as indicated (from Tonndorf, 1970).

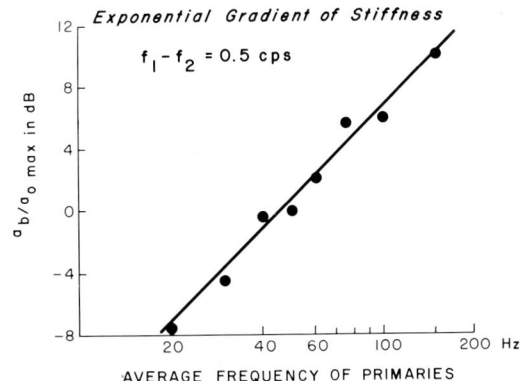

Fig. 7   The relative magnitude of the asymmetrical beat response as a function of the average frequency of the primaries; beat rate constant; partition: <u>exponential</u> gradient of stiffness. The asymmetry was assessed by measuring (a) the amplitude of the beat response in the helicotrema and (b) the amplitude of response to the primaries in the region of the envelope maximum at the instant of maximal displacement. Their ratio ($a_b/a_{o\ max}$) is given in dB (from Tonndorf, 1959a).

metrical response turned out to be a function of the average frequency of the primaries (Fig. 7).

However, the next two experiments showed that the latter finding when expressed in this manner was really misleading. A partition was employed which possessed a <u>linear</u> stiffness gradient, instead of the usual exponential one. Now, the degree of the asymmetrical response was found to be independent of frequency (Fig. 8). Actually, as is seen in Fig. 8, this conclusion was correct only for high frequencies, i.e., for those that did not involve the helicotrema. The presence of the latter complicates matters as will be shown presently.

A series of four partitions was now made. Their stiffness gradients were linear and ranged from zero to three. For one given pair of primaries, the degree of the asymmetrical response increased as a function of the stiffness gradient (Fig. 9).

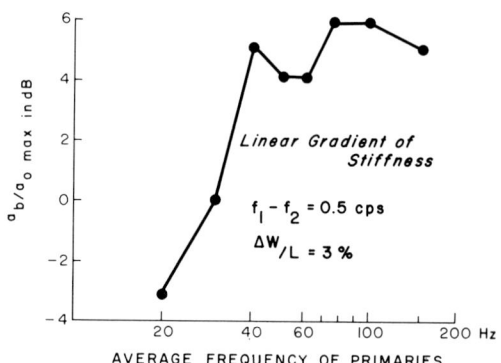

Fig. 8 The relative magnitude of the asymmetrical beat response (for its definition cf. legend of Fig. 7) as a function of the average frequency of the primaries; beat rate constant; partition: <u>linear</u> gradient of stiffness. The steepness of the gradient is expressed by the increment in width of the basilar membrane per unit length ($\Delta W/L$) and expressed in percent, 3% in the present case (from Tonndorf, 1959a).

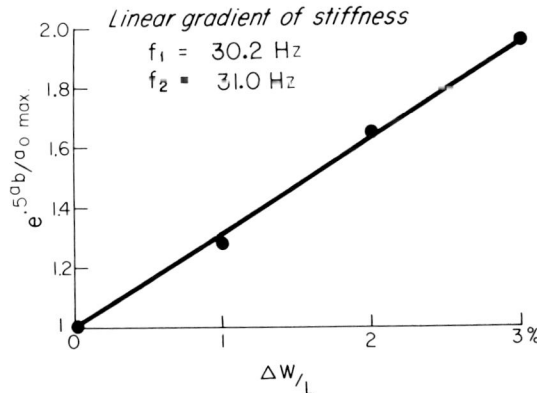

Fig. 9 The relative magnitude of the asymmetrical beat response (for its definition cf. legend of Fig. 7) as a function of linear stiffness gradients for one given pair of primaries. For the exponential expression used, the results fell on a straight line. Note that, when the gradient was zero, there was no asymmetry, i.e., the ratio $\underline{a_b/a_{o\ max}}$ was unity.
(From Tonndorf, 1959a).

As was already mentioned, the degree of the asymmetrical beat response was amplitude-independent. This type of nonlinearity is not encountered in solid systems, but it is characteristic of hydrodynamic ones. It has to do with the fact that viscosity, the force opposing the deformation of fluids, does not approach a limit as does the elastic restoring force of solid structures. Particles simply keep on sliding past one another.

When viscosity of the cochlear fluids was varied, it was seen that the degree of the asymmetrical response increased in proportion to inverse viscosity (Fig. 10). Viscosity, as is recalled, acts mainly in the boundary layer.

Taken together, the experiments underlying Figs. 6 to 10 suggest (a) that the generation of asymmetrical beat responses is a process that is localized in the region of the maximum of the traveling-wave envelope; (b) that its magnitude depends upon the

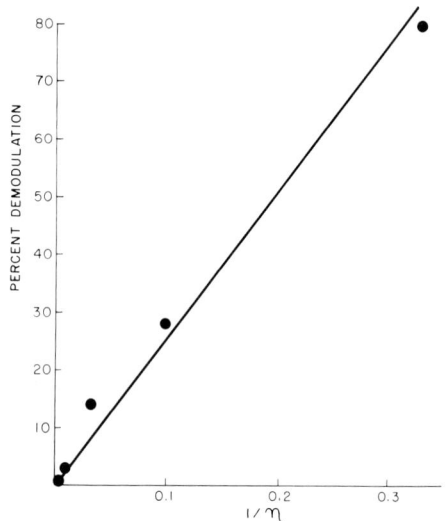

Fig. 10 The magnitude of the asymmetrical beat response (for its definition cf. legend of Fig. 7) as a function of the inverse viscosity of the cochlear fluids. Results are given in linear terms, i.e., in percent (from Tonndorf, 1970).

steepness of the stiffness gradient in that location; and (c) that it is a boundary-layer phenomenon.

This is certainly not the whole story, and we may be able to go a few steps farther. Figure 11 reveals tangible evidence of changes that take place within the boundary layer along the cochlear partition. It shows that the uniform 90° phase relationship between the two vectors of fluid particle motion as illustrated in Fig. 3 was really an oversimplification. There are small phase shifts around the place of the envelope maximum, first in one direction and, beyond that point, in the other one. The occurrence of these phase shifts was restricted to the boundary layer. However, they became more pronounced when viscosity was lowered; but since, in that case, the boundary layer became narrower, the gradient of the phase shift with distance from the partition became steeper.

These phase changes became also more pronounced when

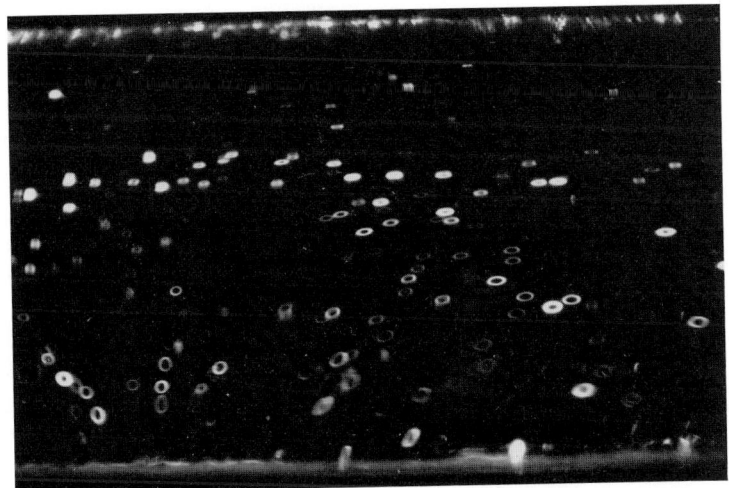

Fig. 11 Particle motion in one scala of a cochlear model in response to a sinusoidal input (photomicrograph). The cochlear windows lie to the left; the outer wall is on top, the partition at the bottom. The point of the envelope maximum is slightly to the right of the center. Note the slight phase shifts between the two vectors of particle motion around the place of the envelope maximum, first in one direction and then, beyond that point, in the other direction. The degree of such phase shifts becomes quickly smaller with distance from the partition, revealing this as a boundary-layer phenomenon. -- The orbits shown were produced by reflection from very fine aluminum particles suspended in the fluid. They were photographed against a dark-field background.

the steepness of the (linear) stiffness gradient was increased as in the experiments underlying Fig. 10. (In that case, of course, the width of the boundary layer remained unaffected.)

Now, one of the effects of making the stiffness gradient steeper is to make a given traveling-wave envelope narrower and its maximum sharper. It is suggested therefore that the changes shown in Figs. 10 and

11 are related to the sharpness of the traveling-wave maximum. This viewpoint is supported by the fact that the changes in Fig. 11 occur in opposite directions on both sides of the maximum. It could also account more fully for the observation (cf. Fig. 7), i.e., that high frequencies are more efficient in generating asymmetrical beat responses than low ones. With increasing frequency, as is well known, the traveling-wave envelopes become shorter and their maxima sharper.

What could be the significance of these phase shifts? I regard the "rectilinear" $90°$ phase relationship between the two vectors of fluid particle motion, as it exists in surface waves on open water, for example, as the ac equivalent of a laminar dc flow. The phase shifts of Fig. 11 then represent rotational effects that take place under the effect of shearing stresses between the partition and the fluids of the boundary layers on each side. Shearing stresses were mentioned in connection with Fig. 4, although, admittedly, the present effects must be considerably more complicated. The vorticity thus postulated is a frequent finding in boundary layers; by definition, its presence implies the introduction of nonlinear factors.

It is suggested that it is this vorticity, which is restricted to the place of the envelope maximum and represents a boundary-layer phenomenon, that is the ultimate cause of the asymmetrical displacements of the cochlear partition.

The point that is not understood at this time is how events that, presumably, arise in a symmetrical manner on both sides of the partition eventually lead to the asymmetry shown in Fig. 5. Some partial rectification must occur that so far has eluded the present attempts of analysis.

It might be added at this point that the observation of asymmetrical fluid motion was not restricted to the case of complex signals. It was also found with single-frequency signals, but only when the intensity was sufficiently high. The evidence will be presented later on.

The helicotrema, as is recalled from Fig. 8, had an adverse effect upon the generation of asymmetrical

responses when low-frequency signals were used. The
explanation lies in the fact that, there is no boundary layer in the helicotrema, and fluid motion is
one-dimensional. The following evidence in support of
this view is being offered: As is shown in Fig. 12,
there is a gradual transition of the two-dimensional
type of fluid motion along the partition to the one-
dimensional form that prevails in the helicotrema.
(It is in this transition that particle orbits once
more appear "tilted".) When fluid viscosity was decreased, the effect of the helicotrema upon fluid motion extended farther in the basal direction. At the
same time, the range of frequency independence of
Fig. 8 became shorter. When viscosity was increased,
both types of changes occurred in an opposite manner.

Some time ago, Békésy had also observed asymmetrical
responses in his cochlear models (pers. comm. 1959).
He felt that its cause might be in the helicotrema
and thus began experimenting with various shapes of
that opening. Results became finally so complex that
he was forced to abandon these experiments. It appears now that Békésy might have affected the generation of asymmetrical responses to low frequency signals by influencing the transition of fluid motion
proximal to the helicotrema.

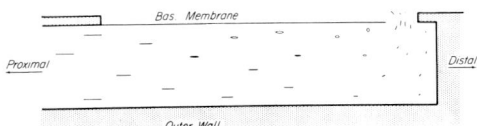

Fig. 12 Fluid motion in one cochlear scala and in
the helicotrema in response to a low-frequency, sine-wave signal (7.5 Hz); viscosity of the cochlear fluids: 30 centipoises,
providing normal damping in the enlarged
model. Note the gradual transition of the
two-dimensional form of particle motion
along the partition to the one-dimensional
form prevailing in the helicotrema. The apparent inclination of particle orbits proximal to the helicotrema is due to the gradual conversion of longitudinal displacements to transversal ones (from Tonndorf,
1959b).

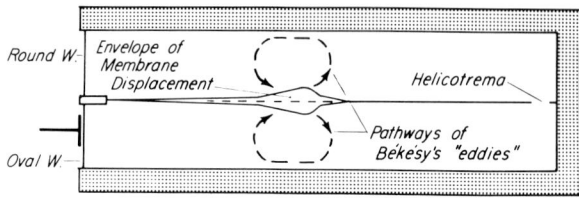

Fig. 13 Schematic outline of Békésy's eddies.

When the input intensity for a given signal exceeds a certain level, two closed-loop fluid streams are set up, one on either side of the partition. These are the cochlear eddies that were first described by Békésy in 1928. As schematically shown in Fig. 13, both eddies are mirror images of each other and are centered about the region of the traveling-wave maximum. Close to the partition, the fluid stream of either eddy runs in the direction of wave travel and returns along the outer wall. As was already mentioned, these two eddies are rectified events and, thus by definition, represent nonlinear phenomena (Zwislocki, 1948). They are superimposed upon the ac particle motion, a point that will be neglected for the time being. The velocity of a given pair of eddies along their respective pathways is not uniform. Fig. 14 shows that the flow accelerates along the partition, only to decelerate sharply at the point where it leaves the partition. Along the return path, there is further deceleration up to the point where the partition is once more reached. At a given place, the flow velocity is reciprocally related to channel width, although there is not really a dead center as Fig. 14 might imply. Toward the center, velocity simply decreases to rather low values. They are true eddies, according to the definition of von Kármán (1954), each having a nucleus of constant vorticity and a vortex-free stream on the outside, the actual "main stream".

With increasing frequency of the signal, as is well known, the traveling-wave envelopes become gradually restricted in length, and so do the eddies. They become smaller both in their longitudinal as well as in their transversal dimensions. The flow velocity, as measured at the point of the envelope maximum, increases with the square of frequency for constant

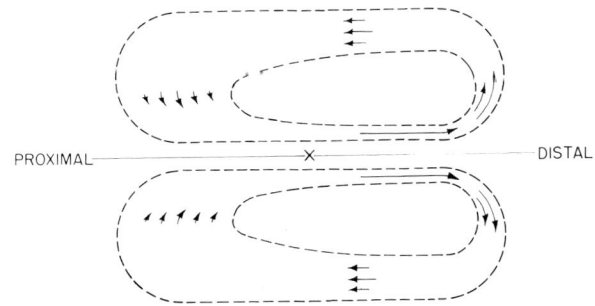

Fig. 14 Streamline pattern of Békésy's eddies (from Tonndorf, 1958b).

signal amplitude. Thus, whereas the revolving fluid volume decreases with frequency, the velocity of such motion increases with it. This finding suggests that the momentum inherent in the eddies might be frequency-independent. However, this relation could be correct only at moderate levels as the revolving fluid volume finally approaches a saturation value (cf. below).

For given signal parameters, the eddy velocity, when measured according to the above criterion, varies with the inverse square of viscosity. This finding suggests once more that the eddies represent a boundary layer phenomenon.

Occasionally in both scalae or even in only one of them, the eddy flow does not immediately get underway when a signal is suddenly switched on. There may be a measureable delay, often of one or more seconds, giving evidence to the effect of static friction. For this reason, it is not surprising to find that the eddies have genuine thresholds. Above threshold, the size of a given eddy, i.e., the revolving fluid volume, increases, at first linearly with signal amplitude, ultimately to approach saturation values. The velocity, once more when measured according to the above criterion, increases with the square of signal amplitude, apparently without reaching an upper limit.

The fact that eddy velocity varies both with the

square of frequency and that of amplitude indicates that it depends upon signal energy. These observations confirm the theoretical predictions of Zwislocki (1948).

The mechanism of the bilateral eddy flow may be explained as follows: Fluid particles of the boundary layer are being propelled by the action of the waves traveling along and displacing the partition. At the basal end, where the waves are relatively low, but fast-moving, this mode of propulsion is not very efficient. However, when waves become steeper, the coupling between the propulsive force and the fluid improves (Kinsman, 1965). Therefore, the eddy stream must gradually accelerate in the direction of wave travel along the partition. Recall that the partition itself is not moving. Across the boundary layer, therefore, velocity must first increase toward the eddy's mainstream, and beyond that, show a negative gradient. However, when such a stream is being accelerated, the difference in velocity across it is reduced, and its channel width becomes narrower (Batchelor, 1967). This is precisely what is seen to occur in the cochlear model.

The return flow is merely passive so as to fulfill the condition of continuity. (There can be no cavitation at the frequencies in question.) Consequently, the flow rate decreases further, and the channel width increases in proportion, up to a point where the loop reaches once more the partition.

Fig. 14 was limited to showing the <u>streamlines</u> of the dc flow. They must be differentiated from the actual <u>pathlines</u> which include the ac particle motion that has so far been disregarded. These pathlines are basically epicycloids, i.e., closed orbits no longer exist. Under the effect of the accelerating eddy motion, these epicycloids are expanding as schematically shown in Fig. 15. Along the return path, they are once more contracting. The orbital velocity of particles is much higher than that of the eddy stream. Thus, because of the eye's long integration time, an observer is under the illusion of seeing closed orbits moving forward in <u>toto</u>. For the sake of convenience, the approximation of "moving orbits" will be maintained in the following.

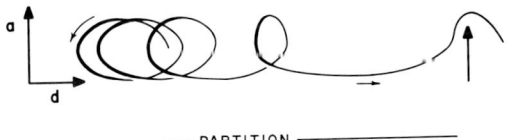

─────── PARTITION ───────

Fig. 15 Pathlines of fluid particles, a-amplitude, d-distance. The superposition of the accelerating dc eddy stream upon the ac particle motion results in "expanding" epicycloids. The direction of particle motion is indicated by arrows. Prolate epicycloids result when dc velocity < ac velocity, and curtate epicycloids result when dc velocity > ac velocity. The vertical arrow on the right indicates the transition from prolate to curtate epicycloids. In the cochlea, the eddy velocity << angular particle velocity. Therefore, only prolate epicycloids can occur (from Tonndorf, 1970).

When the input is raised much higher than the level at which eddies first appear, the moving orbits show some characteristic changes (Fig. 16). Compared to the elliptical shapes of Fig. 11, they flatten out on top and bottom; but their two sides show little, if any alterations.

Reconstructions of such orbits (Fig. 17) reveal the following: The horizontal vectors are unchanged, indicating that displacements of the cochlear windows are still sinusoidal. The vertical vectors are altered in three respects: (1) there is peak clipping on top and bottom; (2) positive and negative displacements are unequal in amplitude; and (3) there is an apparent phase shift, i.e., a slight inclination of the orbits within the boundary layer. The asymmetry and the orbital inclination are identical in sign and place of occurrence to those already described. Thus, they are most likely manifestations of the basic asymmetry of cochlear responses.

With respect to the peak clipping, the question could be raised if it might not represent an artifact of the present model. To answer this question, two different experiments were conducted: (1) As was already mentioned, the eddy velocity varies with the square

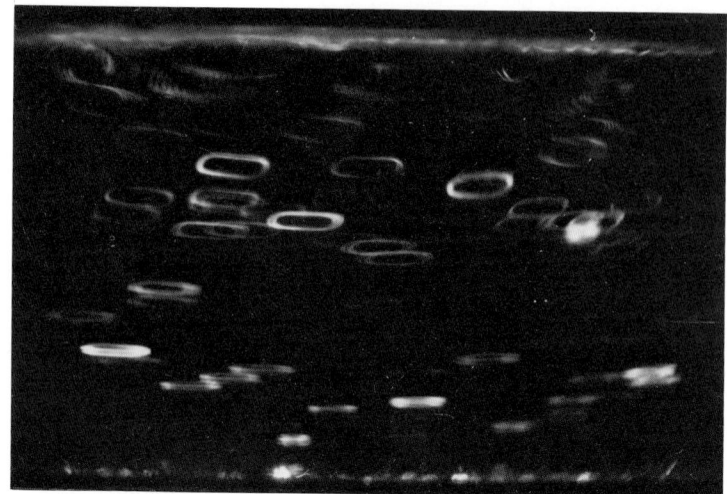

Fig. 16 Particle motion in one cochlear scala in response to a sinusoidal signal in the presence of a strong eddy current (photomicrograph). The partition is on top, but is partially cut off. The region shown is proximal to the place of maximal displacement which would be at least one more frame removed to the right. The brief exposure time permits visualization of epicycloid motion only at the upper right where eddy velocity was relatively high. Compare the shape of these pathways to those occurring below the onset of eddy motion (Fig. 11). See note on method of photographic recording in Fig. 11 (from Tonndorf, 1958a).

of viscosity of the cochlear fluids whereas particle displacement amplitude varies with its linear value. When velocity was systematically altered, it was found that the peak clipping occurred always in a given relation to the onset of eddy motion; it was not related to displacement amplitude. -- (2) A system of fine tubes inserted into the model permitted the induction of eddy-like fluid motions. By means of such "simulated" eddies, peak clipping was produced, once more independent of displacement amplitude.

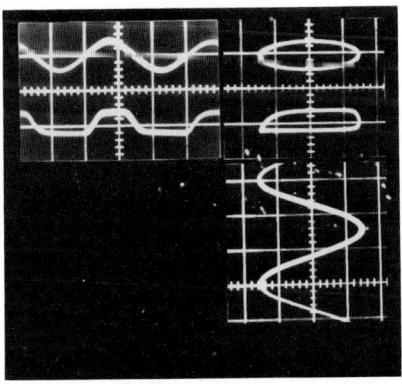

Fig. 17 Reconstruction of particle orbits for a sinusoidal input. Note the undistorted waveform of the longitudinal vector (bottom). Top trace - transversal vector also undistorted; bottom trace - transversal vector distorted, involving peak clipping, asymmetry, and a small phase shift between vectors (from Tonndorf, 1958a).

The results of these experiments strongly suggest that the effects of the eddies upon fluid particle motion are responsible for the generation of the harmonic distortion shown in Figs. 16 and 17. The peak clipping is of course only the end-result of an <u>amplitude-independent</u>, nonlinear process that is initiated at lower levels. The relative insensitivity of the eye to waveform distortion made it difficult to detect it much earlier.

Whenever peak clipping is fully established, the eddy flow becomes quite complex. Inside the large main eddy appear a number of smaller side eddies. However there is never any turbulence as the side eddies are quite stable in time and position, corresponding approximately to the places of higher harmonics of the original signal frequency.

Moreover, each harmonic forms a small amplitude maximum of its own along the partition. This can be verified by means of microscopic observation of the partition and its displacement under appropriate stroboscopic illumination. A stroboscope, as is recalled, is an optical wave analyzer.

The low-pass filter action along the partition affects also the peak-clipped waveform. That is to say, with distance along the partition, particle orbits become once more elliptical, i.e., they gradually lose their high-frequency components.

The formation of cochlear eddies is accompanied by a change in the envelope over the traveling waves. Below the onset of eddy flow, a given envelope maintains its shape as it grows in size with increasing signal amplitude. That is to say, as it becomes higher, it also becomes wider. After the onset of eddy flow, however, the distal slope of the envelope becomes progressively steeper and the maximum sharper (Fig. 18). This latter observation may represent a link between the two types of nonlinear cochlear processes described in the present paper. It is recalled that the degree of asymmetrical responses varied also with the sharpness of the envelope maximum.

When beating signals are raised to levels beyond the onset of eddy motion, the eddy flow is no longer continuous, but speeds up and slows down in synchrony with the beat rate. The flow is fastest at the instant of maximal amplitude, but, in the case of best

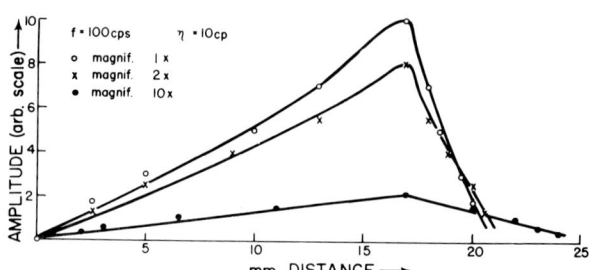

Fig. 18 Traveling-waves envelopes for three different amplitudes of a sinusoidal input signal. The lowermost trace was obtained just below the onset of eddy motion, the two upper ones beyond that point. Note the change in steepness of the distal slopes (from Tonndorf, 1958a).

beats, it stops completely at the instant of zero amplitude. These brief interruptions occur even for relatively fast beat rates. -- These observations make it clear once more that the beat rate is a component of the cochlear response that contains energy, since the eddies were said to be related to signal energy.

When eddies are present, the degree of asymmetry of the "beat" response is no longer independent of amplitude as it had been at levels below the onset of the eddy flow. It varies now with the <u>square</u> of amplitude. The changes from an amplitude-independent event to an amplitude-dependent one must signal the introduction of a new type of distortion product. It is suggested that this represents the appearance of the <u>difference tone</u>. Although difference tones and simple beats happen to have the same frequency value, they must nevertheless result from two different processes.

Lastly, it ought to be mentioned that there was a good correlation between the <u>visible</u> onset of higher harmonics for a systematic series of signal frequencies, as observed in the model, with the <u>audible</u> onset of such harmonics, as determined by Fletcher (1929), provided appropriate frequency differences were taken into account.

The model experiments described in the foregoing demonstrated two forms of nonlinearity. One of them is amplitude-independent, the other one amplitude-dependent. Both of them may occur in essentially the same manner in real cochleas. Since there is hardly a mechanical, hydrodynamical, or electrical system (and that probably includes electrochemical systems as well) that, given a sufficient input, does not produce harmonic distortion, chances are that the occurrence of this form of nonlinearity is not limited to the hydrodynamic domain, and that it may also take place in other parts of the multi-stage cochlear process. With amplitude-independent events, it may be a different matter. Aural beats, as is well known, belong to this class, and so does the $2f_1 - f_2$ combination tone first described by Goldstein (1967). The origin of aural beats, precisely because of their amplitude-independent nature, was long thought to be related to phenomena that have nothing to do with nonlinearities. The classical concept of "neural fusion" is a case in point. Amplitude-independent nonlinearities occur commonly in hydrodynamic systems, and chances are reasonably high therefore that their origin in the cochlea may by-and-large be of the kind described here.

There is one piece of supporting evidence in this regard. J.E. Hind participated in the observations by Perlman (1950) on cochlear traveling waves in guinea pig ears. What struck him most in these experiments was the fact that, as soon as the signals were switched on (which for obvious reasons were on the order of 130 to 140 dB SPL), the entire cochlear partition underwent a large dc displacement toward scala tympani (pers. comm. 1959). This, as may be recalled, is precisely what was found in the present model experiments.

Spoendlin (1971) has reported an electronmicroscopic finding that appears to bear out this evidence. Upon strong acoustic stimulation (SPL >140 dB), the content of hair cells is occasionally either extruded into scala media, or they herniate in the same direction. It follows from simple considerations of the shearing forces involved that, when the displacement towards scala tympani is larger than that towards scala vestibuli, the inward-directed (compressing) shear force on top of the organ is larger than the outward-directed (expanding) force. Thus, the content of these cells may be literally pressed out of them into the lumen of scala media.

There is one possibility that has intrigued the present author for some time, and that concerns the origin of the summating potential (SP). The latter could well represent the electrical manifestation of the mechanical dc shift of the partition. This notion is strengthened by the observation, first made by Davis et al. (1958) and later confirmed by Butler and Honrubia (1963), i.e., that the magnitude and polarity of the SP can be influenced by changes of the differential fluid pressure across the cochlear partition. (The SP has negative and positive components which are thought to be related to its dual origin: inner and outer hair cells (Honrubia and Ward, 1969).)

Summary

The present paper is based on experiments in physical cochlear models. It describes two forms of nonlinearity both of which are hydrodynamic in origin, representing boundary-layer phenomena.

(1) An amplitude-independent nonlinearity that, with suitable signals (beats, missing fundamentals, tone pips, etc.) results in envelope detection along the partition. The underlying phenomenon appears to be localized at the place of maximal displacement of the traveling-wave envelope and is related to the steepness of the stiffness gradient at that point -- and thus to the sharpness of the displacement maximum. It is most likely caused by shearing stresses between the partition and the fluids of the boundary layers on both sides.

(2) An amplitude-dependent nonlinearity that leads to harmonic waveform distortion and eventually to amplitude limitations. The distorted waveform is resolved along the partition in that each harmonic forms a small displacement maximum of its own at a place that corresponds to its actual frequency value. The underlying phenomenon appears to be related to an interaction between Békésy's eddies and fluid particle motion in the boundary layer. Significantly, the revolving fluid volume of the eddies eventually approaches a saturation value. The observation that, with increasing amplitude and under the effect of eddy flow, the maximum of the traveling-wave envelope becomes also sharper may represent a link between the two forms of nonlinearities.

References

Batchelor, G.K. (1967). Fluid Dynamics. Cambridge University Press, Cambridge, England.

Békésy, G. von (1928). Zur Theorie des Hörens: Die Schwingungsform der Basilarmembran. Phys. Z. 29, 793-810.

Békésy, G. von (1947). The variation of phase along the basilar membrane with sinusoidal vibrations. J. Acoust. Soc. Amer. 19, 452-460.

Butler, R.A., and Honrubia, V. (1963). Response of cochlear potentials to changes in hydrostatic pressure. J. Acoust. Soc. Amer. 35, 1188-1192.

Dallos, P., and Linnell, C.O. (1966). Subharmonic components in cochlear-microphonic potentials. J. Acoust. Soc. Amer. 40, 4-11.

Dallos, P., and Sweetman, R.H. (1969). Distribution pattern of cochlear harmonics. J. Acoust. Soc. Amer. 45, 37-46.

Davis, H., Deatherage, B.H., Eldredge, D.H., and Smith, C.A. (1958). Summating potentials of the cochlea. Amer. J. Physiol. 195, 251-261.

Engebretson, A.M., and Eldredge, D.H. (1968). Model of the nonlinear characteristics of cochlear potentials. J. Acoust. Soc. Amer. 44, 548-554.

Fletcher, H. (1929). Speech and Hearing in Communication. D. Van Nostrand Co., New York.

Goblick, T.S., and Pfeiffer, R.R. (1969). Time-domain measurement of cochlear nonlinearities using combination of click stimuli. J. Acoust. Soc. Amer. 46, 924-928.

Goldstein, J.L. (1967). Auditory nonlinearity. J. Acoust. Soc. Amer. 41, 676-689.

Goldstein, J.L., and Kiang, N.Y.S. (1968). Neural correlates of the aural combination tone $2f_1 - f_2$. Proc. IEEE 56, 981-992.

Guinan, J.J., Jr., and Peake, W.R. (1967). Middle-ear characteristics of anesthetized cats. J. Acoust. Soc. Amer. 41, 1237-1261.

Helmholtz, H. von (1863). On the Sensation of Tone. Dover Publications, New York (1954 reprint).

Honrubia, V., and Ward, P.H. (1969). Properties of the summating potential of the guinea pig. J. Acoust. Soc. Amer. 45, 1443-1450.

Kármán, Th. von (1954). Aerodynamics. McGraw-Hill, New York (1963 paperback edition).

Kinsman, B. (1965). Wind Waves. Prentice-Hall, Englewood Cliffs, New Jersey.

Lamb, H. (1879). Hydrodynamics. Dover Publications, New York (1943 reprint).

Lewis, D., and Reger, S.N. (1933). An experimental study of the role of the tympanic membrane and the ossicles in the hearing of certain subjective tones. J. Acoust. Soc. Amer.5, 153-158.

Lowenstein, O., and Wersäll, J. (1959). A functional interpretation of the electron-microscopic structure of sensory hairs in the cristae of the elasmobranch Raja Clavata in terms of directional sensitivity. Nature (London) 184, 1807-1808.

Perlman, H.B. (1950). Observation through cochlear fenestra. Laryngoscope 40, 77-96.

Peterson, L.C., and Bogert, G.P. (1950). Dynamical theory of the cochlea. J. Acoust. Soc. Amer. 22, 369-381.

Spoendlin, H. (1971). Primary structural changes in the organ of Corti after acoustic overstimulation. Acta Otolaryngol. 71, 166-176.

Strutt, J.W., Lord Rayleigh (1877). The Theory of Sound. Vols. 1 and 2, Dover Publications, New York (1945 reprint).

Stumpf, C. (1910). Beobachtungen über Kombinationstöne. Beitr. Akust. Musikwiss. 5, 1-142.

Tonndorf, J. (1956). The analogy between fluid motion within the cochlea and formation of surf on sloping beaches and its significance for the mechanism of cochlear stimulation. Ann. Otol. Rhinol. Laryngol.65, 488-506.

Tonndorf, J. (1957). Fluid motion in cochlear models. J. Acoust.Soc. Amer. 29, 558-568.

Tonndorf, J. (1958a). Harmonic distortion in cochlear models. J. Acoust. Soc. Amer. 30, 929-937.

Tonndorf, J. (1958b). The hydrodynamic origin of aural harmonics in the cochlea. Ann. Otol Rhinol. Laryngol. 67, 754-774.

Tonndorf, J. (1959a). Beats in cochlear models. J. Acoust. Soc. Amer. 31, 608-619.

Tonndorf, J. (1959b). The transfer of energy across the cochlea. Acta Otolaryngol. 50, 174-184.

Tonndorf, J. (1960). Dimensional analysis of cochlear models. J. Acoust. Soc. Amer. 32, 493-497.

Tonndorf, J. (1962). Time-frequency analysis along the partition of cochlear models: a modified place concept. J. Acoust. Soc. Amer. 34, 1337-1350.

Tonndorf, J. (1970). Nonlinearities in cochlear hydrodynamics. J. Acoust. Soc. Amer. 47, 579-591.

Wever, E.G., and Bray, C.W. (1938). Distortion in the ear as shown by the electrical responses of the cochlea. J. Acoust. Soc. Amer. 9, 227-233.

Zwislocki, J. (1948). Theorie der Schneckenmechanik. Acta Otolaryngol. Suppl. 72, 1-76.

Figures 2, 3, 5, 6, 7, 8, 9, 10, 15, 16, 17, 18 reproduced by permission of Journal of the Acoustical Society of America.

Figure 12 reproduced by permission of Acta Oto-Laryngologica (Stockholm).

Figure 14 reproduced by permission of Annals of Otology, Rhinology and Laryngology.

DISCUSSION

PFEIFFER: You said that the frequency scale of your model was different than in the real cochlea. I noticed the effect of the helicotrema in your model started at about 20 or 30 Hz. What does that translate to in the real cochlea?

TONNDORF: 300-400 Hz in a real ear. 50 Hz in my model corresponds exactly to 1500 Hz. When you make a model larger, frequency goes down, and amplitude goes up. Of course, I have also had to use very high driving forces, that is, 130 and 140 dB, which are equivalent to something like 65 to 75 dB, thus I did these experiments at what you might call equivalent physiological levels.

PFEIFFER: What would be the equivalent amplitude at which your eddies start?

TONNDORF: Both the eddy speed and the eddy threshold depend upon frequency. At low frequencies, the eddies start at around 90 dB, in terms of equivalent values upon frequency.

DAVIS: Do you have any closer estimate as to the absolute threshold of the eddies? I also submit the general theorem that "as amplitude increases, non-linearity develops and complexity increases without limit".

TONNDORF: Initially, as I said earlier, it is static friction, which keeps the fluid from moving until the eddy literally breaks through. Very often, in the model at least, the eddies did not appear at the same time in both scalae. With regard to the amplitude you have to realize that when one measures visually, one is only able to cover a range of about 26 dB. In an effort to extend that range somewhat I changed magnification. Thus, the visual detection is not a very reliable method in this respect. I cannot really say, therefore, if the amplitude relationship is linear before the onset of the eddy. After the eddy develops, the relation becomes highly nonlinear.

DALLOS: Dr. Tonndorf, I would not agree with you on the significance of Békésy's eddies. Specifically, what disturbs me is how this phenomenon that is quite apparent in the perilymphatic scalae is being coupled back to the cochlear partition, how it could conceivably create distortions within the partition, and how it could affect stimulation of hair cells. Could you enlighten me on this?

TONNDORF: I think Dr. Zwislocki could answer that better because it was he who corrected an earlier misconception, i.e., that it was the eddy that directly caused the displacements of the sensory hairs. That was a widely held misconception in the 1930's and early 40's. The eddy is an event which takes place in the perilymph and thus, its effect upon the hair cells is only an indirect one, by virtue of its affecting the basilar membrane displacement.

DALLOS: What you are showing and what Békésy has shown is an eddy motion in the perilymph. Now the question is how this eddy motion, this streaming in the perilymph, will distort the cochlear partition. What is the mechanism of this?

TONNDORF: As far as I was able to tell, it is a boundary layer phenomenon, and it is the result of the ac particle motion and the superimposed dc motion. But how the distortion really comes about, I do not know either.

ZWISLOCKI: The chairman has been invited by Dr. Tonndorf to clarify the problem and he would like to do so. The eddies, according to hydrodynamic theory, are not a cause of the distortion of basilar membrane

motion but its result. The distortion stems from the
angle between the inertia force of the fluid and the
restoring force of the membrane, which becomes smaller than $180°$ at sufficiently high amplitudes. The
classical theory assumes that the two forces are
parallel, but they are not exactly so. This leads to
the type of distortion that is seen as eddies. I
would like to call to your attention that the same
thing that happens in the perilymph should happen in
the endolymph, and the theory says that the endolymph
should actually accumulate at the site of maximum
vibration in the cochlea and should increase the mass
of the cochlear duct of this site. Whether or not
this actually happens, I do not think, has been demonstrated.

KLOCKHOFF[1]: In advanced cases of Menière's disease
there is often a flat hearing loss. In these cases a
peroral single dose of glycerine often produces a
transient hearing threshold improvement in the middle frequency range. At the same time there is often
a remarkable improvement of the speech discrimination
score. We assume that these effects are due to a reduction of endolymphatic hydrops by the osmotic route
since glycerine makes the blood hypertonic. Would
such an explanation be in line with the observations
on the hydrodynamics of the inner ear that you have
made on your inner ear model?

TONNDORF: Well, as far as the low frequency loss is
concerned, I would say yes to your question, because
this type of loss has to do with the change in stiffness of the membrane. However, the so-called flat
loss is brought about when the membranes have become
permanently distended. The evidence for this view
point comes from animal experiments of Kimura. In
that case, the problem is not one of a change in
stiffness, but one of a change in mass.

---
[1] Dr. I. Klockhoff
Div. of Audiology
Department of Otolaryngology
Akademiska Sjukhuset
Uppsala
Sweden

AN INVESTIGATION OF POST-MORTEM COCHLEAR
MECHANICS USING THE MÖSSBAUER EFFECT

William S. Rhode

The University of Wisconsin
Madison, Wisconsin
USA

1. Introduction

The possibility of measuring the vibration amplitude of the basilar membrane using the Mössbauer effect has aroused a vigorous interest. Johnstone and Boyle (1967) first made use of this on vibration amplitudes of a size far below the wavelength of visible light. The fact that the "resonance" curves of the basilar membrane motion obtained using the Mössbauer effect at physiological sound levels were considerably sharper than Békésy (1960) had found using very high sound levels offered some hope in resolving the discrepancy between the relatively poor mechanical frequency selectivity of the cochlea and the sharp tuning exhibited by auditory nerve fibers (Kiang, 1965).

The Mössbauer effect is a Doppler phenomenon at the nuclear level which permits the measurement of small velocities, on the order of 0.2 mm/sec. This allows for determination of amplitudes of the order of 20 Å at 10 kHz. In the frequency range around 10 kHz the Mössbauer technique allows measurement of amplitudes 40-60 dB lower that what is possible with light microscopic techniques as that used by Békésy. Measurements can thus be performed at sound pressure levels of 80-100 dB SPL with the Mössbauer effect. Unfortunately, the Mössbauer technique has only a 15-20 dB dynamic range and the possibilities of measuring distortion products are limited.

Two other methods have been used in recent measurements of the vibration of the basilar membrane, the capacitance probe (Wilson and Johnstone, 1972) and fuzziness-detection (Kohllöffel, 1972). These experimental techniques have produced results which are not in complete agreement. While there are a number of differences in experimental circumstances, such as the species of animal used, whether the cochlea is alive or dead, and the location along the cochlear partition at which vibration is measured, these differences must not be used as an excuse to hinder reconciliation of the divergent findings.

A series of experiments was conducted in order to study the effect of death on the vibratory pattern of the basilar membrane. The results of the eight most successful of these experiments contribute to the present interpretation of the differences in basilar membrane vibration during life and death.

2. Methods

The methods used are identical to those already reported (Rhode, 1971) except that the transfer function, or transfer ratio i.e. the ratio between basilar membrane displacement and malleus displacement, was first obtained for the living animal after which the animal was killed via anesthetic overdose and the transfer function then obtained at various time intervals, typically up to seven hours after death.

All experiments were performed in squirrel monkeys anesthetized with Diabutal. The body temperature was maintained at $37.9°C$ throughout the experiment. A calibrated closed acoustic system was used to deliver the stimulus. The surgical approach, made from the dorsal side along the auditory nerve, included a small opening (less than 0.5 mm in diameter) in the scala tympani to permit the placement of the Mössbauer source on the basilar membrane. The Mössbauer source measured either 60 µm × 60 µm × 5 µm or 40 µm × 40 µm × 5 µm; the smaller source weighed about 0.1 µg. After the source was positioned on the basilar membrane, the scala tympani was refilled with fluid and the opening covered (not sealed) with a plastic window. A second source (120 µm × 120 µm × 5 µm) was placed on the umbo of the tympanic membrane to measure the displacement of the malleus.

3. Results

The results of the present study are consistent with the previous results of Rhode (1971) showing the

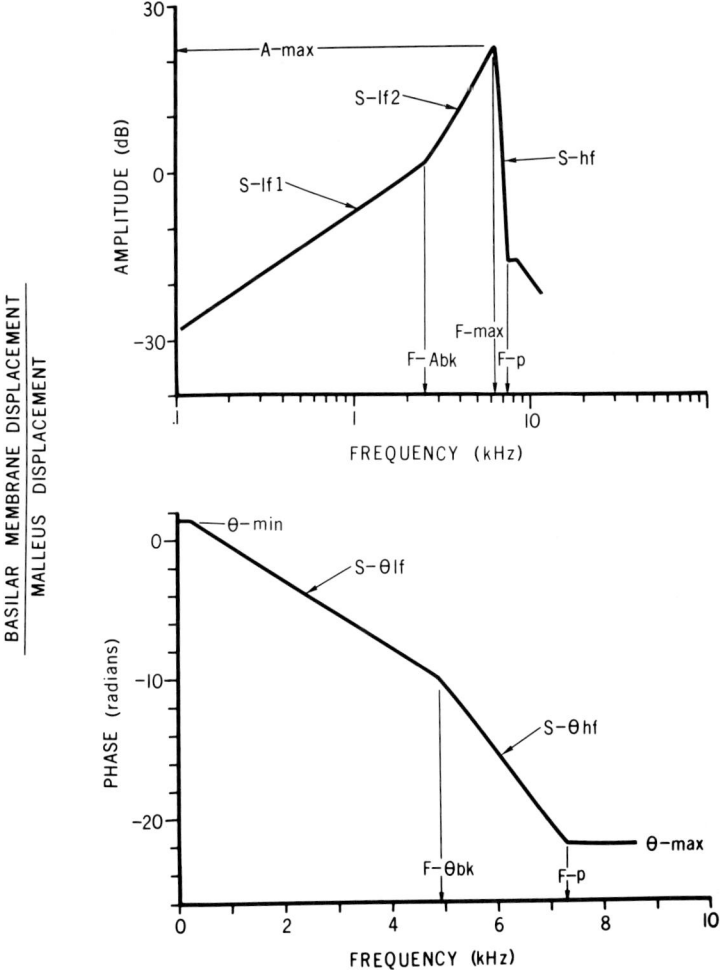

Fig. 1 A schematized transfer ratio for basilar membrane to umbo displacement. The symbols in the figure have the following definitions: A-max - maximum amplitude of the transfer ratio, (db); S-lf1 - low frequency slope near A-max (dB/oct); F-Abk, the intersection of S-lf1 and S-lf2 or the "break" frequency for the magnitude of the transfer ratio (kHz); F-max, the frequency corresponding to the maximum ratio (kHz); F-p, the frequency at which the knee occurs in the magnitude of the transfer ratio (kHz). In the phase (cont'd)

(Fig. 1, cont'd) portion of the transfer ratio for which the frequency scale is linear, the following parameters can be identified; θ-min, the minimum phase difference between the phase of the umbo and the basilar membrane (radians); S-θlf, the low frequency slope of the phase curve; S-θhf, the high frequency slope of the phase curve (radian/ /kHz); θ-max, the maximum phase difference; F-θbk, the frequency at which the two slopes S-θlf and S-θhf intersect; F-p, the frequency at which θ-max first occurs.

transfer function from malleus displacement to basilar membrane displacement. The results are summarized in Fig. 1. Since all the measurements of basilar membrane motion were made in the same region of the cochlea due to anatomical constraints, the frequency which produced the maximum transfer ratio (F-max), was always between 7 and 8 kHz. The other parameters of the amplitude transfer function under these conditions included the low frequency slope, (S-lf1), which was equal to 6 dB/octave, and the second low frequency slope (S-lf2), which averaged about 24 dB/oct. The intersection of the two low frequency slopes was at a frequency (F-Abk), which was typically around 2 kHz. The maximum ratio (A-max) was about 24 dB. The high frequency slope (S-hf) was approximately 100 dB/oct with a wide range of variability (50-150 dB/oct). It was also observed that the high frequency slope did not continue indefinitely but reached a plateau at about 35-45 dB below the peak. Such a plateau has also been reported by Wilson and Johnstone (1972) but with a slower rate of decrease beyond the plateau than found by the present author. The phase difference between the motion of the basilar membrane and that of the malleus at very low frequencies was about +90°. A reasonable approximation for the rest of the phase characteristic could be represented by two line segments. The slope of the first low frequency segment (S-θlf) was between 2.1 and 2.6 rad/kHz; the slope of the second line segment (S-θhf) was between 3.7 and 4.5 rad/kHz. Finally, the phase reached a plateau (θ-max) which was a multiple of radians, either 7, 8 or 9 π. The frequency at which the two line segments intersected (F-θbk) was between 5 and 6 kHz. The lowest frequency at which θ-max was attained (F-p) corre-

sponded to the low frequency edge of the plateau on
the high frequency slope of the amplitude curve.

Besides the above findings, a nonlinearity of the
"saturating" type was discovered. It is limited primarily to the region of the high frequency slope of
the transfer ratio; thus it is on the apical slope of
the displacement envelope of the basilar membrane
(Rhode, 1971). It was observed at the lowest intensities at which the amplitude could be measured with
the Mössbauer method, i.e. 75-80 dB-SPL. This is the
most controversial finding since no other investigator has reported such a pronounced nonlinearity at
any intensity. This nonlinearity is stable and persists even when the small (40 µm x 40 µm x 5 µm)
Mössbauer source is used. It has the effect of shifting F-max toward lower frequencies as intensity is
increased and broadening the peak of the transfer
ratio while decreasing the maximum ratio.

The results of the present study show that the effect
of death upon the vibratory pattern of the basilar
membrane is dramatic. A decrease in the amplitude of
vibration by a factor of 10 over a 10 minute period
immediately after death was observed. The first and
most marked changes occurred for frequencies near
and greater than F-max. One hour after death the
amplitude of vibration at frequencies near F-max decreased by a factor of 100 (Fig. 2). In fact the frequency at which the amplitude "plateau" occurs, F-p,
decreased relative to a value found in the living
preparation.

The transfer functions illustrated in Figs. 2-4 demonstrated the change in vibration of the basilar membrane after death. To ensure that the change in the
transfer ratio was due to changes in the basilar membrane the measurement of the vibration of the malleus
was repeated each time a transfer ratio was taken.
The malleus transfer ratio was constant within ± 3 dB
over the measurement period; therefore changes within the cochlea must have been responsible for the
observed changes in the transfer ratio.

In general, the most marked change in the transfer
ratio occurs within the first hour after death. Fig.
3 illustrates the most marked decrease in the maximum
transfer ratio which was observed, a 20 dB loss over

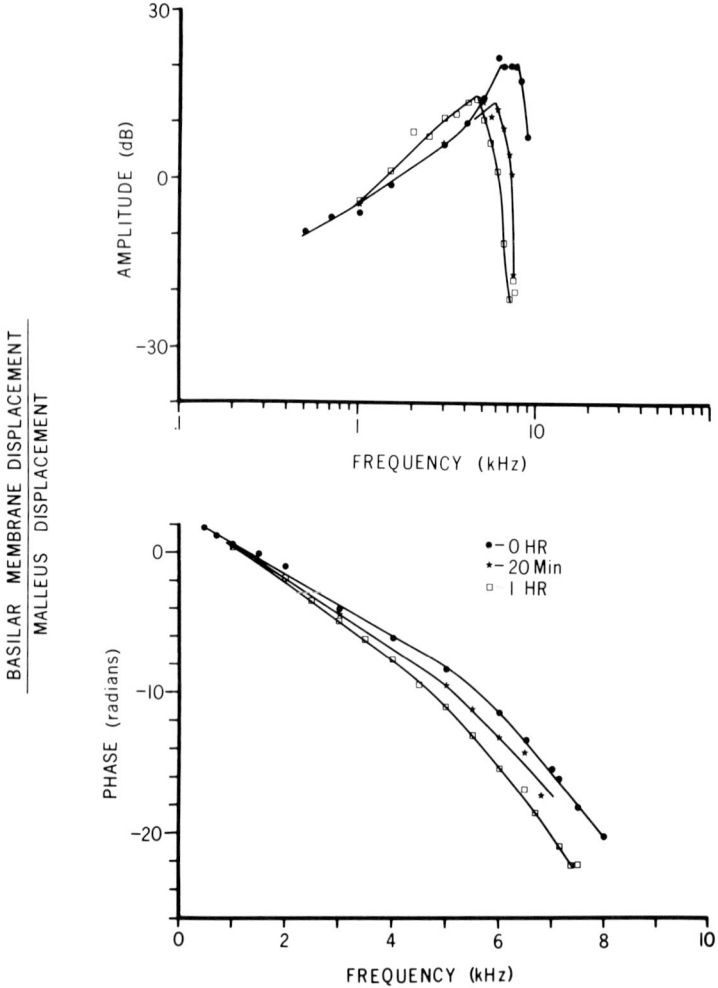

Fig. 2 The basilar membrane/malleus transfer ratio for experiment 72-427. The labels attached to curves indicate the time after death at which data collection began. A separate measurement of the vibration of the malleus was made for each ratio. The legend 0-HR indicates that the data were collected while the animal was alive, 20 min. indicates the data were collected within 20 minutes after death and 1HR indicates the data collection was begun 1 hour after death. The data points for (cont'd)

(Fig. 2, cont'd) the basilar membrane measurements near F-max and beyond were obtained at 80 dB SPL. The remaining measurements were taken at various sound pressure levels and extrapolated which is justified by the linear behavior at these frequencies.

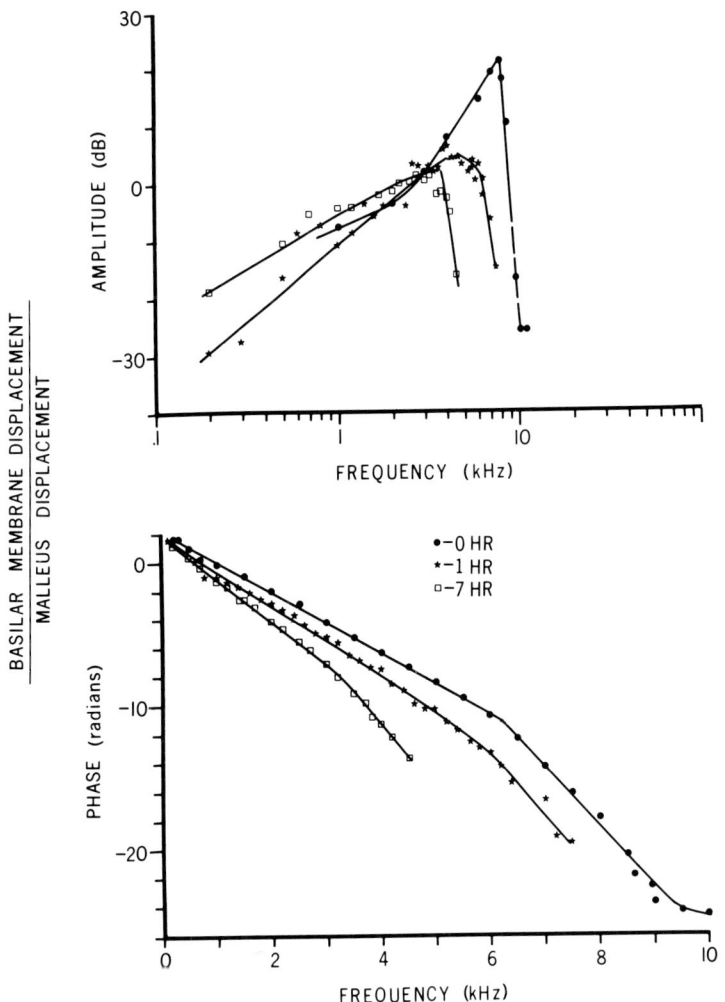

Fig. 3 The basilar membrane/malleus transfer ratio for experiment 72-314. The basilar membrane measurements for frequencies near F-max were obtained at 80 dB SPL while the re- (cont'd)

(Fig. 3, cont'd) maining data points were obtained at other intensities and were extrapolated. The three curves were obtained while the animal was alive (0-HR), 1 hour after death and 7 hours after death.

a 7-hour period after death. The typical loss is 10-15 dB over this same time period during life. Another feature of the transfer ratio after death is that the slope on the low frequency side does not increase as F-max is approached. By six hours after death the low frequency slope has decreased to a nominal 6 dB/oct which is in good agreement with Békésy's results. At low frequencies the transfer ratio is 8-10 dB greater 6 hours after death than before. The high frequency slope decreases in magnitude somewhat, but remains near 90 dB/oct on the average. Further, the frequency of maximum transfer ratio (F-max) is shifted downwards in frequency.

The downward shift in F-max at a particular site along the basilar membrane after death was very small in one experiment for which the results are shown in Fig. 4. In this experiment the animal's body temperature was allowed to cool to room temperature between the measurements 1 hour and 31 hours after death. The results of this experiment along with the experiments in which the animal's body temperature was maintained suggest that maintaining the body temperature at $37.9°C$ may increase the rate at which changes in the mechanical properties of the basilar membrane occur. A more careful study of this needs to be made since the present results can refer to only one experiment in which the animal was not held at $37.9°C$ throughout. An interesting phenomenon that can be observed in Fig. 4 is the increase in the high frequency slope relative to the 1 hour after death ratio! The magnitude of the slope is about 110 dB/oct which is close to the value found at 80 dB SPL in the living preparation.

The phase characteristic also exhibits marked changes as a function of time after death. $S-\theta lf$ increases and $S-\theta hf$ decreases in all experiments except one. The "break" frequency, $F-\theta bk$, also decreases as does θ-max.

In addition to the previously described differences

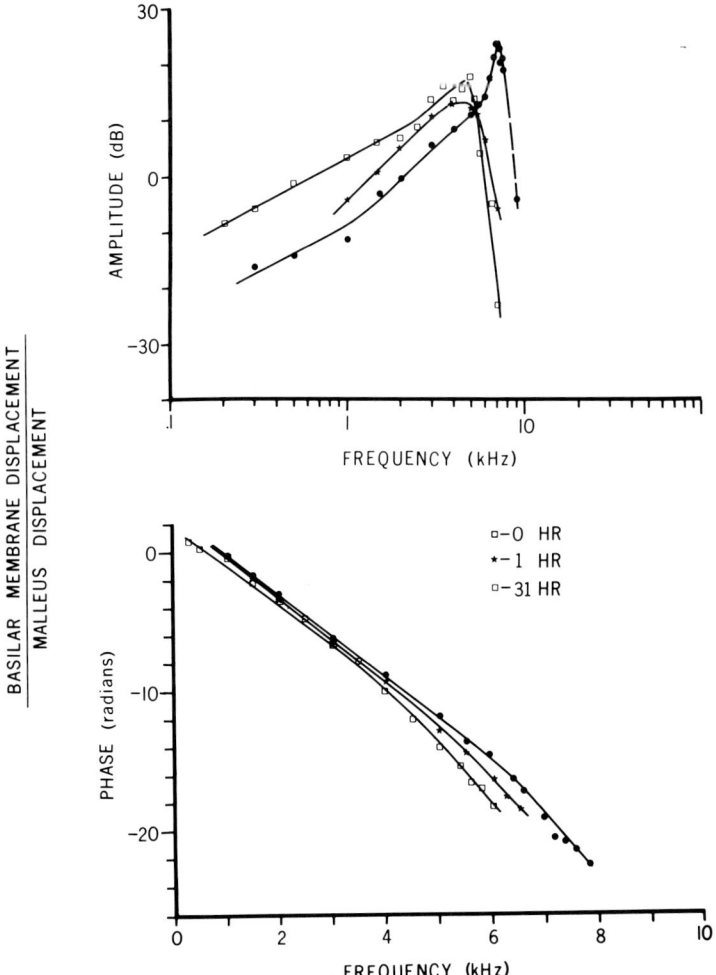

Fig. 4 The basilar membrane/malleus transfer ratio for experiment 72-259. The basilar membrane measurements at frequencies near F-max and beyond were made at 80 dB SPL. The other measurements were extrapolated. The three curves were obtained while the animal was alive (0-HR), one hour after death and 31 hours after death. The body temperature of the animal was not maintained at 37.9°C throughout this experiment but instead allowed to cool to room temperature.

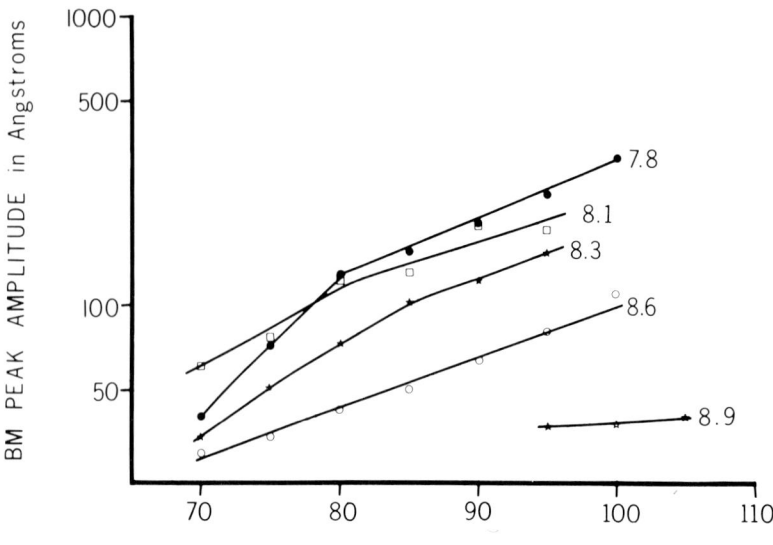

Fig. 5 The basilar membrane displacement as a function of intensity for several different frequencies for experiment 72-314. The data were obtained while the animal was alive.

between the vibration of the basilar membrane in living and dead cochleas, it is interesting to note that the basilar membrane vibrates linearly after the death of the animal. The displacement of the basilar membrane at frequencies corresponding to the region of the high frequency slope of the transfer ratio no longer is dramatically nonlinear as in Fig. 5. The change to linear motion is rapid, occurring within minutes of the animal's death. This explains the one aberrant finding in the previous paper (Rhode, 1971) which reported that in one experiment the basilar membrane was found to vibrate linearly for all frequencies; in this instance the animal died before the measurement of the vibration of the basilar membrane was complete.

In two of the present experiments the eighth nerve was removed while the animal was alive. The effect was similar to that of death. That is, rapid changes (measured in minutes) occurred, with a decrease in the transfer ratio near F-max, a shift in F-max to lower frequencies, and the second slope, S-1f2, becoming equal to S-1f1. The one difference was that the transfer ratio did not increase for low frequencies, indicating that changes in the stiffness of the basilar membrane occur after death while the change in damping of the basilar membrane is dependent on the integrity of the cochlear blood supply. Furthermore, nonlinearity could still be measured at a few frequencies on the high frequency slope of the transfer ratio after the nerve had been removed for 1 hour though over a narrower frequency range and at 105-115 dB SPL.

4. Discussion

The results of the present experiments indicate that the tuning of the basilar membrane is physiologically vulnerable. The change in basilar membrane motion observed after death could be accounted for by changes in the mechanical properties of the cochlear partition. The decrease in the slope, $S-\theta hf$, and the decrease in the amplitude of vibration could be accounted for by an increase in damping. The only difficulty with this interpretation is that the high frequency slope, $S-hf$, did not decrease as much as might be expected for an increase in damping. The increase in displacement at low frequencies could be due to a decrease in stiffness of the basilar membrane.

The preponderance of quantitative measurements of the vibration of the basilar membrane indicates that the membrane vibrates linearly. Békésy (1960), Johnstone and Boyle (1967), Wilson and Johnstone (1972), and Kohllöffel (1972) using stroboscopic illumination, the Mössbauer technique, a capacitance probe and fuzziness detection (laser illumination) respectively, all report linear vibration.

What are the differences in the techniques used by the individual experiments that could be conducive to such differences in results? First of all, the results reported here indicate that within a few hours after death the Mössbauer technique yields results very similar to those obtained by Békésy in cochleas from cadavers except that the magnitude of the high frequency slope is considerably greater in the more recent experiments.

The investigations of Kohllöffel (1972) indicate a continuous change in the vibratory properties of the basilar membrane of the guinea pig after death. The slopes of the amplitude envelope decrease with time and the region of maximum response for a given frequency shifts basally. Moreover, he finds that less pressure is required to reach a given displacement in the region of best response. These changes are compatible with those observed here over a shorter time frame. While the low frequency slope decreased to 5 dB/oct after seven days in the guinea pig, it reached 6 dB/oct after 5-6 hours in the squirrel monkey.

The recent investigation of Evans (1972) indicates that fluid removal has little effect on the tuning curves of auditory fibers of the eighth nerve in guinea pigs. This suggests that removal of fluid from the basal region of the cochlea has little effect on the vibration of the basilar membrane and therefore cannot explain the differences in vibratory behavior between the present results and those of Johnstone et al. (1970) and Wilson and Johnstone (1972).

It is not clear what is producing the nonlinear behavior when the Mössbauer technique is used in squirrel monkeys but it seems to involve some metabolically dependent process. The rapid decrease in the amplitude of vibration and the corresponding disappearance of the nonlinearity in a time frame of minutes could only be explained by some metabolic element of the cochlear partition. The idea that a second "sharp" filter exists in the cochlea whose tuning is physiologically vulnerable is supported by the investigation of Evans (1972). The sharpness of the threshold tuning curves in guinea pigs with pathological cochleas was substantially less than for normal cochleas. In fact, the threshold curves for the nerve fibers with very high thresholds were in substantial agreement with the mechanical data of Johnstone et al. (1970) and Békésy (1960). The present results agree with those of Evans by revealing a physiologically vulnerable filter but differ by demonstrating that this filter affects the motion of the basilar membrane.

The fact that there exists a plateau in the amplitude curve for the basilar membrane displacement while the neural threshold tuning curve for nerve fibers is very steep has been suggested as evidence for a second sharp filter (Wilson and Johnstone, 1972). Fig. 6

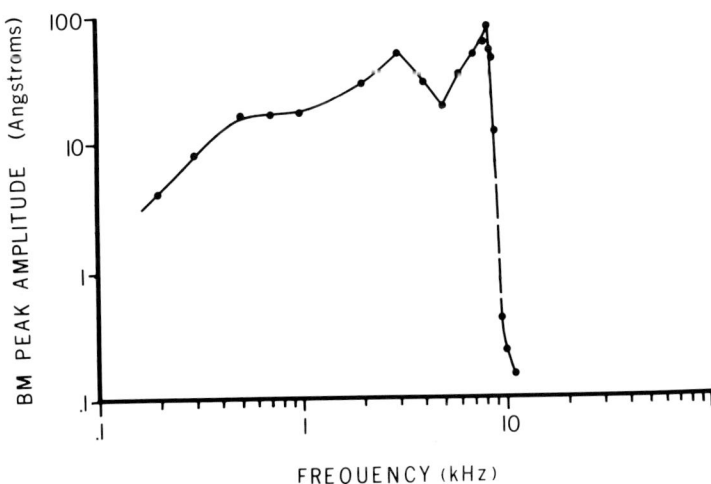

Fig. 6 The displacement of the basilar membrane at 70 dB SPL for experiment 72-314. Only the data points in the vicinity of 7 kHz were obtained at 70 dB SPL. The remaining points are extrapolations from data obtained at higher SPLs.

shows the amplitude of vibration of the basilar membrane at 70 dB SPL. It is obvious that this is quite different from a neural threshold curve for an eighth nerve fiber with a 7 kHz best frequency. But we really do not know how the mechanical curve behaves at lower intensities, although most investigators would probably expect no difference in shape from that at higher SPLs. Whether the nonlinearity observed using the Mössbauer technique persists to much lower SPLs is not known since the Mössbauer technique does not have the necessary sensitivity. If the nonlinearity persists to lower intensities the transfer ratio will appear more similar to the inverted neural threshold curve.

The experimental preparation used here is designed to cause a minimum amount of damage to the cochlea. The opening in the cochlea is very small, the scala tympani is kept filled with fluid, a very small area is studied with the Mössbauer source, and the cochlea is kept alive. Whether these procedural differences can account for the discrepancies between the present results and those of other investigators can be determined only by further study.

Certainly there is a wealth of evidence from physiological and psychoacoustic experiments to indicate the existence of cochlear nonlinearities but this does not necessarily mean that the nonlinearity is mechanical or, more specifically, a result of the motion of the basilar membrane. The cochlear partition involves considerably more than the basilar membrane and its complex structure offers many possibilities for elaborate mechanical and electrical behavior.

Acknowledgments

This research was supported by National Institutes of Health grants RR00249 from the Division of Research Facilities and Resources and NS-06225 from the National Institute of Neurological Diseases and Stroke. My special thanks to Dr. Joseph Hind for a careful reading of this manuscript and to Ms. Betty Hall for typing it.

References

Békésy, G. von (1960). Experiments in Hearing. McGraw-Hill, New York.

Evans, E.F. (1972). Does frequency sharpening occur in the cochlea? Symposium on Hearing Theory 1972, pp. 27-34. IPO Eindhoven, Holland.

Johnstone, B.M., and Boyle, A.J.F. (1967). Basilar membrane vibrations examined with the Mössbauer technique. Science 158, 389-390.

Johnstone, B.M., Taylor, K.J., and Boyle, A.J. (1970). Mechanics of the guinea pig cochlea. J. Acoust. Soc. Amer. 47, 504-509.

Kiang, N.Y.S. (1965). Discharge Patterns of Single Fibers in the Cat's Auditory Nerve. Res. Monogr. 35. M.I.T. Press, Cambridge, Mass.

Kohllöffel, L.U.E. (1972). A study of basilar membrane vibrations II. The vibratory amplitude and phase pattern along the basilar membrane (postmortem). Acustica. 27, 66-81.

Rhode, W.S. (1971). Observations of the vibration of the basilar membrane in squirrel monkeys using the Mössbauer technique. J. Acoust. Soc. Amer. 49, 1218-1231.

Wilson, J.P., and Johnstone, J.R. (1972). Capacitive probe measures of basilar membrane vibration. Symposium on Hearing Theory 1972, pp. 172-181. IPO Eindhoven, Holland.

DISCUSSION

KIANG: Have you considered the possible effects of electromechanical interactions of the cochlear structures with the stainless steel source? Your results are very intriguing, especially the part about the effects of death or destruction of the auditory nerve. Since there are many cochlear potentials that could act on the source and since the system is so very sensitive to small effects, there could be significant interactions. This question can be explored experimentally. If one destroys the nerve in chronic preparations but leaves the cochlear blood supply intact the neural potentials are gone, but the cochlear microphonic potentials remain. The cochlear microphonic potentials and neural potentials both disappear with large doses of kanamycin. In both preparations the animal would be alive and one could see whether the sharp nonlinearities might be absent. Then one might be better able to assess the significance of the changes you get after death.

RHODE: We talked about using the kanamycin preparation for various things. We were worried about the possibility of electrical coupling to the source but we had no real understanding of it.

KIANG: When you removed the nerve, did you check that you did not also hit the blood supply? If so the microphonics as well as the nerve response would disappear.

RHODE: I remove the nerve entirely so I believe that the cochlear blood supply is removed.

DAVIS: I think this apparent relation of the physical properties of the basilar membrane to the metabolic state is a very important contribution to our thinking. We left out that possibility originally in the Békésy era. I do not know whether rigor mortis is a proper analogy here or whether it is a loosening of some kind. Will you kindly recapitulate what you believe to be the physical parameters that have changed? Is it a change of stiffness, is it a change in the stiffness gradient, or is it possibly a difference in the coupling between immediately adjacent elements? I am looking for a model for the sharp slope on the low-frequency side of the response area which gives us a sharp "tail" in the tuning curve.

RHODE: The fact that the amplitude ratio increases after death relative to when the preparation is intact would indicate that there is a lessening in the stiffness of the partition. I have, however, no way of relating that to the individual physical structures.

KOHLLÖFFEL: I wonder whether the disappearance of your nonlinearity after the animal has been killed has something to do with changes in the viscosity of inner ear fluids and components. After all, it is also due to viscous forces that the probe is held in place and is constrained to follow the motion of the membrane. Now in remembering what Dr. Tonndorf has said about viscosity, boundary layers and nonlinearities, it is conceivable that a change in viscosity has a linearizing effect on the probe coupling to the membrane. So it could well be that the whole nonlinear problem is one of viscosity and its influence on the probe coupling to the vibrating membrane. Have you looked at viscosity?

RHODE: No, I have not attempted to control that parameter.

ZWISLOCKI: I would like to back up Dr. Kohllöffel's statement: I feel that viscosity as far as I understand, would make the curves change very nicely as I saw them.

TONNDORF: I do not think this is so much a question

of viscosity here. I would like to come back to the
question that Dr. Davis started. The membranes change
very quickly in their physical properties after death.
You may recall that Békésy reported some twenty years
ago that the tectorial membrane has viscous properties; it is very brittle, i.e. when you take it out
of the organ. However, when you examine it in the
living animal, it is not brittle at all, but highly
elastic. As soon as you open up scala media, things
change, apparently under the influence of the wrong
fluid which is then entering there. These physical
changes of the membrane are probably more important
in this case than the viscosity changes.

RHODE: I agree that some rapid physical change is
probably responsible.

ZWICKER: I agree completely with Dr. Tonndorf's comment that the surrounding is very important for the
tectorial membrane.

EVANS: One of the things that impresses me is the
similarity between the shapes of the frequency response curves in your figures and in the results of
Wilson and Johnstone (1972). That is, an amplitude
response relative to stapes motion with a two-segment
low frequency cut-off of 6 and 24 dB/octave, and a
high frequency cut-off of about 100 dB/octave. The
main difference between your and their data now is
the nonlinearity which you find, which if exploited
(as in my Fig. 1), leads to cut-off of much higher
slopes. There are some differences in the phase behavior, but the striking thing to me is the correspondence between your and their amplitude data.

RHODE: That is right as long as you ignore the nonlinearity and the phase characteristic of Wilson and
Johnstone, which shows at the most about a cycle and
a half difference in phase between the incus and
motion of the basilar membrane.

Reference

Wilson, J.P. and Johnstone, J.R.(1972). Capacitive probe measure of basilar mombrane vibration. Symposium on Hearing Theory 1972, pp. 172-181, IPO Eindhoven, Holland.

A POSSIBILITY FOR SUB-TECTORIAL
MEMBRANE FLUID MOTION

C. R. Steele

Stanford University
Stanford, California
USA

1. Introduction

Very recently several observations and results have been reported which, in my opinion, fit together to form a clear picture of the missing filter between the basilar membrane motion and the neural excitation. I suggest that the missing element is a strong DC component of the sub-tectorial membrane fluid flow. The entire function of the reticular lamina, the spiral sulcus, and the outer hair cells is to establish this directed flow against the cilia of the inner hair cells.

However, my discussion of this flow depends on the recent results from the analysis of a model for the primary basilar membrane motion. So I will summarize these results and show the correlation with the physiological data, before discussing the possibility of significant sub-tectorial membrane fluid motion.

2. Cochlear model

A summary of the analytical and experimental work on cochlear models is given by Tonndorf (1970), in which a clear description of various features of the "traveling wave" and the fluid motion can be found. However, the mechanical model has been lacking, which describes with a reasonable degree of accuracy the fluid-elastic interaction and yet submits to a mathematical analysis of a reasonable degree of simplicity. These seemingly mutually exclusive requirements do appear to be satisfied by a model recently treated (Steele,1973a, 1973b). This model is shown in Fig. 1. The significant feature is actually very simple; the rigid walls of the scalae are tapered.

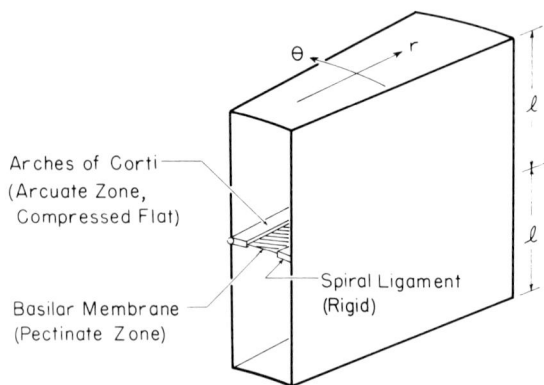

Fig. 1 Cochlear model.

Thus a Fourier series (in θ) can be used for the motions of the basilar membrane and the fluid in the scalae. The soft tissue of the organ of Corti and Reissner's membrane is removed. The viscosity of the fluid is assumed to be 3.8 centipoise. The height ℓ of the model scalae is chosen to be 4 mm, to match the scala area in the cochlea. Only the semi-infinite model is treated; the appropriate end conditions for the helicotrema have not yet been taken into consideration.

Displacement Modes of Organ of Corti

The mass of the organ of Corti is negligible in comparison with that of the fluid, but the appropriate stiffness properties are not so easily resolved. Several investigators have used the static point load results (Békésy, 1960) to calculate the plate bending stiffness of the basilar membrane; but the resulting volume displacement under static pressure is an order-of-magnitude different from the measurement (Békésy, 1960). (See discussion by Zwislocki, 1953.) In recent times the point load results have been ignored for the "long wavelength" cochlear models. However, the wavelengths in the cochlea are most definitely not always "long" in comparison with the cross-section, particularly in the region of maximum displacement, so the question of stiffness must be reopened.

Indeed, Békésy's results for the deflection under

the point load on the basilar membrane, when replotted on a linear scale (Dotson, 1973) clearly show that the arches of Corti have a significant stiffness. Furthermore, the deflection at the inner foot of the arch is relatively significant near the stapes. Thus the three deformation modes shown in Fig. 2 are considered. Mode I is a plate bending of

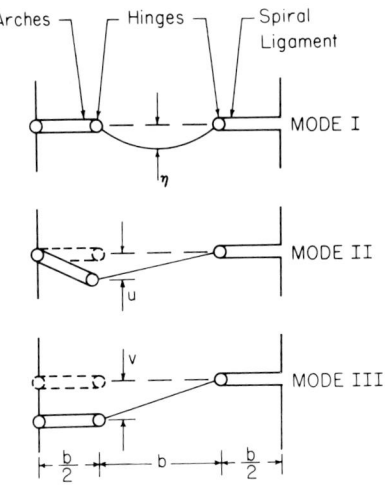

Fig. 2 Deflection modes

the pectinate zone of the basilar membrane; Mode II consists of a rotation of the arches of Corti; Mode III consists of a shearing deflection of the tip of the spiral limbus. The spiral ligament is assumed to be rigid, although, in reality, it will also have some flexibility.

The stiffness parameters are: (Mode I) K, plate bending; Mode II) k, against uniform rotation of the arches, and GJ, against relative rotation between arches, (i.e., torsional stiffness);(Mode III) κ, against uniform displacement, and EI, against bending (in r-direction). Values are chosen so that the model has exactly the behavior under a point load that Békésy measured, and fits the pressure-volume displacement measurement, except near the helicotrema, where the model is only about three times more compliant. Fortunately, the results are not sensitive to a change in stiffness of this magnitude.

The variation in stiffness along the cochlea agrees
qualitatively with the anatomy, i.e., κ and EI are
constant, and K corresponds to a homogeneous plate,
whose thickness is inversely proportional to the
width. I doubt that a simpler structural model can be
found which agrees with Békésy's point load and pressure measurements, and the anatomy.

Now, a very important fact in this: <u>No free parameters remain</u>! The physical features of the model are
clear; the dynamic response results are obtained as
a direct consequence, <u>without</u> any readjustment of the
model properties. Thus the following correlations
with physiological data are not in any way contrived.

<u>Plate Strip in Infinite Fluid</u>

Before discussing the solution for the model in Fig.
1, it should be mentioned that the generation of

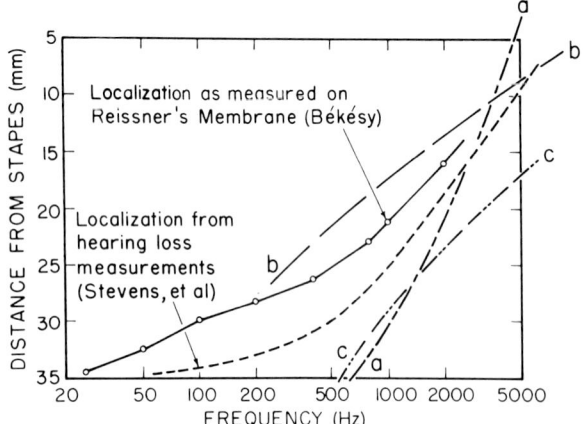

Fig. 3   Locus of transition point for basilar membrane modeled as a tapered plate strip in an
infinite incompressible, inviscid fluid,
with stiffness calculated from Békésy's
measurements:

a) Volume compliance

b) Point load deflection, with assumption
of perfectly flexible arches of Corti

c) Point load deflection, with assumption
of perfectly rigid arches of Corti

traveling waves can be easily explained by consideration of the basilar membrane as a massless tapered plate strip in an infinite, inviscid fluid (Steele, 1973a). The point of transition between almost constant phase and traveling wave motion of the plate is easily determined. The locus of this transition point depends on the frequency, as well as plate width and stiffness as shown in Fig. 3. The actual localization in the cochlea is bounded by these simple limiting considerations. The deviation between curves (a) and (c) is an indication of the importance of Mode III in the basal turn, while the bracketing, through the important frequency range, by curves (b) and (c) of Békésy's observation and the curve of acoustic trauma (guinea pig), which coincides with the integration of difference limens, (Stevens et al., 1935) indicates that the arches do have significant stiffness. Thus we proceed with the analysis of the model in Figs. 1 and 2.

Phase Integral Solution

The solution for the model of Fig. 1 is obtained, for a pure tone excitation at the stapes, in the form of an asymptotic series expansion of a traveling wave

$$\eta(r,t) = \psi(r,\omega)[1 + O(\alpha)] \exp[i(\omega t - P(r,\omega)) - D(r,\omega)] \quad (1)$$

Once the phase function $P = \int \mu dr$ is determined from the "eikonel" equation, the inviscid amplitude function ψ and the damping D due to fluid viscosity are easily determined. Because the taper angle α is so small, the first term of the expansion seems to provide sufficient accuracy. The first approximation to the eikonel equation is

$$\frac{\mu b}{\rho \omega^2} \text{Tanh } \mu \ell = \frac{b^2}{K + EI\mu^4} + \frac{9}{64} \frac{b^4}{k + GJ\mu^2} + \frac{8}{\pi^2 K} \frac{b}{[(\frac{\pi}{b})^2 + \mu^2]^2} \quad (2)$$

For long wavelengths, i.e. $\mu \to 0$, the right-hand-side gives the volume compliance under a static pressure in the scalae. For short wavelengths, the stiffnesses in the r-direction (EI, GJ, K) become significant. On the left-hand-side is the fluid effect. The height ℓ of the scalae appears only in the argument. Thus when $\mu\ell>1$ the behavior is independent of ℓ, i.e. "shortwave", while $\mu\ell<1$ for "longwaves", for which the fluid pressure over a cross-section is essentially constant.

The real root of (2) gives the traveling wave. However, other roots exist which give the solutions needed to satisfy the exact end conditions at the stapes and at the helicotrema.

The impedance at the stapes can be easily calculated from (2). The results for the 1-mode model (i.e., κ = k = ∞), the 2-mode model (i.e., κ = ∞), and the complete 3-mode model are shown on Fig. 4. The low

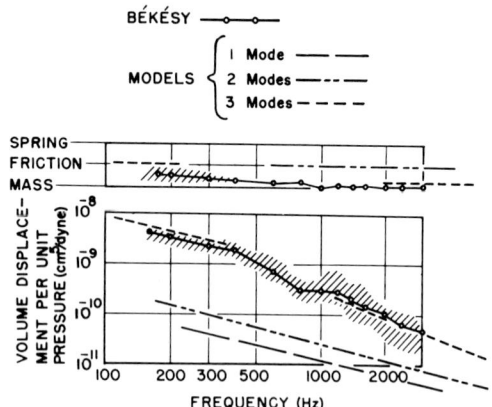

Fig. 4 Impedance of cochlea at stapes.

frequency line for the 3-mode model depends only on κ, i.e., the wavelength at the stapes is "long". But the high frequency line depends only on EI, and the wavelength is "short". Thus for frequencies much over 1 kHz, <u>there are no longwaves in the cochlea</u>. This agrees with the observation (Békésy, 1960) of transverse waves on Reissner's membrane for frequencies over 1 kHz.

Incidentally, the analytical results shown in Fig. 4 are independent of the fluid viscosity, while the envelopes of waves in the cochlea are not. Thus Békésy's use of the independence of the results in Fig. 4 on temperature, to justify subsequent work at room temperature, was not quite correct. However, this viscosity change should not have a particularly severe effect.

Unfortunately, the complete numerical details for the 3-mode model are yet to be worked out. But the following results from the 2-mode model are in such agreement with physiological date that one must conclude that the modes I and II describe a significant part of the mechanical function of the cochlea. Indeed, a conclusion is that the small flexibility of the BM supports, expressed by Mode III, diminishes the high frequency capability. It is clear that the very well-developed spiral ligament and bony shelf found, for example, in bats is intended to eliminate the possibility of Mode III.

Results and Correlations

For the 2-mode model (i.e., with $\kappa \to \infty$) with a stapes excitation of 1 kHz, the traveling wave envelopes are shown in Fig. 5. The important conclusion is that the maximum arch motion u_{MAX}, the maximum basilar membrane displacement w_{MAX}, and the maximum of the angle between the arch and the pectinate zone of the basilar membrane β_{MAX} occur at <u>different locations</u> along the cochlea, although these three kinematic quantities are, to a first approximation, in phase.

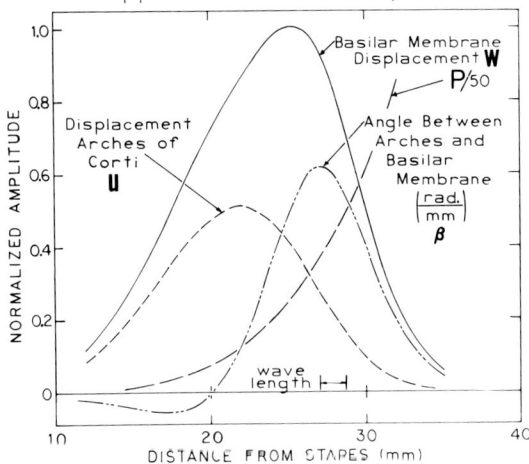

Fig. 5 Envelopes of motion and the phase for 1kHz excitation of 2-mode model.

Békésy observed the motion of Reissner's membrane;

his curve is similar to the arch displacement curve in Fig. 5, while w_{MAX} is near the point for acoustic trauma. The later observation (Békésy, 1960) of a transition from transverse to axial motion of the tectorial membrane also appears in the model. The transverse shearing stress at the hinge has an envelope similar to the total basilar membrane displacement, while the axial shear is similar to the angle discontinuity. The radial shear at the center of the pectinate zone is similar to the curve for arch motion.

On Fig. 6 is shown the locus of u_{MAX}, w_{MAX}, and β_{MAX} with frequency. The curve for w_{MAX} would be similar to Békésy's curve for low frequencies, if the helicotrema end effect solutions were added. However, the

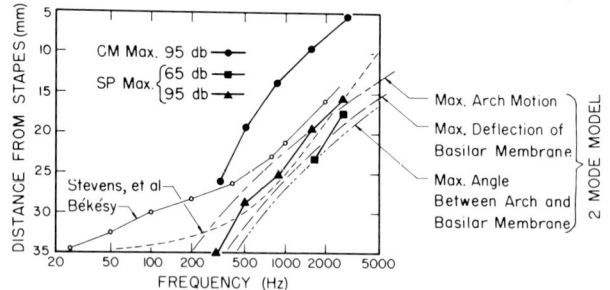

Fig. 6 Cochlear localization; CM and SP data from Honrubia and Ward (1968, 1969).

theoretical curves show the peaks of the main wave generated by the motion of the stapes. If the neural excitation for moderate and high frequencies is due to a "place effect" associated with the maximum of the traveling wave, then it is clear from Fig. 6 that the mechanism of excitation for low frequencies is substantially different. The curve for β_{MAX} reaches the heliocotrema at about 400 Hz, while u_{MAX} is there at about 200 Hz. It seems more than coincidental that Møller (1972) found a limitation of around 300 Hz for the transmission by all nerve fibers of frequency and amplitude modulation, while Simmons and Glattke (1970) found a sharp cutoff at about 500 Hz of the frequency perception of an electrical signal directly on the VIIIth nerve. Thus Fig. 6 shows clearly the transition from the place effect to the direct neural transmission of the low frequencies.

The measurement by Honrubia and Ward (1969) of the spatial distribution of the summating potential is also pertinent. Even though they recorded at only four stations, the properties of the distributions are clear. After rescaling from an 18 to 35 mm cochlea, the locations of the estimated maximum SP for 95 dB is shown on Fig. 6. For a lower intensity level, it is very clear that the maximum shifts; two points for 65 dB are shown on Fig. 6.

The location of the cochlear microphonic maximum is also shown on Fig. 6. Because of the possibility of cancellation of this signal for short spatial wavelengths, it is not clear that this curve should be taken as a true indication of the maximum of this activity. As a matter of fact, the location of the first appearance of CM (Honrubia and Ward, 1968) is near the u_{MAX} curve.

Even though the phase of the traveling wave changes quite rapidly with position (Fig. 5), the variation in phase at a fixed point as the frequency varies is almost linear; Fig. 7 shows the analytical result.

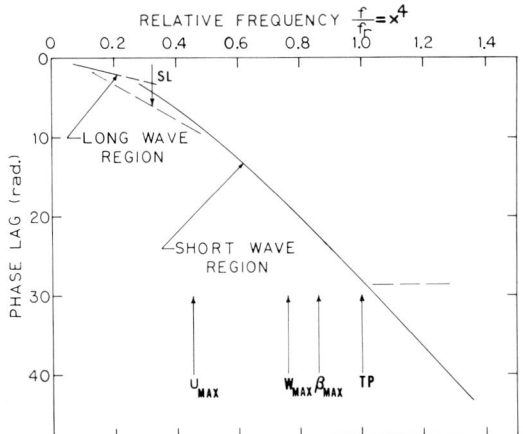

Fig. 7 Phase at fixed point from 2-mode model; for point of w_{MAX} at 7 kHz (i.e. f_r = 8.1 kHz). Arrows show relative frequencies at which u_{MAX}, β_{MAX}, and the transition point arrive. Dashed lines indicate the significant deviation from results of Rhode (1971); the arrow SL shows the relative frequency Rhode found for maximum spiral lamina motion.

With the frequency normalized to the frequency at the transition point (Curve c in Fig. 3) there is the single curve for all frequencies for the short wave region. The slope of the long wave region does depend to some extent on the point. If we consider the point at which w_{MAX} arrives at 7 kHz, then the relative frequencies at which u_{MAX}, w_{MAX}, and β_{MAX} arrive are shown by the arrows in Fig. 7. The phase and slope agree very well with that observed by Rhode (1971) in the neighborhood of w_{MAX}. Rhode also measured the motion of the spiral limbus, and found a maximum amplitude at the relative frequency shown, which is in the middle of the region of disagreement with the 2-mode model result. Thus the second slope observed by Rhode seems to be due to the spiral limbus flexibility, i.e., Mode III. For lower frequencies this should not be as prominent. Indeed, in the results of Anderson et al. (1971) the change in phase of the neural firings with frequency is found to be quite linear.

The phase of the cochlear microphonics also varies almost linearly with frequency. However, the slopes measured by Dallos and Cheatham (1971) fit the "long wave region" curve of Fig. 7. A clearer comparison is shown in Fig. 8, on which the arrival time of the

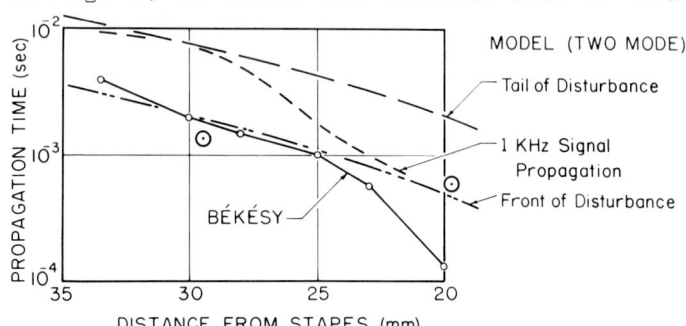

Fig. 8 Click propagation along cochlea; points ⊙ from Dallos and Cheatham (1970) for Guinea pig CM.

front and tail of the disturbance due to a "click" at the stapes is shown. The propagation of the "energy" or "signal" associated with a given frequency (i.e., 1 kHz, Fig. 8) follows the "front" until the point u_{MAX} for that frequency is approached; then the propagation velocity decreases so the curve becomes tangent to the upper envelope which forms the "tail" in Fig. 8. The discrepancy with Békésy's observation at the 20 mm station is due to Mode III, which, according to Fig. 7, would have much less effect on the steady-state phase measurement used by Dallos and Cheatham (1971) for the arrival time estimation indicated in Fig. 8. Thus the 2-mode model is non-dispersive for sufficiently low frequencies, i.e. for frequencies less than that for which u_{MAX} is at the observation point, in agreement with conclusions for the guinea pig cochlea by Nordmark et al. (1969).

A remarkable correlation also occurs with the arrival time (actually the corrected slope of the phase-frequency curve) for single auditory nerve fibers in the spider monkey obtained by Anderson et al. (1971), as shown in Fig. 9. The curves show the arrival time

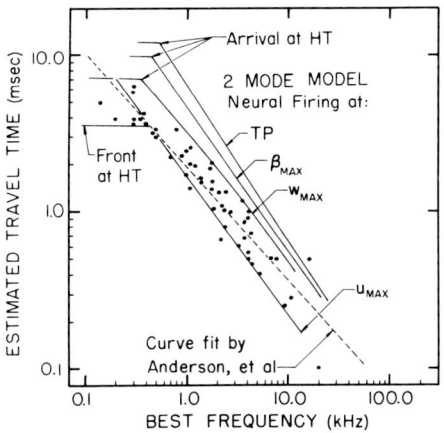

Fig. 9 Data for estimated travel time from Anderson et al. (1971) compared with 2-mode model results.

from the 2-mode model, assuming that the nerve fires at the transition point, at β_{MAX}, at w_{MAX}, and at u_{MAX}. Almost all data points, presumably for 90 dB stimulation, are bounded by the u_{MAX} and w_{MAX} curves. At about 3.7 msec the low frequency front, from Fig. 8, arrives at the helicotrema, which provides the lower bound for the fibers with CF less than 500 Hz. For lower tone intensities the arrival time obtained by Anderson et al. (1971) increases.

Indeed, if the assumption is made that the characteristic frequency is that for which β_{MAX} is at the fiber, then the frequencies, at which the transition point, w_{MAX} and u_{MAX} are at the fiber, are shown by the arrows on the fiber response curve Fig. 10 from Anderson et al. 1971).

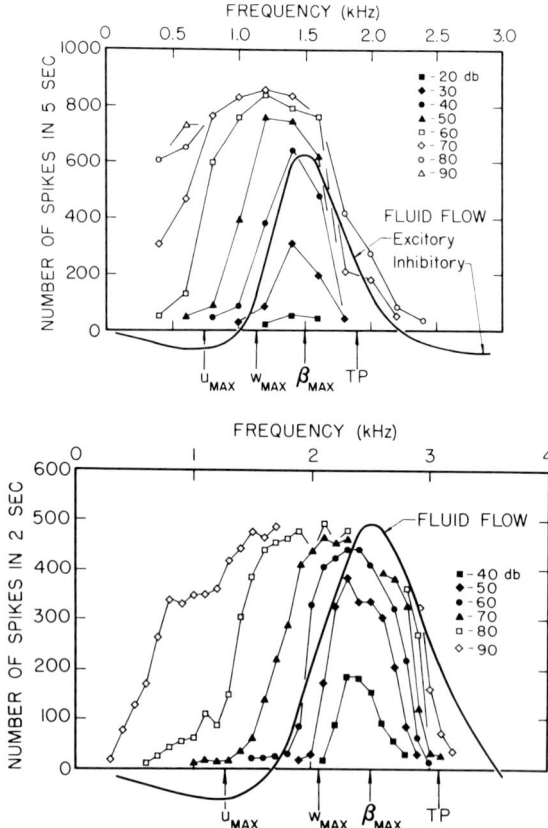

Fig. 10 a & b Single fiber response from Anderson et al. (1971) related to mechanical events from 2-mode model.

Conclusions on the cochlear model

The correlation of the model results with the physiological data is so strong that I must make these conclusions. The model (Fig. 1) does represent the cochlea and the 3 modes of motion in Fig. 2 are significant. From Figs. 6, 9, 10, it seems quite possible that the CF is the frequency for which β_{MAX} is at the fiber. As the tone intensity is increased, the center of neural excitation shifts to w_{MAX} and then toward u_{MAX}.

It is striking that the distance between β_{MAX} and w_{MAX} is about 1 mm, actually ranging from 2.6 mm for 500 Hz to 0.44 mm for 20 kHz. Spoendlin (1971a) has determined the enervation of the cat's organ of Corti. For every inner hair cell, with 20 afferent fibers, there are about two efferents and one afferent, each of which is connected to a group of 10 outer hair cells; for the afferent, however, there is a distance of about 0.6 mm between the point of entry into the organ of Corti and the connection with the outer hair cells. I will, therefore, offer this speculation: the afferent nerves to the outer hair cells respond to the mechanical stimulation associated with w_{MAX}; through the efferent from the central nervous system, we have the control of the activity of the outer hair cells in the region near β_{MAX}.

Since Rhode (1971) did not observe a significant shift in the point of maximum BM motion with increasing intensity, I conclude that the shift shown in Fig. 10 shows transitions in the intermediate mechanism, most recently called for by Evans (1972), between the basilar membrane motion and the excitation of the neural endings.

3. Reticular laminar flow

So we now face the question of what this intermediate mechanism might be. The conventional explanation for the excitation of the hair cells is that the relative displacement of the tectorial and reticular membranes causes a shearing displacement of the cilia. However, the organ of Corti seems rather poorly designed for such a function. The attachment of the cilia of the outer hair cells with the tectorial membrane is extremely delicate, and there appears to be no attachment of the inner cilia. (See, for example, Lindeman et al., 1971.) Furthermore, the inner portion of the tectorial membrane also seems to be very delicate, acting as a soft spring (Fig. 11). If this portion were stiff, Békésy (1960) would have observed a marked phase difference between the tectorial and basilar membranes, with which a shearing excitation would be most effective. For a shearing excitation, the sub-tectorial membrane fluid would merely serve as a lubricant; there would be no need for the large spiral sulcus. My conclusion is that this fluid serves a much more significant function.

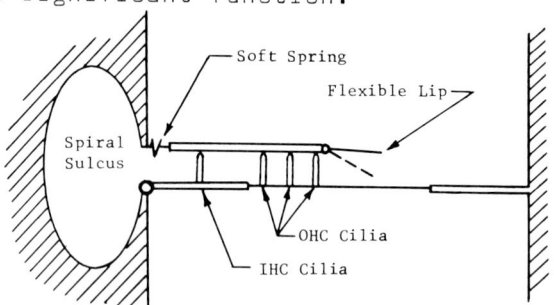

Fig. 11 Possible model for sub-tectorial membrane fluid motion.

From the details of the cochlear anatomy, Neubert (1950) came to the strong conviction that the sub-tectorial membrane fluid flow must be the excitory mechanism. Recently, Zwicker (1972) inserted particles in a pig cochlea and did not see the oscillatory flow suggested by Neubert, but a relatively strong steady flow. This flow was <u>out of the reticular lamina</u> (Zwicker, personal communication). We also have the observation of Spoendlin (1971b) that after noise exposure the early irreversible damage to the inner hair cells consists of a clustering and <u>outward inclination</u> of the cilia.

I, therefore, make the speculation that these observations are related, and that the function of the organ of Corti, under pure tone stimulation, is to establish a <u>directed flow</u> of the sub-tectorial membrane fluid which causes the excitation of the inner hair cells.

Source of Nonlinearity

The next question concerns the source of the nonlinearity which would be necessary for the production of such a directed flow. The Békésy eddy (Békésy, 1960) is well-known. A pair of such eddies also form in the transverse direction (Hallauer, 1973), which are responsible for the accumulation of tympanic lamina cells in the middle of the basilar membrane observed by Spoendlin (1971b). These eddies are, however, due to second order boundary effects (i.e., acoustic streaming) and become significant only at high intensity levels.

The w-shape of the outer hair cell cilia is also a source of nonlinearity. However, a rough calculation indicates that the nonlinearity due to this asymmetric geometry would not be significant until about the 100 dB SPL level. Similarly, the mechanical nonlinearity due to stretching of the basilar membrane is not significant below this level (Hallauer, 1973).

I make the speculation that the source of this nonlinearity is the outer lip (Marginal Zone) of the tectorial membrane. I consider the long controversy (Lindeman et al., 1971, Lim, 1972) over the details of the connections to be evidence that the lip is extremely delicate and flexible. Békésy (1960) found that the lip had almost no resistance while the central portion is stiff. Thus I propose the model of the tectorial membrane in Fig. 11.

Consider a to-and-fro motion of the reticular lamina fluid past this lip. For sufficiently small amplitudes the behavior is linear, but since the lip is so flexible, the flow amplitude does not have to be very large before a significant nonlinear valving action takes place. The lip offers little resistance to the outward flow, but, with the inward flow, closes and restricts the flow. The result is a directed flow against the cilia of the inner hair cells.

Such a mechanism fits perfectly with the results of Lindeman et al. (1971). The outer edge of the tectorial membrane in the new-born kitten is firmly attached to the Dieters' cells. Even though the organ of Corti appears mature two to three weeks after birth, the detachment of the tectorial membrane edge occurs at about five weeks, the age at which the kitten apparently attains normal hearing. Lindeman et al. (1971) report that even when the attachment is firm, the spacing of the fibers would allow fluid flow in and out of the reticular lamina. Thus the lip must be free in order to perform the proper valving action necessary for auditory function.

Viscous Flow Between Parallel Plates

The analysis of the tectorial membrane model of Fig. 11 has only begun, so the hard mathematical facts that might remove the preceding suggestions from the category of speculation are not available. However, a simple consideration does increase the plausibility.

The thickness of the reticular lamina is small in comparison with the viscous boundary layer. Therefore, the inertial forces are negligible in comparison with the viscous forces in the motion of the reticular laminar fluid. This means that the flow follows the basilar membrane motion <u>with no time delay</u>.

The equation for viscous flow between parallel plates is Laplace's equation. We now consider a point source of this steady flow. Since no fluid is lost or gained, this is a point "pump" or doublet. The resulting flow is shown in Fig. 12. Now imagine a row of inner hair cells on the dotted line of Fig. 12. In the center region the inner hair cell cilia would be exposed to a strong outward pressure, while out of this central region there would be a much weaker inward flow.

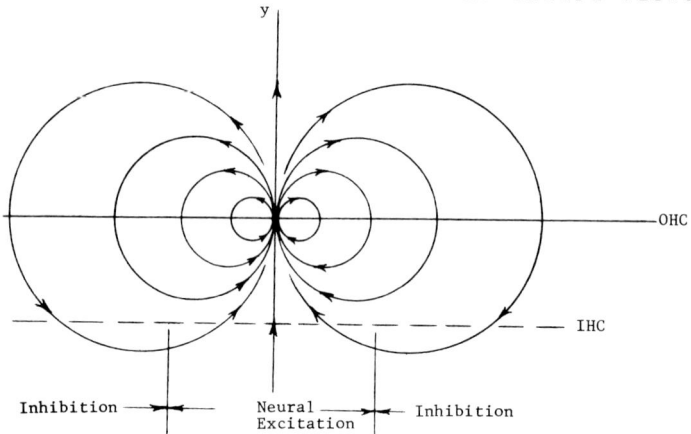

Fig. 12   Viscous flow between parallel plates due to point pump (doublet).

Thus the function of the inner hair cells is almost the same as in the vestibular apparatus. The outward flow causes depolarization, with an increase in neural firing rate, while the inward flow causes hyperpolarization, with an inhibition of firing rate. Indeed, many of the SP distribution curves obtained by Honrubia and Ward (1969) show such a distribution. In addition, the two-tone inhibition shown by Sachs and Kiang (1968) is easily explained by this flow.

To explicitly demonstrate the plausibility of such a mechanism, consider the distribution of doublets shown in Fig. 13. along the x axis of Fig. 12. The

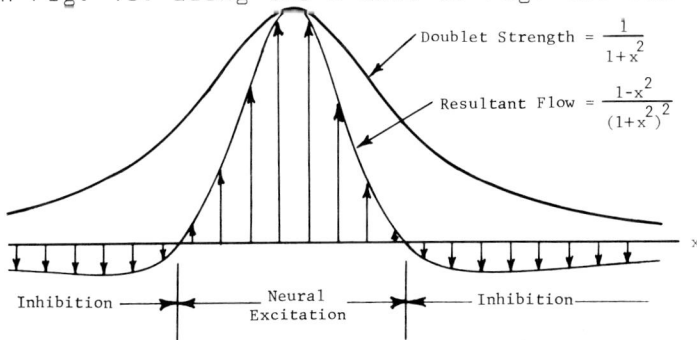

Fig. 13. Fluid velocity caused by line of doublets.

resultant flow velocity distribution (Fig. 13) changes direction when the doublet strength is only one-half its maximum value. Even though the pumping action has a broad distribution, the neural excitation is sharply restricted. Let us assume that this directed pumping is proportional to the curve for $|\beta|$ in Fig. 5, which reasonably fits (except at 20 mm) the doublet strength distribution of Fig. 13. Thus the neural excitation for 1 kHz would be from about 24 to 31 mm from the stapes. Or if we consider a fixed point, the flow velocity would have the variation with frequency shown in Figs. 10a and b for points with β_{MAX} at 1.5 and 2.5 kHz, respectively. In Fig. 10a, the distribution fits the neural recording of Anderson et al. (1971) at the 40 dB level, while the distribution in Fig. 10b very roughly fits the 60 dB level curve. If the pumping is assumed to be proportional to the w curve of Fig. 6, the resulting flow velocity distribution roughly fits the 80 dB level curves of Fig. 10a and b. The flow should change directions at about the frequency at which w is half its maximum value, which is at about 1.5 CF. This gives the vertical asymptotes shown on the tuning curves in Fig. 14 from Evans (1972), which match well with the data in the middle frequency range. Thus consideration of the flow offers a good reason for having tuning curves with infinite slope.

The nonlinear mechanism producing a directed flow would also exert a significant nonlinear forcing of the basilar membrane. Thus the addition of the tec-

85

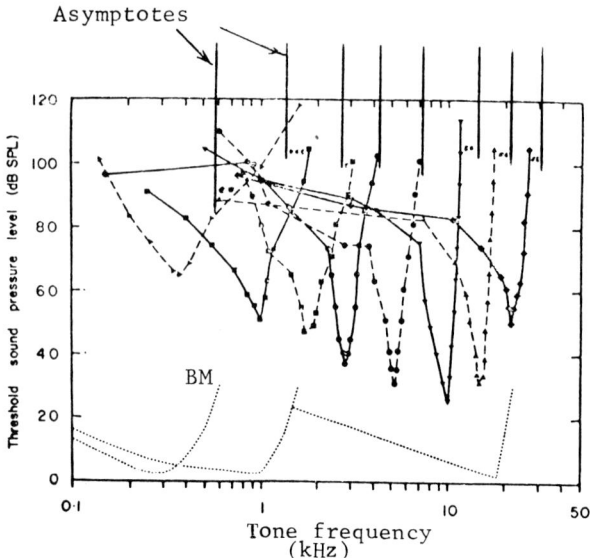

Fig. 14 Tuning curves from Evans (1972) with estimated vertical asymptotes, assuming reversed flow at $w_{MAX}/2$ and CF at β_{MAX}.

torial membrane of Fig. 11 would necessitate a reanalysis of the basic basilar membrane motion. The nonlinearity observed by Rhode (1971) could be caused by exactly this process, as well as the somewhat steeper high-frequency slope of the neural firing rate, compared with the rough estimate of the fluid velocity distribution in Figs. 10a, b.

4. Conclusion

The correlation of the results from the analysis of the basilar membrane model of Figs. 1, 2 with the physiological data is too strong to be considered as coincidental. This model does describe the basilar membrane behavior. The conclusion is that Békésy (1960) is correct; Rhode (1971) is correct; all of which is very compatible with the neurological data of Anderson et al. (1971), the summating potential data of Honrubia and Ward (1968), and the cochlear microphonic result of Dallos and Cheatham (1971).

The mathematical results have not yet been obtained for the tectorial membrane model of Fig. 11. However, the notion of an induced directed flow in the retic-

ular lamina seems to provide a simple explanation of
the missing sharpening mechanism between the basilar
membrane and the neural excitation, which is consistent with phyciological data. There is certainly
enough promise to warrant a further effort to place
this notion on a more substantial analytical basis.

5. Summary

The recently obtained analytical results for the
"pure tone" and "click" excitation of a cochlear model are briefly summarized. These results are shown
to be in substantial agreement with the available
physiological data. Much remains to be quantified,
but a reasonably coherent picture of the basic basilar membrane motion is offered, which involves the
consideration of independent flexibility of the
arches of Corti and the pectinate zone of the basilar
membrane, as well as the support at the tip of the
spiral limbus.

The focus is, however, on the missing filter between
the basilar membrane motion and the neural excitation. It is suggested that, due to a valving action
of the flexible lip of the tectorial membrane, a directed flow of the sub-tectorial membrane fluid
against the inner hair cells is established. This
notion fits with recent physiological observations,
and is supported by preliminary analytical calculations.

Acknowledgement

A portion of this study was supported by the Bio-
Medicine Institute, University of Zürich, Zürich,
Switzerland.

References

Anderson, D.J., Rose, J.E., Hind, J.E., and Brugge,
J.F. (1971). Temporal position of discharges in
single auditory nerve fibers within the cycle
of a sine-wave stimulus: frequency and intensity
effects. J. Acoust. Soc. Amer. 49, 1131-1139.

Békésy, G.v. (1960). Experiments in Hearing, pp. 420,
467-468, 476, 489-497. McGraw-Hill, New York.

Dallos, P., and Cheatham, M.A. (1971). Travel time in the cochlea and its determination from cochlear-microphonic data. J. Acoust. Soc. Amer. 49, 1140-1143.

Dotson, R. (1973). Cochlear model with transient excitation. Thesis. Stanford Univ., Palo Alto, Calif. (In preparation).

Evans, E.F. (1972). Does frequency sharpening occur in the cochlea? Symposium on Hearing Theory 1972, pp. 27-34. IPO Eindhoven, Holland.

Hallauer (1973). Nonlinear mechanical behavior of inner ear. Thesis. Stanford Univ., Palo Alto, Calif. (In preparation).

Honrubia, V., and Ward, P.H. (1969). Properties of the summating potential of the guinea pig's cochlea. J. Acoust. Soc. Amer. 45, 1443-1450.

Honrubia, V., and Ward, P.H. (1968). Longitudinal distribution of the cochlear microphonics in side the cochlear duct (guinea pig). J. Acoust. Soc. Amer. 44, 951-958.

Lim, D.J. (1972). Fine morphology of the tectorial membrane. Arch. Otolaryngol. 96, 199-215.

Lindeman, H.H., Ades, H.W., Bredberg, G., and Engström, H. (1971). The sensory hairs and the tectorial membrane in the development of the cat's organ of corti. Acta Otolaryngol. 72, 229-242.

Møller, A.R. (1972). Coding of amplitude and frequency modulated sounds in the cochlear nucleus of the rat. Acta Physiol. Scand. 86, 223-238.

Neubert, K. (1950). Die Basilarmembran des Menschen und ihr Verankerungssystem. Z. Anat. 114, 539-588.

Nordmark, J.O., Glattke, T.J., and Schubert, E.D. (1969). Waveform preservation in the cochlea. J. Acoust. Soc. Amer. 46, 1587-1588.

Rhode, W.S. (1971). Observations of the vibration of the basilar membrane in squirrel monkeys using the Mössbauer technique. J. Acoust. Soc. Amer. 49, 1218-1231.

Sachs, M.B., and Kiang, N.Y.S. (1968). Two-tone inhibition in auditory-nerve fibers. J. Acoust. Soc. Amer. 43, 1120-1128.

Simmons, F. Blair, and Glattke, T.J. (1970). Some electrophysiological factors in volley-pitch perception by electrical stimulation. In: Sensorineural Hearing Loss (G.E.W. Wolstenholme and J. Knight, eds.), pp. 225-240. J. & A. Churchill, London.

Spoendlin, H. (1971a). Degeneration behavior of the cochlear nerve. Arch. Klin. Exp. Ohr.-Nas.-Kehlk. Heilk. 200, 275-291.

Spoendlin, H. (1971b). Primary structural changes in the organ of corti after acoustic overstimulation. Acta Otolaryngol. 71, 166-176.

Steele, C.R. (1973a). Cochlear mechanics. In: Handbook of Sensory Physiology, Vol. 5, The Auditory System. (W.D. Keidel and W.D. Neff, eds.) Springer, Berlin. (In press).

Steele, C.R. (1973b). Behavior of the basilar membrane with pure tone excitation. J. Acoust. Soc. Amer. (In press).

Stevens, S.S., Davis, H., and Lurie, M.H. (1935). The localization of pitch perception on the basilar membrane. J. Gen. Psychol. 13, 297-315.

Tonndorf, J. (1970). Cochlear mechanics and hydro-Dynamics. In: Foundations of Modern Auditory Theory (J.V. Tobias, ed.), Vol. 1, pp. 203-250. Academic Press, New York.

Zwicker, E. (1972). Investigation of the inner ear of the domestic pig and the squirrel monkey with special regard to the hydrodynamics of the cochlear duct. Symposium on Hearing Theory 1972, pp. 182-185. IPO Eindhoven, Holland.

Zwislocki, J. (1953). Review of recent mathematical theories of cochlear dynamics. J. Acoust. Soc. Amer. 25, 743-751.

DISCUSSION

SPOENDLIN: If I understood you correctly, in mode number three, the arch region moves as a whole and not as a hinge and you said that this movement is more important in the basal turn than in the apical turn. On anatomical grounds, I find it difficult to explain this because in the basal turn, the inner pillars are placed directly on the bone of the tympanic lip of the osseous spiral lamina and hence this structure cannot possibly move as a whole. This is so both in the cat and the guinea pig cochlea.

STEELE: Both of these animals have a higher upper frequency limit than the human ear, for which there is, I believe, more of a distance between the bone edge and the inner pillars. Von Békésy did find a finite pillar, which I have used to compute the stiffness. The bone edge itself will have some flexibility.

TONNDORF: I would like to caution you a little against regarding all bones as being extremely stiff. You mentioned the bat. In that animal, the apical portion of the basilar membrane is a thin plate of bone, and it does vibrate. There bony plates are so thin that they behave much like membranes. On the spiral ligament i.e., on the opposite side, the anchorage with some fibers going up and some fibers going down, is probably much stiffer, but I do think that the spiral lamina ossia is capable of flexing to some extent.

DALLOS: I would like to agree with the importance which you attach to fluid streaming between tectorial membrane and reticular membrane. In a recent dissertation from our laboratory, Dr. Billone (Billone, 1972) has gone through similar computations to yours, and has shown a very significant streaming component. Some of the results on inner versus outer hair cell differences seem to bear out the importance of this streaming which apparently is instrumental in stimulating inner hair cells. There is one item that I would like to caution you against, however. The cochlear microphonic produced by the inner hair cells in animals in which we have removed the outer hair cells with kanamycin is considerably lower than normal; but, so is the summating potential. In other words, the inner hair cells that are stimulated by streaming are not stimulated exclusively by a dc component but also by an ac component of similar magnitude. I shall present some of these results tomorrow.

KOHLLÖFFEL: You stress the importance of dc-flow as stimulus to the receptor cells. I do not understand how any dc process could account for the phase-locking one observes in the auditory fibers.

STEELE: To the dc component of flow (Figs. 12, 13) will be added an ac component, which follows the basilar membrane motion and is large enough to cause the neural phase-locking (Fig. 9).

GRIFFIN: Speaking as a partisan of bats, I am delighted to see that they are coming into basic auditory neurophysiology. But I would like, as a zoologist, to enter a caution against the thinking that all bats are alike. Furthermore most other small mammals that do not echolocate also have rather good high frequency hearing. As I recall from the work of Ada Pye there are some very complicated anatomical differences which I at least have never been able to correlate with the kinds of sounds made.

STEELE: I am aware that different bats have different properties; but a common characteristic of those with high frequency echolocation capability seems to be an unusually well-developed support of the basilar membrane.

ZWICKER: As I mentioned at the Eindhoven Symposium, we have observed some of these sub-tectorial membrane fluids motions and I would like to add a little bit

more to what you said about inhibitory and excitatory
fields. You have shown a symmetrical curve. We have
observed that the flow is unsymmetrical and that the
eddies produce a flow along the basilar membrane from
the windows to the helicotrema. This means that we
have a flow not directly in radial direction but in
the direction which has a certain angle toward the
helicotrema which is very similar to the direction of
the fibers of the tectorial membrane.

STEELE: That is indeed interesting. These calculations of the flow are, of course, quite preliminary.
There are most definitely significant mechanical
features of the cochlea which I have not yet considered.

ZWISLOCKI: Thank you very much, Dr. Steele. Unfortunately for theoreticians, there are so many experimental results today to choose from that one can
agree with almost anything.

Reference

Billone, M. (1972). Mechanical stimulation of coch-
    lear hair cells. Thesis. Northwestern Univ.
    Evanston.

OBSERVATIONS OF THE MECHANICAL DISTURBANCES ALONG
THE BASILAR MEMBRANE WITH LASER ILLUMINATION

L.U.E. Kohllöffel

Eaton-Peabody Laboratory of Auditory Physiology
Massachusetts Eye and Ear Infirmary
Massachusetts Institute of Technology
Cambridge, Massachusetts
USA

Introduction

With the progress in the research on the activity of
the auditory nerve and of higher levels of the auditory system, it becomes increasingly more important
to have a clear quantitative understanding of cochlear mechanics. Not only does this concern - more
broadly speaking - the development of concepts in
formulating input-output models of auditory data
processing but it also concerns - more specifically -
the development of techniques that allow direct
intracochlear stimulus control. Such a control is
essential, for instance, in any eventual future experimental study of the multiple stages of intracochlear signal transformation. For several decades
the direct optical work of von Békésy (1960) on basilar membrane vibrations stood practically alone in
the field, and his results were complemented by research on the cochlear microphonic potential (Tasaki
et al., 1952) that revealed certain qualitative similarities between aspects of this potential and the
travelling wave pattern established by von Békésy.
Quite recently this situation has changed and the
experimenter is now in a position of choose from a
set of newly developed techniques that have been
successfully employed in the study of basilar membrane vibrations. It is probably fair to say that
none of these new techniques is as yet "ideal" and
that certain shortcomings have to be accepted for all
of them. Considering the minute size and large dynamic range of the membrane deflections and the relative inaccessibility of the intracochlear spaces,

this is not surprising.

The Mössbauer technique has been adapted by Johnstone et al. (1970) for intracochlear use. In talking of a shortcoming, one could emphasize that it is, in the strict sense, an indirect method. The technique monitors the velocity of a probe placed on the basilar membrane while leaving the problem of how well membrane motion is coupled to the probe unanswered. In the event of conflicting data, this feature may turn out to be an important one. Wilson and Johnstone (1972) used a capacitive technique rather elegantly to monitor basilar membrane deflection. Apart from the relatively large size of their capacitive probe, it may be considered a disadvantage that the membrane has to be fairly dry for the procedure. On the corresponding side of cochlear microphonic recordings, quite a different technique (Kohllöffel, 1971) evolved based on the theoretical work of Whitfield and Ross (1965) to throw light on the excitatory pattern along the basilar membrane. The cochlear microphonic distribution is measured with a multiple electrode array, and it is shown to be the spatially filtered image of the electrical activity along the organ of Corti. The results of this technique are quantitatively consistent with mechanical measurements. The disadvantage of the multiple electrode technique is due to its being indirect which becomes particularly evident when dealing with cochlear microphonic distributions that - on closer inspection - carry a certain ripple structure (see Kohllöffel, 1971). Although there are many different ways in laser optics to measure vibrations, only some will prove suitable for intracochlear use. One such method is fuzziness-detection which we shall report on now. This technique and the obtained results have been described in a more detailed fashion in a previous publication (Kohllöffel, 1972 a,b,c) than is possible here.

Methods

In the experiments a 10m W laser (Scientifica, B.22, wavelength $0.6328\,\mu m$) was used to illuminate the exposed part of the basilar membrane, and measurements were done by observing through a Zeiss otoscope the changes in membrane appearance with stimulus variation. The study was carried out in the basal part of the guinea pig's cochlea, and the basilar membrane was exposed and viewed from the side of scala tympani. Two different exposures were chosen. For the investigation of vibratory reponses in the living condition the membrane was approached in the very basal, stapedial region, and airborne sound was delivered in a closed system to the eardrum where the sound pressure was monitored. In the other approach the cochlea was removed from the skull and the membrane was exposed so as to be visible from about 3 to 8 mm from the basal end. The preparation was immersed in a fluid-filled tank and sound pressure generated by a hydrophone was hydraulically coupled with a steel tube directly into the vestibule. In both instances measurements were done on successive days after death to follow up the changes in membrane response characteristics. The technique to be described is contactless; it is not necessary to deposit any probing material on the membrane and furthermore the fluid above the examined membrane region is no obstacle for measurements. In mentioning these attractive features it may be also emphasized that it is, of course, still necessary to open the cochlear space to expose the basilar membrane for the optical technique to work.

The speckled appearance of laser illuminated objects is a well-known phenomenon. Very recently several schemes based on speckle patterns to measure surface vibration have been proposed, some of which offer advantages for certain applications over holographic techniques (see, for instance, Butters and Leendertz, 1971; Archbold et al., 1970; Eliasson and Mottier, 1971). The present technique is particularly suited for studies of basilar membrane vibrations. It is, in my opinion, certainly much simpler than holography since it was during a rather frustrating attempt to use real-time holographic interferometry in the inner ear that I developed it.

The specks on the basilar membrane arise due to the interference of the coherent light backscattered from neighboring points. When the membrane - being a narrow strip constrained in motion on the side of the spiral ligament and the spiral lamina - is set into vibration, it undergoes deformations mainly in the transverse direction that alter the phase relationships of the backscattered light which in turn results in a change of the configuration of specks. Such changes can easily be observed when the membrane is slowly driven, say at frequencies below 10 Hz where the slow speckle motions give a clear impression of the up and down movements of the membrane. At higher frequencies one cannot follow the changes of individual specks, the transition between different speckle patterns being too rapid and instead one observes a blurring, smearing-out of the speckle pattern - the membrane appears fuzzy. Fuzziness becomes noticeable at amplitudes around 0.05 μm (Kohllöffel, 1972 a), and thus membrane regions vibrating at this threshold value or above can be distinguished from regions that vibrate with smaller amplitudes since those regions appear unblurred.

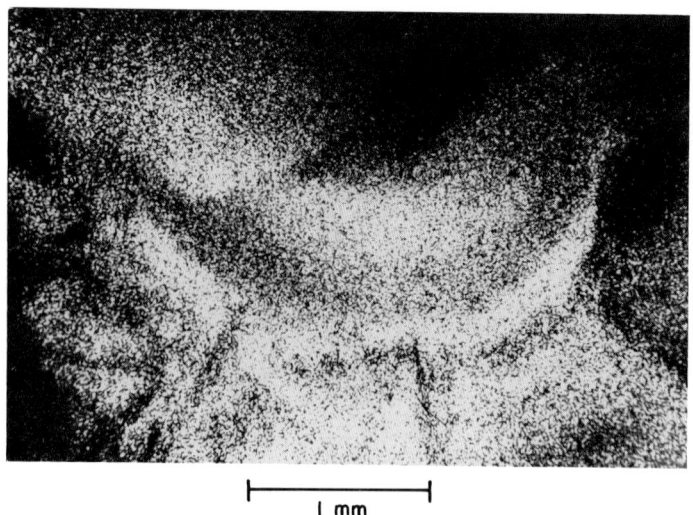

Fig.1 Photograph of basilar membrane taken under continuous laser illumination with the preparation immersed in the hydraulic tank filled with mammalian Ringer solution four days after death of the guinea pig. The basilar membrane is the dark half-ring shaped structure in the middle part of the picture. The membrane is visible from the tympanic side from approx. 4 mm (left, basal) to 8 mm (right, apical) measuring from the basal end. The black stripes radiating from the membrane are distance markers scratched into the dental

cement that covers the bottom part of the
preparation. In this photograph the basilar
membrane is stationary. The membrane is
covered with similar well-defined specks
as the surrounding areas of bone and dental
cement. (From Kohllöffel, 1972a).

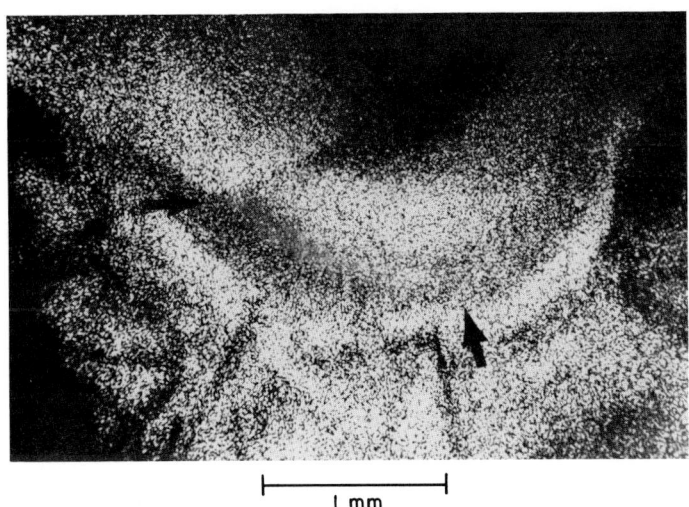

|← 1 mm →|

Fig.2 Photograph of same preparation as in Fig.1
taken under continuous laser illumination
(compare with Fig.1 where fuzziness is absent).
The membrane is driven by the hydrophone at
12 kHz and V_{THB} + 30 dB, i.e. 30 dB above the
level where fuzziness became noticeable in the
region of best response. Fuzziness is visible
from the extreme basal part of the exposure
(left arrow) up to the region marked by the
right arrow which is the threshold region
where fuzziness becomes just noticeable in
this case. In this location the membrane vibrates with an amplitude 30 dB below the
amplitude level of the basally located region
of best response. Note the change in "degree
of fuzziness" from left to right, i.e. from
regions of larger to regions of smaller amplitude. (From Kohllöffel, 1972a).

The photographs in Figs. 1 and 2 were taken under
continuous laser illumination with the preparation
mounted in the hydraulic tank. The basilar membrane
is the half-ring shaped structure in the middle
region of the photographs, and it is visible here
from the tympanic side from about 4 mm (left, basal)
to 8 mm (right, apical) measuring from the extreme
basal end. In Fig. 1 the membrane is stationary and
it is covered with similar well-defined specks as
the surrounding areas of bone and dental cement.
Fig. 2 shows the membrane driven at 12 kHz, and
one can see the resulting region of fuzziness extending over part of the exposed length of membrane
(left arrow to right arrow). The region of best
response for 12 kHz is located in the basal region
and consequently fuzziness is more readily noticeable there than in the more apical regions, which
are regions of progressively smaller amplitude. It
is apparent from Fig. 2 that according to the different amplitudes one obtains different "degrees of
fuzziness", or different degrees of loss of contrast,
and one may indeed try to base vibration analysis on
a continuous scale of fuzziness. However, in the
present technique measurements are based on the observation of the threshold regions where fuzziness
becomes just noticeable. Such a region is indicated
by the right arrow in Fig. 2.

With fuzziness-detection we obtain the distribution
of the regions of best response, i.e. the cochlear
frequency-space map, simply by locating under continuous laser illumination for different stimulus
frequencies the regions where fuzziness appears
first with stimulus level increase. Also, under continuous illumination we obtain the amplitude distributions of the vibratory patterns. In this case we
observe at a fixed frequency the spread of fuzziness
- i.e. the spatial shift of the region of just
noticeable fuzziness - in the apical and basal direction from the region of best response for stepwise increases in stimulus level. For instance, in
the 12 kHz example of Fig.2 the stimulus level is set
at V_{THB} + 30 dB, i.e. 30 dB above the level at which
fuzziness appeared in the region of best response.
The threshold location (marked by right arrow) therefore indicates the apical region of the 12 kHz pattern that vibrates 30 dB below the level of the
maximum region. With the spatial amplitude distribu-

tion and the frequency-space map known, we can deduce
the frequency response curve of the basilar membrane.
However, the frequency response curve of a given
point along the membrane can also be measured directly. To this end we monitor at different frequencies
the stimulus level (e.g.pressure at the eardrum) required to produce just noticeable fuzziness in the
observed region. Fuzziness-detection can thus be
used in two different ways to measure response characteristics; the one proceeds in the space domain,
the other in the frequency domain.

By incorporating stroboscopic techniques, fuzziness-
detection can be extended beyond the simple determination of amplitude which is done under continuous
illumination. Measurement of the phase relationships
along the membrane is possible when the scene is
synchronously illuminated with laser flashes of
finite duration. During the illumination intervals
the vibrating membrane deforms slightly, motions
being relatively larger in regions of greater velocity than in those of smaller velocity. Regions of
relatively greater velocity are those where the illumination interval straddles the time of zero-crossing
and consequently regions of zero-crossing will appear
fuzzy at relativly lower pressures than regions of
peak-excursion. Under such stroboscopic illumination
we therefore obtain fuzzy-islands along the membrane
which indicate regions of zero-crossing and they are
spaced 180° apart in phase. The interspaced regions
of peak-excursion may be investigated by slowly
changing stimulus level and observing the resulting
speckle motion which indiciates whether the local
motion has been optically arrested during the deflection towards scala tympani or scala vestibuli.

When we compare the pressure levels required to
evoke just noticeable fuzziness in a given region
for the cases of illumination during peak-excursion,
zero-crossing and for continuous illumination, we
obtain some idea of the linearity of basilar membrane deflections. For linear motion these level
differences appear to be mathematically predictable
(Kohllöffel, 1972 a) so that systematic deviations
of measured values from predicted ones may be due
to nonlinear effects. In order to investigate for
the presence of dc-effects of membrane motion, one
slowly varies the stimulus level while searching for

a corresponding slow speckle motion which would appear superimposed on the fuzzy regions. This can be done with continuous or stroboscopic illumination. In the latter case one concentrates attention to regions of zero-crossing.

Results

Fig. 3 shows some of the results measured five days after death in a preparation kept in mammalian Ringer solution in the hydraulic tank.

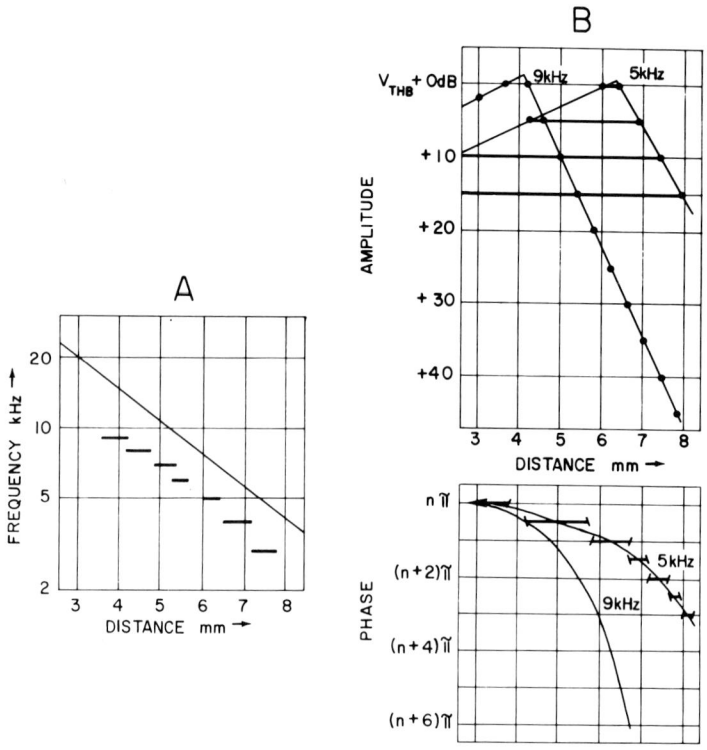

Fig.3 Typical example of response patterns measured in a normal preparation (Preparation was kept in the hydraulic tank in mammalian Ringer solution. Measurements were taken five days after death of animal.) Ordinate is distance along the basilar membrane.
A. Regions of best response (black bars) are

given for different stimulus frequencies. The line is a section of Greenwood's cochlear frequency-space map shown for comparicon. The regions of best response closely follow a straight line and the preparation is therefore called normal.
B. Amplitude patterns measured at 5 and 9 kHz. For the 5 kHz case the black bars indicate the detected extension of fuzziness along the membrane at different stimulus levels beginning with V_{THB} + 0dB, the level at which fuzziness appeared in the region of best response. Note: the 9 kHz pattern has a steeper apical slope than the 5 kHz pattern.
Phase patterns measured under stroboscopic illumination at 5 and 9 kHz. For the 5 kHz case, bars indicate detected regions of peak excursion. As shown, there are two sets of complementary bars since two phases of illumination different by 90° were used. The arrow indicates that the basalmost region did not terminate with the basal end of the exposure. The basal phase value $n\pi$ is not known in absolute terms from the experiment, and the two phase curves should therefore only be compared with respect to their shapes. Note: Beyond the region of maximum amplitude the phase curve assumes a straight course as is well shown in the 9 kHz example.

Fig. 3A displays the distribution of the regions of best response with the black bars denoting the regions where fuzziness appeared first with increasing pressure at different stimulus frequencies. The solid line is drawn according to the cochlear frequency-space map given by Greenwood (1961) for the guinea pig. For fresh preparations - those in the living state and those shortly after death - the regions of best response fall directly onto this line (Kohllöffel, 1971), but for older preparations, like the present one, they fall below the line (Kohllöffel, 1972 b,c). With the age of a preparation, regions of best response shift towards the basal end - a phenomenon that I have called the "first effect of aging". As one can see, the distribution of the best response regions very closely follows the slope of Greenwood's curve, and we can therefore use his value of 2.25 mm for the spatial shift of the location of maximum amplitude per octave change in frequency to convert data from the space domain into the frequency domain and vice versa. Preparations like the one in Fig. 3A where the arrangement of the regions of best response can be closely approximated by a straight line are called "normal". With the fuzziness-detection method, membrane motion was found to be linear and dc-effects were absent in normal preparations.

In Fig. 3B the amplitude and phase patterns at 5 and 9 kHz are given for the above preparation. In the 5 kHz case bars are drawn into the graphs in order to remind us of the way in which these curves were obtained. The bars in the amplitude plot denote the length of the fuzzy region along the membrane detected under continuous illumination, and one can see the increase in length in both the apical and the basal direction as the stimulus level is increased above V_{THB} + 0dB, the level at which fuzziness became noticeable in the region of best response. In the phase plot, bars denote regions of peak-excursion which were detected under strohoscopic illumination. There are two sets of complementary bars because the phase of illumination relative to the stimulus signal was different by $90°$ for the two sets during the measurement. In each set successive bars along the membrane denote regions $180°$ out of phase others. The phase plot is obtained by drawing a line free-hand through the middle of the bars. In the plots the phase begins in the basal part of the exposed region with $n\pi$, where n is an arbitrary number.

The amplitude patterns show the characteristic triangular shape, in this case with a flat basal slope of 1.8 mm per 5 dB, i.e. the fuzzy threshold region shifts basalward by 1.8 mm per 5 dB increase in stimulus level. While the basal slope value is the same for the 5 and the 9 kHz pattern, the value for the steep apical slope is not. The steeper 9 kHz slope amounts to 0.4 mm per 5 dB and the 5 kHz slope amounts to 0.5 mm per 5 dB. In deducing the corresponding slopes of the frequency response curves, we arrive at a low frequency slope of 6.2 dB per octave in both cases and a high frequency slope of 28 dB per octave and 22 dB per octave for the 9 kHz and 5 kHz case respectively. The increase in steepness of the apical slope with increasing stimulus frequency was consistently seen in normal preparations.

The phase plots take a curved course approximately up to the region of maximum amplitude corresponding to a progressive reduction of wavelength as this region is approached from the basal end. Beyond this region, however, the phase curve straightens and consequently the wavelength assumes a constant value.

It was one of the intentions of this study to observe the changes in response characteristics with time after the animal's death. Several changes were found and they occurred in a slow, continuous fashion. Fig. 4 illustrates these effects of aging for three different preparations either in the frequency domain, as in Fig 4A, or in the space domain, as in Fig. 4B and C. In Fig. 4A the frequency response curves are plotted for a point on the basilar membrane approximately 1.5 to 1.7 mm from the basal end. Curves are given in terms of the sound pressure at the eardrum required to produce just noticeable fuzziness at the observed point. In the living condition (curve 0.) the observed point has a best frequency of 28 kHz, a value which is in close agreement with Greenwood's cochlear frequency-space map. According to the first effect of aging, the best frequency drops so that three days after death (curve 3.) a value of 19 kHz has been reached. In the living state the low frequency slope is approximately 7 dB octave and the high frequency slope is approximately 130 dB per octave. With time after death, slopes become continuously flatter and three days after death the low frequency slope is approximately 4.5 dB per octave, the high frequency slope being approximately 46 dB per octave. The flattening of slopes is called the second effect of aging. The third effect of aging is the drop in the pressure level required to evoke fuzziness in the region of best response, the effect being well shown in Fig. 4A.

These three effects of aging are also clearly demonstrated in Fig. 4B where the 8 kHz spatial amplitude pattern of a preparation mounted in the hydraulic tank is given for three, five and seven days after death. One can see the basal shift of the region of best response (first effect), the flattening of the slopes (second effect), and the drop in pressure level (third effect) which leads here to an upward shift since the levels of the later curves are referred to V_{THB3}, the level that produced fuzziness in the region of best response three days after death.

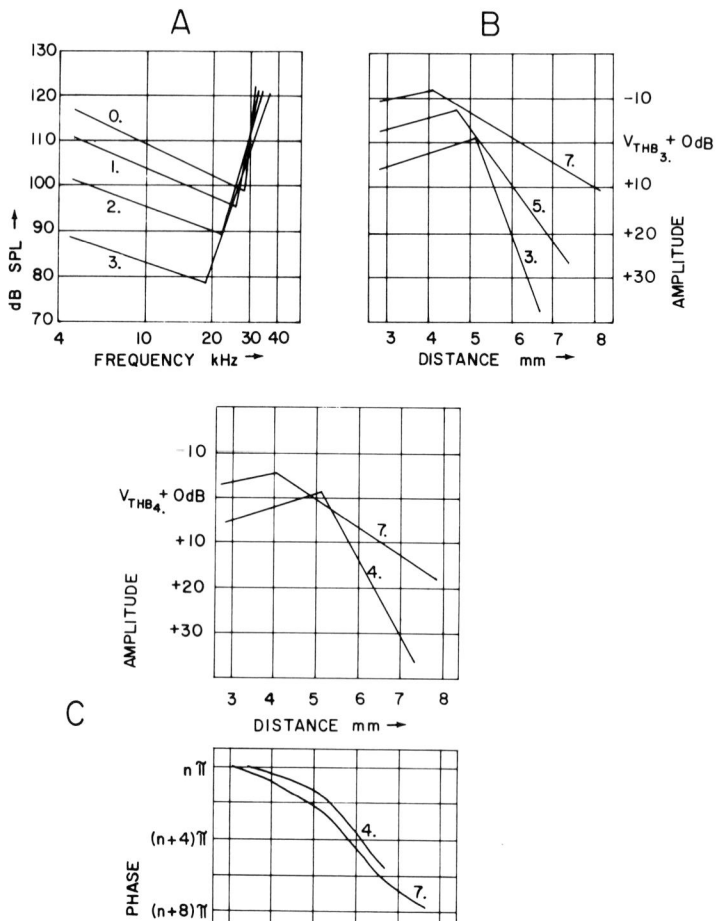

Fig.4 Illustration of the effects of aging in three different preparations.
A. Frequency response curves of a point 1.5 to 1.7 mm away from the basal end. The curves give the required sound pressure level at the eardrum to evoke fuzziness in the observed

region at different frequencies. Curves were measured in the living state (0.) and one (1.), two (2.) and three (3.) days after doath. Note: Drop in the best frequency - from 28 kHz (0.) to 19 kHz (3.) - first effect of aging. Flattening of slopes - second effect of aging. Drop in pressure level - third effect of aging.
B. 8 kHz amplitude distribution along the basilar membrane measured three (3.), five (5.) and seven (7.) days after the animal's death. (Preparation was mounted in the hydraulic tank and it was kept in mammalian Ringer solution.) Pressure levels are referred to V_{THB3}. + 0 dB, the level at which fuzziness appeared in the region of best response three (3.) days after death. Note: Basal shift of the region of best response (first effect), flattening of slopes (second effect), and pressure drop (third effect).
C. 9 kHz amplitude and phase distribution along the membrane measured in a third preparation four (4.) and seven (7.) days after death. (Preparation was kept in mammalian Ringer solution in the hydraulic tank.) In the amplitude plot, pressure levels are referred to V_{THB4}. + 0 dB, i.e. the level at which fuzziness appeared in the region of best response four days after death. Note: Amplitude patterns show effects of aging as A and B. However, phase curves show practically no change in shape over the region where both curves have been measured. Thus the relation between amplitude and phase pattern changes with time after death and the regions of maximum amplitude and constant wavelength move apart (fourth effect of aging).

Fig. 4C is meant to illustrate the fourth effect of aging, and it displays the 9 kHz amplitude and phase curves four and seven days after death of a preparation also mounted in the hydraulic tank. While there is a drastic change in the amplitude patterns, thoro is practically no change in the shape of the phase patterns. Thus the relation between the amplitude and the phase curves changes with time after death and we find in older preparations the region of

constant wavelength relatively more apical to the region of maximum amplitude than in fresher preparations. This is called the fourth effect of aging.
- In older preparations the phase pattern was measured over a greater length of exposed membrane (Kohllöffel, 1972 b),and such measurements revealed that the straight part of the phase curve does not continue indefinitely but that the curve starts to bend again indicating an increase in wavelength in the apical region of the vibratory pattern. This is well shown in the seventh-day curve of Fig. 4C.

The apical increase in wavelength reminds one of certain interesting features of the frequency response curves measured by Rhode (1971) and Wilson and Johnstone (1972). These authors found a region of constant amplitude and phase response above the best frequency. In this respect no conclusive results are as yet available from the present study for reasons that have to do with the stimulus generation and with limitations in the flexibility of the strobing equipment. In the case of stimulus delivery to the external ear we also observed a "constant" response region (Kohllöffel, 1972 c); however, the corresponding sound pressure at the eardrum was around 120 dB and the middle ear is known to generate strong subharmonics at this level (Dallos and Linnell, 1966). In the case of hydraulic stimulation we also observed some "tailing off" in the amplitude patterns (Kohllöffel, 1972 b); however, this occurred at levels 40 to 60 dB above V_{THB}, the threshold level for fuzziness in the region of best response. Unfortunately, at such high levels the hydrophone began to introduce cavitation.

So far we have dealt with the response in normal preparations. What about the abnormal cases? The study of such cases is particularly interesting because on the experimental side it allows one to develop a certain intuitive understanding of the effects of different kinds of injuries on the response patterns; on the theoretical side such a study furnishes data to test the predictive power of cochlear models. Fig. 5 shows some amplitude patterns from an abnormal preparation. The insert depicts schematically the rather complicated injury which happened accidentally during the exposure of the basilar membrane. There was a 'hole' in the

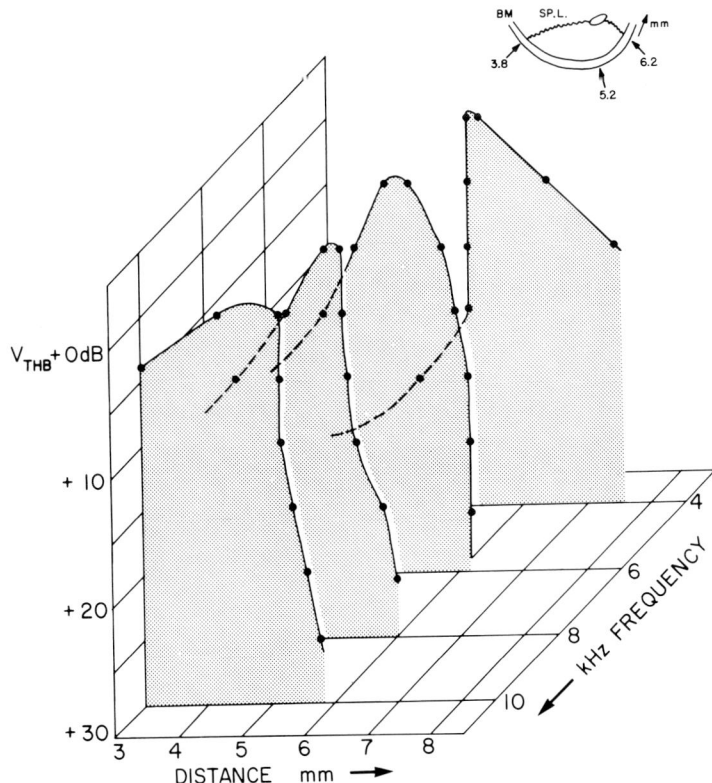

Fig.5   Amplitude distributions along the basilar membrane measured at different frequencies one day after death in an abnormal preparation. (Preparation was kept in mammalian Ringer solution in the hydraulic tank.) The insert displays schematically the injury as it could be seen with the aid of a Zeiss otoscope. The spiral lamina (SP.L.) showed a crack running from the 3.8 to the 6.2 mm location of the basilar membrane (B.M.). There was also a hole in SP.L. extending approximately from 5.2 to 6.2 mm along the membrane. Note: Regions of best response accumulate around 5 mm. Amplitude patterns are irregular and extremely steep slopes occur. The 4 kHz pattern has over part of the dynamic range an infinitely steep basal slope and a flat apical slope.

spiral lamina extending along a corresponding segment of basilar membrane for approximately 1 mm, from about 5.2 to 6.2 mm. Furthermore, a crack across the spiral lamina was visible, and it terminated at 3.8 and 6.2 mm along the membrane. There was, however, no direct fluid passage from scala vestibuli to scala tympani other than via the helicotrema. This was determined by pressing stain through the cochlear canals. It can be seen at once in Fig. 5 that the resulting response patterns deviate clearly from the normal triangular shape and that extremely steep slopes can be obtained. All regions of best response for the stimulus frequencies used occur in the area around 5 mm - such crowding of regions of best response was found to be typical for abnormal preparations with discontinuities in the mechanical impedance along the cochlear canals. Crowding usually occurred slightly basal to the location of the discontinuity. The most interesting feature of Fig. 5, however, is the 4 kHz amplitude pattern where the standard triangular shape appears reversed over part of the dymnamic range; there is an extremely-infinitely-steep basal slope and a flat apical slope.

Fig. 5 illustrates another point that is relevant in quite a different context. In view of the sharp tuning of auditory-nerve fibres, one may be led to question the reliability of direct measurements of basilar membrane vibrations. One may doubt whether such measurements are able to detect steep slopes. This question was accentuated since Rhode (1971) found rather steep slopes on the low frequency side of the basilar membrane frequency response curve in the squirrel monkey. It is evident from Fig. 5 that with fuzziness-detection one can measure steep slopes - basal and apical - provided such slopes do occur.

Discussion

Fuzziness-detection was introduced as a technique that allows the study of basilar membrane vibrations by direct observation. Measurements were carried out in the basal turn of the guinea pig's cochlea and the resulting features of the vibratory patterns were found to be in quite satisfactory agreement with those furnished by alternative techniques (Johnstone et al., 1970; Kohllöffel, 1971; Wilson and Johnstone, 1972). It turned out that the response patterns undergo continuous changes with time after the animal's death. As regards the underlying changes of membrane properties, it has been suggested (Kohllüffel, 1972 b) that an overall drop in membrane stiffness which leaves the stiffness relations along the membrane rather unaffected is probably the predominant factor. It may be remembered in this context that Tonndorf (1969) observed a flattening of the amplitude envelope in studies of cochlear models when the stiffness gradient of his artificial membrane was reduced. A flattening of the amplitude curve was described here as the second effect of aging.

With fuzziness-detection a substantial gain in sensitivity is achieved over von Békésy's method which was based on conventional optics. However, the required basilar membrane displacements are still in the upper part of the ear's dynamic range and this may limit the scope of possible applications of fuzziness-detection in future intracochlear studies. Directness, simplicity and speed are the outstanding features of this method which makes it an extremely useful tool for intracochlear work.

Acknowledgements

The work described here was done while I was at the Neurocommunications Research Unit, University of Birmingham, Great Britain. I am most grateful to Dr. I.C. Whitfield, Director of the Neurocommunications Research Unit, for his interest and criticisms during the course of the study. The work was supported by the Science Research Council, Great Britain.

I want to thank Miss S.A. Mrose from the Eaton-Peabody Laboratory of Auditory Physiology for help in the preparation of the illustrations.

References

Archbold, E., Ennos, A.E., and Taylor, P.A. (1970). A laser speckle interferometer for the detection of surface movements and vibration. In: Optical Instruments and Techniques (J.H. Dickson, ed.), pp. 265-275. Oriel Press, Newcastle upon Tyne.

von Békésy, G. (1960). Experiments in Hearing. McGraw Hill, New York.

Butters, J.N., and Leendertz, J.A. (1971). Speckle pattern and holographic techniques in engineering metrology. Optics and Laser Technology 3, No. 1, 26-30.

Dallos, P.J., and Linnell, C.D. (1966). Even-order subharmonics in the peripheral auditory system. J. Acoust. Soc. Amer. 40, 561-564.

Eliasson, B., and Mottier, F.M. (1971). Determination of the granular radiance distribution of a diffuser and its use for vibration analysis. J. Opt. Soc. Amer. 61, 559-565.

Greenwood, D.D. (1961). Critical bandwidth and the frequency coordinates of the basilar membrane. J. Acoust. Soc. Amer. 33, 1344-1356.

Johnstone, B.M., Taylor, K.J., and Boyle, A.J. (1970). Mechanics of the guinea pig cochlea. J. Acoust. Soc. Amer. 47, 504-509.

Kohllöffel, L.U.E. (1971). Studies of the distribution of cochlear potentials along the basilar membrane. Acta Oto-Laryngol. Suppl. 288.

Kohllöffel, L.U.E. (1972a). A study of basilar membrane vibrations I. Fuzziness-detection: a new method for the analysis of micro-vibrations with laser light. Acustica 27, 49-65.

Kohllöffel, L.U.E. (1972b). A study of basilar membrane vibrations II. The vibratory amplitude and phase pattern along the basilar membrane (post-mortem). Acustica 27, 66-81.

Kohllöffel, L.U.E. (1972c). A study of basilar membrane vibrations III. The basilar membrane frequency response curve in the living guinea pig. Acustica 27, 82-89.

Rhode, W.S. (1971). Observations of the vibration of the basilar membrane in squirrel monkeys using the Mössbauer technique. J. Acoust. Soc. Amer. 49, 1218-1231.

Tasaki, I., Davis, H., and Legouix, J.P. (1952). The space-time pattern of the cochlear microphonics (guinea pig), as recorded by differential electrodes. J. Acoust. Soc. Amer. 24, 502-519.

Tonndorf, J. (1969). Hydrodynamic distortion in the cochlea. Trans. Amer. Otol. Soc. 57, 38-49.

Wilson, J.P., and Johnstone, J.R. (1972). Capacitive probe measures of basilar membrane vibration. Symposium on Hearing Theory 1972, pp. 172-181. IPO Eindhoven, Holland.

Whitfield, I.C., and Ross, H.F. (1965). Cochlear-microphonic and summating potentials and the outputs of individual hair-cell generators. J. Acoust. Soc. Amer. 38, 126-131.

DISCUSSION

TONNDORF: Dr. Zwislocki, earlier, after Dr. Rhode's paper you raised the question: What was really changing here? I think Dr. Kohllöffel has given us a hint, namely one of his phase curves indicates that the stiffness gradient becomes less steep. Is that also your interpretation?

KOHLLÖFFEL: I would say that the changes indicate a drop in membrane stiffness and stiffness gradient; there will however be relatively little change in the stiffness profile, i.e., the stiffness relations along the membrane.

TONNDORF: Your phase curve flattens out and that means a lessening of the stiffness gradient.

KOHLLÖFFEL: Well, two points indicate directly that the stiffness is affected and these are the basal shift of the region of best response (first effect of aging) and the reduction in the required pressure to drive the membrane (third effect of aging). If we take Zwislocki's (1948) notation for illustration and denote with

$$S = \frac{1}{C_0} \exp(-\beta x)$$

the stiffness along the membrane (along x), then I think $\frac{1}{C_0}$ - the absolute stiffness - drops. This implies, of course, that the stiffness gradient

$$(-\frac{\beta}{C_0} \exp(-\beta x))$$

will also drop. It is interesting that Dr. Tonndorf's investigations have shown a flattening of the amplitude distribution for reduced stiffness gradients which lends support to the present interpretation. A drop in the stiffness gradient would explain the observed flattening effect in the preparations (second effect of aging).

Zwislocki (1948, equation 58) found an equation for
the distribution of the best response regions where β
determines the slope of the distribution. Since in my
studies this slope did practically not change, I assume that β did not change, either. This is why I am
saying that the stiffness profile, the stiffness relations along the membrane do not change, or at any
rate much less than the absolute stiffness.

EVANS: You have mentioned the plateau which Rhode as
well as Wilson and Johnstone (1972) found in the
phase determinations. Both have also found amplitude
plateaus, that is, the high frequency cut-off is
steep for 30 to 40 dB and then it flattens out drastically. Did you see that yourself?

KOHLLÖFFEL: I saw something like an amplitude plateau
in both preparations, the living one and the dead;
however, I am not sure whether these plateaus were
not entirely due to nonlinearities. In the case of
normal stimulation via the eardrum the "plateau" appeared around 120 dB SPL, where we know that the
middle ear generates subharmonics (Kohllöffel, 1972c).
For hydrophone stimulation "plateaus" appeared at
pressure levels where the hydrophone produced cavia-
tion (Kohllöffel, 1972b).

FEX: What limits the resolution of the technique to
500 Å?

KOHLLÖFFEL: The wavelength of the light.

GREEN: At the peak of those tuning curves, your sound
pressure levels are of the order of 100 dB, so as you
go down the tuning curve, they are going up to 130,
140, is that right?

KOHLLÖFFEL: Yes, but I do not go above 120 dB because
of subharmonics.

GREEN: For the older preparations, you can get good

measurements of the linearity, from 70 dB SPL up to
100 dB SPL. Are they parallel and do they agree with
Rhode's measurements?

KOHLLÖFFEL: I think there is rather good agreement
between Rhode's measurements and my own as regards
the post-mortem situation, taking into account that
is, that measurements were done in different species.
As far as linearity is concerned I would like to
refer you to Kohllöffel (1972a, b) where it is shown
that fuzziness-detection allows for a linearity check.
I have done such checks only in post-mortem preparations and membrane motion appeared to be linear. It
maybe interesting to mention that in normal preparations I could not find any dc displacements.

MICHELSEN: I just have a technical comment. Recently,
a more sensitive laser method has been developed (described in my paper), which allows you to measure a
vibration amplitude of 50 Å. This method is a direct
one and does not involve the use of a computer.

KOHLLÖFFEL: With fuzziness-detection as with holographic techniques you are limited by the wavelength
of the light used. Both kinds of techniques give you
a "whole field" appreciation of the vibratory event
in the observed scene. If one is not interested in
this whole field effect one can use more sensitive
techniques, e.g. the laser-doppler shift. But then
you have to do measurements point by point along the
membrane.

FEX: In living animals, are your measurements disturbed by movements from pulsation and from respiration?

KOHLLÖFFEL: No, I did not notice that.

References

Kohllöffel, L.U.E. (1972a). A study of basilar membrane vibrations I. Fuzziness-detection: a new
method for the analysis of microvibrations with

laser light. Acustica 27, 49-65.

Kohllöffel, L.U.E. (1972h). A study of basilar membrane vibrations II. The vibratuiy amplitude and phase pattern along the basilar membrane (postmortem). Acustica 27, 66-81.

Kohllöffel, L.U.E. (1972c). A study of basilar membrane vibrations III. The basilar membrane frequency response curve in the living guinea pig. Acustica 27, 82-89.

Wilson, J.P., and Johnstone, J.R. (1972). Capacitive probe measure of basilar membrane vibration. Symposium on Hearing Theory 1972, pp. 172-181. IPO Eindhoven, Holland.

Zwislocki-Moscicki, J. (1948). Theorie der Schneckenmechanik. Acta Oto-Laryngol., Suppl. 72.

CONCLUDING REMARKS

Jozef J. Zwislocki

Syracuse University
Syracuse, New York
USA

First of all, I would like to congratulate the organizers of the symposium on their skillful arrangement of this session's papers. Perhaps you noticed that theoretical and experimental contributions were perfectly interlaced. In this respect, we should realize that Dr. Tonndorf's paper was a theoretical one, since even a mechanical model of the cochlea is a theoretical model.

Instead of reviewing the specifics of today's session, which would appear to me quite superfluous, I would like to make a more general statement which I prepared in advance and which concerns the state of the art in cochlear research.

Perhaps research on cochlear mechanics may be divided into three periods: before Békésy, during Békésy, and after Békésy. In the first period, most of the mechanically important anatomy of the cochlea had become known. Otherwise, research on this intriguing organ had been performed almost exclusively in the armchair. I am sure, a study of the research of that period would be revealing with respect to human imagination. It would reveal, among other things, how fallible this imagination is. Not one of the many theories then proposed had succeeded in predicting accurately the wave pattern that Békésy discovered.

Békésy radically changed the mores of the field. He substituted well controlled experiments for vague theorizing. While, before Békésy, scientists only suspected what went on in the cochlea, now we know at least in principle. Békésy's era was not an era for petty detail; it was an era for discovery of fundamental phenomena. During it, we learned that sound produced traveling waves in the cochlea, and that they vanished before reaching the apex; that these waves reached an amplitude maximum at a location dependent on sound frequency -- close to the oval window for high frequencies and close to the apex for the low ones. We also learned that the maximum was not produced by the resonance of the basilar membrane, as Helmholtz thought, but resulted from an interaction between the mechanical impedance of the cochlear duct and the surrounding perilymph. We learned further that the wave pattern in the cochlea was very stable and, in particular, did not depend on the channel through which sound reached the cochlea. During the same time, we learned that not the sound pressure but the motion of the basilar membrane excited the cochlear hair cells. Of course, most of these things that we learned, Békésy taught us.

Now, we are in the post-Békésy period and seem to know what goes on in the cochlea but are not sure how much. Science in all its fields begins with qualitative description, progresses to fundamental laws, and ends with nearly exact quantification. After that, science tends to become applied science. Cochlear science appears to have reached the third period and is somewhat on the crossroads, as I believe, we may have noticed today. We do not really know the exact values of the physical constants that control cochlear waves. What is the exact value of the compliance of the basilar membrane under natural conditions? How great is its phylogenetic variation? Does it vary much within one animal species? What is the damping of the basilar membrane? What is its effective mass? How much does the mass of the endolymph affect the basilar membrane motion? Is the phase lag at the vibration maximum the same for all mammals, or does it vary among species? These are only a few examples of quantitative questions that need answering before we can devise quantitatively accurate models of cochleas, and before we can accurately specify the stimulus for the hair cells. No quick answers can be expected. They will require great expertise and good theoretical understanding. The latter will be particularly important when direct measurements will not be possible. Cochlear mechanics occupies a really interdisciplinary position in science, and hardly anybody has an appropriate background for it. Physiologists usually lack the requisite mathematics, mathomaticians are rarely versed in physiology, and neither are expert in hydrodynamics.

It is certain that the third cochlear chapter is far from being closed but, I believe, we should realize that we are in it. It seems to me that the time for proposing and solving fundamental differential equations has passed. What we now need are accurate measurements. They are the prerequisite for more accurate models.

I hope, you will agree with me that we had an interesting session. It reviewed for us the Békésy era, and gave us a taste of what the post-Békésy era will be like. Now, I would like to thank the speakers for their excellent contributions.

II
COCHLEAR MORPHOLOGY

THE NORMAL ORGAN OF CORTI

C. Angelborg and H. Engström

University Hospital
Uppsala
Sweden

1. Introduction

The organ of Corti, also called organon spirale according to international nomenclature, has been the subject of very many recent studies, and the main features of its structure are well known (Figs. 1 and 2).[1]

One of the basic requirements for a study of the detailed structure is a reliable technique of preparation. In this field methods for electron microscopy have proved of great value. It is today possible to use such well standardized fixation, embedding and sectioning procedures that we can count upon reproducible results. The transmission electron microscope has proved to be of excellent value for the study of the inner ear (Engström and Wersäll, 1953, 1958, Engström et al., 1962, 1966, Wersäll et al., 1954, 1961, 1965, Spoendlin, 1966, 1970, Smith, 1956, 1967, Kimura, 1966, Iurato, 1967, Iurato et al., 1971, Engström and Ades, 1973) and recently the scanning electron microscope has added to our knowledge about surface structures in the inner ear (Lim, 1969, 1972, Engström, 1970, Engström et al., 1970, Bredberg, et al., 1972). The development of new techniques for histochemistry has also been of great importance for our understanding of the functional properties of the inner ear sensory regions. In the following a general survey of some of the inner ear structures in mammals will be given, with the main emphasis on the inner and outer hair cells and some of the supporting structures. It is here assumed that the basic features of the organ of Corti are known.

---

[1] In this chapter, all figures appear at the end, an arrangement necessitated by the nature of the text.

2. The sensory cells

The inner and outer hair cells form two distinct and spatially separated groups of receptors in the organ of Corti. Most of the basic information about the arrangement of these cells in animals and man was beautifully described by Retzius (1884) and Held (1926). Some of the beautiful illustrations made by Retzius have only recently, almost a century later, been surpassed.

The inner hair cells (Figs. 2, 3) form one single row axially of the inner pillar cells. They have a round or oval surface provided with sensory hairs, a slightly bent neck and an ovoid cell body which at its lower half contacts nerve endings of different kinds. In Fig. 5 a schematic drawing shows the main features of the cells. At the surface there is a well developed cuticle which in the center is rather thick. In a small area the cuticle is absent and at least in many species we have found a basal body, the remains of a kinocilium present during embryonic life (Bredberg et al., 1972). During embryonic life all sensory and supporting cells have a kinocilium on their upper surface, which in the human embryo is very large and distinct. This kinocilium disappears to a great extent during the later part of fetal life and only small vestiges remain. In adult man and in the animals we have studied only a small basal body or a short vestige remains in the cuticle-free area at the surface.

All sensory cells in the inner ear are provided with large numbers of sensory hairs on their upper surface. This is the reason why they are generally called hair cells. In earlier publications several authors have counted the number of hairs and given descriptions of their lengths and diameters (Iurato, 1961, Engström et al., 1962). It is today clear that the lengths and diameters vary not only among individual coils of the cochlea but also within a single cell. In general the most peripheral row has the longest hairs and then they become gradually reduced in length and diameter in the axial hair rows (Fig. 4). This is especially the case in the inner hair cells. There are 2-4 rows of hairs on each inner hair cell and the first row is much longer and coarser than the following ones. The last row of hairs has

no actual length; they remain only as tiny rootlets
in the cuticle.

Each hair consists of a rootlet which is cylindrical
and inserted in a lighter area in the cuticle. The
rootlet continues in the hair proper as a central
core which only reaches to the lower half of the hair.
It is then diffusely lost in the stroma of the hair.
In surface sections through the cuticle rootlets can
be found in several rows on each cell. This is even
more evident in outer hair cells (Fig. 8). The region
close to the inner pillar cells has one portion where
there is no cuticle and this region corresponds to
the area where there was a kinocilium during embryonic
life. In many animals we have observed a basal
body in this region. Its significance is obscure.

The cytoplasm of the inner hair cell is very rich in
endoplasmic reticulum and this is especially true
for the infracuticular and supranuclear regions. We
usually distinguish one infracuticular, one supranuclear and one infranuclear portion in both inner
and outer hair cells.

In the inner hair cell the infracuticular region contains large numbers of mitochondria and many smooth
and granulated profiles (Figs. 5, 27). There is quite
a difference between inner and outer hair cells in
the cytoplasmic differentiation and the endoplasmic
reticulum of inner hair cells is very richly developed. In the region where a basal body is found several lysosomes and also several mitochondria can be
seen. The mitochondria are rounded, or oblong but
never very long like the mitochondria along the vertical sides of the outer hair cells (Fig. 17).

The Golgi complexes are moderately well developed;
there are no lamellated bodies as there are in outer
hair cells.

In both inner and outer hair cells there is a system
of thin tubules or filaments which appear at the infracuticular region and continuo all the way through
the cells down to the synaptic areas in the infra
nuclear region. These filaments have certain resem-
blance to the neurotubuli which are described by
Spoendlin (this volume) in the afferent nerve fibers
of the organ of Corti. They were seen by several au-

thors but first described separately by v. Ilberg (1969). They have been discussed in several publications from our group.

Multivesicular bodies are found in the supranuclear portion where the Golgi complexes are also generally found.

The nucleus of the inner hair cell is round, larger than the nucleus of outer hair cells and its chromatin network is also usually denser.

The infranuclear portion has an endoplasmic reticulum (Fig. 28) which is less developed than in the supranuclear portion. However, this region contains a group of mitochondria in close relation to granulated membranes often forming an almost spherical agglomeration below the nucleus. After stimulation with intense noise and also after damage by ototoxic antibiotics we have found this spherical group of mitochondria to be very prominent.

The plasma membrane of the inner hair cell is rather smooth. The cell is partly surrounded by supporting cells, partly by nerve endings and fluid spaces. At the surface the cuticle is surrounded by the reticular membrane from inner pillar cells, inner phalangeal cells and border cells. The last type of cells are provided on their surface with large numbers of microvilli (Fig. 3). Along the "vertical" surfaces of the inner hair cells, inside the plasma membrane there is one single layer of discontinuous membranes. The multilayered systems of lamellae observed in the outer hair cells of some species have never been seen in inner hair cells.

At their basal end the inner hair cells are in contact with afferent and efferent nerve endings. The afferent endings often have very dense synaptic regions and well developed synaptic bars or bodies. The efferent endings are of moderate size. They often have a subsynaptic cistern inside the plasma membrane of the hair cell. While the nerve endings of outer hair cells usually contact only the lowest portion of the cells, those found on inner hair cells can be found, especially axially on the cells, even above the level of the nucleus. Many of the efferent endings form axo-axonic synapses below the inner hair cells (cf Spoendlin's paper, this volume).

The outer hair cells form three, four or five rows outside the outer pillar cells. They are separated from each other by extensions from the pillar cells and the phalanges of the Deiters´ cells. They form a very regular geometric pattern in mammals. This has been repeatedly described before but was especially well clarified by Engström et al. (1966). In human ears it was carefully studied by Bredberg (1968) who could show that during embryonic life the development followed the regular pattern observed in mammals. With increasing age the regular pattern started to deteriorate into rather pronounced irregularities. In old age many outer hair cells disappeared, due to aging or to damage to the cells. The cells have a cuticular plate inserted in the reticular lamina of the organ of Corti. This surface is flat or slightly upwards bulging. The stereocilia or sensory hairs are inserted with their rootlets in the cuticle and these rootlets reach to the lower level of the cuticle and sometimes even through the cuticle to the infracuticular region. During embryonic life mammalian outer hair cells have a very long kinocilium but this kinocilium disappears and only a basal body remains in a cuticle free region. In some monkeys and also in some other mammals we have observed by scanning electron microscopy that small, vestigial kinocilia may remain.

As in the inner hair cells, we distinguish in outer hair cells an infracuticular, a supranuclear and an infranuclear region. The infracuticular region contains large numbers of oblong mitochondria, lysosomes and a rich endoplasmic reticulum. The lysosomes increase in size and numbers with old age, and also in animals exposed to intense noise. Especially the region below the basal body seems to become rich in lysosomes. This is a very interesting region as the basal body is a residue of the kinocilium, a structure which has been very much discussed, especially in relation to the function of vestibular sensory cells and in relation to the morphological and functional polarization of the side-line organs of fishes and other animals.

The supporting cells surrounding the hair cells have many microvilli on their upper surface. Very few such microvilli are found on the outer hair cells and they seem not to have any very close relation to the infracuticular region. In the supporting cells the microvilli send extensions down into the interior of the cells.

The outer hair cells are cylindrical with a rounded lower end, where afferent and efferent nerve endings form synaptic contacts. At the lower end the outer hair cells are also surrounded by Deiters´ cells, which form cupshaped sockets for the bases of the hair cells. The peripheral plasma membrane of the outer hair cell is very smooth, with few irregularities in normal cells. In damaged cells the form may vary considerably and occasionally degenerating cells can also be found in cochleas supposed to be normal. Occasional macrophages are also found between the cells in normal organs of Corti. These become numerous in damaged cochleas. On the inner side of the plasma membrane along the vertical sides of the hair cells from one to several layers of discontinuous membranes can be seen (Fig. 17). In man and in those monkeys we have studied these membranes form only one or two layers, whereas in the guinea pig they may form five to seven layers. Each membrane has a thickness of about 300 Å. They consist of an outer denser layer with a thickness of 60-70 Å and a central less dense structure with an irregular middle, denser membrane. The multilayered arrangement continues in the guinea pig down to the nuclear level (Fig. 18) and from there on there is only a single layer. In man and monkeys there is one layer only in both the supranuclear and the infranuclear portion.

Recently we have repeatedly found a few of these membranes also along the upper, free surface of the hair cells in the region close to the basal body. The function of these membranes is not known but it is evident that they are closely related to the glycogen as will be discussed later.

It should also be pointed out that no membranes of this kind are ever found in regions where afferent nerve endings form synaptic contacts with the hair cells. At efferent endings on the other hand, subsynaptic cisterns are regularly found but they seem to differ a little from the membranes just described.

Inside the discontinuous membranes rather long, slender mitochondria are abundant (Fig. 17), indicating high enzymatic activity along these membranes. Likewise many mitochondria are seen along the lamellated bodies found on the border between the infracuticular and the supranuclear portions. These rounded or flat bodies are formed by membranes of a similar nature to the peripheral ones. In both the peripheral membranes and the lamellated bodies many variations from typical membranes of the type just described to one single dense layer may be observed (Fig. 19). A large portion of the outer hair cell above the nucleus is almost free of any cytoplasmic organelles. In the fixed specimen this part is usually very rich in granules. These are regarded as glycogen granules by us. It is well known that the outer hair cells are rich in glycogen, especially in the supranuclear region but glycogen can also be found below the nucleus. In this infranuclear region the cells contain many mitochondria and a rather rich endoplasmic reticulum. In this region we can also recognize many of the tubular filaments which were described in inner hair cells. They begin close to the cuticle and especially the basal body region. They follow the peripheral region of the cells and end close to the nerve endings, often close to afferent synaptic regions. In the afferent regions there are also found many invaginations and vesicles with a spiny outer structure usually described as coated invaginations or coated vesicles. They were described by Engström (1965) in vestibular cells and by Wersäll (1968) in cochlear hair cells. They are very numerous in cochlear hair cells. They seem to become much more developed in animals exposed to high intensity noise. They are only present at afferent endings. At efferent endings there is a thin subsynaptic cistern.

The infranuclear region is of utmost interest in many ways and especially because this is the region where nerve endings of afferent and efferent nature form synaptic contacts with the outer hair cells. It has been shown repeatedly by several authors (cf Engström et al., 1966) that there is a spatial difference in form and size of the two types of endings. This influences the structure of the hair cells also. In regions of afferent synapses we find coated invaginations (Fig. 34) and synaptic bars (Fig. 23). At efferent endings there are subsynaptic cisterns. In in-

ner hair cells rounded synaptic bodies are common;
in outer hair cells there are usually synaptic bars
only.

The nucleus of the outer hair cell is round or ovoid
with a fine chromatin network (Fig.21). Modifications
in volume of the nucleus after sound stimulation have
been described by Beck (1965). These changes have
also been reported by other authors as resulting from
noise exposure and ototoxic drugs (cf. Wersäll's
paper, this volume).

The outer hair cells vary in length and also to a
certain extent in structure in the different coils.
In general they are shorter at the basal end, increasing in length towards the apex. However, a difference
in length can be seen also in the same region as an
example, the third row outer hair cells in the upper
coils of the guinea pig cochlea are considerably
longer than the first row cells. The functional significance of this is not known. There are many other
different characteristics among hair cells from different coils. The angle in the W-shape of the hairs
is very different, being large at the base (about
120°) and small (about 60°) at the top. The most significant difference between the hair cells is, however, the great difference in nerve ending mass between base and top. This can be seen very clearly
when comparing Figures 34 A and B. The large granulated endings in B are from the lower end of a guinea
pig cochlea.

3. The supporting cells in the organ of Corti

The sensory cells in the cochlea have received a considerable interest during the years but many fewer
studies have been made of the supporting cells. In
general they have been ascribed a supporting function
and they have received rather superficial interest
from the point of view of other possible functions.
In studies by Angelborg (to be published) it has been
shown that there is good reason to believe that they
have other interesting functions as well and we shall
describe them in the following.

The outer and inner hair cells reach from the surface
down into the interior of the organ of Corti but they
do not reach to the basilar membrane. The region between the basilar membrane and the hair cells is fil-

led by the supporting cells and fluid spaces.

The supporting cells are when located from the inner sulcus cells: inner border cells, inner phalangeal cells, inner and outer pillars, Deiters´ cells, Hensen's cells and Claudius´ cells. The latter are followed by the outer sulcus cells and in the basal coil there are also a special group of cells called Boettcher cells.

The surface of the organ of Corti has recently been carefully described by Lim (1969) and by Bredberg <u>et al</u>. (1972), and it has been shown, as was known before, that all the supporting cells, except the pillar cells at their upper free surface are provided with large numbers of microvilli. Especially the border cells (Fig. 3) and the Hensen cells are covered by numerous microvilli. The presence of large numbers of microvilli indicates that the cells increase their upper surface enormously, either for an improved exchange with endolymph or for some kind of attachment to the tectorial membrane. All the supporting cells also have one kinocilium during embryonic life but this hair degenerates in man at a rather early embryonic age and disappears almost completely. Vestiges may, however, remain also in adult man.

The cells of the inner sulcus are very "light" cells with very few mitochondria and a little developed endoplasmic reticulum. <u>The inner border cells</u> are tall irregular cells which reach from the basilar membrane to the surface where they form a thin line of cells axially of the inner hair cells. They are very richly provided with microvilli at the surface. The basal portion of the cells below the nucleus is adjacent to the entering nerve fibers. The infranuclear portion is very rich in mitochondria and differs in this respect from the other supporting cells. The supranuclear portion of the cell contains much fewer mitochondria, but close to the surface several, partly osmiophilic, granules appear. These granules seem to increase with age in man and also in animals.

The rich agglomeration of mitochondria at the basal end of these cells and the rich cover of microvilli at the surface as well as the close relation to the inner hair cells makes it probable that they have an important nutritional function.

The inner phalangeal cells form one single row of slender cells reaching from the basilar membrane to the surface, where one phalanx stands between two inner hair cells. They are also provided with microvilli but not at all as richly as the border cells. It is very common to see one centriole very near the surface and another centriole immediately below. From these centrioles cross-striated fibrils reach down into the cell (Fig. 32). We have not been able to describe exactly the inner phalangeal cells and we are not certain if they contain the fibrillar components we describe in the Deiters´ cells and in the pillar cells.

The pillar cells. According to Retzius the human cochlea contains 3,500 inner and 12,000 outer hair cells. The number of inner pillars is 5,600 and of outer pillars 3,850. These pillars are in direct contact with many of the sensory cells. They form a very conspicuous system of a presumably mainly supporting nature and they also form a very important part in reticular membrane in which the upper portion of all the sensory cells is enclosed.

The pillar cells were beautifully and best described by Held (1926). Electron microscopy showed that the pillar cells contained large numbers of fibrillar structures (Engström and Wersäll, 1953) and these fibrils were counted and described by several authors. Angelborg and Engström, (1972) could demonstrate a very characteristic arrangement of two kinds of filaments in both pillar cells (Fig. 30) and Deiters´ cells. These filaments have quite different size and form. There is one thicker tubelike type with a diameter of 275 Å and a wall thickness of 60 Å. We called them tubular filaments in contrast to the other, thin solid micro-filaments which have a diameter of only 60 Å. The pillar cells have a footplate, a middle portion and a head portion. The complicated arrangement of the heads of inner and outer pillars is in good agreement with the description given by Held.

The Deiters´ cells have a lower portion reaching from the basilar membrane to the base of an outer hair cell and a slender process which runs obliquely to another hair cell and ends in a "phalanx" (Figs.

12-17). The lower portion of the Deiters' cell forms
a cup shaped formation close to the nerve endings of
the outer hair cell and contacts the surface of the
hair cell very firmly (Figs. 21, 22, 24). The pillar
cells and the Deiters' cells are very important participants in the formation of the reticular membrane
(Figs. 14, 15, 16). The Deiters' cells contain a thin
strand of tubular filaments and microfilaments. They
start close to the basilar membrane where a little
basal cone of cementlike nature and some mitochondria
also are found. The fibrils are usually eccentrically
located in the cells. Some of the fibrils reach to
the base of the hair cells but another bundle goes
through the slender process to the phalanx where it
fans out to insert itself in the reticular membrane
(Fig. 13).

The Hensen cells form the next group outside the outer
tunnel. These cells are high columnar, with a little
developed endoplasmic reticulum. At the surface the
cells are richly provided with microvilli. In rodents
it is very common to find lipid-like granules in the
Hensen cells of the upper coils. In osmic acid fixed
specimens they are easily recognized. There has been
much discussion as to what extent the tectorial membrane is in contact with the Hensen cells. It seems
probable that the contact before birth is very wide
but when hearing begins the contact is loosened and
only small strands reach the tectorial membrane to
the Hensen cells.

The organ of Corti is resting on the basilar membrane
which has been thoroughly described by Iurato (1962).
The membrane separates the footplates of the supporting cells from the perilymph. It is possible to discern two different parts of the basilar membrane; the
pars tecta under the tunnel reaching to the outer
pillar and the pars pectinata extending from the
outer pillar to the spiral ligament.

The basilar membrane consists mainly of extracellular
material. There is a homogenous part of ground substance in which there are fibrillar strands, one in
pars tecta, two in pars pectinata. In the homogenous
layers a few cells may be seen (Fig. 33). The cells
of the organ of Corti are not in direct contact with
the basilar membrane as there is a thin basement membrane between the intercellular substance of the mem-

brane and the plasma membrane of the supporting cells. On the tympanic side of the basilar membrane are the mesothelial cells which are called the tympanic border cells or the cells of the tympanic covering layer. These cells are spindle shaped with very long slender parallel processes which overlap.

This arrangement can be clearly seen in scanning electron microscopy (Bredberg et al., 1972). The cells are bathed in perilymph which is in direct contact with the lower homogenous layer of ground substance in the basilar membrane. Recently some authors (v. Ilberg, 1968, Duvall and Sutherland, 1972) have reported an almost free passage of small tracer particles (thorium dioxide and horseradish peroxidase) through the basilar membrane up to the spaces and the cells in the organ of Corti. If there is a free communication through the basilar membrane to the extracellular fluid in the organ of Corti, (the Cortilymph (Engström, 1960)), that fluid ought to be the same as perilymph.

In our own experiments with thorium dioxide, we have observed the tracer between the cells of the tympanic border and noticed high phagocytic activity in these cells. The particles are further seen in the basilar membrane, but only in the homogenous layers, never in the fibrillar strands. The number of tracer particles found in the basilar membrane is dependent on the amount of tracer substance used. When small doses are injected into the cerebrospinal fluid, the substance will very soon reach the perilymph via the cochlear aqueduct and the tracer is taken up by the mesothelial cells and some particles are also seen in the basilar membrane. We have not seen any tracer in the cells of the organ of Corti when only small amounts (0.05-0.10 ml) of Thorotrast (R) are administered in the way mentioned above, even though there is a high concentration of tracer particles in the perilymph and in the mesothelial cells below the basilar membrane. It has become quite clear that these cells have a high phagocytic activity and may act to deter unwanted material from reaching the basilar membrane and the organ of Corti.

In Fig. 33 thorium dioxide particles are seen in the basilar membrane after direct administration into the perilymph. There is a concentration gradient and no tracer substance is seen above the basilar membrane, which also seems to be a hindrance to at least the Thorotrast (R) particles.

Acknowledgements

This study has been supported in part by the Swedish Medical Research Council Project No. 12X-3156, by the NASA Grants No. NGR 52-028-003 and No. NGR 52-028-004, and by the University of Uppsala.

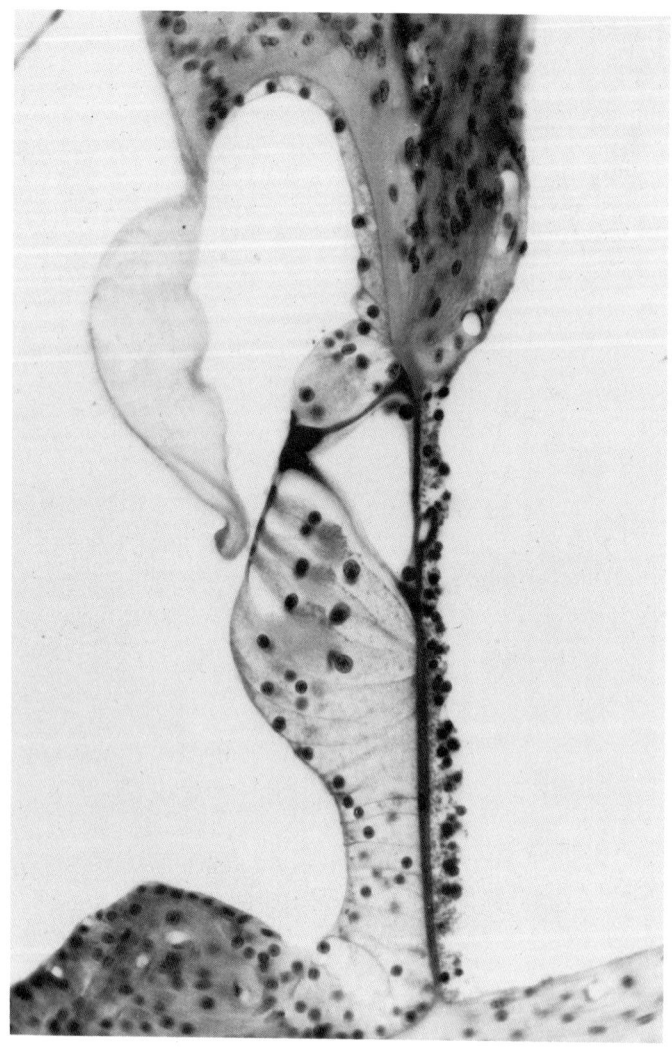

Fig. 1 Organ of Corti, middle coil. The sensory cells are seen surrounded by the supporting cells resting on the basilar membrane. Below the basilar membrane the very interesting layer of mesothelial cells is seen. Cat. × 290.

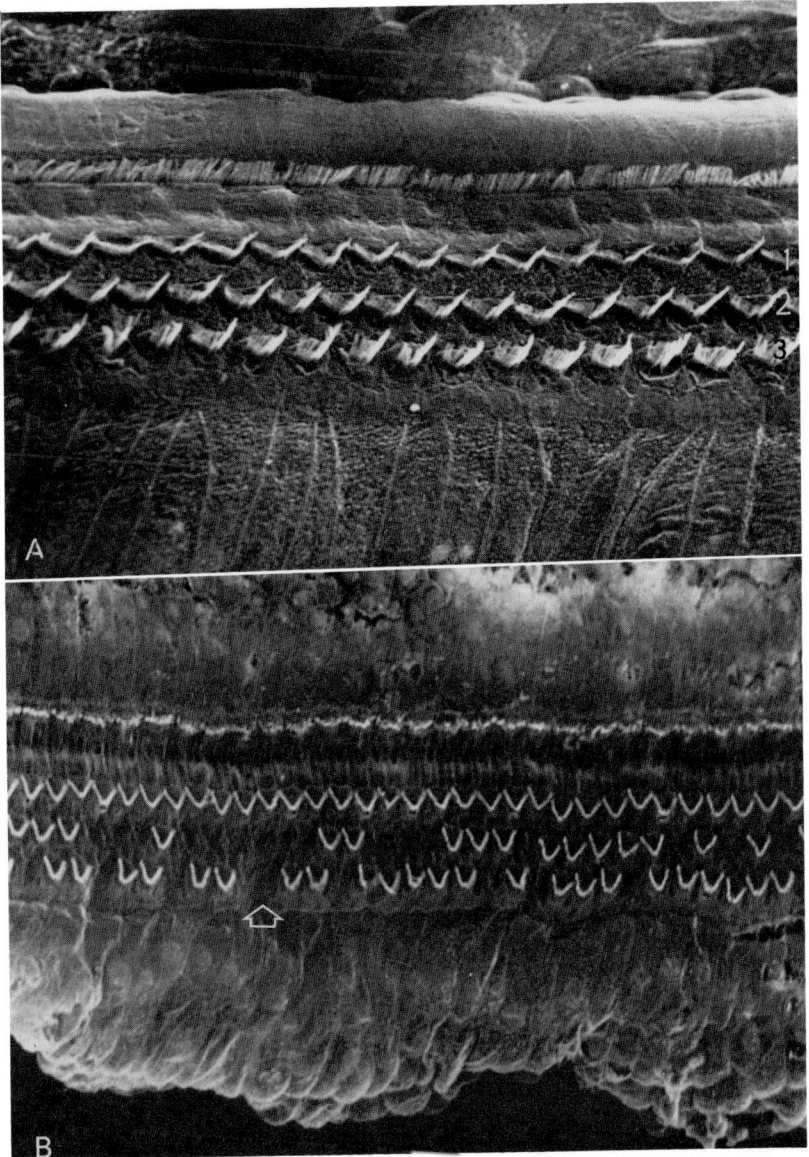

Fig. 2. A. The organ of Corti as seen in scanning electron microscopy. One row of inner hair cells (IHC) and three rows of outer hair cells (1,2,3) are seen. The sensory cells are regularly arranged.

(cont'd)

(Fig. 2, cont'd)

B. Some of the sensory cells in the second and third row are missing (arrow). This animal has been exposed to noise from a starting pistol. Guinea pig. SEM.

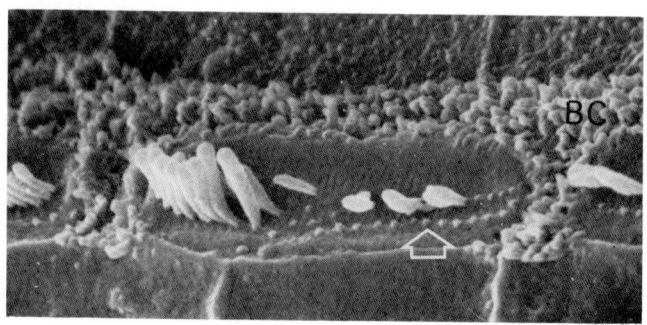

Fig. 3 Inner hair cell. The oblong surface of the inner hair cell with the hair is seen. Some of the hairs have been torn away during the preparation and the insertions in the cuticular membrane can be seen (arrow).

BC is a border cell with many microvilli.

Macaca fascicularis. SEM.

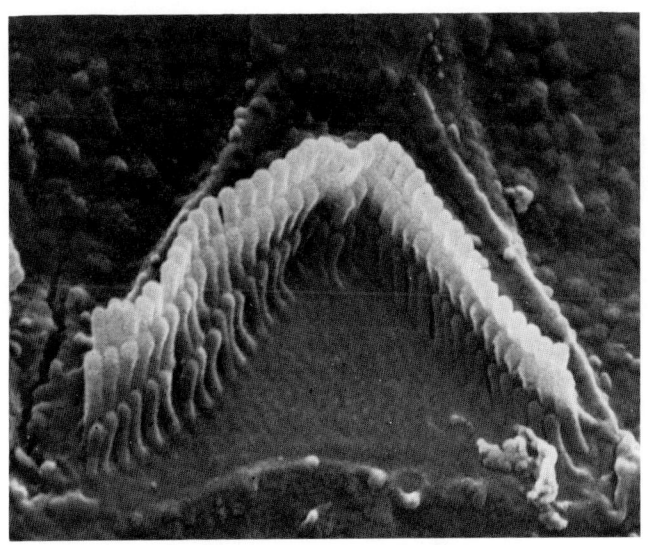

Fig. 4 M or W-formation and three rows of hairs on an outer hair cell. In the first, uppermost row, the hairs are longer and a little coarser. The length of the hairs is gradually reduced in the second and third row. The surface of the hair cell is fairly smooth compared to the surface of the surrounding supporting cells where microvilli can be seen.

Macaca fascicularis. SEM.

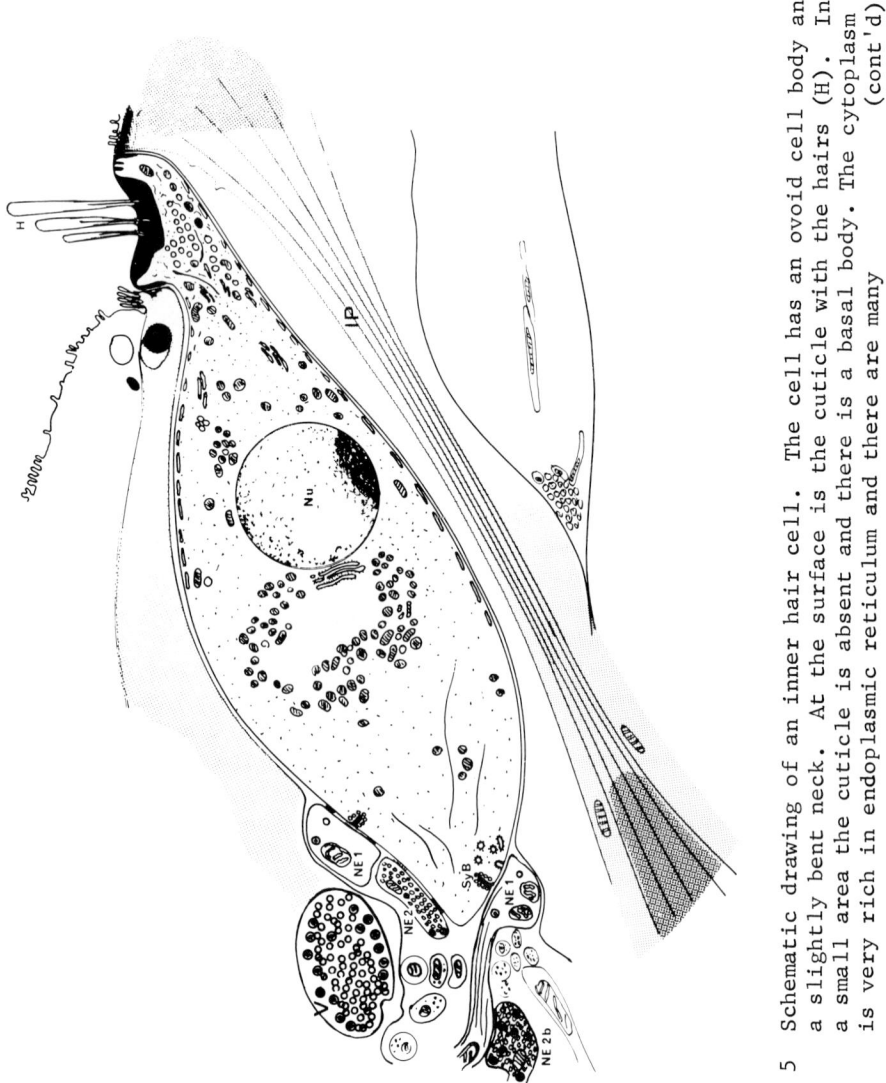

Fig. 5 Schematic drawing of an inner hair cell. The cell has an ovoid cell body and a slightly bent neck. At the surface is the cuticle with the hairs (H). In a small area the cuticle is absent and there is a basal body. The cytoplasm is very rich in endoplasmic reticulum and there are many (cont'd)

(Fig. 5, cont'd) mitochondria which in the infranuclear portion often form an almost spherical agglomeration. The nucleus (Nu) is round, larger than the nucleus of the outer hair cell. Inside the plasma membrane along the "vertical" surfaces there is one single layer of discontinuous membranes. Afferent (Ne 1) and efferent (Ne 2) nerve endings are in contact with the inner hair cell at its basal end.

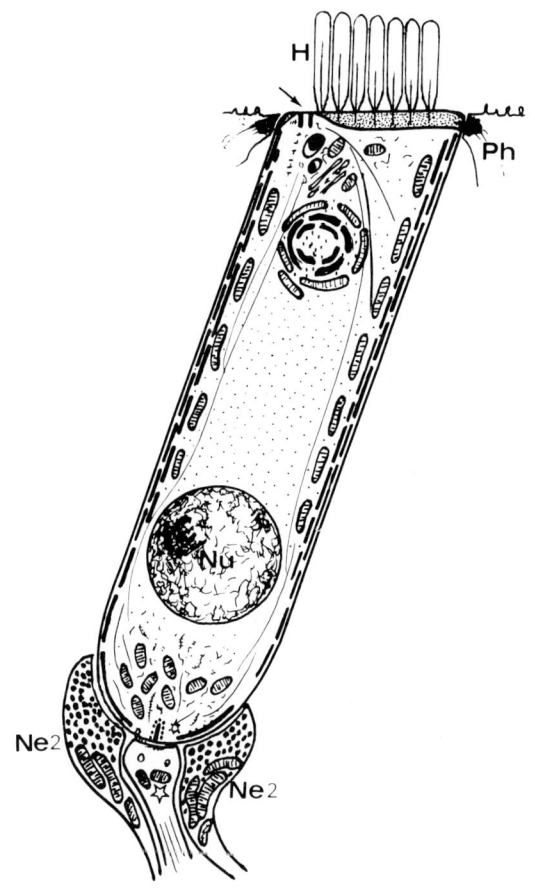

Fig. 6 Schematic drawing of an outer hair cell. The hair cell is cylindrical with a rounded lower
(cont'd)

(Fig. 6, cont'd) end. At the surface there are hairs (H) with their rootlets inserted in the cuticular plate. Below the surface are mitochondria and lysosomes. Along the vertical sides of the hair cell there are discontinuous membranes and mitochondria. Below the infracuticular region there is one lamellated body with mitochondria. In the central part of the cell in the supranuclear portion, the small dots indicate the presence of glycogen particles. The nucleus (Nu) is in the lower portion of the cell and below the nucleus is the infranuclear region where a synaptic bar is seen adjacent to the afferent nerve ending (star). On both sides of the afferent nerve ending there are efferent endings (Ne 2). The phalanx of a Deiters' cell (Ph) is attached to the sensory cell at its surface. The small arrow at the surface indicates a basal body.

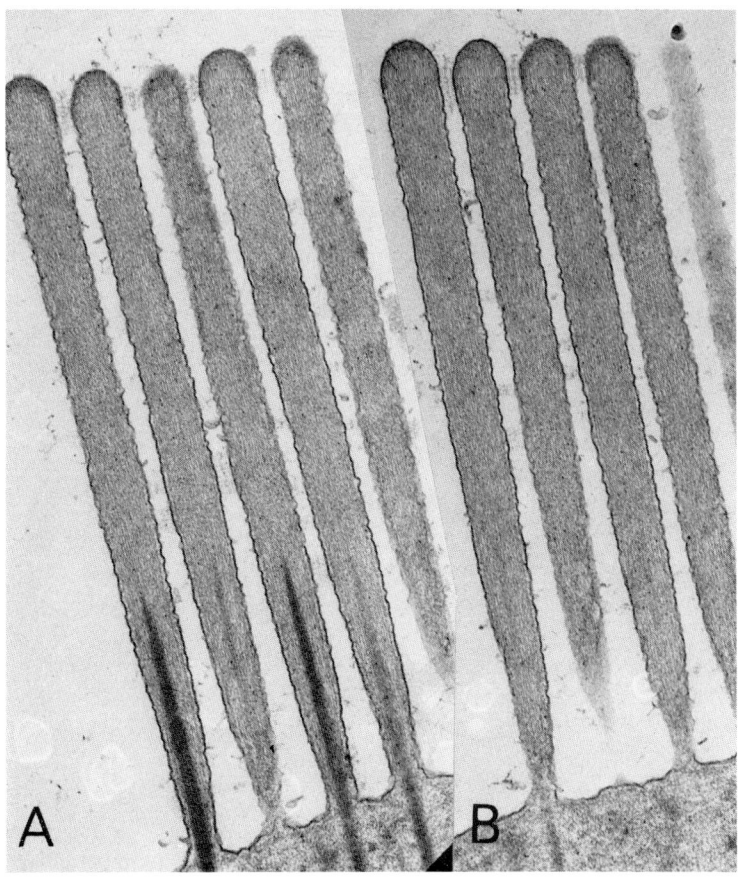

Fig. 7 A and B. Hairs on an outer hair cell seen in two different sections. The typical cylindrical sensory hairs protruding from the surface are shown. In the basal portions of the hairs the dense central core and the rootlet going down into the cuticle are seen. It is also possible to see the longitudinal arrangement of macromolecules inside the sensory hair.

Guinea pig. TEM. (A) × 32200, (B) × 30500.

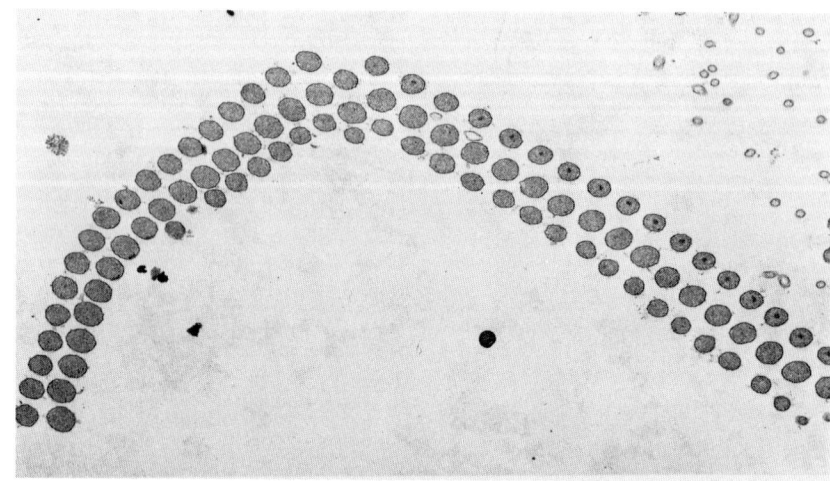

Fig. 8   Cross sectioned hairs on an outer hair cell. Three rows of hairs can be seen. They have the typical M or W arrangement. In the hairs of the first, uppermost, row there is a central core. This is reaching higher up in the first row than in the second and third rows. The hairs of the first row are longer then the hairs in the other rows.

Guinea pig. TEM. x 14000.

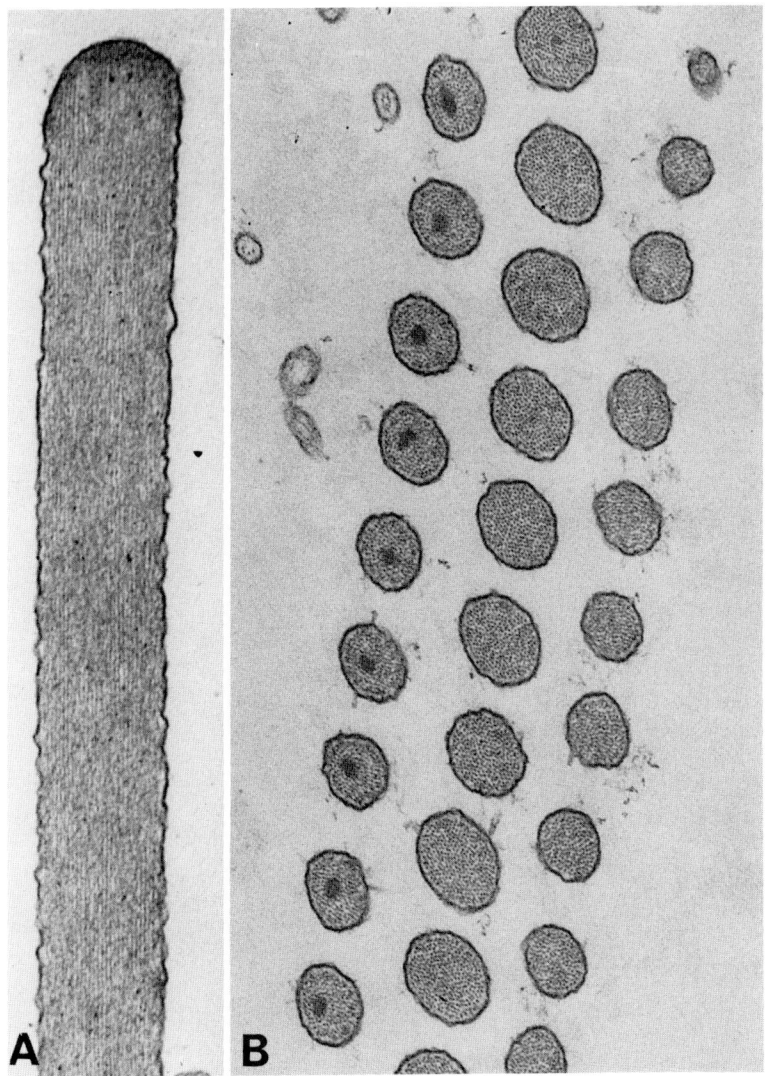

Fig. 9 A. Longitudinal section through a hair from an outer hair cell. It is possible to see the longitudinal macromolecules arranged in parallel all the way from the basal part of the hair to its tip where the darker area indicates the area of attachment (cont'd)

(Fig. 9, cont'd) to the tectorial membrane.

B. Cross sectioned hairs of an outer hair cell. There are three rows of hairs and in the left row is seen a denser core in the center of the hairs. Many cross-sectioned macromolecular fibrils are seen inside the hairs.

Guinea pig. TEM. (A) × 58000, (B) × 52500.

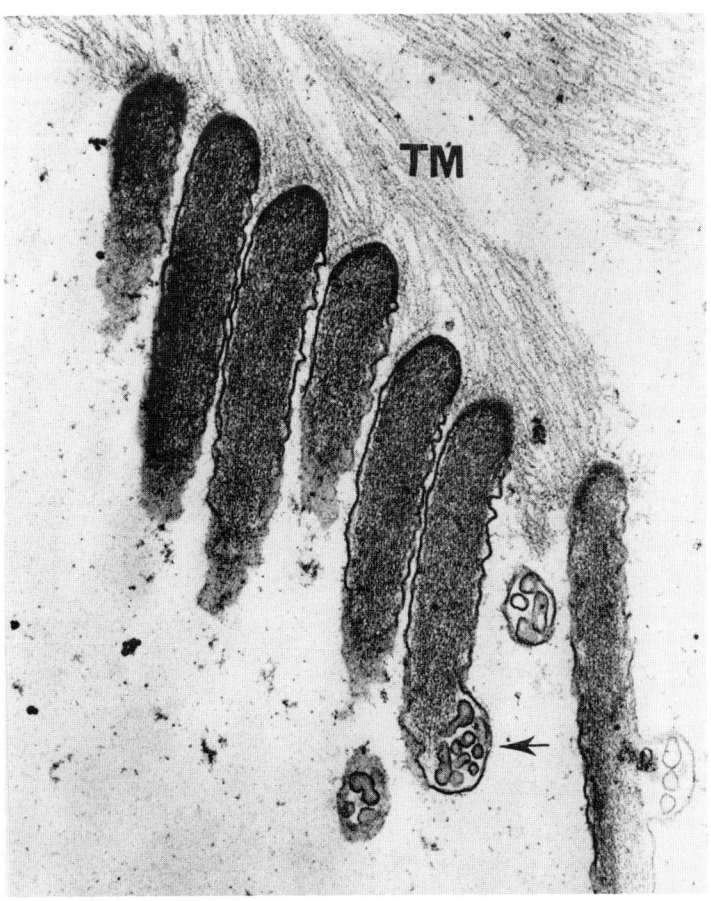

Fig. 10 Upper ends of hairs on an outer hair cell. The attachment between the hairs and the tectorial membrane is seen. The rounded tips of the hairs are in close contact with the tectorial membrane. There is a darker reinforcement almost like a halo over the tip of the hairs and the micellar fibrils in the tectorial membrane are attached to this darker substance. The arrow indicates one of a few blebs on the hairs. This is a normal animal but blebs of this kind appear both in normal and pathological (cont'd)

(Fig. 10, cont'd) animals.
Guinea pig. TEM. X 30500.

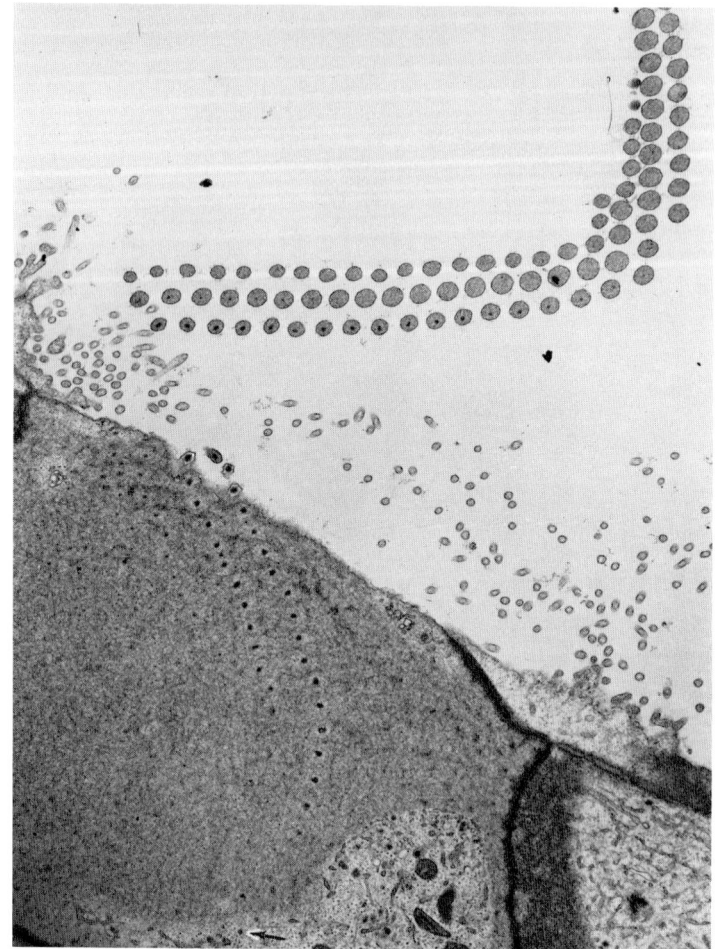

Fig. 11 Section through the cuticular plate below, and the hairs over, the surface of an outer hair cell. The plane of section is slightly oblique in relation to the surface and it is possible to see how the rootlets of the hairs are inserted in the cuticle. The lowest hair rootlets even seem to penetrate below the cuticular plate (arrow). In the upper part of the picture cross-sectioned (cont'd)

(Fig. 11, cont'd) hairs are seen with a denser core in the first row of hairs. At the side of the sensory cell many microvilli are seen emanating from supporting cells.
Guinea pig. TEM. X 12000.

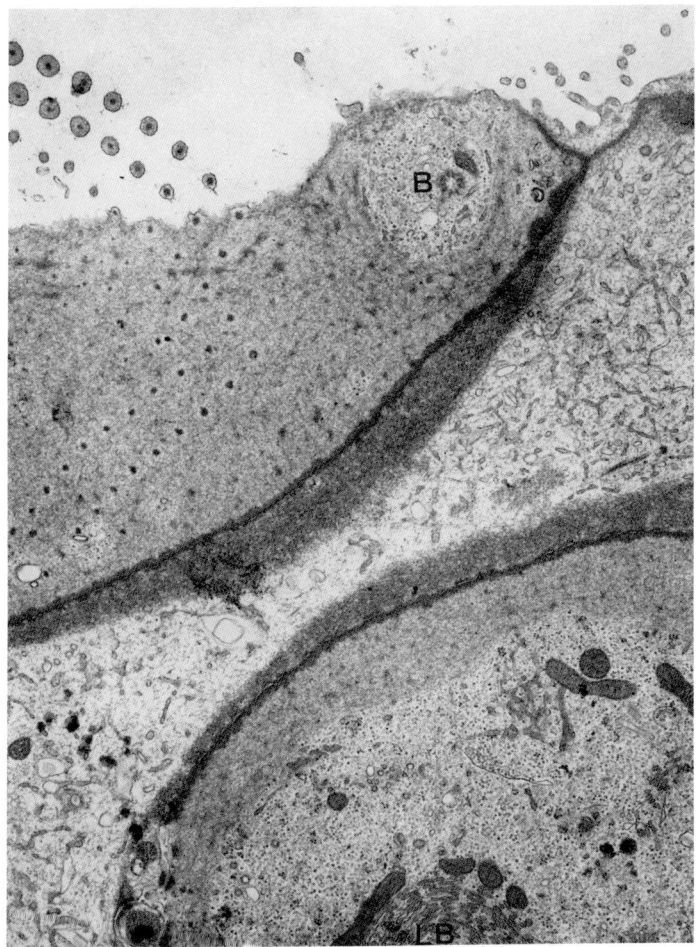

Fig. 12 Section through the surface of two outer hair cells and the phalanx of a Deiters' cell. In the upper cell is seen the basal body (B). The hairs are partly sectioned over the surface partly through their rootlets. (cont'd)

(Fig. 12, cont'd) It is possible to discern the M-shape in the arrangement of the hairs. A slightly lighter zone is seen around the rootlets at their insertion in the cuticular plate. The lower sensory cell is sectioned below the cuticle but a little rim of the cuticle is still seen around the cell in contact with the supporting cell. In the lower right corner a lamellated body (LB) surrounded by mitochondria is seen. Between the two hair cells there is the phalanx of a Deiters cell. The darker reinforced areas belong to the reticular membrane.

Guinea pig. TEM. X 18700.

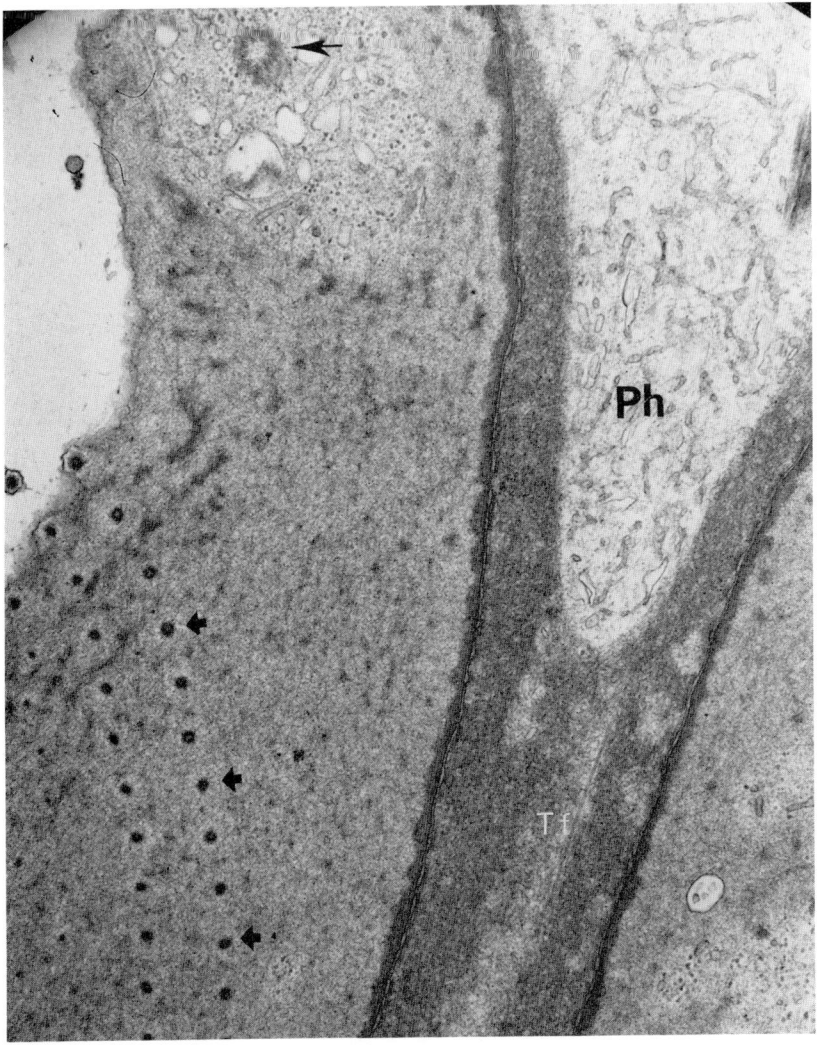

Fig. 13 This picture represents a higher magnification of a section corresponding to fig. 12. The hair rootlets are seen inserted in the cuticle. The rootlets of the first row (small arrows) are slightly thicker than the rootlets in the other rows. The upper arrow indicates the basal body in the cuticle free area. The phalanx of a Deiters´ (cont'd)

(Fig. 13, cont'd) cell (Ph) is seen between the sensory cells. It can be observed that both the hair cells and the supporting cell have a small dark region close to the cell membrane. This denser membrane seems to be a reinforcement of importance in relation to the reticular membrane. It can also be discerned how a few tonofibrils pass into the reticular membrane (Tf).

Guinea pig. TEM. X 32000.

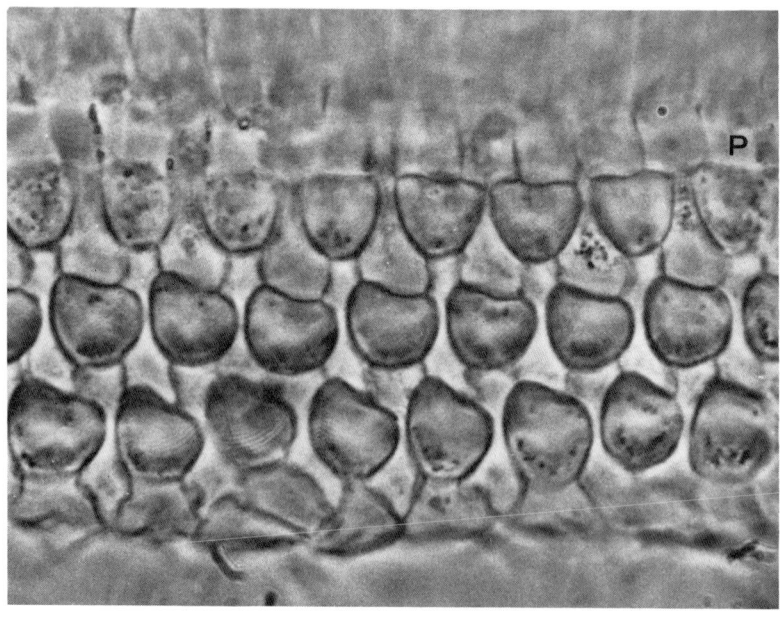

Fig. 14 Surface specimen of the organ of Corti. Three rows of outer hair cells and their supporting cells are seen. P indicates the pillar heads.

Rabbit. Phase contrast. X 1320.

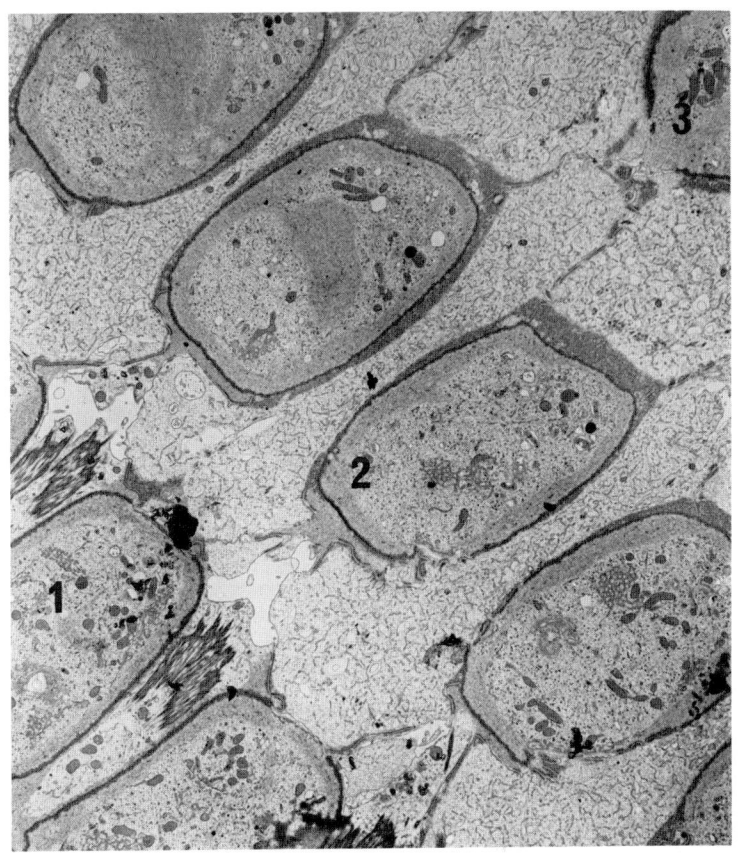

Fig. 15 Surface section through the organ of Corti. 1, 2, and 3 indicate the first, second and third row of the outer hair cells. The supporting cells are seen between the hair cells forming a very regular framework. The phalangeal shape of the processes of the Doiters' cells between the cells in the second row is very evident.

Guinea pig. TEM. x 7000.

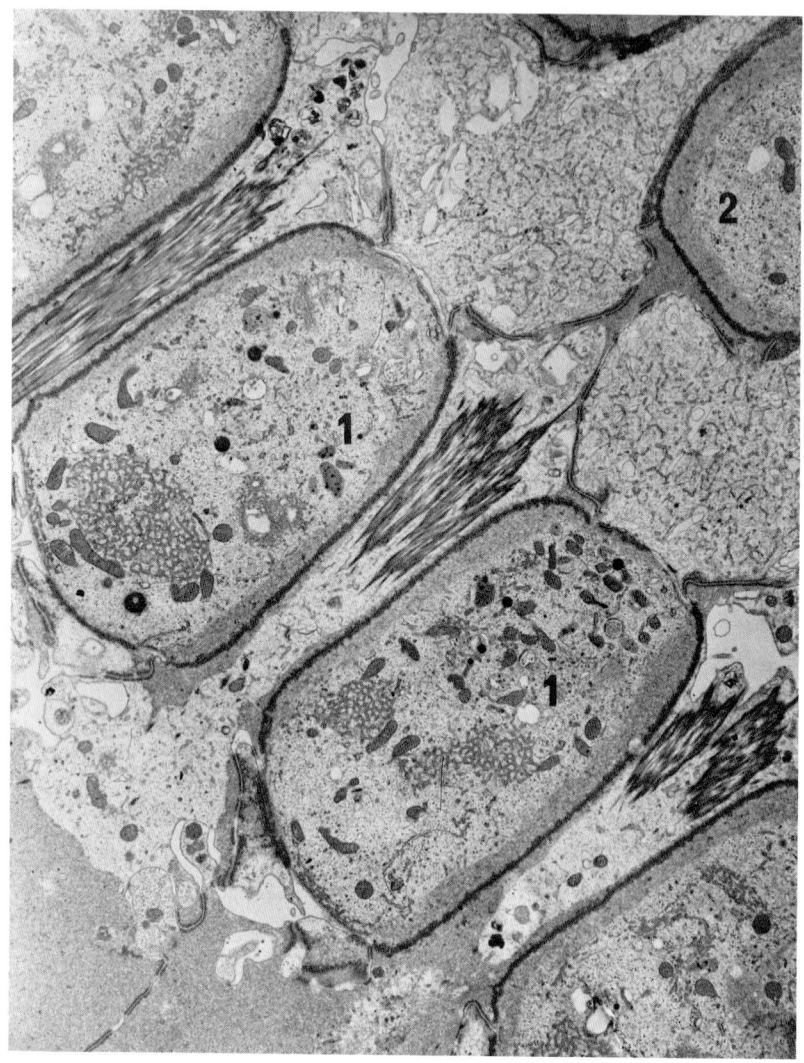

Fig. 16 Section through the organ of Corti as in Fig. 15. In this case the cell is sectioned slightly deeper just below the cuticular plate and several lamellated bodies are seen in the infracuticular region. In this region mitochondria and intracytoplasmic organelles can be seen. Between the hair cells in the first row the outer portions of the (cont'd)

(Fig. 16, cont'd) outer pillars are seen.
These prolongations, the outer oars, contain
a large number of tonofibrils.
Guinea pig. TEM. × 7500.

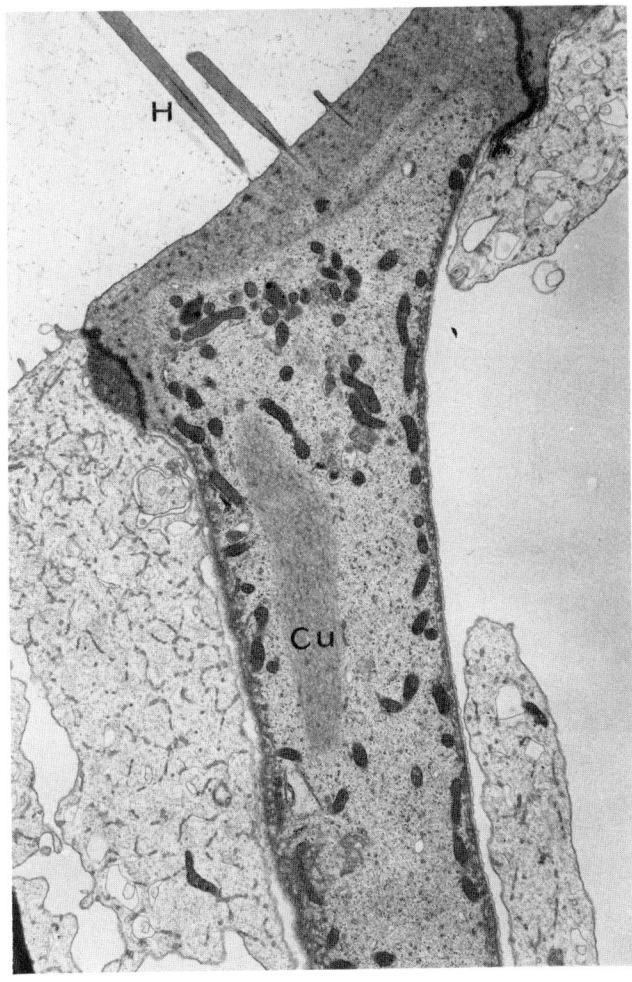

Fig. 17 Longitudinal section through the upper part
of an outer hair cell. It is possible to see
the cuticular plate with hairs (H) at its
surface. In the infracuticular region several
mitochondria and lysosomes are seen. The
cuticle has a long prolongation down into
the interior of the cell (Cu).   (cont'd)

(Fig. 17, cont'd) Along the outer vertical membranes of the cell many discontinuous membranes and mitochondria can be seen.

Guinea pig. TEM. x   8900.

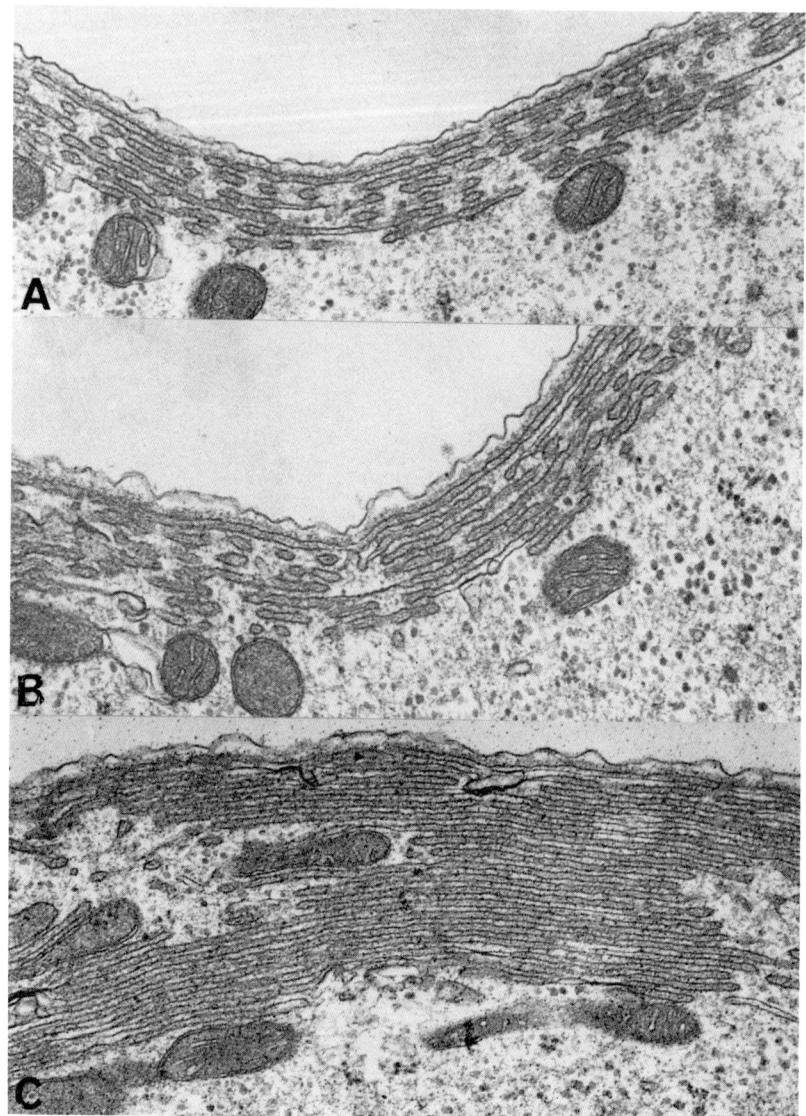

Fig. 18 A, B and C represent different outer hair cells with discontinuous membranes (cont'd)

(Fig. 18, cont'd) along their surfaces. In A and B a few layers of membranes, in C many membranes are seen.

Guinea pig. TEM. A x 42000, B x 43000, C x 39200.

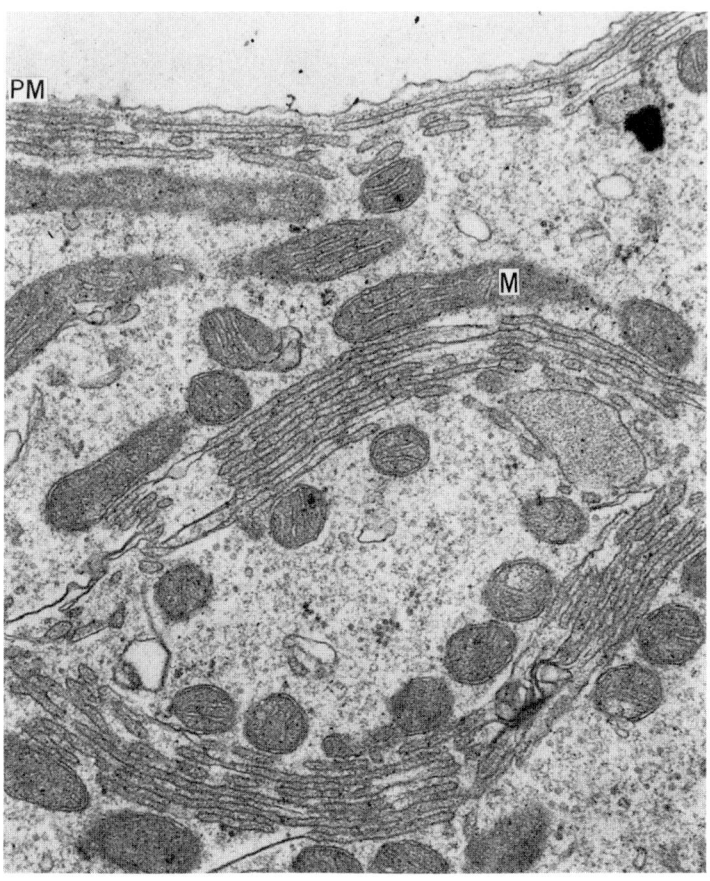

Fig. 19 Section through an outer hair cell. PM indicates the plasma membrane inside which are a few layers of discontinuous membranes and some mitochondria (M). In the lower part of the cell there is a lamellated body of typical nature with several layers of membranes surrounded by and containing mitochondria. In one part of the lamellated body (cont'd)

(Fig. 19, cont'd) an inclusion with distinct osmiophilic membrane can be seen.

Guinea pig. TEM. x 35500.

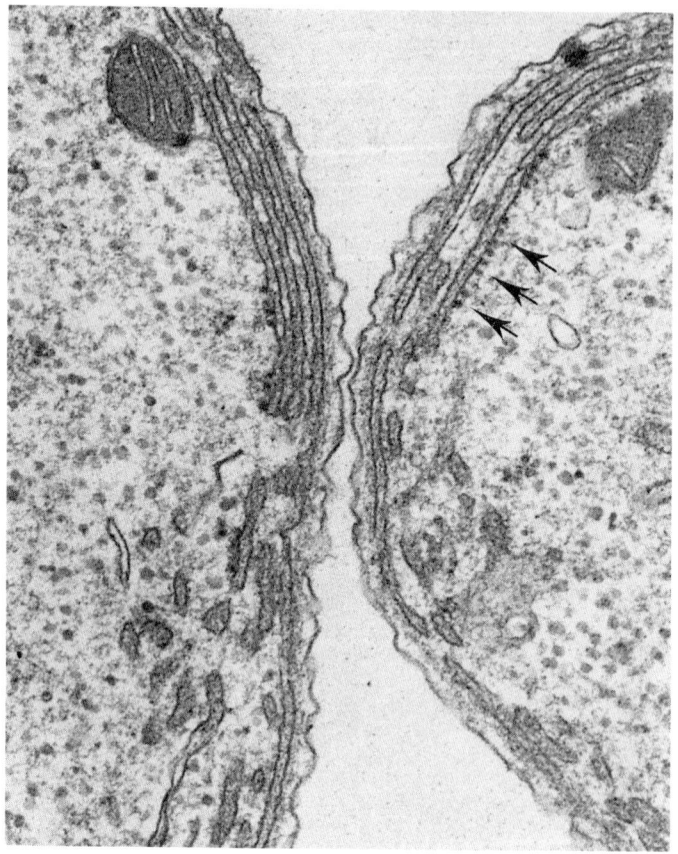

Fig. 20 Parts of two adjacent cross-sectioned outer hair cells. Inside the plasma membrane both sensory cells contain a few layers of lamellated membranes. The arrows indicate ribosome-like particles on the inside of the lamellated membrane. This could indicate that the membranes belong to the endoplasmic reticulum. In each membrane there is a denser outer line and a lighter zone in the middle. In the center of the light zone an irregular denser line can be seen.

Guinea pig. TEM. x 29500.

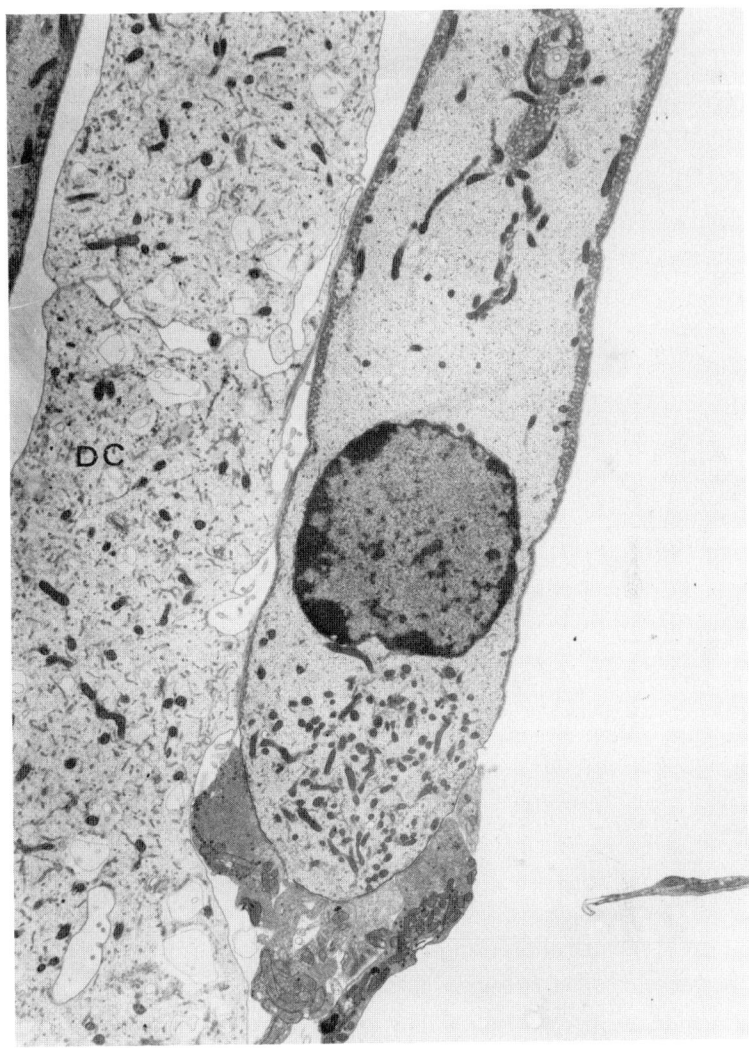

Fig. 21 Middle and lower part of an outer hair cell
of the first row. The nucleus is situated in
the lower portion and above it is a light
area containing a large number of glycogen
granules. Higher up in the hair cell there
are a few lamellated bodies and some mitochondria. Around the vertical sides in the
supranuclear region the cell is (cont'd)

(Fig. 21, cont'd) provided with discontinuous membranes. Inside these membranes there are many mitochondria. In the infranuclear portion, many mitochondria are arranged in a group corresponding to what has been called Retzius´ body. The agglomeration of mitochondria indicates a high enzymatic activity in this part of the cell. Below the cell afferent and efferent nerve endings form synaptic contacts with the cell. To the left of the cell there is a Deiters´ cell (DC).

Guinea pig. TEM. x 6100.

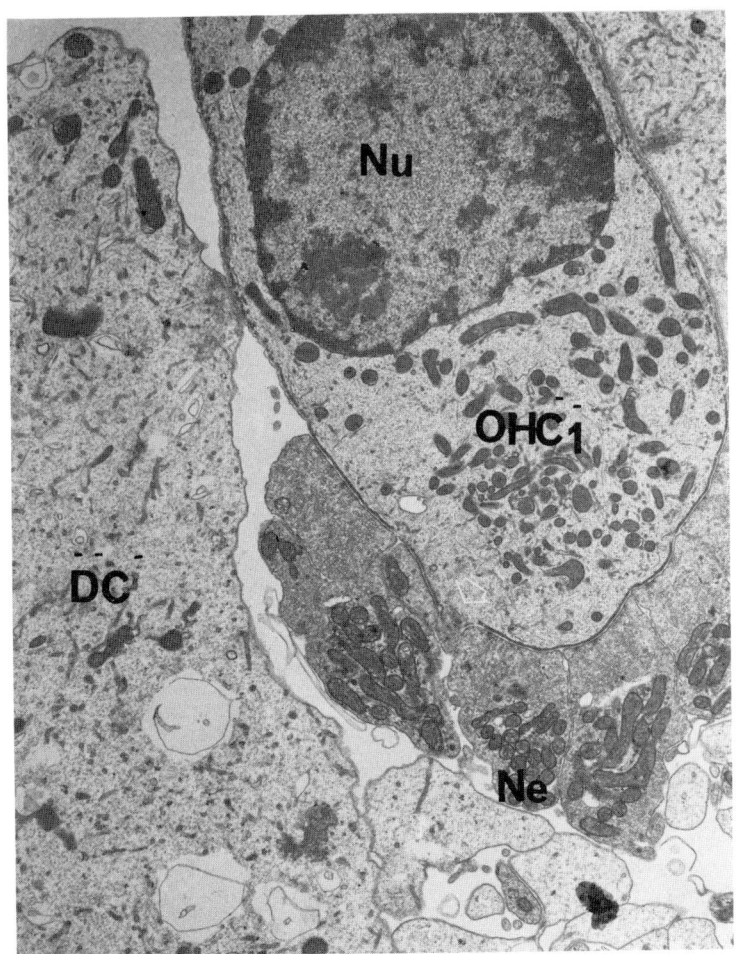

Fig. 22 Lower portion of an outer hair cell in the first row (OHC_1). The nucleus (Nu) is dark and slightly compressed, presumably due to the preparation procedure. In the infranuclear region, many mitochondria are clustered. The nerve endings (Ne) surround the base of the cell and a lighter zone at the plasma membrane (arrow) corresponds to the position of an afferent ending. DC indicates a Deiters' cell.

Guinea pig. TEM. × 15300.

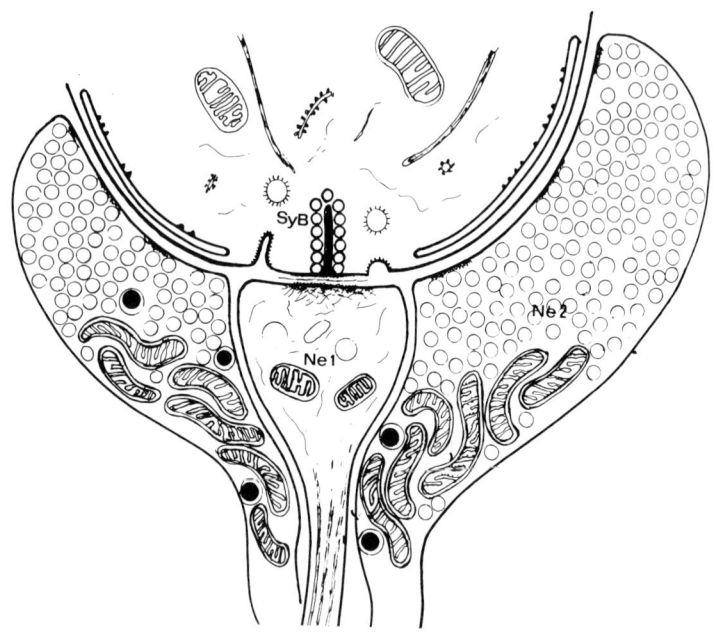

Fig. 23 Schematic drawing of the synaptic area of an outer hair cell, showing a synaptic bar (SyB) consisting of a dark rod surrounded by vesicles, presumably containing transmitter substance. Below the synaptic bar the afferent endings (Ne 1) form a synaptic contact with the sensory cell. On both sides efferent endings (Ne 2) are seen. They contain large numbers of synaptic vesicles and also some dense cored vesicles and mitochondria.

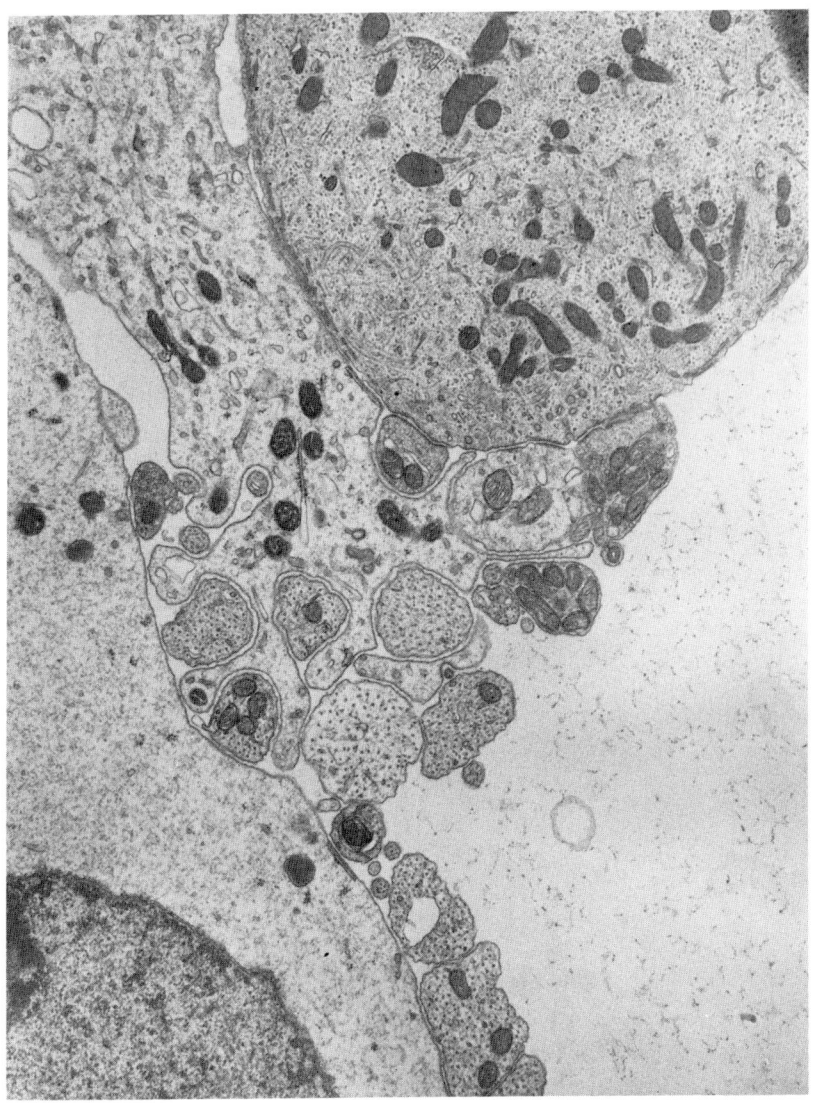

Fig. 24   Lower portion of an outer hair cell from the third row. In this case only small nerve endings contact the hair cell and below the cell several afferent and efferent nerves can be seen.
Guinea pig. TEM. x   17700.

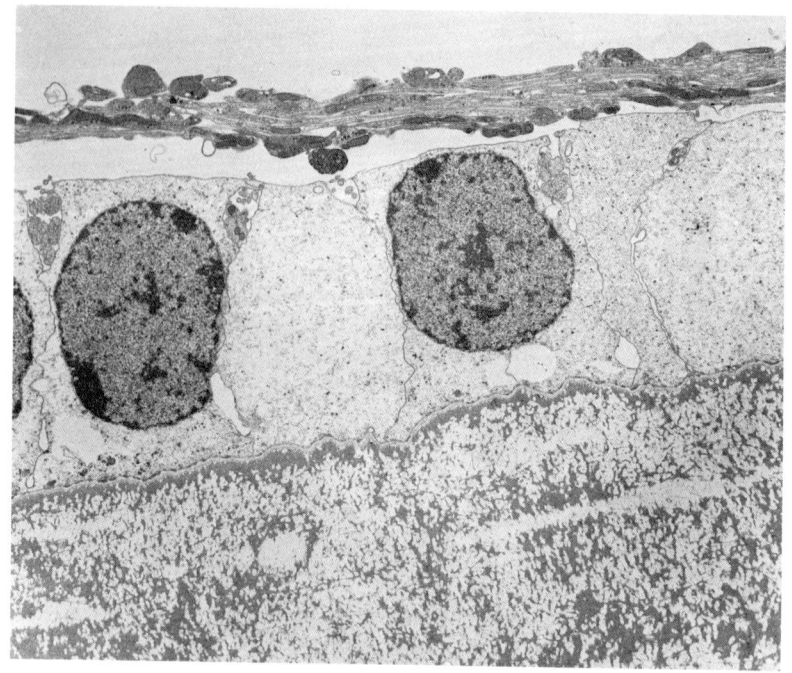

Fig. 25 Section through inner pillar cells and the spiral tunnel bundle. This nerve bundle has been longitudinally sectioned to show the beaded appearance of the fibers. These beads contain large numbers of synaptic vesicles, mainly of the clear type and also many dense cored vesicles of a large size. Between the individual pillar cells several afferent fibers can be seen.

Guinea pig. TEM. x 25000.

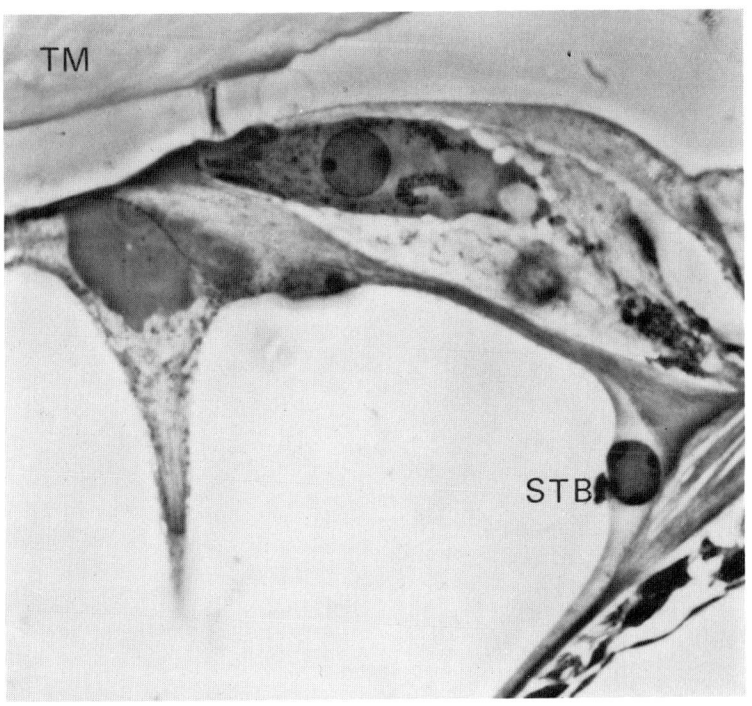

Fig. 26 Inner hair cell, pillars and tectorial membrane. The tectorial membrane (TM) is seen just above the hairs of an inner hair cell. Inside the hair cell the nucleus and the nucleolus can be seen. In the cytoplasm, especially in the infranuclear region, groups of mitochondria are observed. Below the nucleus they form two groups. Often there is seen a rounded ball shaped formation of mitochondria. The inner pillars often have nuclei at two different levels, at the base or close to the head. The spiral tunnel bundle (STB) is also visible.

Guinea pig. Phase. X 1230.

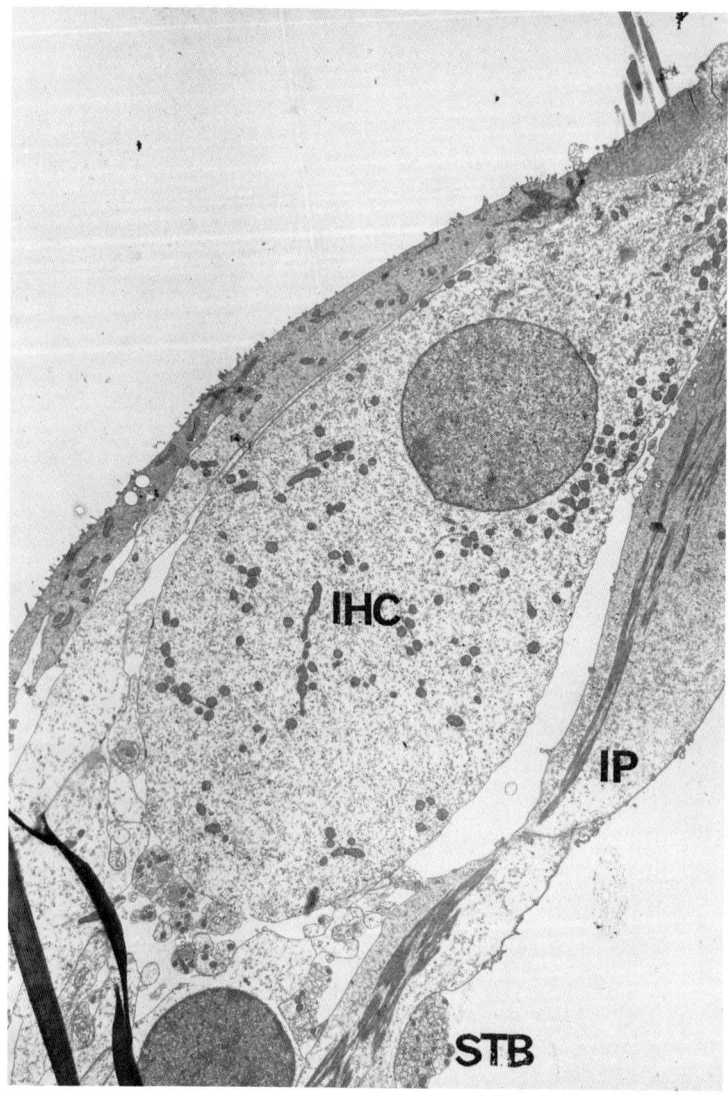

Fig. 27 Inner hair cell with its cuticular plate, a bent neck and an oblong rounded cell body. The endoplasmic reticulum is better developed in the inner hair cell than in the outer. Especially in the infracuticular region the reticulum forms a very well developed system. Nerve endings are in (cont'd)

(Fig. 27, cont'd) contact with the hair cell, especially at its base but also along the sides. Both afferent and efferent endings are in direct contact with the hair cell.

Guinea pig. TEM. × 2800.

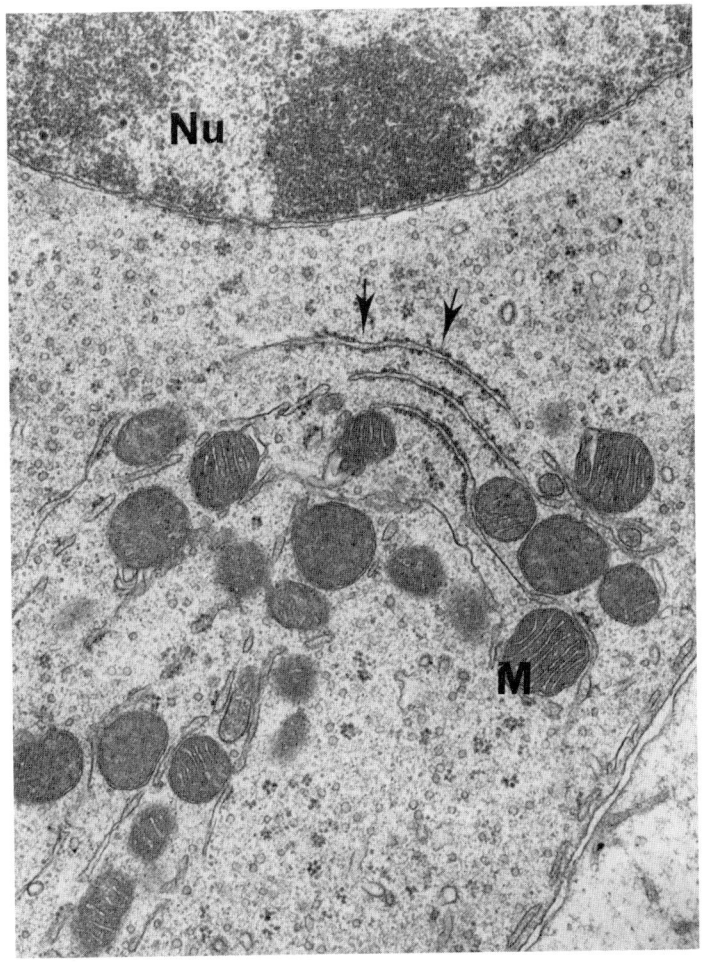

Fig. 28 Infranuclear region of an inner hair cell. Below the nucleus (Nu) there is a group of mitochondria (M) in close contact with endoplasmic reticulum (arrows) with ribosomes along their surfaces. This is a constant finding in the inner hair cells. (cont'd)

(Fig. 28, cont'd) Ribosomes in rosette-like formations or clusters can be seen in the cytoplasm where there also is a rich endoplasmic reticulum.

Guinea pig. TEM. x 33600.

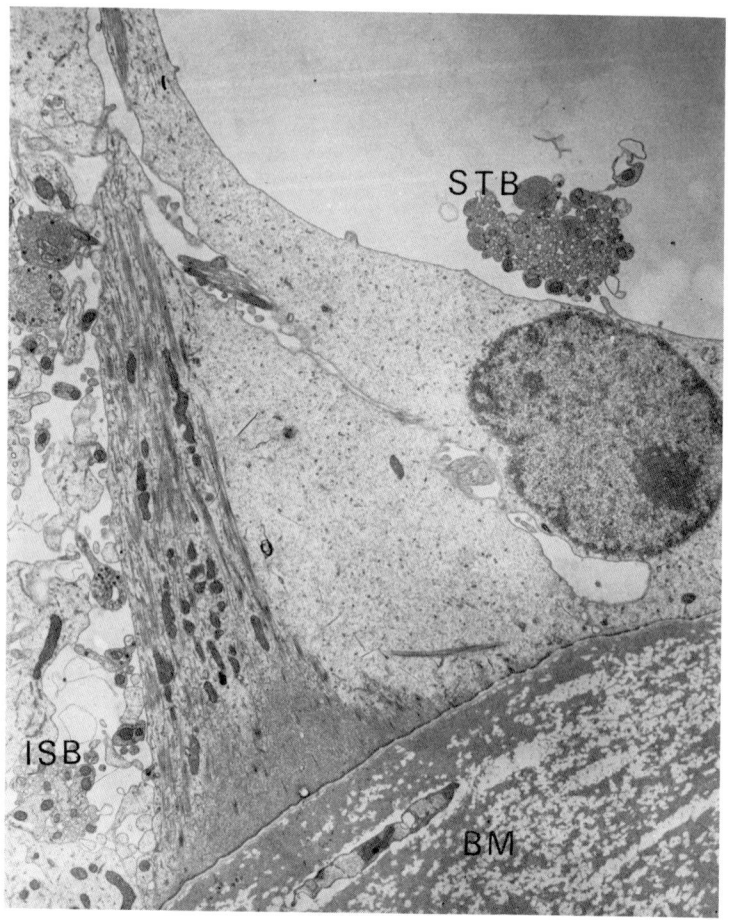

Fig. 29 Base of an inner pillar cell. It can be seen how the nucleus of the inner pillar cell usually is located close to the basilar membrane (BM). The tonofibrils of the pillar cells consist of two different types as described by Angelborg and Engström (1972). They reach from the basilar mem- (cont'd)

(Fig. 29, cont'd) brane to the top of the pillar and are closely attached to the basilar membrane by a cement-like structure. There are several mitochondria both in the lower and upper portion of the pillar cell. ISB indicates the inner spiral bundle containing both afferent and efferent fibers. This section goes through two pillars between which nerve fibers are seen. STB represents the spiral tunnel bundle and in this bundle a large number of beads containing clear and dense cored vesicles are also seen.

Guinea pig. TEM. x 6000.

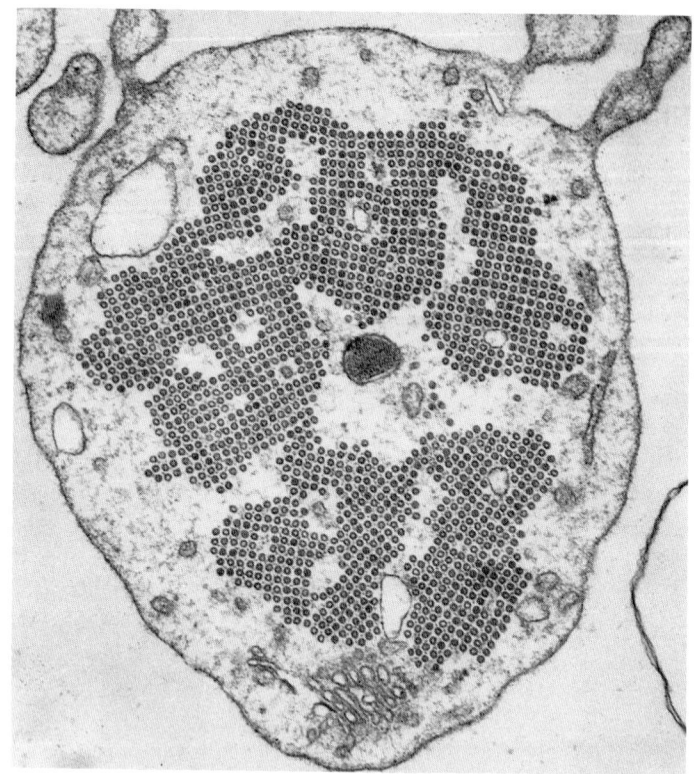

Fig. 30 Cross sectioned outer pillar showing the typical arrangement of the fibrils in the central portion of the pillar. In both pillar cells and Deiters' cells of mammals, we have found two kinds of tonofilaments. The one kind is a tubular filament with a diameter of about 275 Å and a wall-thickness of the tube of about 60 Å. The other filamental structure which we have named microfilament has a diameter of approximately 60 Å. Both kinds of fibers seem to reach from the basilar membrane to the reticular framework at the top of the organ of Corti. This pillar contains 1,556 tubular filaments and considerably more microfilaments. The position of this pillar was approximately one and a quarter coil from the base.

Guinea pig. TEM. × 37500.

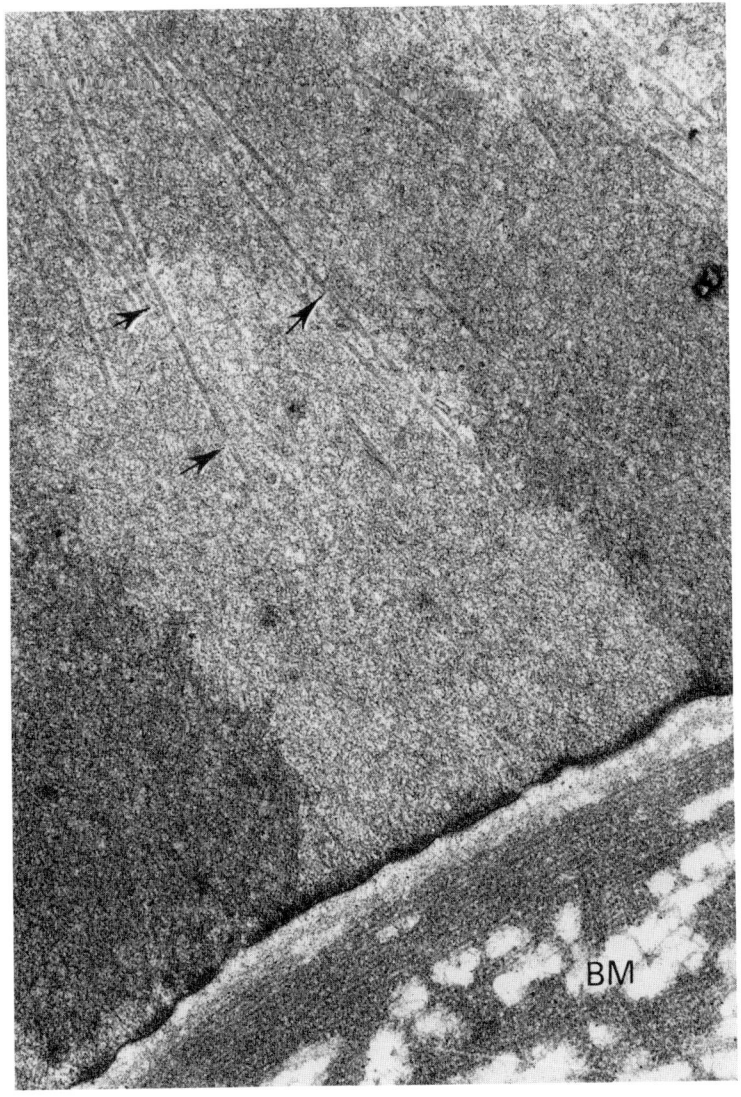

Fig. 31 Basal cone of an outer pillar cell. The basal cone is attached to the basilar membrane (BM) and it consists of a rather opaque, very finely fibrillar material with a denser portion in direct contact with this cement-like structure. A few tubular filaments (arrows) and many solid (cont'd)

(Fig. 31, cont'd) microfilaments are inserted in both. The beginning of the tubular filaments seems to be in the form of very thin fibrils which form a tube.

Guinea pig. TEM. × 45000.

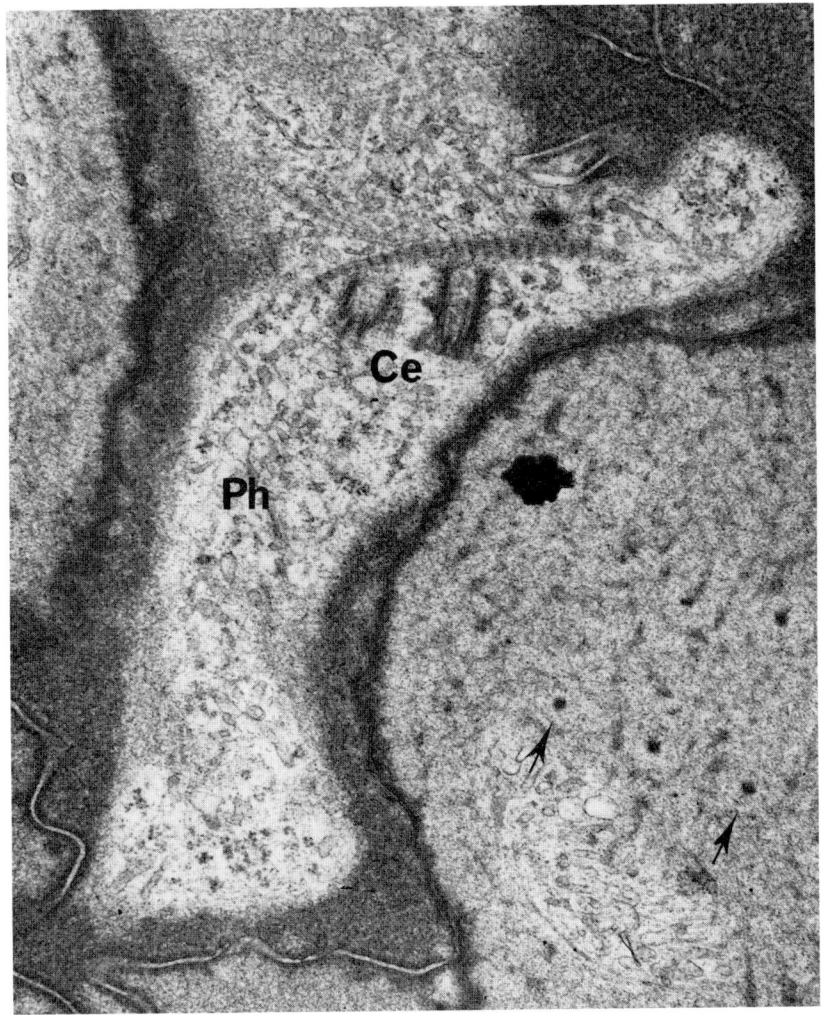

Fig. 32 Phalangeal cell (Ph) between two inner hair cells. In the hair cell the arrows indicate the rootlets of some hairs. In the phalanx two centrioles (Ce) and striated fibers can be seen.

Guinea pig. TEM. x 28700.

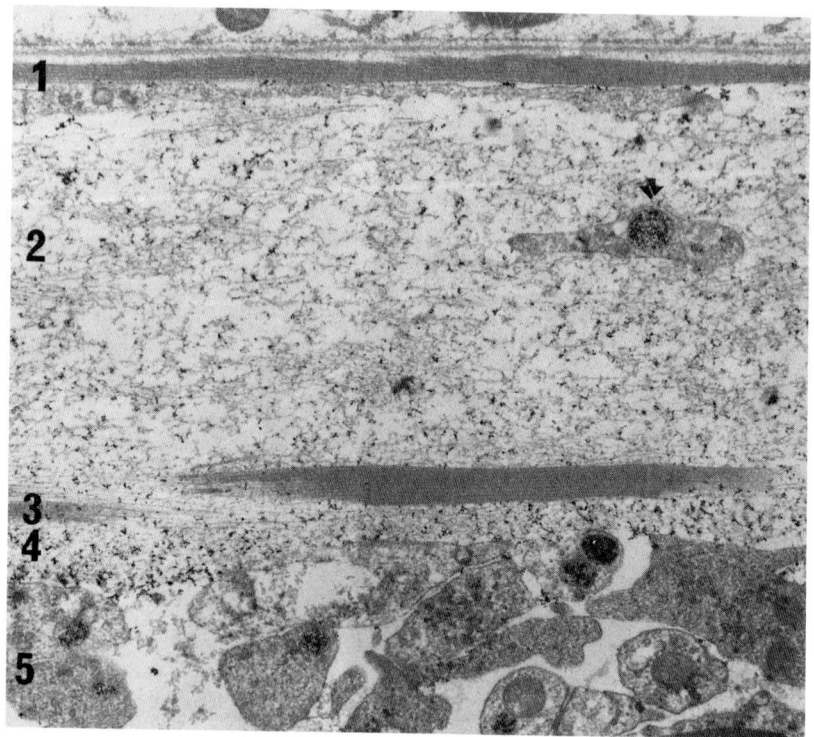

Fig. 33 Section through the basilar membrane. This part of the membrane belongs to the pars pectinata where there are two fibrillar layers (1 and 3) and two homogenous layers (2 and 4). Below the basilar membrane there are mesothelial cells (5) with a high phagocytic capacity. In this animal thorium dioxide in the form of Thorotrast (R) has been injected into the perilymph. The small black dots represent Thorotrast particles, with a diameter of approximately 50-100 Å. A cluster of particles is seen in a lysosome (arrow) in a cell in the upper homogenous layer. There is no Thorotrast in the fibrillar layers and a concentration gradient is seen, with a higher concentration in the layer nearest the perilymph.
Guinea pig. TEM. × 17300.

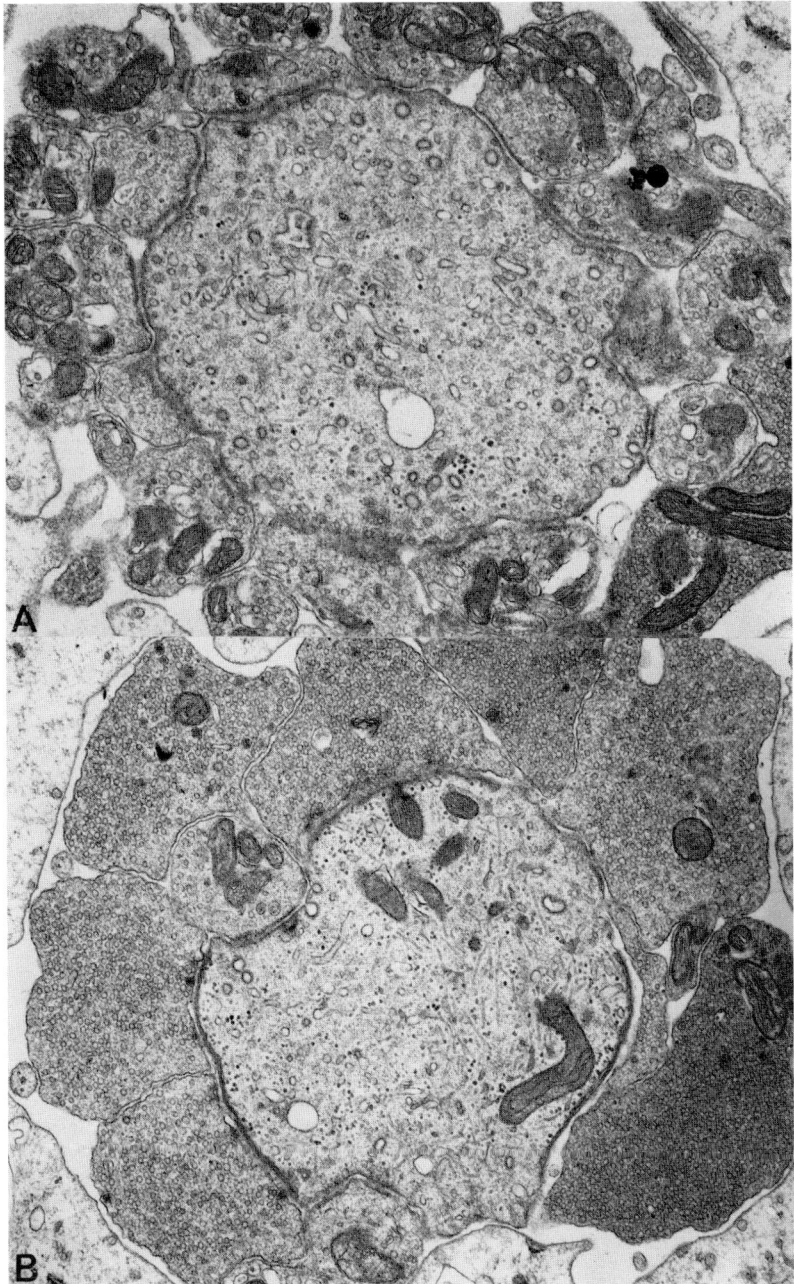

Fig. 34 (cont'd)

(Fig. 34 A and B, cont'd) Cross-section of the lower end of an outer hair cell from the third row. There are many afferent endings and the plasma membrane of the hair cell is richly irregular, forming coated invaginations and coated vesicles. Such invaginations are common at afferent endings, but they do not occur at efferent endings. This can also be seen in B which is from the basal end of a first row outer hair cell. The very large efferent endings have a subsynaptic cistern, here seen as a dense line. The afferent endings have well developed coated invaginations.

Guinea pig. TEM. A × 24500, B × 22000.

References

Ades, H.W., and Engström, H. (1972). Inner ear studies. Acta Otolaryngol. Suppl. 301.

Angelborg, C., and Engström H. (1972). Supporting elements in the organ of Corti. Acta Otolaryngol. Suppl. 301, 49-60.

Beck, C. (1965). Biochemie des Ohres. In: Hals-Nasen-Ohren-Heilkunde Band III/Teil 1 (J. Berendes, R. Link and F. Zöllner, eds.). Georg Thieme, Stuttgart.

Bredberg, G. (1968). Cellular pattern and nerve supply of the human organ of Corti. Acta Otolaryngol. Suppl. 236.

Bredberg, G., Ades, H.W., and Engström, H. (1972). Scanning electron microscopy of the normal and pathologically altered organ of Corti. Acta Otolaryngol. Suppl. 301, 3-48.

Duvall, A.J. III., and Sutherland, C.R. (1972). Cochlear transport of horseradish peroxidase. Ann. Otol. Rhinol. Laryngol. 81, 705-713.

Engström, H. (1960). The cortilymph, the third lymph of the inner ear. Acta Morphol. Neer. Scand. 3, 195-204.

Engström, H. (1965). Elektronenoptische Histologie des Innenohres. In: Hals-Nasen-Ohren-Heilkunde Band III/Teil 1 (J. Berendes, R. Link, and F. Zöllner, eds.). Georg Thieme, Stuttgart.

Engström, H. (1970). The first-order vestibular neuron. In: Fourth symposium on the role of the vestibular organs in space exploration. 123-135. NASA SP-187.

Engström, H., and Wersäll, J. (1953). Structure of the organ of Corti. I. Outer hair cells. Acta Otolaryngol. 43, 1-10.

Engström, H., and Wersäll, J. (1958). Structure and innervation of the inner ear sensory epithelia. Int. Rev. Cytol. 7, 535-585.

Engström, H., and Ades, H.W. (1973). The ultrastructure of the cochlea. In: <u>Ultrastructure of Animal Tissue and Organs.</u> (In preparation).

Engström, H., Ades, H.W., and Hawkins, J.E. (1962). Structure and functions of the sensory hairs of the inner ear. <u>J. Acoust. Soc. Amer.</u> <u>34</u>, 1356-1363.

Engström, H., Ades, H.W., and Andersson, A. (1966). <u>Structural pattern of the organ of Corti.</u> Almqvist & Wiksell, Stockholm.

Engström, H., Ades, H.W., and Bredberg, G. (1970). Normal structures of the organ of Corti and the effect of noise induced cochlear damage. In: <u>Sensorineural Hearing Loss.</u> (G.E.W. Wolstenholme and J. Knight, eds.), pp. 127-156. J & A. Churchill, London.

Held, H. (1926). Die Cochlea der Säuger und der Vögel, ihre Entwicklung und ihre Bau. In: <u>Bethes's Handbuch der normalen und pathologischen Physiologie. Rezeptionsorgane.</u> <u>11</u>, 467-534.

Ilberg, C. von (1968). Elektronenmikroskopische Untersuchungen über Diffusion und resorption von Thoriumdioxyd an der Meerschweinschenschnecke. 4. Basilar membran und Cortisches Organ. <u>Arch. Klin. Exp. Ohr.-Nas.-Kehlk. Heilk.</u> <u>192</u>, 384-400.

Ilberg, C. von (1969). Tubuläre Strukturen in äusseren Haarzellen. <u>Arch. Klin. Exp. Ohr.- Nas.- Kehlk. Heilk.</u> <u>194</u>, 408-442.

Iurato, S. (1961). Submicroscopic structure of the membranous labyrinth. II. The epithelium of Corti's organ. <u>Z. Zellforsch.</u> <u>52</u>, 259-298.

Iurato, S. (1962). Submicroscopic structure of the membranous labyrinth. III. The supporting structure of Corti's organ (basilar membrane, limbus spiralis and spiral ligament). <u>Z. Zellforsch.</u> <u>56</u>, 40-96.

Iurato, S. (1967). <u>Submicroscopic structures of the inner ear.</u> Pergamon Press, Oxford.

Iurato, S., Luciano, L., Pannese, E., and Reale, E. (1971). Histochemical localization of acetylcholinesterase (AChE) activity in the inner ear. Acta Otolaryngol. Suppl. 279.

Kimura, R.S. (1966). Hairs of the cochlear sensory cells and their attachement to the tectorial membrane. Acta Otolaryngol. 58, 390.

Lim, D.J. (1969). Three dimensional observation of the inner ear with the scanning electron microscope. Acta Otolaryngol. Suppl. 255, 1-38.

Lim, D.J. (1972). Fine morphology of the tectorial membrane. Its relationship to the organ of Corti. Arch. Otolaryngol. 96, 199-215.

Retzius, G. (1884). Das Gehörorgan der Wirbeltiere. II. Das Gehörorgan der Reptilien, der Vögel und der Säugetiere. Samson & Wallin, Stockholm.

Smith, C.A. (1956). Microscopic structure of the utricle. Ann. Otol. Rhinol. Laryngol. 65, 450-469.

Smith, C.A. (1967). Innervation of the organ of Corti. In: Submicroscopic structure of the inner ear (S. Iurato, ed.), pp. 107-131. Pergamon Press, Oxford.

Spoendlin, H. (1966). The Organization of the Cochlear Receptor. Advances in Oto-Rhino-Laryngology 13. Karger, Basel-New York.

Spoendlin, H. (1970). Auditory, vestibular, olfactory and gustatory organs. In: Ultrastructure of the peripheral nervous system and sense organs (Bischoff, ed.), pp. 173-263. Georg Thieme, Stuttgart.

Wersäll, J., Engström, H., and Hjort, S. (1954). Fine structure of the guinea pig macula utriculi. Acta Otolaryngol. Suppl. 116, 298-303.

Wersäll, J., Hilding, D., and Lundquist, P.-G. (1961). Ultrastruktur und Innervation der cochlearen Haarzellen. Arch. Klin. Exp. Ohr.- Nas.- Kehlk. Heilk. 178, 106-126.

Wersäll, J., Flock, Å., and Lundquist, P.-G. (1965). Structural basis for directional sensitivity in cochlear and vestibular sensory receptors. Cold Spring Harbor Symp. Quan. Biol. 30, 115.

Wersäll, J. (1968). Efferent innervation of the inner ear. In: Structure and functions of inhibitory neuronal mechanisms. (C. von Euler, S. Skoglund, and U. Söderberg, eds.) pp. 123-139. Pergamon Press, Oxford.

DISCUSSION

TONNDORF: Dr. Engström, you stated that you do not think that cortilymph and perilymph are the same. You know we discussed this some 10 years ago and I thought that your work and that of Vosteen had settled the question. I would like for you to elaborate on the statement that you made a few minutes ago.

ENGSTRÖM: It stated in that paper (Engström, 1960) that while awaiting further evidence, we should regard it as a separate fluid and I called it cortilymph. And then v. Ilberg and the Vosteen group came with such nice evidence that I thought now it was settled that it was perilymph. We have repeated their experiments now and have come to the conclusion that the question still is open.

ZWICKER: What animal and what kind of fixation were used to show the connection between the hairs and the tectorial membrane?

ENGSTRÖM: We have used a whole set of animals in the laboratory, rats, mice, guinea pigs especially, squirrel monkeys to a great extent and we have seen about the same in all animals. The fixation was from the beginning osmic acid and nowadays we work mainly with glutharaldehyde-osmic acid fixation.

References

Engström, H. (1960). The cortilymph, the third lymph of the inner ear. Acta Morphol. Neerland. - Scand. 3, 195-204.

v. Ilberg, C. (1968). Elektronenmikroskopische Untersuchungen über diffusion und resorption von thoriumdioxyd an der meerschweinchenschnecke. 4. Basilar-membran und Cortisches organ. Arch. Klin. Exp. Ohr-, Nas- Kehlk, Heilk, 192, 384-400.

THE INNERVATION OF THE COCHLEAR RECEPTOR

H. Spoendlin

ORL Klinik, Kantonsspital
Zürich
Switzerland

The transformation of acoustic information into nerve activities is achieved in several steps, each of which is bound to certain structures in the cochlea and is entirely dependent of their structural characteristics. The terminal unmyelinated portions of the cochlear nerve fibers in the organ of Corti and their endings and interconnections are the morphological substrate of the coding of the acoustic message in the cochlea (Figs. 1, 4). Any stimulus integration

Cochlea	Mech. analysis	Travelling waves
Sensory cells	Mech.-electric transduction	Microphonics
Nerve endings, Terminal unmyelinated nerve branches	Coding of acoustic information	Generator potential ?
Myelinated nerve fibres	Transport to CNS	Action potential

Fig. 1 Schematic representation of the different steps of information transformation in the cochlea.

most probably is only possible in these unmyelinated terminal nerve portions whose response is a graded potential before the information is digitalized in all-or-nothing spikes at the initial segment of the neurons. Ample electrophysiological information is available on the receptor potentials and the nerve action potentials, whereas very little is known of the important step in-between, the coding in the nerve endings and terminal unmyelinated nerve fibers.

Three types of nerve fibers, the afferent neurons of the cochlear nerve, the efferents and the adrenergic fibers participate in the innervation of the cochlear receptor. Whereas the afferent and efferent fibers are directly involved in the coding process, the adrenergic innervation most probably has a more general influence on the receptor rather than a specific action on coding.

As shown with the histochemical method of Falck et al. (1962)(Spoendlin and Lichtensteiger, 1966, Spoendlin, 1967, Ross, 1971, Spoendlin, 1972b) the adrenergic innervation of the cochlea consists of a perivascular and a blood-vessel independent system (Fig. 2). The latter forms a loose terminal plexus in the

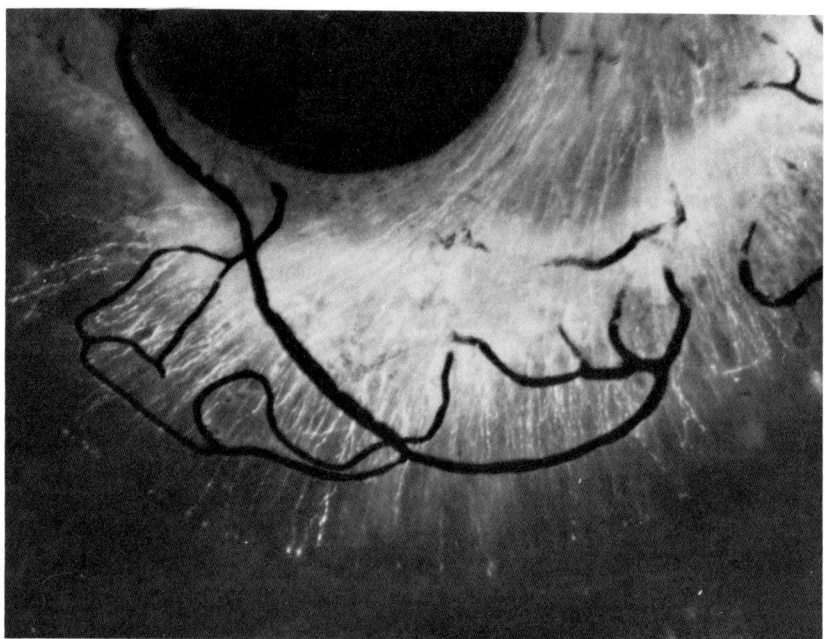

Fig. 2 Combined demonstration of the blood-vessel-independent adrenergic innervation (cont'd)

(Fig. 2, cont'd) in the apical turn of a cat cochlea by the method of Falck et al. (1962) and indian ink injection of the blood vessels. It is clearly seen that most fluorescent nerve fibers run independently from the blood vessels, (From Spoendlin, 1967).

area of the habenula, originates in the superior cervical ganglion and probably reaches the inner ear by the way of facial anastomosis. The unequivocal electron microscopic demonstration and precise determination of their actual endings have not been possible so far. An accumulation of dense core vesicles in nerve fibers and endings, as seen especially after glutaraldehyde fixation in the inner spiral plexus, does not prove adrenergic fibers, since such vesicles are also found in efferent and afferent nerve terminals (Figs. 5, 11).

There have been various attempts to demonstrate the influence of the sympathetic nerve supply on the cochlear function (Seymour and Tappin, 1953, Beickert et al., 1956, Vasilev, 1963) but these have not produced any really convincing evidence.

An abundant efferent nerve supply of the organ of Corti has been demonstrated in many animals (Iurato, 1962, Kimura and Wersäll, 1962, Spoendlin and Gacek, 1963, Smith and Rasmussen, 1963). The initial argument as to whether all of the surprisingly large and numerous vesiculated nerve endings at the outer hair cells (Figs. 5, 6, 7) and most inner spiral fibers belong to the olivocochlear efferent system could be settled by the demonstration of the complete disappearance of all these fibers and endings after selective and total transection of the olivocochlear bundle in the vestibular root or nerve (Figs. 3, 8) (Spoendlin, 1966, 1969b, 1970). Furthermore we were able to show that all upper tunnel radial fibers, the only tunnel crossing fibers visible in light microscopy, also disappeared completely after section of the olivocochlear bundle (Spoendlin, 1969a)(Fig. 3). The conclusion that all those tunnel crossing fibers belong to the efferent innervation was not easily accepted although there is not much reasonable way to escape the experimental evidence.

The efferent nerve supply of the organ of Corti

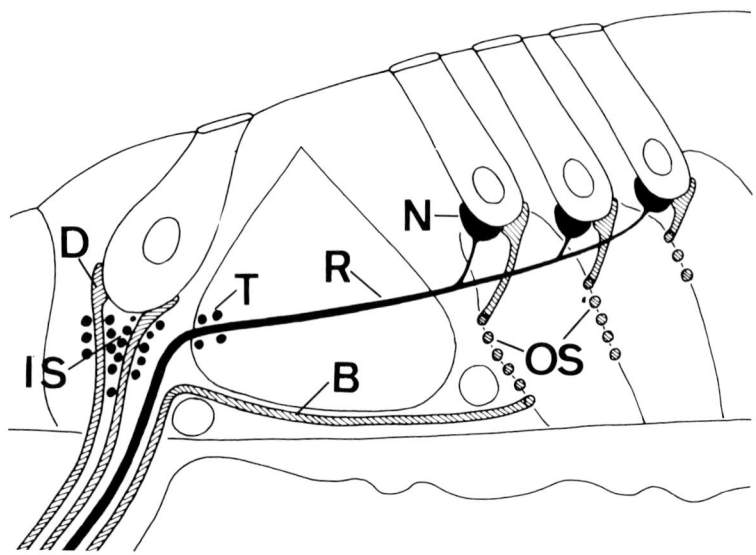

Fig. 3 Schematic representation of the principle nerve fiber tracts in the organ of Corti. All fibers in full black are efferent. Radial dendrites to the inner hair cells (D), inner spiral fibers (iS), tunnel spiral fibers (T), upper tunnel radial fibers (R), basilar fibers (B), outer spiral fibers (OS) and nerve endings at the base of the outer hair cells (N)(compare Fig. 4).

starts with about 500 fibers in the olivocochlear bundle (Rasmussen, 1960), which in the cochlea forms the intraganglionic spiral bundle and finally becomes in the organ of Corti the inner spiral bundle consisting of 50-200 small fibers (Figs. 3, 4, 9). The upper tunnel radial fibers include a total of about 8000 fibers of varying diameters from 0.3-1.5 µ and finally there are the approximately 40,000 vesiculated nerve endings at the base of the outer hair cells. From these numbers extensive ramifications of the efferent fibers are quite evident. In the basal turn each outer hair cell is provided with 6-8 efferent nerve endings (Fig. 5), a number which is gradually reduced towards the cochlear apex especially in the second and third rows of outer hair cells where the nerve endings disappear entirely in the upper turns.

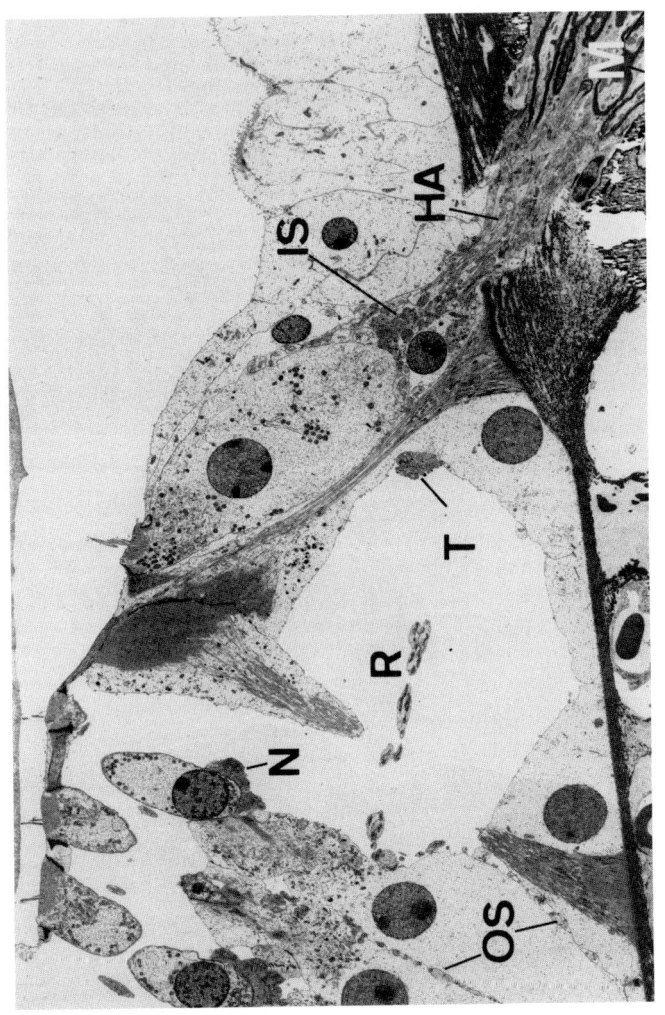

Fig. 4 Low magnification EM-picture of the organ of Corti of the guinea pig in the basal turn. Habenular opening (HA) where the myelinated nerve fibers (M) lose their myelin sheaths and penetrate into the organ of Corti. Inner spiral fibers (IS), tunnel spiral fibers (T), upper tunnel radial fibers (R), outer spiral fibers (OS), nerve endings at the base of the outer hair cells (N) (compare Fig. 3).

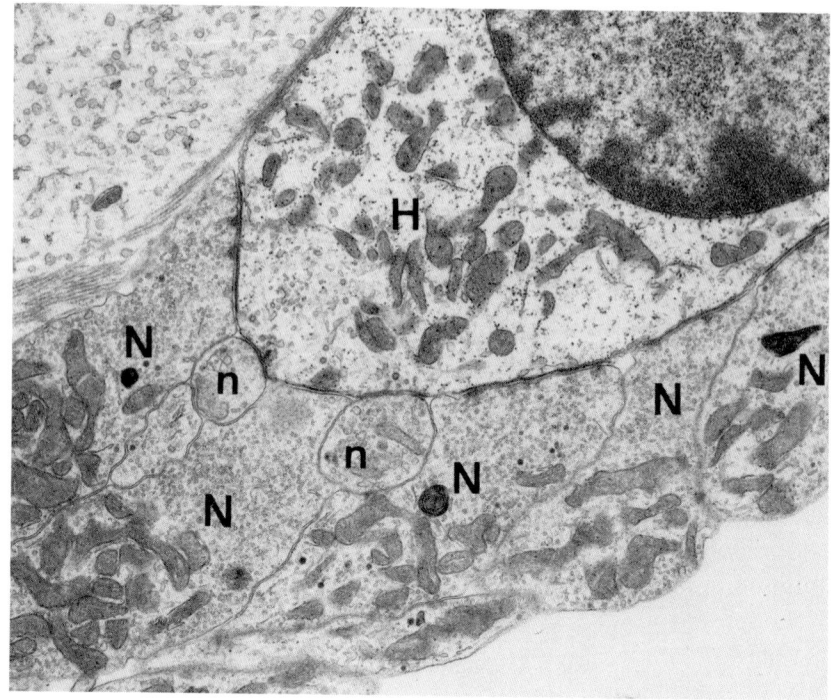

Fig. 5 Base of a first row outer hair cell (H) of the basal turn of a guinea pig. There is a surprisingly large number of large efferent nerve endings (N) and only very few afferent terminals between them (n) presenting some synaptic structures. The efferent endings show frequent synaptic vesicle-condensations at the membrane facing the hair cell and very rarely only towards the afferent nerve endings and fibers. Several dense core vesicles are seen within the efferent nerve endings.

After degeneration of the efferent fibers no significant reduction of the outer spiral fibers is found, indicating a predominantly radial distribution of the efferent fibers which after crossing the tunnel ramify and innervate a group of adjacent outer hair cells (Figs. 6, 7, 38). The efferents of the inner spiral fibers however expand spirally over a considerable, not yet determined, distance.

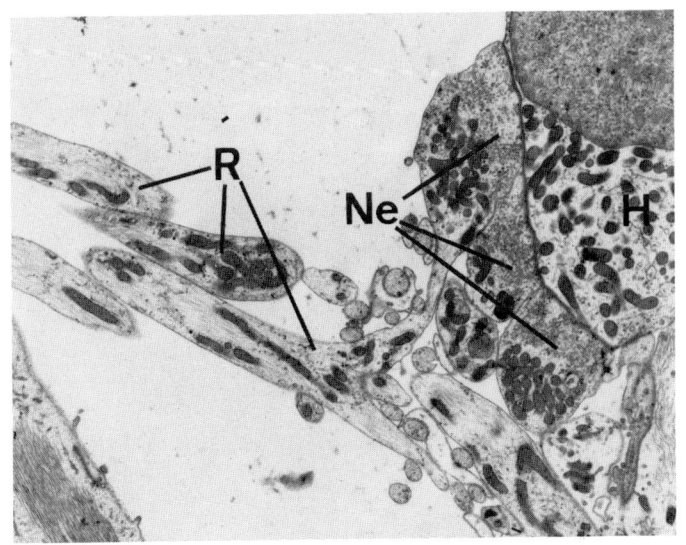

Fig. 6   The upper tunnel radial fibers (R) which are all efferent are usually large. They divide into several branches after crossing the tunnel and form the large efferent nerve endings (Ne) at the base of the outer hair cells (H). The distribution of these fibers is predominantly radial.

According to Rasmussen (1960) 3/4 of the efferent fibers originate in the contralateral and only 1/4 in the homolateral superior olivary complex. Judging from the very few remaining intraganglionic spiral fibers in the cat after midline lesions with degeneration of only the contralateral fibers the percentage of homolateral fibers is even considerably smaller (Fig. 10/b). After selective elimination of the contralateral olivocochlear bundle almost all vesiculated nerve endings at the outer hair cells and about 50 % of the inner spiral fibers disappeared in the cat (Fig. 10a)(Spoendlin, 1969b) in contrast to

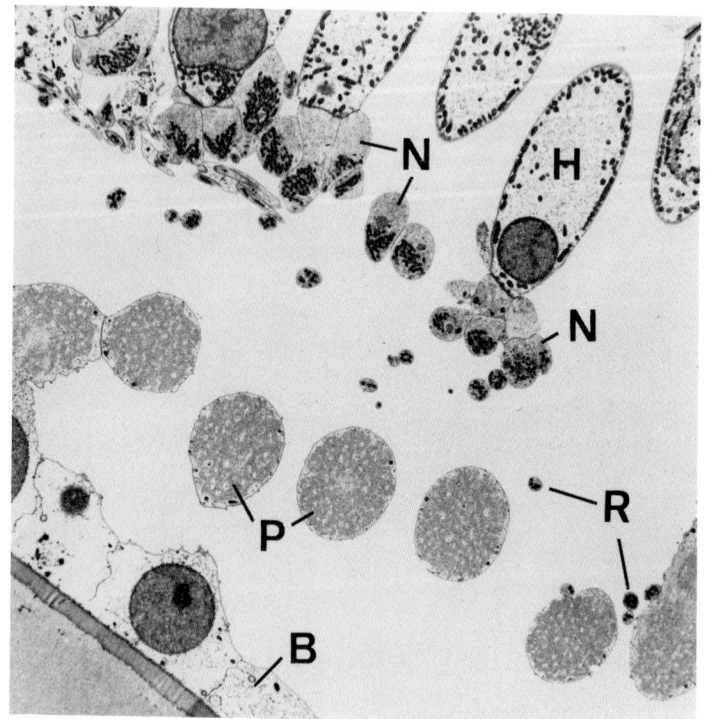

Fig. 7 Longitudinal section through the area of the outer pillars (P) and first row outer hair cells (H). It is clearly seen how the large upper tunnel radial fibers approach the base of the outer hair cells and form the efferent nerve terminals (N). The afferent basilar fibers (B) are very small and hardly seen at this low magnification.

Iurato's (1964) findings in the rat, where all inner spiral fibers seemed to belong to the homolateral system. This indicates some species differences.

The efferents of the inner and outer hair cell regions differ not only in caliber and distribution pattern but also in their synaptic connections. At the level of the outer hair cells morphological evidence of synapses, such as condensation of vesicles at the presynaptic membrane and postsynaptic cisternae is found almost exclusively between nerve ending and sensory cell (Fig. 5) and at the level of the inner hair cells almost exclusively between vesicle filled enlargements and afferent radial fibers from the inner hair cells (Fig. 11)(Spoendlin, 1969b). (In rodents there seem to be more exceptions to this rule, in so much as some efferents might also contact the

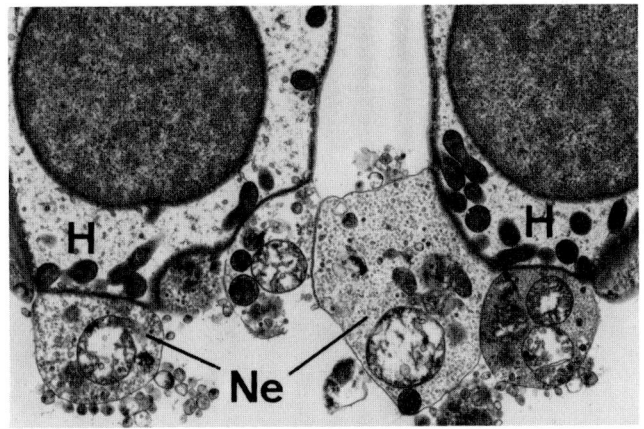

Fig. 8   A base of two outer hair cells (H) 4 days after transection of the olivocochlear bundle in the vestibular nerve. The large efferent nerve endings (Ne) are obviously in full degeneration.

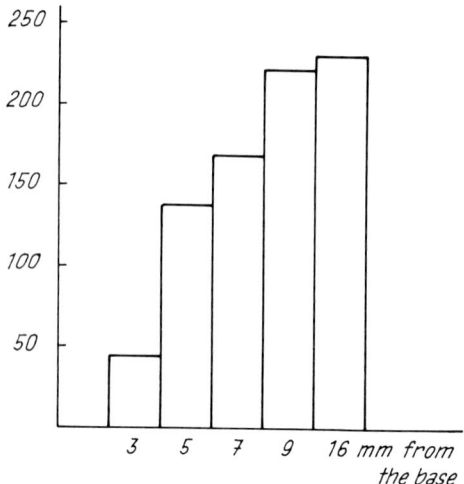

Fig. 9 Number of internal spiral fibers in different parts of the cochlea in the cat (From Spoendlin, 1969b).

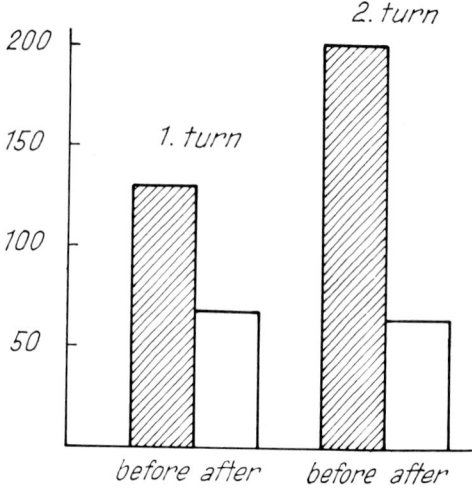

Fig. 10 a Average number of internal spiral fibers before and after transection of the crossed olivocochlear bundle (average of six ears (From Spoendlin, 1969b).

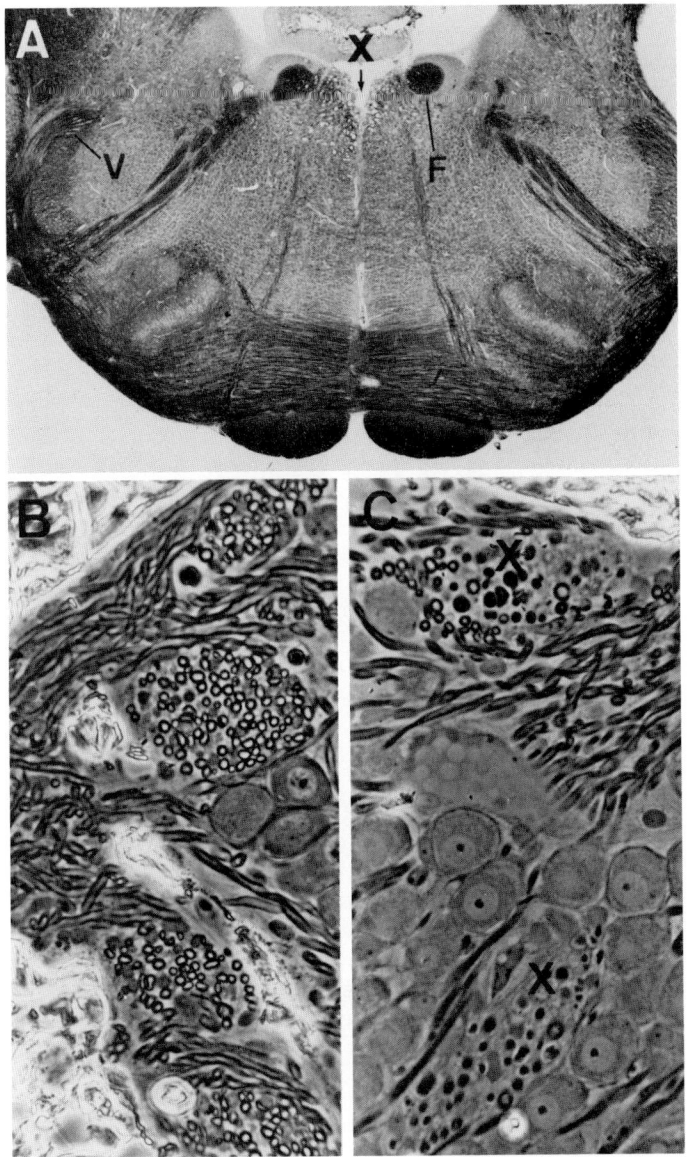

Fig. 10/b Transection of the crossed olivocochlear fibers in the cat by means of a "midline lesion".

  A: Section through the brain stem (cont'd)

(Fig. 10/b, cont'd) showing the lesion in the midline (X) between the colliculi faciales (F). Vestibular root (V).

B: Intraganglionic spiral bundle of a normal animal. A great number of myelinated nerve fibers run in several fasciculi along the peripheral contour of the spiral ganglion.

C: Situation a few weeks after transection of the crossed olivocochlear fibers in the midline of the brain stem as shown in A. The great majority of all myelinated nerve fibers of the intraganglionic spiral bundle has degenerated (X).

inner hair cells and some synapses might exist between efferent and afferent fibers at the level of the outer hair cells). We would therefore expect the influence of the efferents to be presynaptic directly on the outer hair cells and postsynaptic on the afferent dendrites from the inner hair cells (Fig. 12).

The afferent nerve distribution in the organ of Corti, as studied after elimination of the efferent innervation, is again basically different for inner and outer hair cells. Since we know that all upper tunnel radial fibers belong to the efferent system, the basilar fibers are the only afferent fibers leading to the outer hair cells (Fig. 3). Counted at the level of the outer pillars (Fig. 15) we found an average of one basilar fiber penetrating between two pillar feet, which amounts to the surprisingly small total number of 2000-3000 for the whole cochlea (Spoendlin, 1969a). This means that only about 5 % of all 50,000 cochlear neurons are associated with the outer hair cells, an observation which needs further evidence. The other 95 % of the cochlear neurons are presumably associated with the inner hair cells. In fact reconstructions of the habenula and inner hair cell region in the cat with eliminated efferents confirmed directly the predominant afferent innervation of the inner hair cells. Of 20 afferent fibers entering the organ of Corti 18-19 lead directly unbranched to the nearest inner hair cell and only 1 or 2 fibers turn outwards to the outer hair cells (Spoendlin 1969a, b)(Figs. 13, 16).

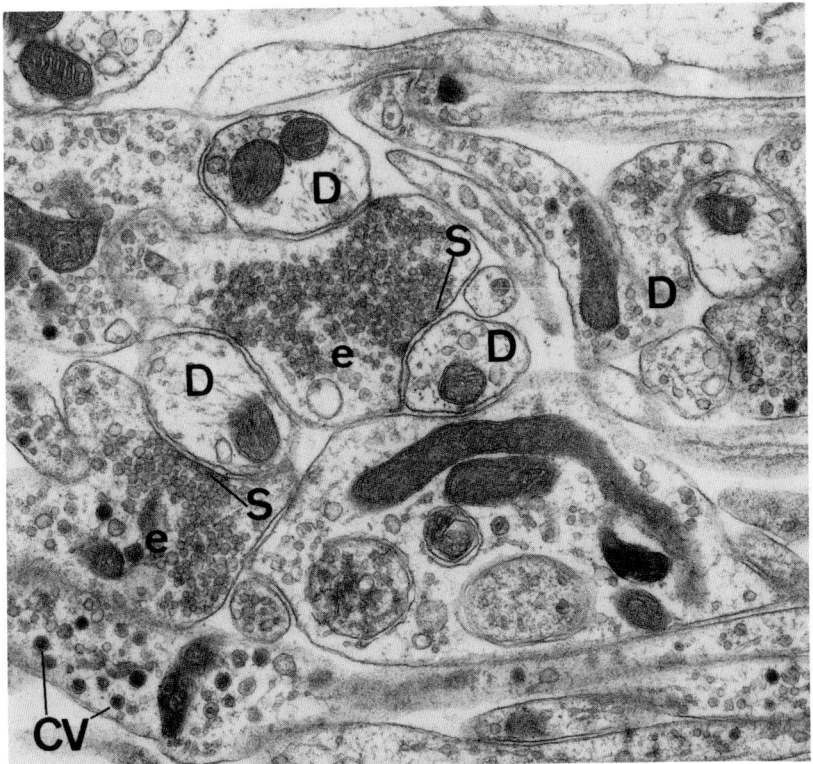

Fig. 11 Horizontal section through the inner spiral plexus. Efferent and afferent nerve fibers are intimately intermingled. The afferent dendrites to the inner hair cells (D) are cross-sectioned. The efferent fibers of the inner spiral bundle show numerous enlargements (e) filled with synaptic vesicles which are frequently condensed at the membrane facing an afferent dendrite. Such a condensation of synaptic vesicles (S) might be taken as evidence for synaptic activity. Dense-core vesicles (CV) are frequently observed within these efferent fibers as well as sometimes in the efferent and afferent nerve terminals at the outer hair cells. Their mere presence probably does not prove an adrenergic nerve fiber.

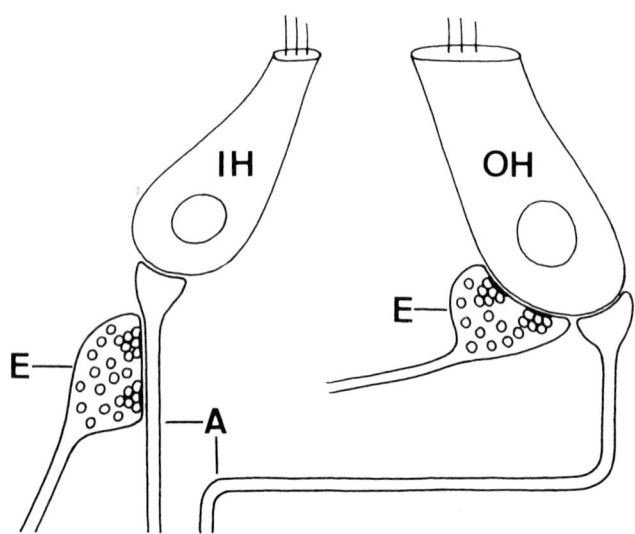

Fig. 12   Schematic representation of efferent synaptic connections in the organ of Corti of the cat. At the outer hair cells (OH) synaptic contacts are almost exclusively with sensory cells and at the inner hair cells (IH) only with the afferent dendrites (A). Efferent endings (E). (From Spoendlin, 1969b).

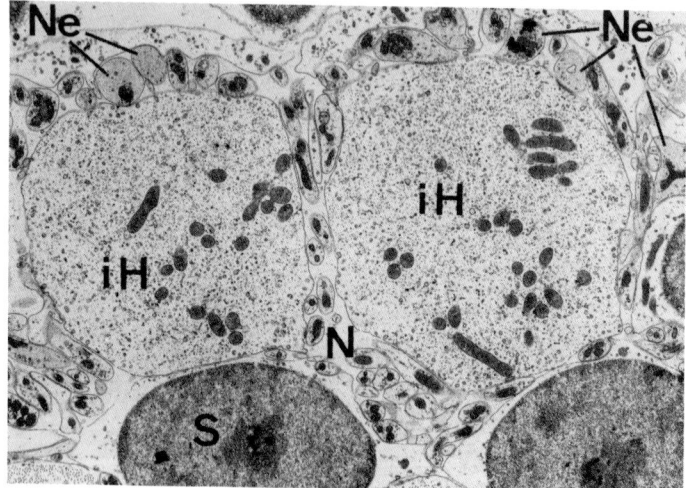

Fig. 13   Horizontal section through two inner hair cells (iH) surrounded by numerous afferent radial nerve fibers (N) and their   (cont'd)

(Fig. 13, cont'd) nerve endings (Ne). Nucleus of a supporting cell (S). (cf. Fig. 16).

In order to avoid all possible errors which might occur in degeneration experiments we counted and compared in normal animals all nerve fibers entering the organ of Corti through the habenula and all nerve fibers, efferents and afferents, crossing the tunnel (Fig. 17)(Spoendlin, 1972a). Regardless of whether the number of fibers was related to the number of pillars or to a certain length of the cochlear duct as measured by the width of the grid holes in the electron microscope (Fig. 18) we obtained essentially the same figures. Of 3500 fibers entering the organ of Corti per mm length in the first turn only 500 cross the tunnel, which corresponds to a ratio of 6/1 between total nerve supply to the inner and outer hair cells. Since the basilar fibers are about 1/2-1/3 of all tunnel crossing fibers (Fig. 20) the total afferent nerve supply of the outer hair cells is only about 5 % of all afferent neurons entering the organ of Corti. The total innervation density varies greatly along the cochlea. It is highest in the upper basal turn and rapidly reduced on either side of the peak (Fig. 19).

The number of fibers in the osseous spiral lamina does not increase from the spiral ganglion to the habenula, excluding important ramifications in this region (Spoendlin, 1972a).

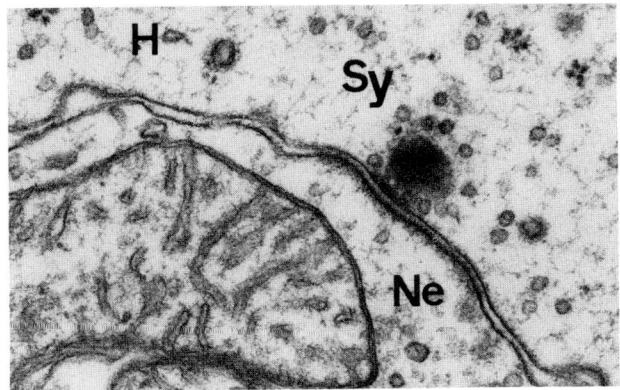

Fig. 14   Typical synaptic complex (Sy) between an afferent nerve terminal (Ne) and an inner hair cell (H).

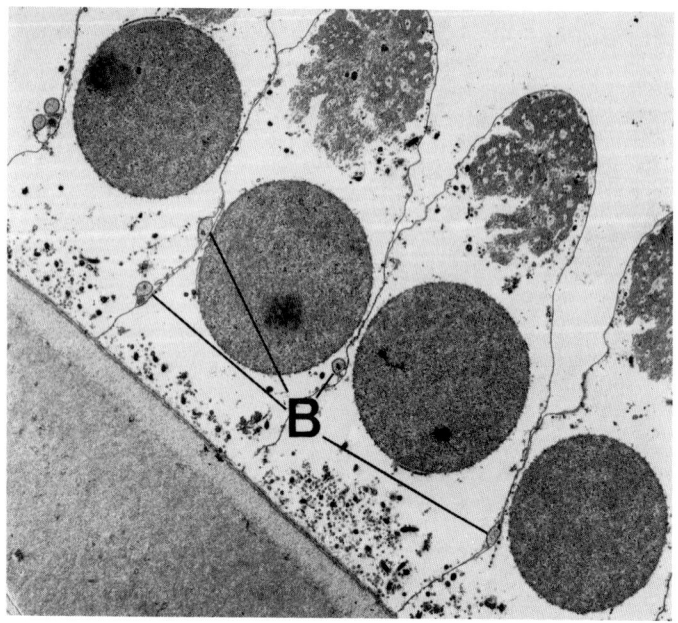

Fig. 15 Longitudinal section through the base of the outer pillars showing the basilar fibers penetrating between the pillar cells. There is normally an average of one basilar fiber running between two pillars. This preparation actually comes from an animal in which the cochlear nerve has been cut several months previously. These basilar fibers do not degenerate; they remain in normal numbers.

Each inner hair cell is innervated by about 20 afferent unbranched strictly radial neurons (Figs. 13, 16, 38) whose small endings usually form one synapse with the hair cell (Fig. 14). The afferents to the outer hair cells take a long spiral course as outer spiral fibers between the Deiter cells before they send their terminal collaterals to the hair cells (Figs. 4, 31, 38). On the basis of the fact that all outer spiral fibers are the continuation of the basilar fibers, that there is an average of one basilar fiber per outer pillar and that we find about 100 outer spiral fibers at any given place we can conclude that the outer spiral fibers extend spirally

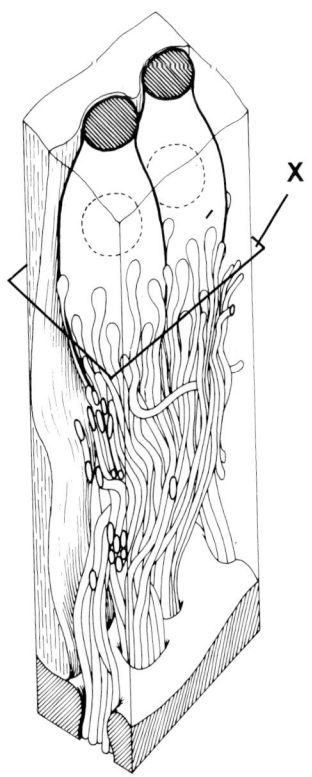

Fig. 16 Reconstruction of two inner hair cells of an animal in which the efferent nerve fibers have been eliminated. A great majority of all afferent dendrites run directly radial to the nearest inner hair cell and end there with a single ending. Only about 5 % of these fibers turn outwards between the inner pillars to reach the outer hair cell region. At X the approximate sectional plan of Fig. 13 is shown.

over an average distance of 100 pillars corresponding to 0.6-0.7 mm (Spoendlin, 1968). In the last 200 µ of its course each fiber sends collaterals to about 10 outer hair cells and each hair cell in the basal turn is provided with about 4 afferent endings of different neurons according to the principle of multiple innervation (Spoendlin 1969b). Just recently this

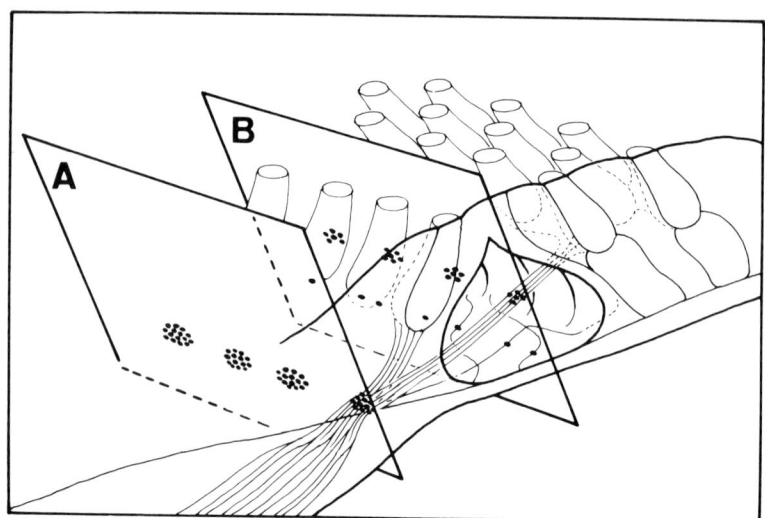

Fig. 17 For fiber counts in normal animals the sectional plans shown as A and B were used (see Figs. 18-20).

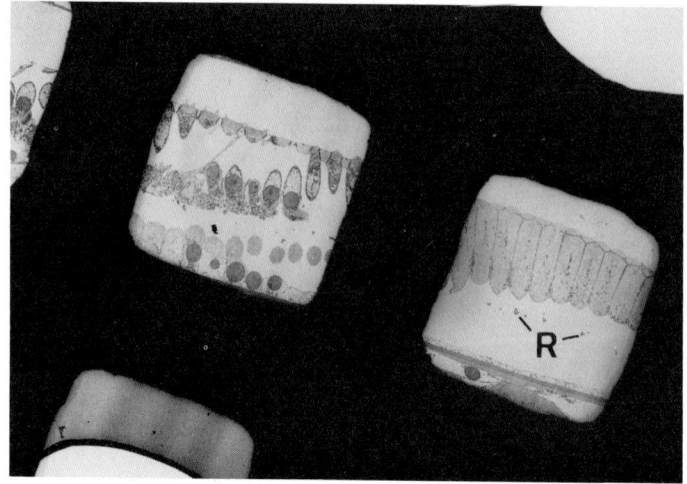

Fig. 18 A large tangential section through the tunnel and the outer hair cell region (on the left) on a 200-mesh grid. The gridholes vary only ± 5 % in diameter and therefore can be used to measure the length of the area where the fibers are counted.

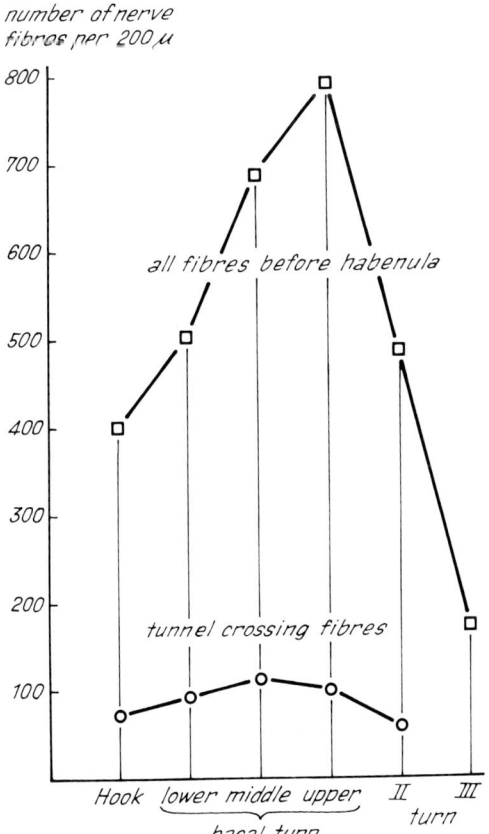

Fig. 19 Total numbers of nerve fibers in normal animals over a distance of 200 µ for different turns. It is quite evident that a great majority of all fibers stay within the area of the inner hair cells and only a small portion (1/7) cross the tunnel to reach the outer hair cells. The total innervation density reaches a clear maximum at the upper basal turn (from Spoendlin, 1972a).

extention and arrangement of outer spiral fibers has been confirmed by Smith (1972) in the rat by direct visualization of single fibers in light microscopic preparations.

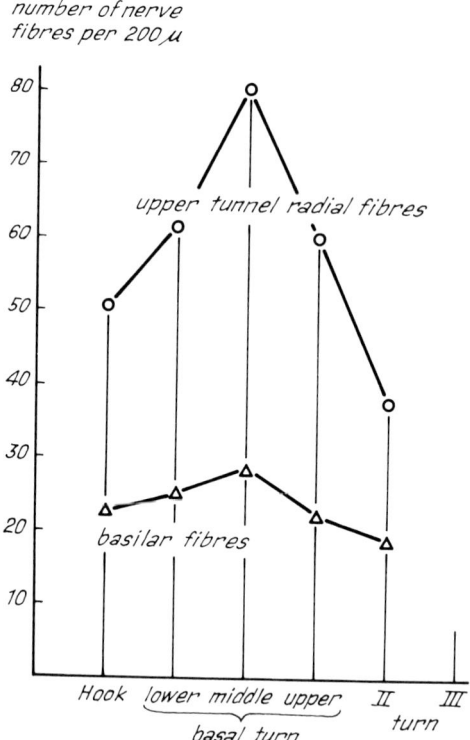

Fig. 20 Relative numbers of upper tunnel radial fibers and basilar fibers which in the middle basal turn amount to about 1/3 of all tunnel crossing fibers. (From Spoendlin, 1972a).

In general terms there is an enormous divergence of 1 hair cell to 20 neurons in the inner hair cell-system and a considerable convergence of 10 outer hair cells to 1 afferent neuron in the outer hair cell-system. Thus, as we have seen, the fiber distribution for inner and outer hair cells follows characteristic principles: The distribution pattern of the efferents is spiral for the inner and radial for the outer hair cells whereas the afferents are arranged radially for the inner and spirally for the outer hair cells (Spoendlin, 1966)(Fig. 38).

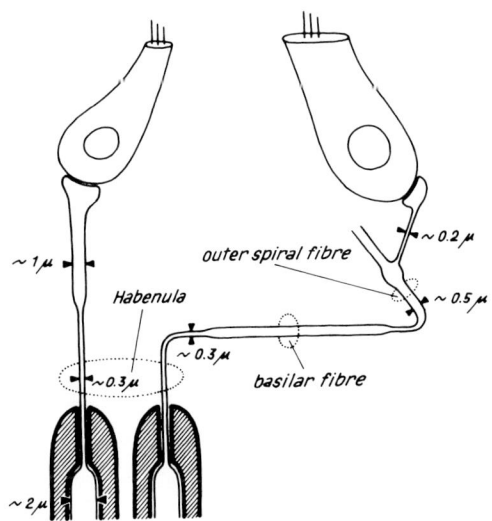

Fig. 21 Average diameters of the afferent nerve fibers in the organ of Corti of the cat. (From Spoendlin, 1969b).

The caliber of the afferent fibers is subject to considerable variation in their course in the organ of Corti (Fig. 21). The dendrites to inner hair cells are the largest, with an average diameter of 1 μ, whereas the outer spiral fibers are in the range of 0.5 μ. At all places where the fibers have to pass narrow passages, especially in the habenular openings, the caliber of all fibers is markedly reduced. Such a rapid reduction of fiber size and, as a consequence, of the capacity of the axon membrane might be important for the creation of spikes and determination of the initial segment which most probably is situated in the area of the habenula or just below it at the beginning of myelin sheaths.

The only place where afferents and efferents of the outer and inner hair cells are closely related is the area just above the habenula, where the fibers lie side by side without any sort of sheath (Fig. 22). We have never found morphological evidence for synapses between these fibers. Whether a functional interaction can occur at such places, not on a synaptic but on an electric basis, remains an open question. Inside the habenula down to the beginning of the mye-

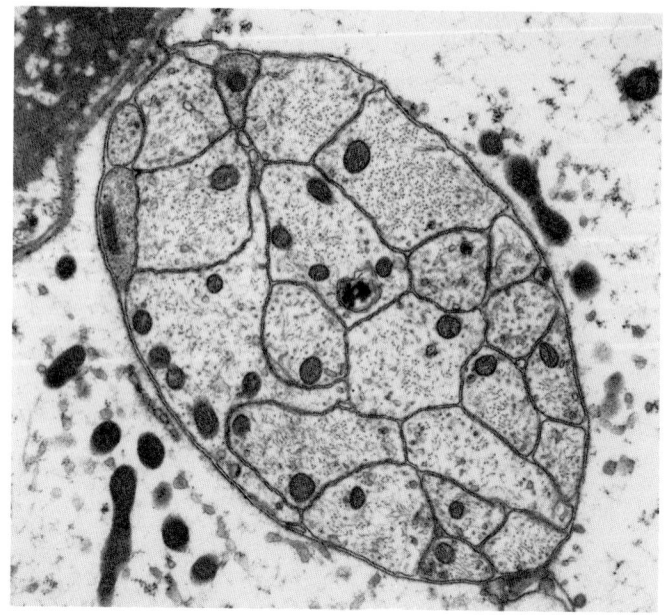

Fig. 22 Nerve bundle immediately above the habenula perforata. The nerve fibers of different calibers are closely adjacent to each other but no morphological evidence for synaptic contacts between the fibers has been found.

line sheath all fibers are surrounded by the processes of a single special satellite cell, whose function is unknown (Spoendlin, 1969b).

The basic difference in the innervation patterns of outer and inner hair cells brings up the question as to whether the afferent neurons associated with outer and inner hair cells are also different in other respects.

It has been known for a long time that the cochlear neurons including the spiral ganglion cells degenerate completely after transection of the statoacoustic nerve in the inner acoustic meatus, whereas most vestibular neurons survive. This is not too surprising considering the spinal nerves of which only about 50 % undergo retrograde degeneration after section of the spinal root or nerve (Ranson, 1905, Andres, 1961 a, b). Two types of bipolar neurons seem therefore to

exist in the spinal as well as in the statoacoustic
nerves. One type is subject to retrograde degeneration and the other type resists.

More recently we found that even in the cochlear nerve some neurons survive and a certain number of ganglion cells remain scattered throughout the spiral
ganglion after total transection of the cochlear nerve (Fig. 23)(Spoendlin, 1971, 1972a). The electron
microscopic evaluation of these remaining ganglion

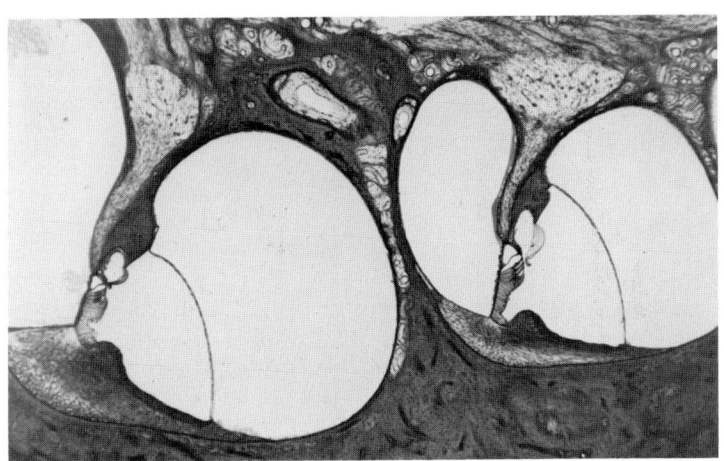

Fig. 23   Two turns of a cat cochlea six months after
transection of the cochlear nerve in the inner acoustic meatus. A large majority of all
spiral ganglion cells have disappeared. However a few ganglion cells remained scattered
throughout Rosenthal's canal in all turns.
(From Spoendlin, 1972a).

cells revealed that many of them are morphologically
quite different from the majority of spiral ganglion
cells, which undergo retrograde degeneration (Fig.
24). The latter, Type I ganglion cells are myelinated,
have a large light round central nucleus with a pronounced nucleolus and their cytoplasm contains mainly large quantities of ribosomes (Fig. 27). The other
surviving type II ganglion cell is smaller, non-myelinated, with an eccentric, lobulated nucleus with a
small nucleolus and the cytoplasm contains less ribosomes but many fibriles of the type of neurofilaments
(Figs. 25, 27).

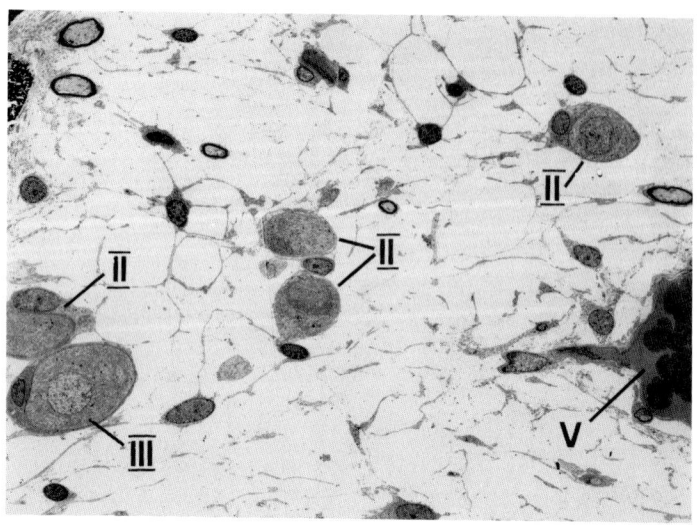

Fig. 24 Low magnification EM-picture of a group of surviving type II and one type III ganglion cell. In normal animals this ganglion would be densely packed with type I ganglion cells. A blood vessel (V) at right.

Two different types of ganglion cells in the acoustic ganglion have also been described by Rosenblith and Palay (1961) in the goldfish, by Rosenblith (1962) in the rat and by Kellerhals et al.(1967) in the guinea pig. In the normal cat with an intact ganglion cell population it is rather difficult to find these small ganglion cells scattered between great numbers of densely packed large type I ganglion cells (Fig. 27).

The axons of these type II neurons are unmyelinated at the beginning but often become myelinated at a certain distance from the cell body (Spoendlin, 1971). Occasionally the myelin sheaths begin very close to the unmyelinated perikaryon (Fig. 28).

About half of these surviving ganglion cells resemble morphologically more the type I ganglion cells with a thin myelin sheath, only a few neurofilaments in the cytoplasm and a rounded nucleus (Fig. 26). Although their morphological distinction from the type I gang-

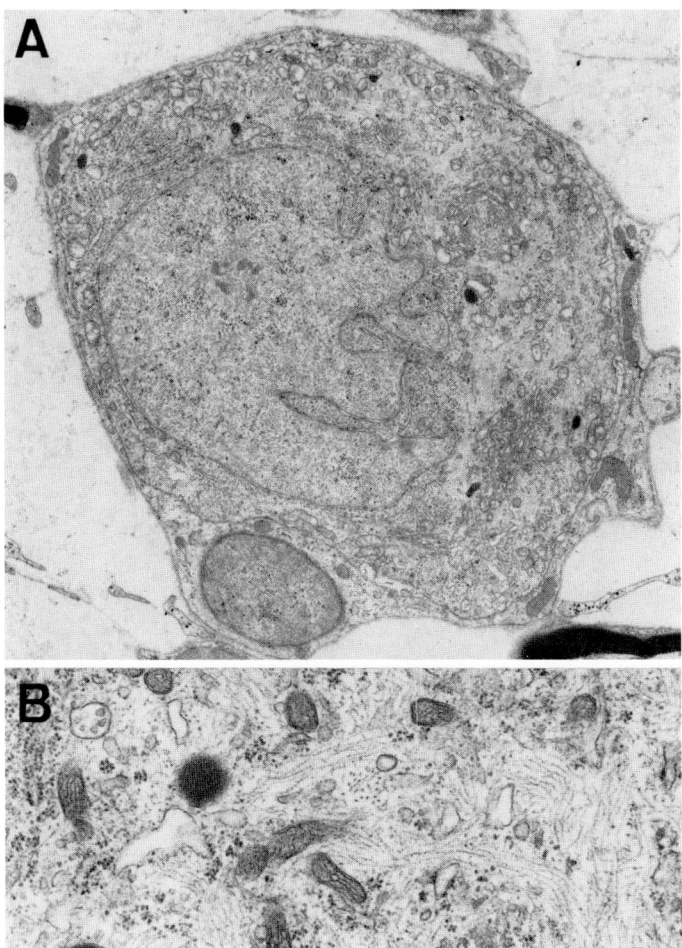

Fig. 25 A: Type II ganglion cell with a lobulated nucleus with only a very faint nucleolus and a cytoplasm containing relatively few ribosomes but a lot of fine neurofibrils and Golgi membranes. The ganglion cell is unmyelinated.

B: Detail of a cytoplasm of such a type II cell showing many neurofilaments in the cytoplasm.

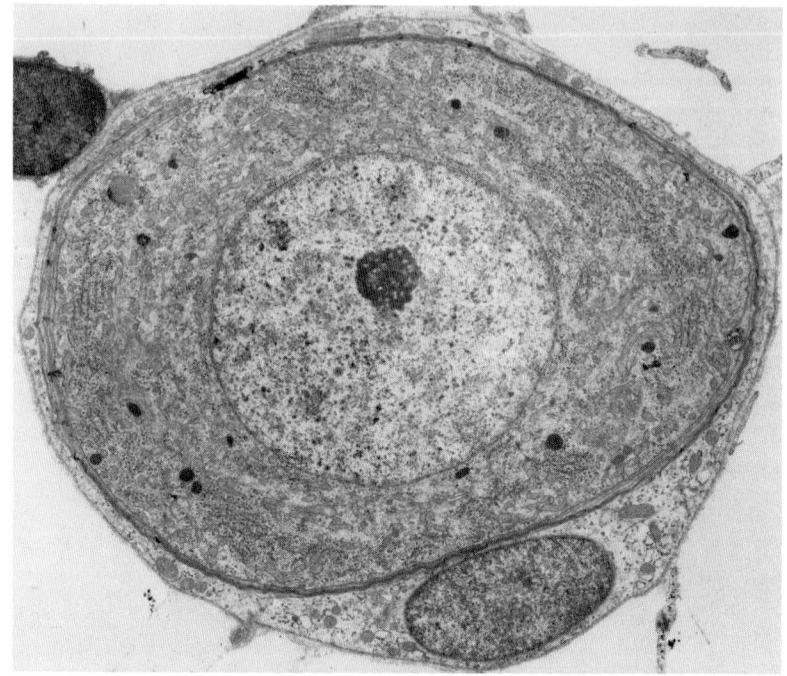

Fig. 26 Surviving ganglion cell of type III which resembles very much the regular type I ganglion cell. However the myelin sheaths of this cell are much thinner than those of type I cells.

lion cells is not very clear it is justified to consider them on the basis of their resistance against retrograde degeneration as a special, type III, ganglion cell.

The type II and III ganglion cells represent only about 5 % of the entire ganglion cell population in the spiral ganglion, a number which corresponds nicely with the afferent neurons associated to the outer hair cells, i.e. 5 % of all afferent nerve fibers of the cochlea (Fig. 29).

Some years ago Spoendlin and Gacek (1963, 1965) made the strange observation that in spite of what they thought to be a practically total degeneration of the spiral ganglion after sectioning of the cochlear nerve the afferent fibers to the outer hair cells and their nerve endings showed no signs of degeneration and remained unchanged in normal numbers (Fig. 31). No reasonable explanation was found for this observa-

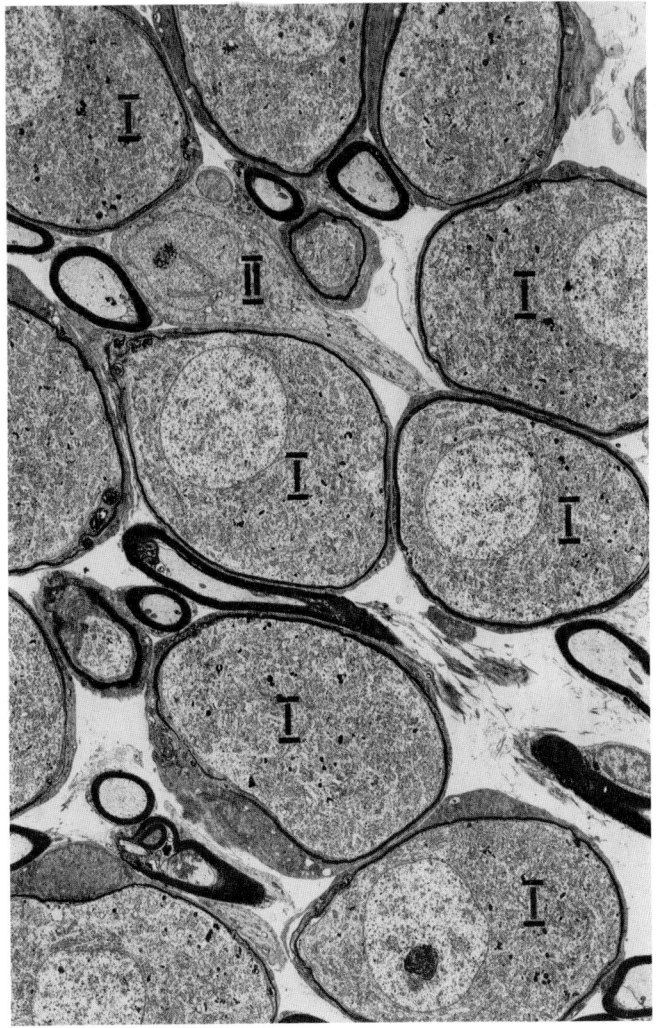

Fig. 27   Low magnification of a portion of a normal spiral ganglion with a great number of type I ganglion cells and only the type II ganglion cell squeezed in between.

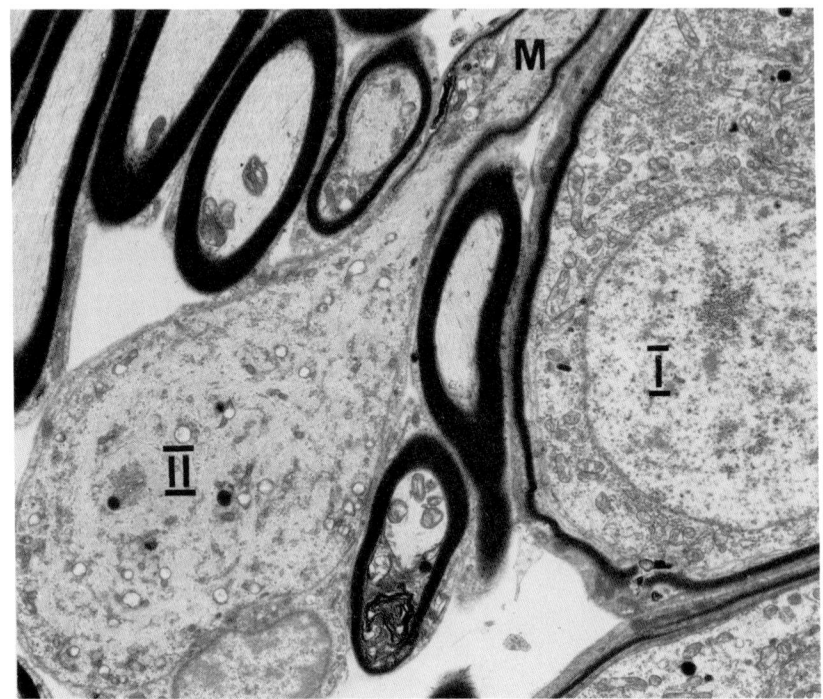

Fig. 28 Sometimes the unmyelinated type II ganglion cells send out axons which become myelinated (M) very close to the ganglion cell body. A ganglion cell of type I is seen at right.

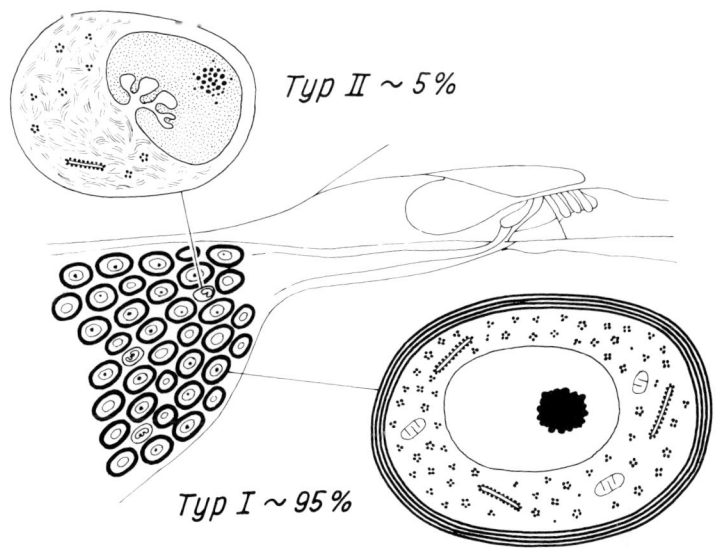

Fig. 29 Schematic representation of the two types of ganglion cells in the spiral ganglion and their relative percentage. (From Spoendlin, 1971).

tion, which therefore was neglected as being unrealistic. Today, since we know of the surviving 5 % type II and III neurons it is tempting to correlate these neurons with the afferent nerve fibers associated to the outer hair cells (Spoendlin, 1971, 1972a). In fact the remaining myelinated nerve fibers can be followed through the osseous spiral lamina to the habenula (Fig. 32) where they enter the organ of Corti. Here the majority takes a short spiral course in a basalward direction before they penetrate between the inner pillars (Fig. 33), cross the tunnel as basilar fibers and reach the outer hair cells in the usual way (Fig. 38).

Very few of these surviving neurons behave differently. After the habenula they appear to be unusually large and divide into two large branches, one of which runs spirally apicalwards and the other basalwards, sending collaterals with typical synaptic contacts to a group of about 10 inner hair cells (Figs.

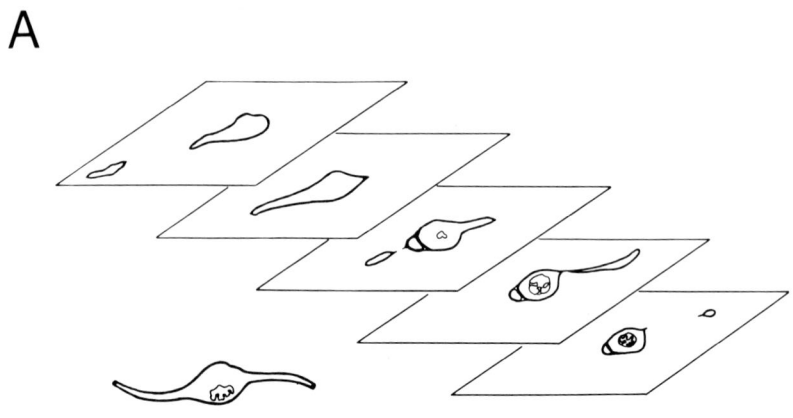

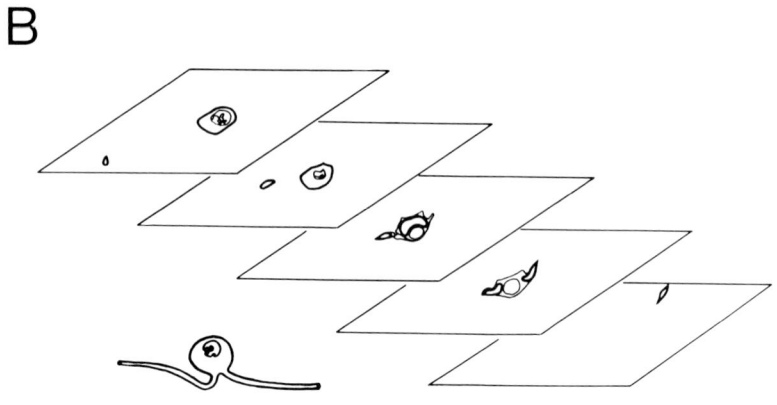

Fig. 30 Two examples of reconstructions of type II ganglion cells on the basis of serial sections. A gives an example of a bipolar neuron whereas B gives an example of a pseudomonopolar cell.

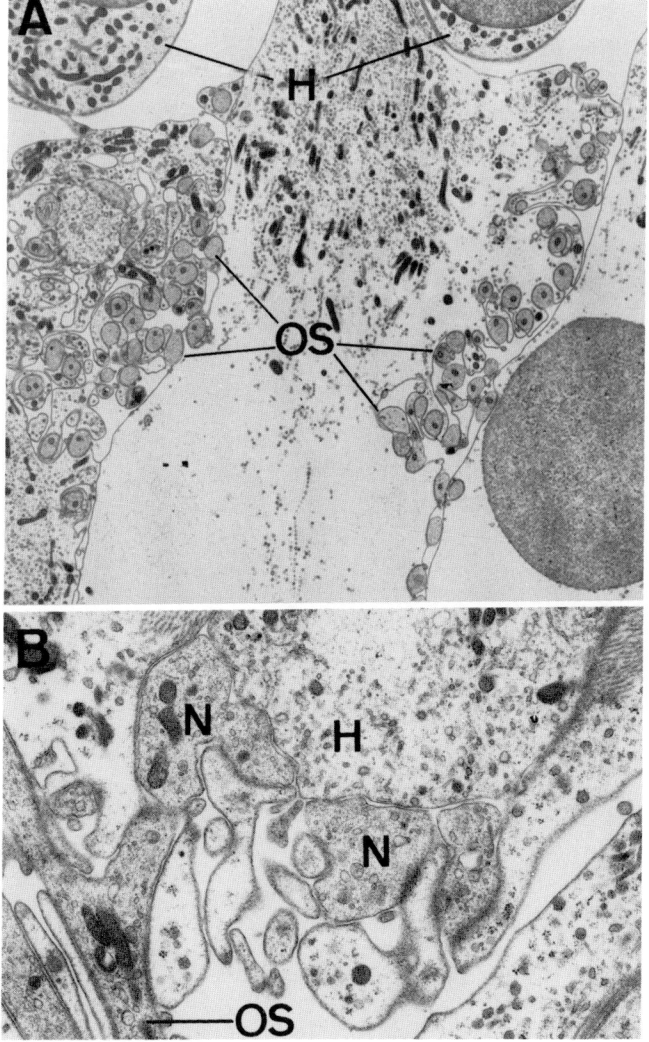

Fig. 31 The organ of Corti of a cat six months after the transection of the cochlear nerve. The number of the outer spiral fibers (OS) below the outer hair cells (H) appears to be normal and the nerve fibers show no sign of degeneration. The afferent nerve endings (N) at the base of the outer hair cells (H) are of normal appearance and are present in full numbers.

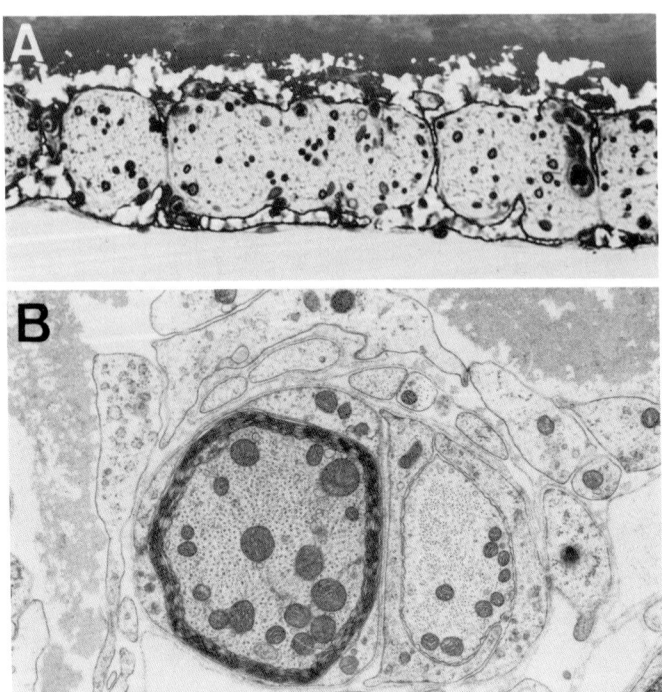

Fig. 32 A: Tangential section through the osseous spiral lamina of a cat with complete degeneration of type I ganglion cells in the spiral ganglion after transection of the 8th nerve. A certain number of myelinated nerve fibers scattered throughout the osseous spiral lamina is still present.

B: Two of surviving nerve fibers immediately before the habenula perforata. The fiber to the left still has its myelin sheath whereas the fiber to the right already has lost it. The axoplasm contains many neurofilaments and neurotubules without signs of degeneration.

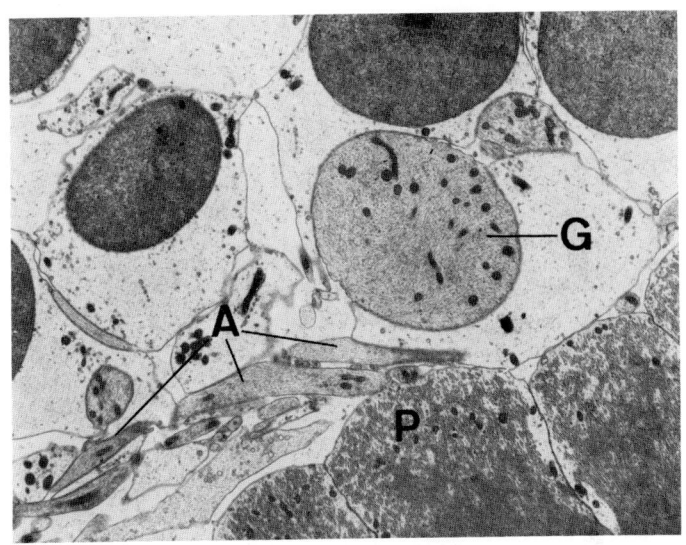

Fig. 33   Tangential (longitudinal) section through
           the area below the inner hair cells im-
           mediately after the habenula in an animal
           where all type I spiral ganglion cells
           have disappeared. Most of the remaining
           nerve fibers take a short spiral course
           after they have entered the organ of Corti
           (A) before they penetrate between the in-
           ner pillars to reach the outer hair cells.
           At larger intervals giant axons (G) are
           usually found.

33, 34). Such a giant neuron is only found in about
every tenth habenular opening and their estimated
total number amounts to approximately 0.5 % of all
afferent cochlear neurons (Figs. 35, 38)(Spoendlin,
1971, 1972a). On a numerical basis it would be possible for these giant axons to belong to the type III
ganglion cells, but this for the time being remains
an assumption.

In order to get more precise information on the axons
of the type II neurons we made reconstructions of
some of these cells on the basis of serial sections
(Fig. 30A/B). Only some are bipolar, others are pseudomonopolar or really monopolar, giving off one
single large axon which divides into two branches

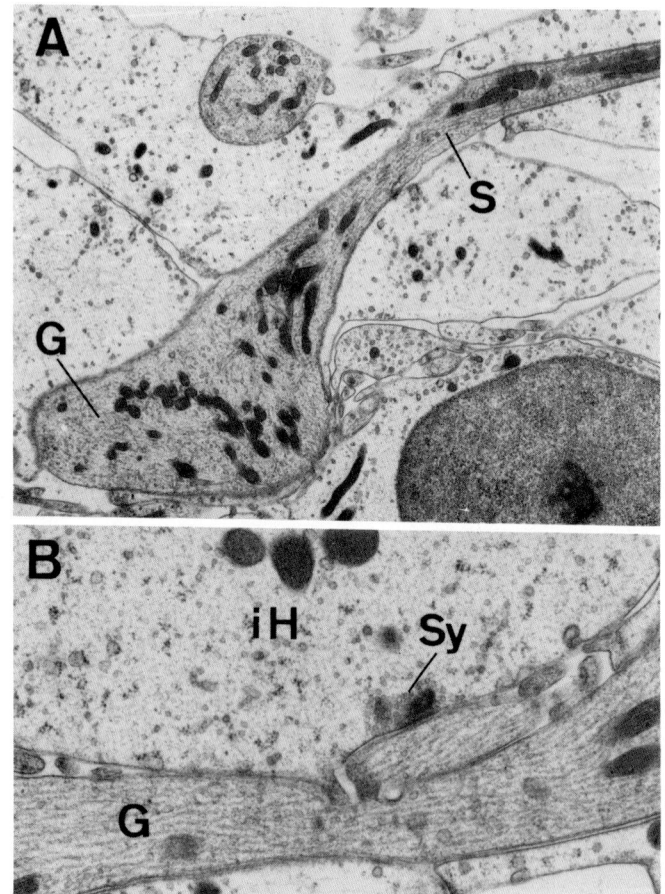

Fig. 34 A: Giant axon (G) giving off a branch in the spiral direction (S).

B: The giant axon branch (G) passes close to the base of an inner hair cell (iH). Sometimes synaptic complexes (Sy) with the inner hair cells are seen.

only at a certain distance from the cell body. Frequently the off-going axons are rather tortuous. At least many of these neurons seem to be connected to the CNS by axons through the cochlear nerve. Sections through the cochlear nerve central to the spiral ganglion in animals in which only the type II and III

ganglion cells remained always show a certain number
of intact myelinated nerve fibers.

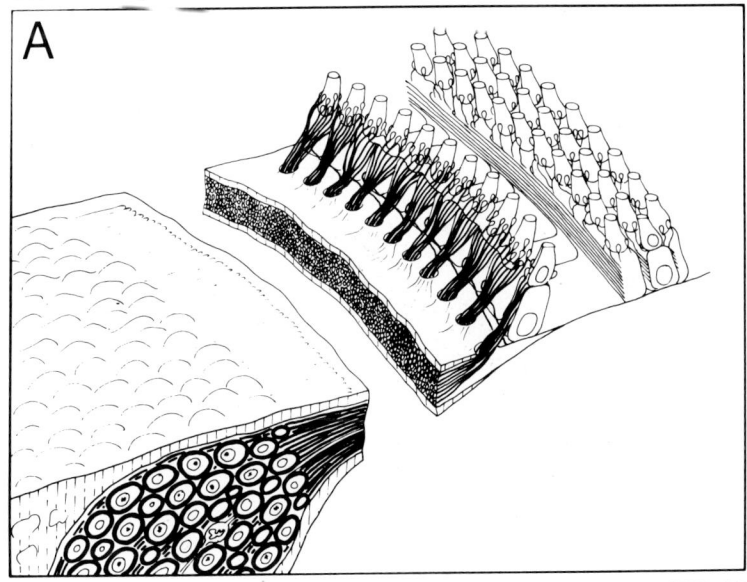

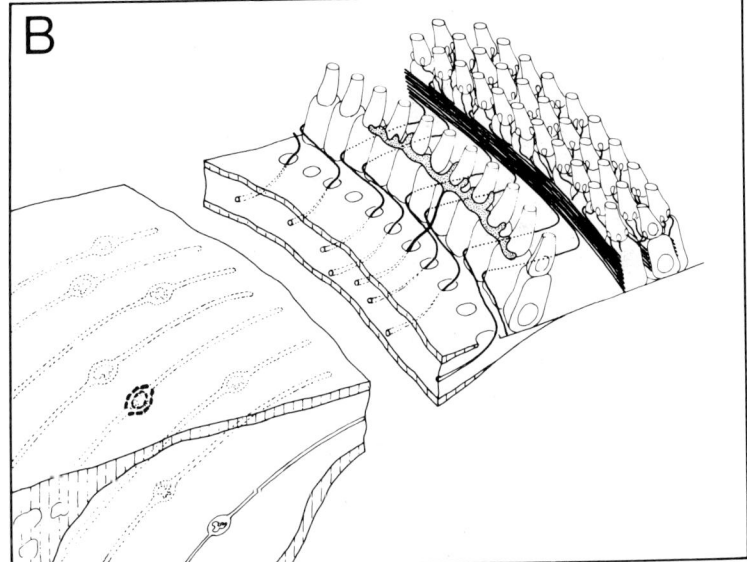

Fig. 35 Schematic representation of the afferent innervation pattern of the organ of Corti in
a normal animal in (A) and after (cont'd)

(Fig. 35, cont'd) elimination of the type I neurons (B). The overwhelming mass of radial dendrites from the type I neurons to the inner hair cells masks the other fibers at this level. In B the neurons associated with the outer hair cells are more clearly seen and only here do the giant neurons of the inner hair cells really appear. These giant axons might be related to the somewhat larger type III ganglion cells.

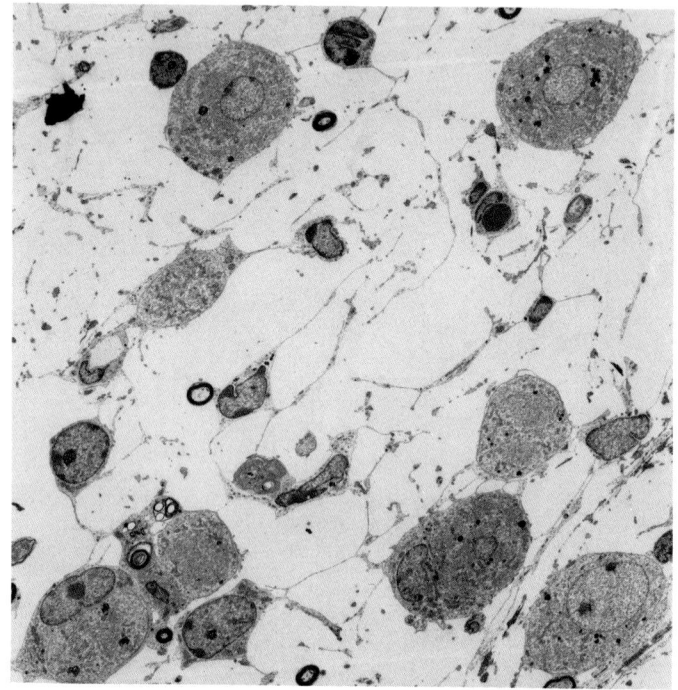

Fig. 36 Low magnification of a spiral ganglion of a guinea pig which has been exposed to high intensity noise 14 months ago. The organ of Corti has been completely destroyed in the basal and second turn. Retrograde degeneration in such places, where the organ of Corti has completely disappeared, does not affect all ganglion cells. The surviving ganglion cells are all unmyelinated of type II.

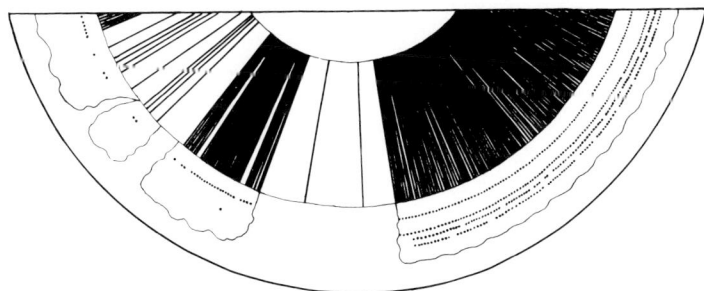

Fig. 37 Schematic representation of the findings in a second turn of a guinea pig four months after an acoustic trauma which destroyed greater portions of the organ of Corti. In the central area where the organ of Corti is completely missing only very few nerve fibers remain. On the left side almost all sensory cells are present and the nerve fibers show a normal density. In the right area where only the inner hair cells are left, the nerve fiber density is almost the same as in the left normal area. When the inner hair cells are partly gone (far left) there is a marked decrease in density of nerve fibers in the osseous spiral lamina.

Retrograde degeneration is, of course, also induced when the afferent neurons are damaged on the other side of their ganglion cell by destruction of the organ of Corti by acoustic trauma. We exposed guinea pigs repeatedly to 130-140 dB white noise which leads to a complete, immediate destruction of the organ of Corti in the lower turns (Spoendlin and Brun, 1973). After survival times up to 14 months there are always some remaining regularly distributed nerve fibers and spiral ganglion cells in spite of a completely missing organ of Corti in the respective cochlear turn (Fig. 36). In the electron microscope practically all remaining ganglion cells appeared to be of the unmyelinated type II, which in the guinea pig represents a somewhat higher percentage of the total ganglion cell population than in the cat. Thus the type II ganglion cell seems to resist retrograde degeneration in both directions.

All the presented observations provide evidence for a numerically far predominant afferent innervation of

the inner hair cells, being in fact associated with
about 95 % of the cochlear neurons. This view receives
further support from some findings in cochlear pathology. Following acoustic traumatic damage of the organ of Corti certain areas of the cochlea might end
up with a permanent complete loss of outer hair cells
and an essentially intact set of inner hair cells. In
such areas with only the inner hair cells left almost
no retrograde degeneration is found. The nerve fiber
density in the osseous spiral lamina as well as the
spiral ganglion cell population is only slightly reduced (Fig. 37).

Discussion

The innervation pattern of the organ of Corti as presented above (Fig. 38) undoubtedly outlines some basic
principles of the function of the system. The coding
of the acoustic input most probably occurs to a great

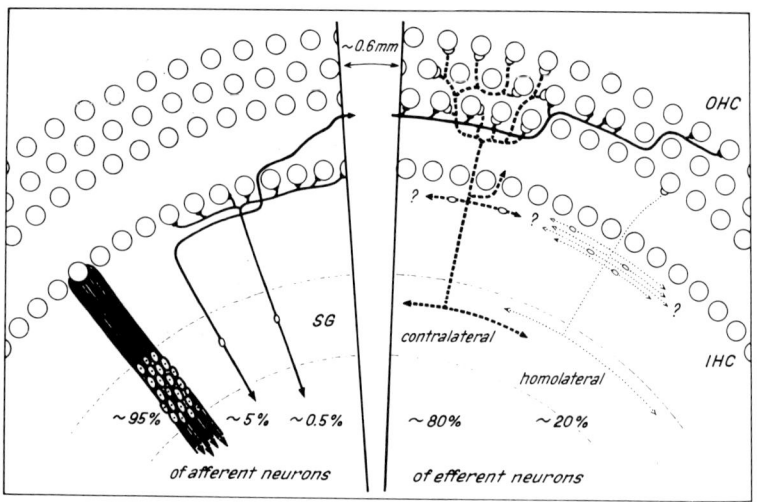

Fig. 38   Summarizing schema of the innervation pattern of the organ of Corti of the cat on the
basis of the present knowledge. (From
Spoendlin, 1971).

extent in these peripheral unmyelinated nerve branches
and their endings. Evans (1969) gives clear evidence
that the travelling wave pattern as recently measured
by Johnstone et al. (1967), Rhode (1971) and Wilson
and Johnstone (1972) can not explain to full extent
the sharpening of the frequency response in the coch-

lea and that a metabolically vulnerable mechanism probably is responsible for this additional sharpening. This process might well be located in the terminal nerve branches and endings. A very important feature of the innervation pattern is the association of ≃ 95 % of the cochlear neurons to the inner hair cells, which allots them probably a very important quantitive role in the process of hearing. For the general functional implications of the innervation pattern of inner and outer hair cells the reader is referred to earlier publications (Spoendlin, 1966, 1969a, 1970, 1971, 1972a).

In this connection an interesting study of Altmann (1972) should be mentioned. On the basis of the known physiological mechanisms of membranes, synapses and spike initiation and on the assumption that the acoustic receptor consists only of a simple inner hair cell system, Altmann elaborated a mathematical model of the coding mechanism. By simulating in this mathematical system the same experimental conditions as used by Kiang (1965) in his experiments on the discharge pattern of the primary auditory neurons, he obtained exactly the same spike-histograms as found by Kiang. This means that Kiang in his experiments most probably recorded essentially from neurons associated with the inner hair cells and that his results reflect mainly the coding mechanisms of the inner hair cell-system.

The next important question is, of course, what is the role of the outer hair cell-system in the cochlear receptor? In view of the pronounced convergence of the outer hair cell pathways it is tempting to attribute them a higher sensitivity because of the possibility of spatial summation. The electrocochleogram as measured by Aran et al. (1969) tends to support such a view (Portmann, 1972) although Kiang was never able to find two populations of cochlear neurons with significantly different thresholds. Pfeiffer(pers. comm) has shown very recently electrophysiological evidence for the presence of a small percentage, about 5 %, of cochlear neurons with a significantly different behavior from the majority of cochlear neurons.

Another more revolutionary concept attributes to the outer hair cell system the role of a monitor of the whole receptor rather than a function of transmitting information to the CNS (Lynn and Sayers, 1970). This however would necessitate the possibility of functional interrelations between the outer and inner hair cell systems, for which so far no structural substrate, such as synaptic connections between fibers from outer and inner hair cells, has been found. There might however be a possibility that these fibers can directly electrically interfere with each other in the area immediately above the habenula where all fibers run densely packed together (Fig. 22). A connection of the same neuron to the inner as well as outer hair cell, as it has frequently been postulated, can practically be excluded at least for the 95 % type I afferent neurons to the inner hair cells, which degenerate selectively after transection of the cochlear nerve. Whether and how the efferent system could be involved in such mechanisms is again an open question.

Although clear evidence for an inhibitory action of the efferents on the afferent nerve activity exists (Desmedt, 1962, Fex, 1962, Wiederhold, 1970, Wiederhold and Kiang, 1970) no satisfactory explanation of the main function of the efferents in the cochlear receptor has been found. This main function is undefined despite a number of observations and postulations on the functional role of the efferents, such as an effect on adaptation (Leibbrandt, 1965) and masking (Trahiotis and Elliot, 1970), stabilization of threshold (Johnstone, 1968) or prevention of wastage of chemical transmitter in the outer hair cells (Davis, 1968). The basic difference of the efferents to the outer and inner hair cells most probably expresses also a different functional significance. The enormous, in comparison to the afferent nerve supply apparently overdimensioned, efferent nerve supply to the outer hair cells would go along with a concept of more of a monitoring role of the outer hair cell system. Whatever the role of the efferents might be it is bound to be important in the view of the enormous representation of efferent fibers and endings in the organ of Corti.

With respect to the type II spiral ganglion cells, which remain after section of the cochlear nerve, the possibility that they might be autonomic ganglion cells has to be taken into consideration. It is very unlikely that they belong to the sympathetic nervous system, because, as we have seen earlier, the adrenergic nerve fibers originate in the superior cervical ganglion (Spoendlin and Lichtensteiger, 1967) and no noradrenaline containing ganglion cells have been found in the region of the spiral ganglion (Ross, 1971). On the other hand Ross (1969) described in a histochemical study cholinergic multipolar ganglion cells in the proximity of the intraganglionic spiral bundle of the rat, which could at least partly correspond to our type II ganglion cells. However our type II cells are scattered regularly throughout the entire spiral ganglion and many of them seem to have axons which become myelinated after a certain distance from the perikaryon. The type II cells we were so far able to reconstruct were either bipolar or unipolar but never multipolar. The remaining myelinated fibers, after degeneration of the 95 % type I ganglion cells proximal or distal to the spiral ganglion, must reasonably be connected to some of the remaining ganglion cells in the spiral ganglion, since other ganglion cells in the cochlear nerve do not seem to exist. The fact that the ganglion cells show an acetylcholinesterase reaction does not mean they are necessarily autonomic. In spite of all these reasons we cannot exclude the possibility that some of the type II ganglion cells belong to the autonomic cholinergic nervous system.

References

Altmann, A. (1972). Modellierung von Nervenfunktionen bei spezieller Anwendung auf den primären Hörnerv. Thesis. ETH, Zürich.

Andres, K.H. (1961a). Untersuchungen über den Feinbau von Spinalganglien. Z. Zellforsch. 55, 1-48.

Andres, K.H. (1961b). Untersuchungen über morphologische Veränderungen in Spinalganglien während der retrograden Degeneration. Z. Zellforsch. 55, 49-79.

Aran, J.-M., Portmann, Cl., Delaunay, J., Pelorin, J., and Lenoir, J. (1969). L'électro-cochléogramme: méthodes et premiers résultats chez l'enfant. Rev. Laryng. (Bordeaux) 90, 615-634.

Beickert, P., Gisselsson, L., and Löfström, B. (1956).
Der Einfluss des sympathischen Nervensystems
auf das Innenohr. Arch. Klin. Exp. Ohr.- Nas.-,
Kehlk.-Heilk. 168, 495-507.

Davis, H. (1968). Contribution to discussion. In:
Hearing Mechanisms in Vertebrates. (A.V.S. de
Reuck and J. Knight, eds.) pp. 119, 305. Chur-
chill, London.

Desmedt, J.E. (1962). Auditory-evoked potentials from
cochlea to cortex as influenced by activation
of the efferent olivo-cochlear bundle. J. Acoust.
Soc. Amer. 34, 1478-1496.

Evans, E.F. (1969). Narrow "tuning" of cochlear nerve
fibre responses in the guinea pig. J. Physiol.
206, 14P-15P.

Falck, B., Hillarp, N.-A., Thieme, G. and Torp, A.
(1962). Fluorescence of catecholamines and related compounds condensed with formaldehyde.
J. Histochem. Cytochem. 10, 348.

Fex, J. (1962). Auditory activity in centrifugal and
centripetal cochlear fibres in cat. Acta Physiol.
Scand. 55, Suppl. 189, 5-68.

Iurato, S. (1962). Efferent fibers to the sensory
cells of Corti's organ. Exp. Cell. Res. 27,
162-164.

Iurato, S. (1964). Fibre efferenti dirette e crociate
alle cellule acustiche dell'organo del Corti.
Atti. Soc. Ital. Anat. 72, 60.

Johnstone, B.M., and Boyle, A.J.F. (1967). Basilar
membrane vibration examined with the Mössbauer
technique. Science 158, 389-390.

Johnstone, B.M. (1968). General discussion. In:
Hearing Mechanisms in Vertebrates (A.V.S. de
Reuck and J. Knight, eds.), p. 299, Churchill,
London.

Kellerhals, B., Engström, H., Ades, H.W. (1967).
Die Morphologie des Ganglion spirale cochleae.
Acta Oto-Laryngol. Suppl. 226, 1-78.

Kiang, N.Y.S. (1965). Discharge Patterns of Single
Fibers in the Cat's Auditory Nerve. Res. Monogr.
35, pp. 84-92. M.I.T. Press, Cambridge, Mass.

Kimura, R., and Wersäll, J. (1962). Termination of
the olivo-cochlear bundle in relation to the
outer hair cells of the organ of Corti in guinea
pig. Acta Oto-Laryngol. 55, 11-32.

Leibbrandt, C.C. (1965). The significance of the
olivo-cochlear bundle for the adaptation mechanism
of the inner ear. Acta Oto-Laryngol. 59,
124-132.

Lynn, P.A., and Sayers, B.McA. (1970). Cochlear innervation,
signal processing and their relation
to auditory time intensity effects. J. Acoust.
Soc. Amer. 47, 525-532.

Portmann, M. (1972). Discussion to H. Spoendlin. In:
Innervation densities of the cochlea. Acta
Otol. Rhinol. Laryngol. 73, 235-248.

Ranson, S.W. (1905). Retrograde degeneration in the
spiral nerves. J. Comp. Neurol. Psychol. 16, 1.

Rasmussen, G.L. (1960). Efferent fibers of the cochlear
nerve and cochlear nucleus. In: Neural
Mechanisms of the Auditory and Vestibular
Systems (G.L. Rasmussen and W.F. Windle, eds.),
pp. 105-115. Charles C. Thomas, Springfield,
Ill.

Rhode, W.S. (1971). Observations of the vibration of
the basilar membrane in squirrel monkey using
the Mössbauer technique. J. Acoust. Soc. Amer.
49, 1218-1231.

Rosenblith, J., and Palay, S.L. (1961). The fine
structure of nerve cell bodies and their myelin
sheaths in the eighth nerve ganglion of the
goldfish. J. Biophys. Biochem. Cytol. 9,
853-877.

Rosenblith, J. (1962). The fine structure of acoustic ganglia in the rat. J. Cell. 12, 329-359.

Ross, M.D. (1969). The general visceral efferent component of the eighth cranial nerve. J. Comp. Neurol. 135, 453-478.

Ross, M.D. (1971). Fluorescence and electron microscopic observations of the general visceral, efferent innervation of the inner ear. Acta Oto-Laryngol. Suppl. 286, 1-18.

Seymour, J.C., and Tappin, J.W. (1953). Some aspects of the sympathetic nervous system innervation in relation to the inner ear. Acta Oto-Laryngol. 43, 618-635.

Smith, C.A., and Rasmussen, G.L. (1963). Recent observations on the olivo-cochlear bundle. Ann. Otol. Rhinol. Laryngol. 72, 489-506.

Smith, C.A. (1973). Preliminary observations on the terminal ramifications of nerve fibres in the cochlea. Acta Oto-Laryngol. (In press).

Spoendlin, H., and Gacek, R. (1963). Electron microscopic study of the efferent and afferent innervation of the organ of Corti in the cat. Ann. Otol. Rhinol. Laryngol. 72, 660-686.

Spoendlin, H., and Gacek, R. (1965). Survival of the peripheral dendrites after section of the cochlear nerve. Proc. Int. Congr. of Neuropathol., 5th Excerpta Med. Found. Int. Congr. Ser. No. 100, 926-934.

Spoendlin, H., and Lichtensteiger, W. (1966). The adrenergic innervation of the labyrinth. Acta Oto-Laryngol. 61, 423-434.

Spoendlin, H. (1966). The Organization of the Cochlear Receptor. Karger, Basel-New York.

Spoendlin, H., and Lichtensteiger, W. (1967). The sympathetic nerve supply to the inner ear. Arch. Klin. Exp. Ohr.- Nas.- Kehlk. Heilk. 189, 346-359.

Spoendlin, H. (1967). The innervation of the organ of Corti. J. Laryngol. Otol. 81, 717-738.

Spoendlin, H. (1968). Ultrastructure and peripheral innervation pattern of the receptor in relation to the first coding of the acoustic message. In: Hearing Mechanisms in Vertebrates, (A.V.S. de Reuck and J. Knight, eds.), pp. 89-119. Churchill, London.

Spoendlin, H. (1969a). Innervation patterns in the organ of Corti of the cat. Acta Oto-Laryngol. 67, 239-254.

Spoendlin, H. (1969b). Structural basis of peripheral frequency analysis. In: Frequency Analysis and Periodicity Detection in Hearing (R. Plomp and F.G. Smoorenburg, eds.), pp. 2-36. Sijthoff, Leiden, The Netherlands.

Spoendlin, H. (1970). Auditory, vestibular, olfactory and gustatory organs. In: Ultrastructure of the Peripheral Nervous System and Sense Organs. Atlas of Normal and Pathologic Anatomy (by J. Babel, A. Bischoff (ed.) and H. Spoendlin), pp. 173-306. Georg Thieme, Stuttgart.

Spoendlin, H. (1971). Degeneration behaviour of the cochlear nerve. Arch. Klin. Exp. Ohr.- Nas.- Kehlk. Heilk. 200, 275-291.

Spoendlin, H. (1972a). Innervation densities of the cochlea. Acta Oto-Laryngol. 73, 235-248.

Spoendlin, H. (1972b). Autonomic nerve supply to the inner ear. Symposium on Vascular disorders and hearing defects at Johns Hopkins Univ. in Baltimore. (In press).

Spoendlin, H., and Brun, J.-P. (1973). Relation of structural damage to exposure time and intensity in acoustic trauma. Acta Oto-Laryngol. (In press).

Trahiotis, C., and Elliot, D.N. (1970). Behavioral investigation of some possible effects of sectioning the crossed olivo-cochlear bundle. J. Acoust. Soc. Amer. 47, 592-596.

Vasilev, A.I. (1963). The significance of the superior cervical sympathetic ganglion for the auditory function of the cochlea. Zh. Ushn. Nos. Gorl. Bolez. 3, 59-62.

Wiederhold, M.L., and Kiang, N.Y.S. (1970). Effects of the electrical stimulation of the crossed olivocochlear bundle on single-auditory-nerve fibres in the cat. J. Acoust. Soc. Amer. 48/4, (II) 950-965.

Wiederhold, M.L. (1970). Variations in the effects of electric stimulation of the crossed olivocochlear bundle on cat single auditory-nerve-fiber responses to tone bursts. J. Acoust. Soc. Amer. 48/4, (II) 966-977.

Wilson, J.P., and Johnstone, J.R. (1972). Capacitive probe measure of basilar membrane vibration. Symposium on Hearing Theory 1972, pp. 172-181. IPO Eindhoven, Holland.

Figure 2 reproduced by permission of Journal of Laryngology and Otology, Headley Bros. Ltd., Ashford, England.

Figures 9, 10a, 12 and 21 reproduced from FREQUENCY ANALYSIS AND PERIODICITY DETECTION IN HEARING edited by R. Plomp and F.G. Smoorenburg, 1969, by permission of Sijthoff, Leiden, The Netherlands.

Figures 19, 20, and 23 reproduced by permission of Acta Oto-Laryngologica (Stockholm).

Figures 29-38 reproduced by permission of Archiv für Klinische und Experimentelle Ohren-, Nasen- und Kehlkopfheilkunde.

DISCUSSION

EVANS: I would like to hear Prof. Spoendlin's comments on the problem of getting information down the outer spiral fibers, in view of their long length (approx. 0.6 mm) and their small diameter (approx. 0.5 µm). I understand that the length constant is something of the order of 10 µ. Would you consider the possibility of spike propagation in the spiral fibers? Secondly what does your engineer mean by "analog integration" in his model of the innervation of inner hair cells?

SPOENDLIN: Spatial integration is very unlikely since all nerve fibers are unbranched with a single synaptic connection to the inner hair cells. The locus of spike initiation is not known for sure. From a morphological point of view it is most likely in the area of the habenula. It can, however, not be excluded that the afferent fibers from the outer hair cells have the possibility of spike propagation in their long spiral course in the outer spiral fibers.

EVANS: And it is on that basis that he gets the multiple peaks in the post-stimulus time histograms (PSTH's) of the responses to click stimuli?

SPOENDLIN: Yes. The PST histogram peaks are mainly the consequence of the stimulus frequency and intensity, the temporal integration in the unmyelinated peripheral nerve segments and of the spike threshold at the initial segment.

EVANS: What is taken as the mechanical input to this system? Von Békésy's data suggest that the basilar membrane is so heavily damped that its impulse response could not account for the multi-peaked click PSTH's observed at the cochlear nerve level. On the other hand, there are results by Robles et al. (1972) and Wilson and Johnstone (1972), which suggest that the basilar membrane is less damped and that it can give an oscillatory impulse response of many cycles. Therefore I am very interested to know what mechanical input in particular your engineer used.

SPOENDLIN: A tonotopical organization of the cochlea as well as a characteristic threshold-frequency relation of each neuron to be studied is assumed. The mechanical input therefore is defined by the frequency, intensity and duration of the stimulus and indirectly affected by the characteristic frequency of the nerve fibers. For further detail I have to refer you to Dr. Altmann's thesis.

KOHLLÖFFEL: Would you say that the only conceivable place for interaction between information from outer and inner hair cells is the habenula? Do you thereby exclude that there could be ganglion cells which are connected to inner and outer hair cells? Could the interaction not occur in Rosenthal's canal?

SPOENDLIN: We have evidence against substantial branching in the osseous spiral lamina. If we count the number of fibers close to the spiral ganglion and at the habenula and compare the distance, we do not find significant changes of number of fibers. So we can exclude a substantial ramification of the afferent neurons in this course from the spiral ganglion to the habenula.

MICHELSEN: You said that the radial and spiral dendrites run very closely together, but that you never found any connections between them. How much have you looked?

SPOENDLIN: In my large sections, I have seen hundreds of these. I must add here that I do not exclude electrical interferences among closely related fibers.

ZWISLOCKI: I would like to come back to Dr. Evan's

argument concerning the long distance between the outer hair cells and where the spikes are presumably generated. I wonder if it would be possible to have a compromise and have a partially regenerative system. I think such things happen in the stimulus. In the retinular cells, potential changes have been found that seem to involve a regenerative process but are of normal longer duration that axonal spikes.

SPOENDLIN: With our present knowledge on the electrophysiology of these unmyelinated small nerve fibers, we cannot reach a conclusion. If the fibers electrophysiocally behave as electronic conductors the decrement with distance would in fact be too large.

ENGSTRÖM: In your picture of inner hair cells with the inner spiral bundle, I saw a large amount of dense, coarse vesicles with a diameter of more than 800 Å. I have seen similar in our own pictures and we have devoted much interest to them. Those are present just in an area which differs from the others in the inner spiral bundle. Can you comment on those?

SPOENDLIN: I have of course also considered a special significance of these large dense coarse vesicles. I do not think there is evidence enough to prove that these fibers are adrenergic.

ENGSTRÖM: They are over 800 Å and then they are not adrenergic?

SPOENDLIN: They could be. The only thing we know is that these fibers disappear when we cut the olivo-cochlear fibers completely in the vestibular nerve.

ENGSTRÖM: You do not believe that they are a kind of precursors for the enormous amount of synaptic vesicles that we need in the efferent system?

SPOENDLIN: This is very possible, but I think they belong to the olivo-cochlear efferent system.

References

Altmann, A. (1972). Modellierung von Nervenfunktionen bei spezieller Anwendung auf den primären Hörnerv. Thesis. ETH, Zürich.

Robles, L., Rhode, W.S., and Geisler, C.D. (1972). Proc. Meet. Acoust. Soc. Amer., 84th, A9.

Wilson, J.P., and Johnstone, J.R. (1972). Capacitive probe measure of basilar membrane vibration. Symposium on Hearing Theory 1972, pp. 172-181. IPO Eindhoven, Holland.

PROBLEMS AND PITFALLS IN STUDIES
OF COCHLEAR HAIR CELL PATHOLOGY

Jan Wersäll

Karolinska Hospital and
King Gustav V Research Institute,
Stockholm
Sweden

1. Introduction

Friedmann et al. (1963), Hilding and House (1964), Kimura et al. (1964) and Lundquist et al. (1971) have demonstrated that some information about the fine structure of labyrinth hair cells and their pathology on the ultrastructural level can be obtained from human material. Most studies on cochlear hair cell pathology are done on material from experimental animals.

Studies on hair cell pathology purport to learn the effect of aging, genetically induced damage, toxins and trauma on the hair cell as such. An equally important reason for studying hair cell pathology is to correlate the extent of hair cell damage to the effect on the physiology of the cochlear receptor. Although the principle of frequency localization in the cochlea as carefully analyzed by Békésy (1960) is generally accepted, the complicated innervation pattern of the cochlea makes an analysis of the effect of various patterns of hair cell damage on cochlear function extremely important.

Light microscopic studies on fixed, decalcified and celloidin embedded material (Guild, 1921, Schuknecht, 1953) are valuable with regard to temporal bone material especially from humans and have given us much information about cochlear diseases in man. Light microscopic findings can serve as a basis for a rough correlation between the general pattern of hair cell degeneration and cochlear physiology. There is, however, little or no possibility to make a more detailed analysis of structural changes within the hair cells with this method. The surface specimen technique originally introduced by Retzius (1884) was further developed by Neubert (1954) and systemized by Engström et al. (1964, 1966). This technique involves dissected undecalcified pieces of the cochlear duct suspended in glycerol on glass slides which are viewed from the surface by means of a phase contrast microscope. It gives a far better preservation of the material and makes possible a systematic analysis of the number of present or missing cells in the organ of Corti, which is valuable information in studies on the effect of noxious agents on the organ of Corti.

Histochemical changes in the cochlear hair cells under various conditions have been demonstrated in frozen sections or undecalcified material embedded in wax or epon (Ishii et al., 1968). This is a more reliable method for studying histochemistry than electron microscopical methods which are mostly poorly controlled biochemically, although some steps forward have been taken in this respect.

Fine structural changes in the cochlear hair cells have been demonstrated after acoustic trauma by Spoendlin (1958, 1962, 1971), by Engström and Ades (1960), by Beagley (1965), Stockwell et al. (1969), Ishii et al. (1969), Duvall and Quick (1969), and Lim and Melnick (1971). Genetically induced hair cell degeneration was studied by Kikuchi and Hilding (1965), in the shaker-I mice, by Anderson et al. (1968) in the dalmatian, and by Ernstson (1971, 1972) in the waltzing guinea pig. An analysis of the hair cell damage on the ultrastructural level was made by Duvall and Wersäll (1964) after streptomycin intoxication, by Lundquist and Wersäll (1966) after kanamycin intoxication, by Lundquist and Wersäll (1967) and Ylikoski et al. (1973) after gentamycin intoxication.

The aim of the present paper is to describe some characteristic changes in hair cell morphology caused by genetic defects and exogenous noxious agents and to indicate some problems and pitfalls in methods used to correlate morphological and physiological data in partly damaged cochleas.

2. Material and methods

The material from the waltzing guinea pig is taken

from a strain bred in our laboratory and derived
from a group of waltzing guinea pigs donated to the
laboratory by the National Institutes of Health, Baltimore,
U.S.A. This strain has recently been carefully
studied and its genetics, cochlear physiology and
pathology described by Ernstson at our laboratory
(1970, 1971, 1972).

The hearing tests were performed with a method developed
and described by Anderson and Wedenberg (1965)
for guinea pigs. All specimens were fixed in 1 % or
2 % buffered osmium tetroxide solution and embedded
in epon. Each cochlea was divided through the modiolus
with a thin saw. Each half cochlea was split with
a razor blade in such a way that each half coil was
contained in a block-shaped section of more than 100
µ including the whole cochlear duct. The round window
part of the cochlea was taken separately. All the
specimens were mounted with the tectorial membrane
side up on glass slides in epon without cover glass.
They were studied with a Zeiss light microscope
which had an optical system (according to Nomarski)
for interference contrast microscopy through a water
lense 40 x. Each hair cell in the cochlea was counted
and missing and present cells were marked in a diagram,
a so-called cytocochleogram (Engström et al.,
1964, 1966). An averaged cytocochleogram was made in
which groups of five cells from the same row of hair
cells were counted. When more than three cells were
missing the hair cell group was marked as missing.
When less than three cells were missing the group was
marked as present. The study of antibiotic damage in
the paper is based on studies by Lundquist and Wersäll
(1966), and by Ylikoski et al. (1973). The method
of studying cytocochleograms from epon embedded specimens
is slightly modified from the description given
by Ernstson (1971). Selected parts of the epon mounted
specimens from the cochlear coils were remounted, cut
and studied in a Siemens electron microscope.

3. Cochlear hair cell damage in waltzing guinea pigs

The genetically induced deafness in the adult waltzing
guinea pig is the result of a progressive degeneration
of the hair cells in the organ of Corti
(Ernstson 1970, 1971, 1972). The degeneration starts
in the upper part of the basal coil and the lower
part of the second coil and progresses basally as

well as apically. In the newborn, a certain distortion can already be seen in the hair bundles of some cells in the epon embedded material mounted for surface studies in the interference contrast microscope. Otherwise the organ of Corti in these animals appears normal. When successively older animals are studied, a progressive hair cell degeneration can be followed. The third row of outer hair cells is the first to show signs of degeneration followed by the second and first row of outer hair cells and last the inner hair cells. The gross morphological effect of this degeneration is easily visualized in the light or interference contrast microscope. Beginning as a scattered disappearance of sensory cells, the degeneration of the hair cells in the organ of Corti gradually becomes complete. Nerve fibers and ganglion cells degenerate when all sensory cells are gone.

Electron microscopic studies of late embryos or newborn waltzers demonstrate that hair cells showing grossly normal appearance in the light microscope have undergone significant changes in their tops. The sensory hairs show various degrees of fusion which is the result of two or more sensory hairs coming into close contact. Appearing first as bridges between the hairs, this fusion later affects the hair plasma membrane in such a way that two or more bundles and axial filaments form one giant hair. Finally the whole hair bundle can form an irregular ball shaped protrusion from the cell surface. The cuticle protrudes over the cell surface and minute ruptures of the cell membranes can be observed (Figs. 1-4).

Some of the hair cells showing deformities also have irregular fiber formations in the supranuclear part of the cytoplasm. An increase in dark bodies subcuticularly and a degeneration in some mitochondria are also often found.

During the further stages of degeneration the fenestrated membranes of the Hensen body and those along the inside of the plasma membrane become dilated. Multiple ruptures appear along the side of the hair cell. Swelling or pycnosis of the nucleus appears and a complete disintegration of the sensory cell is finally found. Part of the debris is apparently taken up by supporting cells forming inclusion bodies in these cells.

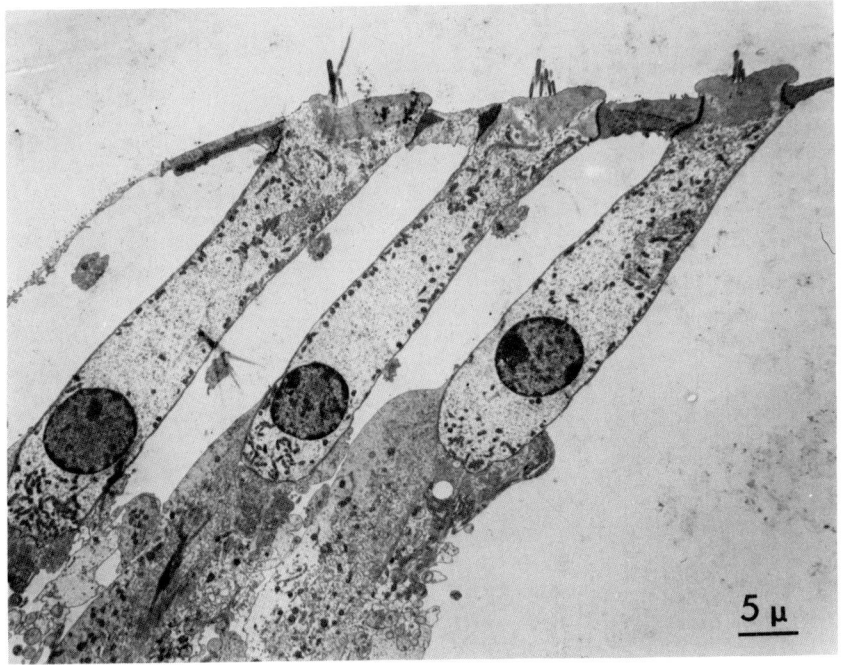

Fig. 1 Electron microscopic survey of outer hair cells from the second coil in the organ of Corti of a newborn waltzing guinea pig. The specimen appeared normal in the light microscope. The electron microscopic picture reveals, however, a protrusion of the cuticle of the outer hair cells and a starting hair fusion.

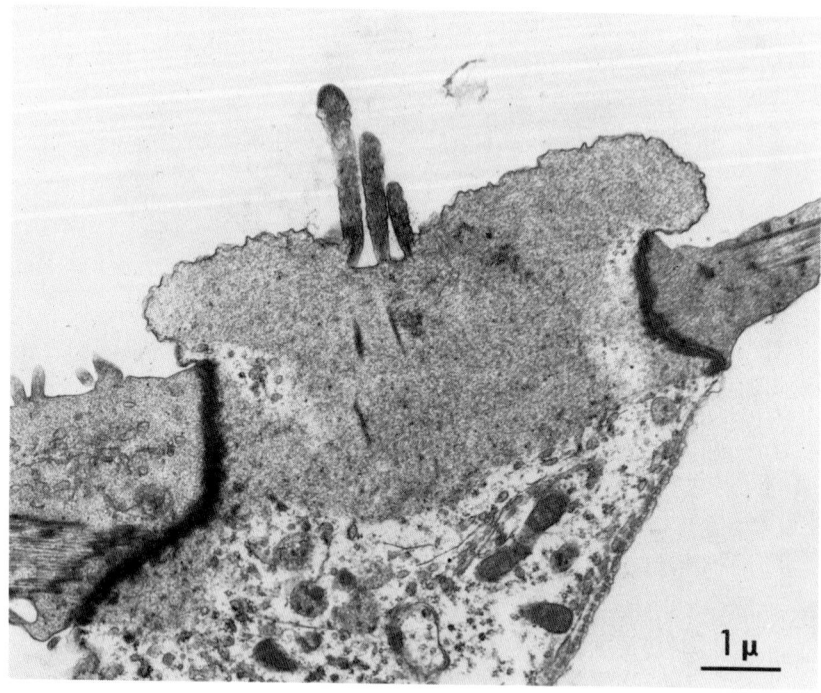

Fig. 2 Higher magnification of the hair bearing end of an outer hair cell from the same area of the organ of Corti as demonstrated in Fig. 1. Observe the extensive protrusion of the cuticle as well as increased amount of filamentous material under the cuticle.

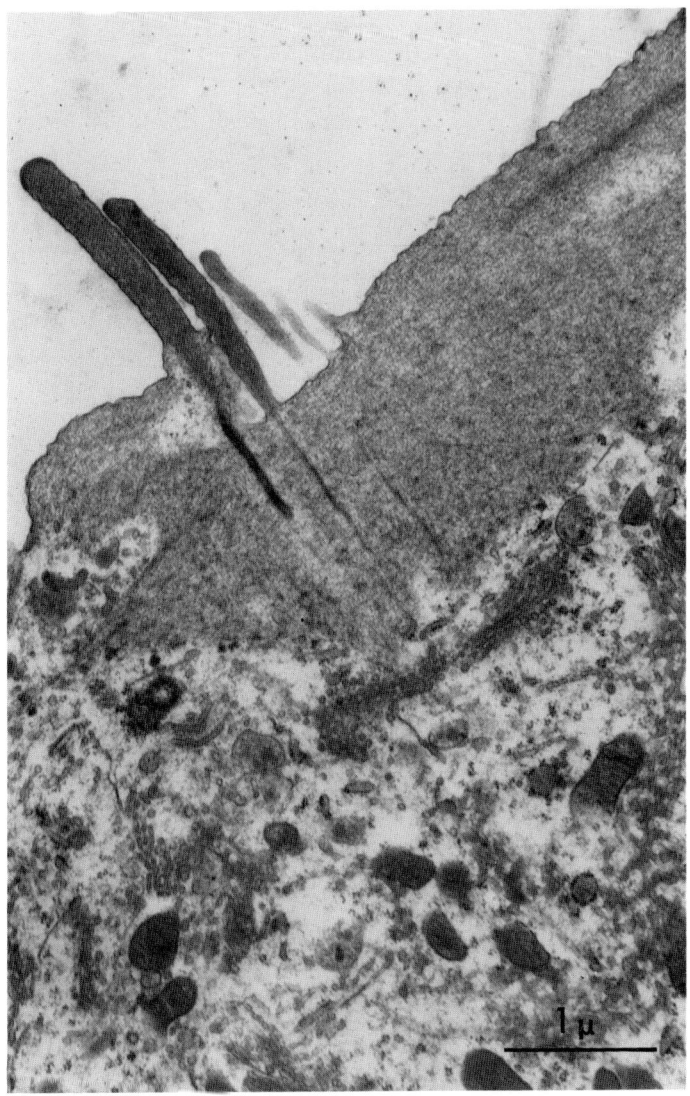

Fig. 3 Starting hair fusion in an outer hair cell from a waltzing guinea pig.

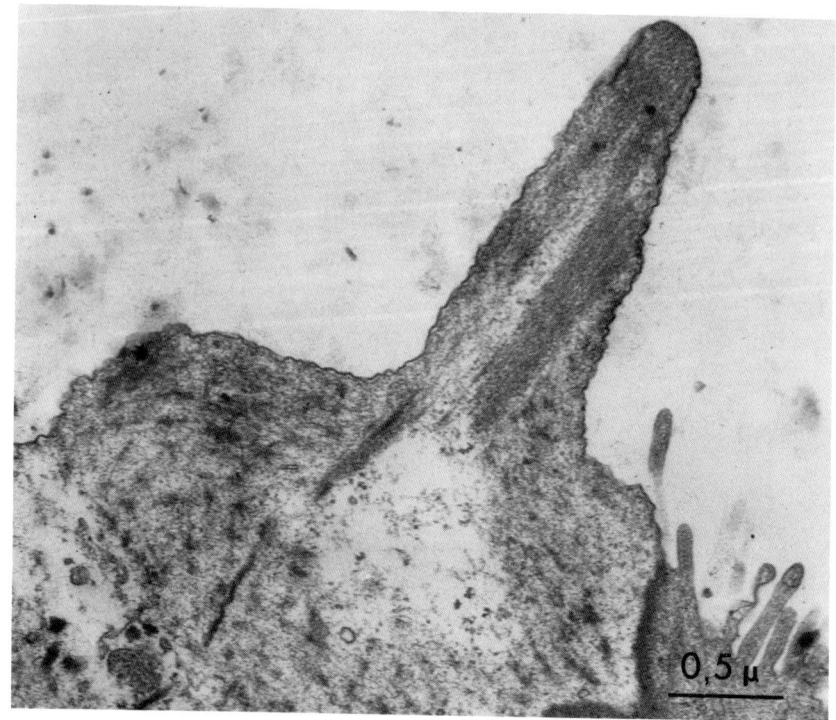

Fig. 4   Giant hair formed by fusion of several sensory hair in an inner hair cell from the organ of Corti in a waltzing guinea pig.

4. Antibiotic induced hair cell damage

A cytocochleogram of cochleas from animals treated with cochleotoxic antibiotics in progressively larger doses will give a gross picture of the various stages of degeneration of cochlear hair cells. The early stage as appearing in the cochleogram after neomycin, kanamycin, or gentamycin intoxication, can be described as a scattered degeneration of hair cells. This degeneration starts in the first row of outer hair cells; that is the hair cell row closest to the tunnel of Corti (Fig. 5). Later it engages the two other rows of outer hair cells and last the inner hair cells (Fig. 6). The first scattered degeneration is the most pronounced in the upper part of the basal

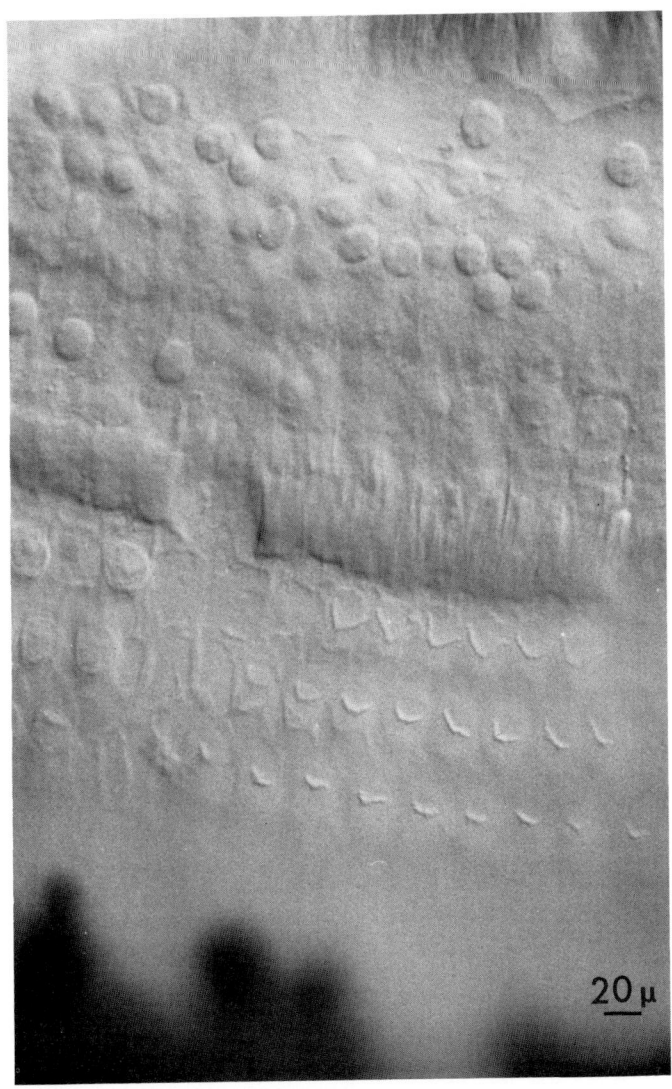

Fig. 5 Thick section of epon embedded cochlear duct observed from the surface. Scattered degeneration with a few missing outer hair cell in the third coil of the cochlea. The guinea pig had been treated with gentamycin 100 mg base for 17 days.

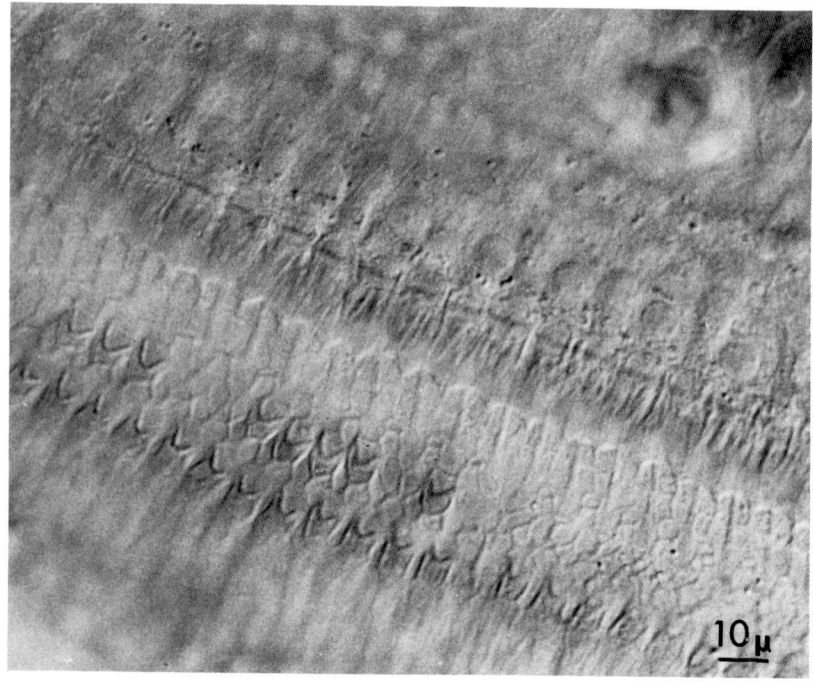

Fig. 6 Area of the organ of Corti from the same cochlea taken from the second coil showing advanced hair cell degeneration in the first and second row of the outer hair cells.

coil and the basal part of the second coil and more slowly in apical direction (Figs. 7, 8). A complete degeneration appears early in the most basal part of the basal coil and then spreads apically. There is always an area of varying length which contains a scattered degeneration between the totally degenerated areas and that with a normal or nearly normal hair cell population. The degeneration pattern is slightly different when a small dose of the antibiotic is given for a prolonged time as compared to a larger dose of a more potent antibiotic for a short length of time. In the latter case a more localized area of destruction is found in the basal coil with little scattered degeneration in other parts of the cochlea.

Electron microscopic studies of the organ of Corti taken a few days after the last injection of an oto-

MECHANISMS IN HEARING

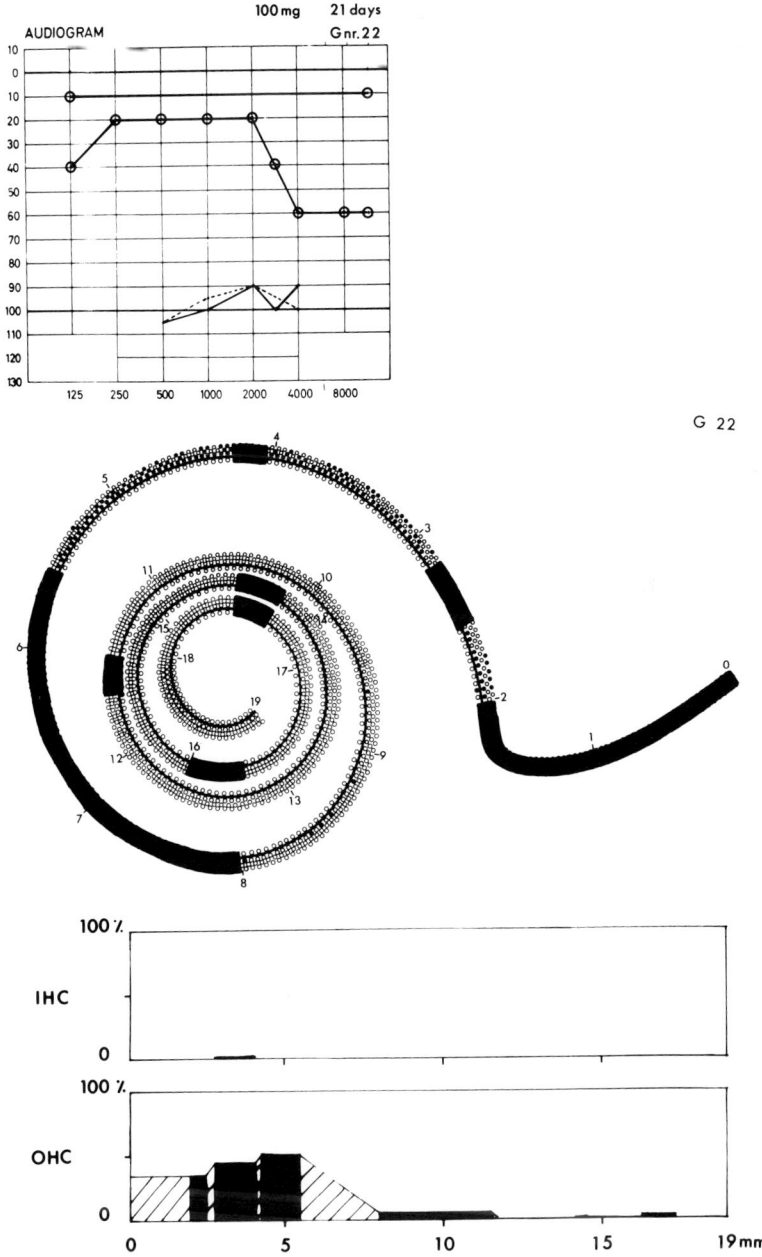

Fig. 7

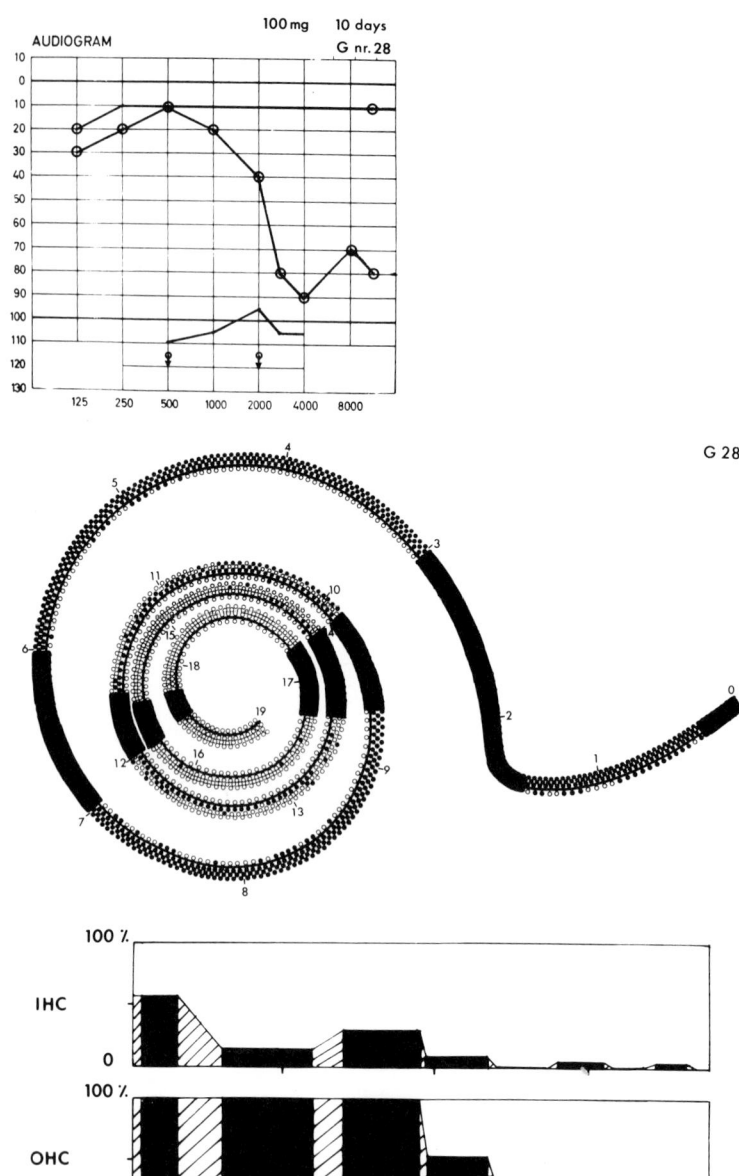

Fig. 8

Fig. 7. 8 Audiogram taken with the Anderson-Wedenberg method, average cytocochleogram from the whole cochlea and percentage distribution of destroyed cells in the cochlea. Audiogram: Continuous line before treatment with antibiotic. Line and circles after treatment.

Lower diagram illustrates threshold for Preyer reflex before treatment (whole line) and after treatment (dotted line).

Average cytocochleogram: Totally dark areas, parts destroyed at preparation.

Open circles: Present cells. Closed circles: Missing cells. Percentage diagram: Dark areas missing cells; Hatched areas: Parts of the organ of Corti destroyed at preparation.

toxic antibiotic will reveal cytoplasmic changes in the hair cells which do not appear in the light microscope or at least do not appear in the cytocochleogram. These changes include increase in the dark bodies under the cuticle. Some of these particles are nearly spherical with dense and less dense areas, others are lamellated and some of them are undoubtedly destroyed mitochondria (Figs. 9, 10). A fibrous material appears in the supranuclear part of some cells. A decrease in the ribosomal content of the cell is a later finding often coinciding with a widening of the interspace between the layers of the fenestrated membranes along the sides of the hair cells. A disorganization of the hair pattern is seen in late stages of degeneration and is most easily observed with the scanning electron microscope (Fig. 11). It is remarkable how well preserved the cuticle and the hairs might be in a cell with advanced cellular protoplasmatic disintegration.

A pronounced swelling of the nucleus of the cell is followed by multiple ruptures of the plasma membrane. Finally the cell undergoes a disintegration leaving the debris of the cell in many cases lying at the site of the hair cell in the fluid of the Nuel's space, before it completely disappears.

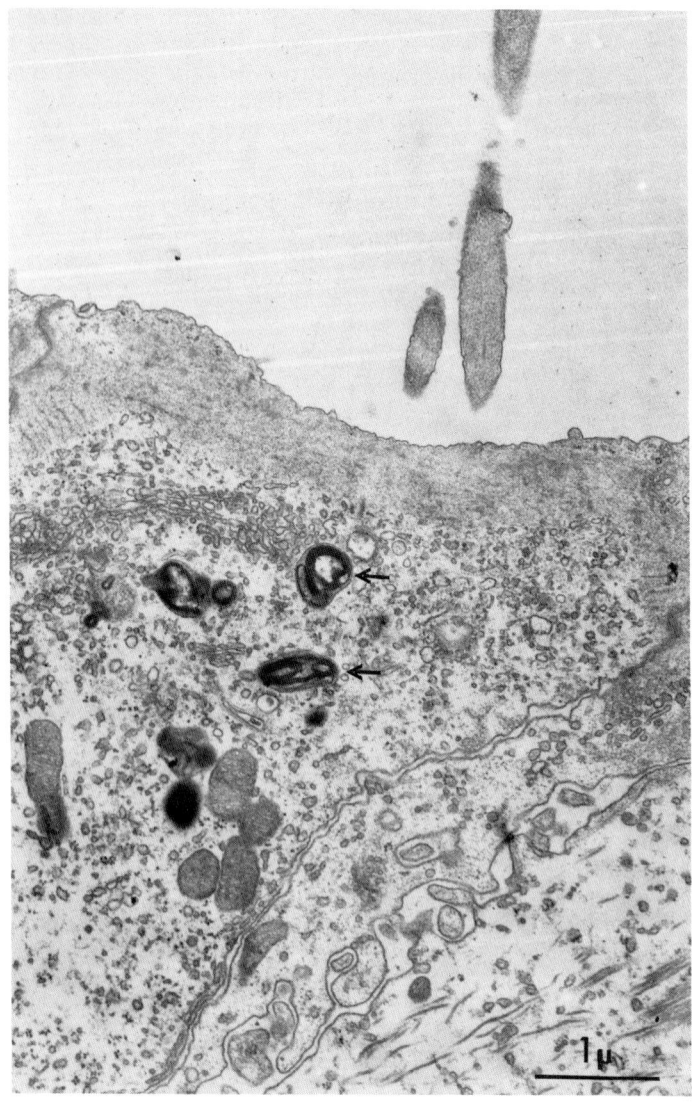

Fig. 9 Apical part of an inner hair cell from a gentamycin treated animal showing early signs of degeneration with formation of lamellated bodies in the subcuticular region (Arrows). Electron micrograph.

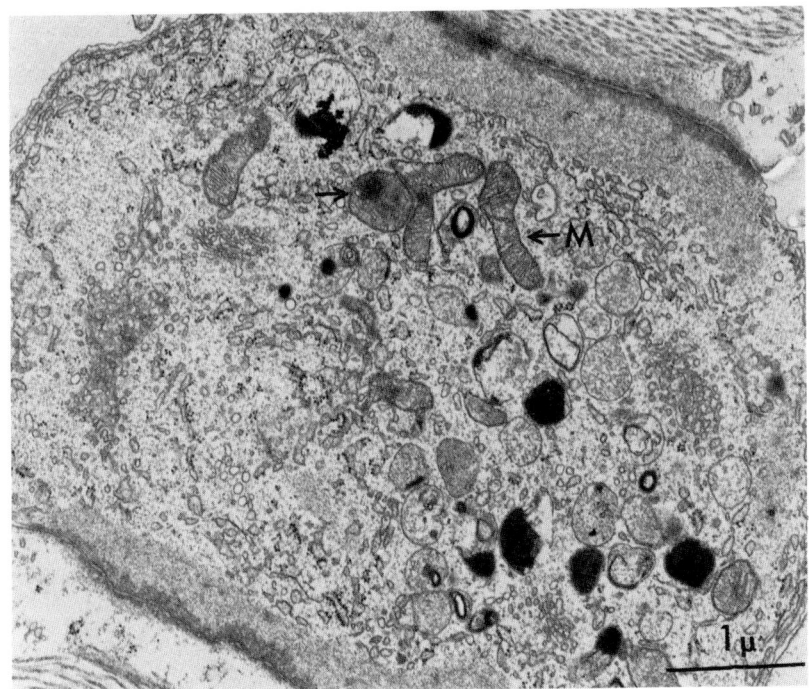

Fig. 10 Section cut parallel with the surface and slightly below the cuticle demonstrating early degeneration of mitochondria M with formation of dark accumulations in the mitochondria causing destruction of the mitochondria in a cochlea from a guniea pig treated with gentamycin. Serial sections through the cell demonstrated that the hair bearing end otherwise appeared normal whereas neighboring cells were completely degenerated. Electron micrograph.

Hair cell degeneration after acoustic trauma has been studied by Spoendlin (1958, 1962, 1971), Engström and Ades (1960), Beagley (1965), Stockwell et al. (1969), Duvall and Quick (1969) and Lim and Melnick (1971). The pathological changes in this type of degeneration include several of those described above for cells damaged in other ways. The hair cells in some cases show a distortion or a ballooning of the hair bearing surface. Increases in the lamellated bodies, the so-called Hensen's bodies and in dark inclusion bodies

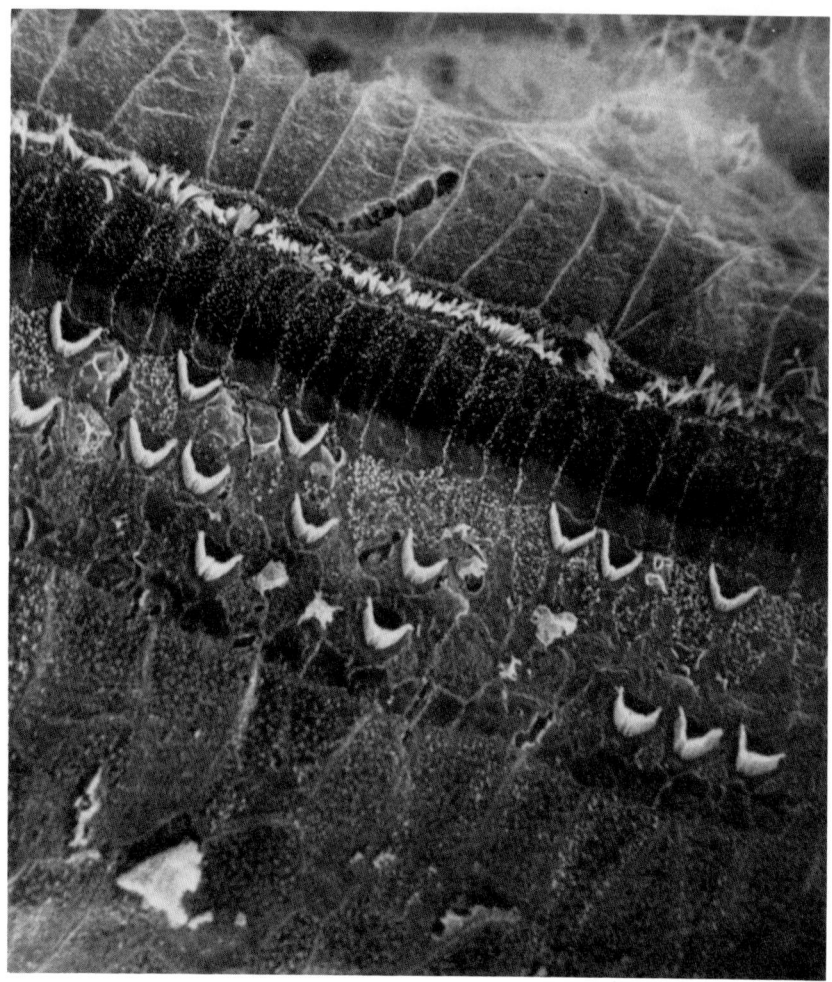

Fig. 11 Scanning electron microscope picture from the second coil of the cochlea from an animal treated with gentamycin. Some outer hair cells have disappeared. The hair bundles of other hair cells have disintegrated. Other hair bundles are well preserved. Some inner hair bundles are destroyed but most of them are intact.

on the subcuticular area have been described. At an early stage, Lim and Melnick (1971), who used a combination of scanning and transmission electron microscopy, found blebs on the surface of the hairs. In some cells the cuticular plate had softened and the cuticle was indented or bulging, sometimes squeezed out into the scala media.

In cells with a more advanced degeneration vesiculation appeared in the cytoplasm which apparently leads to a rupture and disintegration of the cells.

5. Correlation between physiology and pathology in the cochlea

One important goal in experiments on cochlear damage in animals has been to relate the degree of damage of the hair cells to the cochlear function especially with regards to the localization of pure tone reception within the cochlea.

Elliot (1961) studied the effect of partial nerve sectioning on pure tone hearing and pitch discrimination in cats. He found remarkably good hearing after degeneration of a large percentage of nerve fibers and hair cells in the apical part of the cochlea. He also studied the effect on pure tone hearing in conditioned cats exposed to intense sound at frequency of 7000 cycles/sec. The pure tone hearing was correlated to the degeneration of sensory cells as studied in a reconstruction of serial sections from embedded material. In one animal the hearing was normal, above 4000 cycles/sec although a profound hair cell degeneration was found in the basal 10 mm of the cochlea. On the other hand one cat with a drop of hearing to the 100 dB level above 4000 cycles/sec had normal ganglion cells and hair cells within the whole cochlea as revealed by microscopy. Elliot writes about this animal "we believe that the hearing losses are due to structural alterations in the organ of Corti which interfere with excitation phenomena but are not detectable by light microscopy". Stebbins et al. (1969) destroyed the hair cells of the basal part of the organ of Corti in five monkeys and found a good correlation between the spread of the damage in the basal coil and the hearing loss where presently accepted theories of frequency localization in the cochlea were taken into account.

The studies by Ernstson (1972) on waltzing guinea pigs showed a poor correlation between cytocochleograms and hearing in the conditioned guinea pig. The same was true in many patients studied by Bredberg (1968). Their audiograms were taken prior to death and compared to temporal bone cytocochleograms as studied after death.

It was clearly demonstrated by Ernstson (1971, 1972) that the sometimes poor correlation between hearing and cytocochleogram in the waltzing guinea pig was dependent on the inability to observe the first morphological signs of progressive hair cell degeneration in the light microscope. With the electron microscope, several structural changes were demonstrated which indicated a cellular degeneration of such a degree that it could be of physiological significance.

In our experiments we have examined the pure tone hearing threshold in guinea pigs after antibiotic intoxication with the Anderson-Wedenberg method (Anderson and Wedenberg 1965). One ear was destroyed surgically before antibiotic treatment (Ylikoski et al., 1973). A cytocochleogram was made of the whole cochlea from each animal and selected areas from each coil of the cochlea were later studied in the electron microscope.

Many animals showed normal or close to normal hearing within frequencies from 500-8000 cycles/sec even when large areas of the basal coil showed scattered degeneration among the outer hair cells. A severe hearing loss in frequencies below 2000 cycles/sec was found when both outer and inner hair cells were destroyed (Figs. 7, 8). When the same specimen was studied with the light and electron microscope it was found that cells which appeared normal in the interference contrast microscope often showed cytological signs of cell degeneration in the electron microscope. When the animal was killed soon after the last injection of the antibiotic the discrepancy between the light microscopic and electron microscopic picture was more pronounced than when the animals were left alive several weeks after the end of the antibiotic treatment. In the latter case most of the severely damaged cells died and disappeared from the specimen before the animal was killed. It is thus essential that the animals remain alive six to eight weeks after exposure to trauma or toxins before an analysis of the morphology and a correlation between morphology and function are attempted.

6. Conclusion

When cochlear pathophysiology is to be probed, several observations from past experience must be kept in mind. Some sensory cells within the organ of Corti will die and disappear after a certain length of time, when the cochlear sense organ is exposed to trauma of sufficient severity. Some signs of degeneration can only be visualized in the electron microscope. It is possible that some cells can be damaged physiologically without visible cytological changes.

Acknowledgements

The author acknowledges the support from the Swedish Medical Research Council Grant No. 12X-720-08A, and the research funds of the Karolinska Institute.

References

Anderson, H., and Wedenberg, E. (1965). A new method for hearing tests in the guinea pig. Acta Otolaryngol. 60, 376-393.

Anderson, H., Henricson, B., Lundquist, P.-G., Wedenberg, E., and Wersäll, J. (1968). Genetic hearing impairment in Dalmatian dog. Acta Otolaryngol. Suppl. 232, 1-34.

Beagley, H.A. (1965). Acoustic trauma in the guinea pig. II. Electron microscopy including the morphology of cell junctions in the organ of Corti. Acta Otolaryngol. 60, 479-495.

Békésy, G. v. (1960). Experiments in Hearing. McGraw-Hill, New York.

Bredberg, G. (1968). Cellular pattern and nerve supply of the human organ of Corti. Acta Otolaryngol. Suppl. 236.

Duvall, A.J., and Wersäll, J. (1964). Site of action of streptomycin upon inner ear sensory cells. Acta Otolaryngol. 57, 581-598.

Duvall, A.J., and Quick, C.A. (1969). Tracers and endogenous debris in delineating cochlear barriers and pathways. An experimental study. Trans. Amer. Otol. Soc. 57, 21-37.

Elliot, D. (1961). The effect of sensory neural lesions on pitch discrimination in cats. Trans. Amer. Otol. Soc. 49, 139-156.

Engström, H., and Ades, H.W. (1960). Effect of high-intensity noise on inner ear sensory epithelia. Acta Otolaryngol. Suppl. 158, 219-229.

Engström, H., Ades, H.W., and Hawkins, J.E., Jr. (1964). Cytoarchitecture of the organ of Corti. Acta Otolaryngol. Suppl. 188, 92-99.

Engström, H., Ades, H.W., and Anderson, A. (1966). Structural pattern of the organ of Corti. Almqvist & Wiksell, Stockholm.

Ernstson, S. (1970). Heredity in a strain of the waltzing guinea pig. Acta Otolaryngol. 69, 358-362.

Ernstson, S. (1971). Cochlear morphology in a strain of the waltzing guinea pig. Acta Otolaryngol. 71, 469-482.

Ernstson, S. (1972). Cochlear physiology and hair cell population in a strain of the waltzing guinea pig. Acta Otolaryngol. Suppl. 297.

Friedmann, I., Cawthorne, T., McLay, K., and Bird, E.S. (1963). Electron microscopic observations on the human membraneous labyrinth with particular reference to Méniéres disease. J. Ultrastruct. Res. 9, 123-138.

Guild, S.R. (1921). A graphic reconstruction method for the study of the organ of Corti. Anat. Res. 22, 141-157.

Hilding, D.A., and House, W.F. (1964). An evaluation of the ultrastructural findings in the utricle in Méniéres disease. Laryngoscope 74, 1135-1148.

Ishii, T., Ishii, D., and Balogh, K. (1968). Lysomalenzymes in the inner ears of kanamycin treated guinea pigs. Acta Otolaryngol. 65, 449-458.

Ishii, D., Takahashi, T., and Balogh, K. (1969). Glycogen in the inner ear after acoustic stimulation. Acta Otolaryngol. 67, 573-582.

Kikuchi, K., and Hilding, D.A. (1965). The defective organ of Corti in shaker-1 mice. Acta Otolaryngol. 60, 287-303.

Kimura, R.S., Schuknecht, H.T., and Sando, I. (1964). Fine morphology of the sensory cells of the organ of Corti of man. Acta Otolaryngol. 58, 390-408.

Lim, D.J., and Melnick, W. (1971). Acoustic damage of the cochlea. A scanning and transmission electron microscopic observation. Arch. Otolaryngol. 94, 294-305.

Lundquist, P.-G., and Wersäll, J. (1966). Kanamycin induced changes in the cochlear hair cells of the guinea pig. Z. Zellforsch. 72, 543-561.

Lundquist, P.-G., and Wersäll, J. (1967). The ototoxic effect of gentamicin. An electron microscopic study. In: Gentamicin, pp. 26-46. First International Symposium. Schwabe & Co., Basel.

Lundquist, P.-G., Flock, Å., and Wersäll, J. (1971). Raster- und Electronen-Mikroskopie des menschlichen Labyrinths. Mschr. Ohrenheilk., 105/7, 285-300.

Neubert, K. (1954-55). Experimentelle Erfassung der Aspsechgebiete im Innenohr. Berichte der Physikalisch-Medizinischen Gesellschaft zu Würzburg. Neue Folge 67, 92-100.

Retzius, G. (1884). Das Gehörorgan der Wirberthiere. II. Das Gehörorgan der Reptilien, der Vögel und der Säugethiere. Samson & Wallén, Stockholm.

Schuknecht, H.F. (1953). Techniques for study of cochlear function and pathology in experimental animals; Development of anatomical frequency scale for cat. Arch. Otolaryngol. 58, 377-397.

Spoendlin, H. (1958). Submikroskopische Veränderungen am Cortischen Organ des Meerschweinchens nach akustischer Belastung. Pract. Oto-Rhino-Laryngol. 20, 197-214.

Spoendlin, H. (1962). Ultrastructure of the organ of Corti in normal and acoustically stimulated animals. Ann. Otol. Rhinol. Laryngol. 71, 657-677.

Spoendlin, H. (1971). Primary structural changes in the organ of Corti after acoustic overstimulation. Acta Otolaryngol. 71, 166-176.

Stebbins, W.C., Miller, J.M., Johnsson, L.-G., and Hawkins, J.E., Jr. (1969). Ototoxic hearing loss and cochlear pathology in the monkey. Trans. Amer. Otol. Soc. 57, 110-128.

Stockwell, C.W., Ades, H., and Engström, H. (1969). Patterns of hair cell damage after intense auditory stimulation. Ann. Otol. Rhinol. Laryngol. 78, 1144-1168.

Ylikoski, J., Wersäll, J., and Björkroth, B. (1973). Hearing loss and cochlear pathology in gentamycin intoxicated guinea pigs. J. Infec. Dis. (In press).

III
COCHLEAR PHYSIOLOGY

"THE COCKTAIL HOUR BEFORE THE SERIOUS BANQUET"

H. Davis

Central Institute for the Deaf
St. Louis, Missouri
USA

I shall begin by a generalization from observing symposia and their operation over a number of years. I have decided that the usual method of organizing a symposium is to make a list of the important people in the field and invite them to come and repeat the stories that have made them important. New material does appear because these important people, in the intervals between trips to congresses and symposia and committee meetings, do actually do additional experiments, although usually in the familiar pattern. The result is a collection of facts, of stories, and perhaps even a set of answers with or without a clear set of questions appropriate to the answers. Now I do not have any new facts so I have amused myself by assembling instead a set of questions to which I do not have the answers but which interest me. In fact I hope by posing the questions to obtain some of the answers from the rest of you. Actually, some answers were suggested yesterday.

To stimulate your thoughts I shall offer some fanciful hypotheses, half in earnest, half in jest. First, has anyone a model for mechanical excitation in receptors such as hair cells or the pacinian corpuscle? The pacinian corpuscle (Fig. 1) is disarmingly simple. There is the neuron, ending with a dendritic non-myelinated terminal covered by layers of connective tissue, like an onion, around it; the connective tissue can be peeled off and the central non-myelinated core exposed. This structure is excited when it is deformed mechanically. There it is, but how is it done? I mean, at the molecular level. We recognize four kinds of sensitivity and receptive structures: the first is

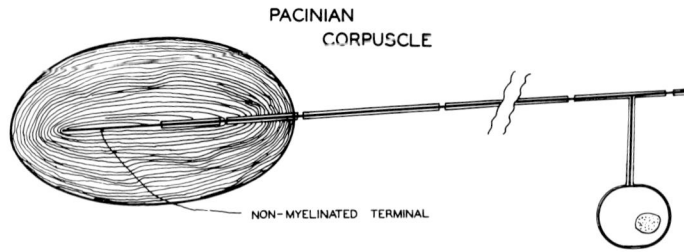

Fig. 1 A pacinian corpuscle. (Davis, 1961). (By permission of the American Physiological Society).

electrical, as in the axon; the second is a great variety of chemical sensitivities; the third is sensitivity to heat and cold; and the fourth is mechanical sensitivity. The least understood is mechanical sensitivity. When the sensitive membrane is compressed or stretched, whichever it is, does distortion of the membrane simply open up pores of molecular dimensions and let the potassium current or the sodium current flow? How much must these pores open?

The anatomical complexity in the organ of Corti is greater than in the pacinian corpuscle! Here (Fig. 2) is the latest version of my theoretical scheme for excitation (cf. Davis, 1965). In the middle of the figure, just below where it says "endolymphatic space", there is a hypothetical variable resistance. This is the place where I look for a change in the permeability of a membrane. Such a variable resistance could be the basis of the receptor potential in the ear, namely the cochlear microphonic; but now how is it that the cochlear microphonic can be symmetrical, positive and negative? The arrangement of cilia on the hair cells is systematically unsymmetrical and excitation occurs only in one half of the vibratory cycle. Unlike the electrical output of the hair cells of lateral line organs, the cochlear microphonic is symmetrical (at moderate intensities), and furthermore, it is linear over a dynamic range of 60 dB or more. I have said more than once that I believe that the most difficult problem in our model-making here is to provide for the tremendous dynamic range of

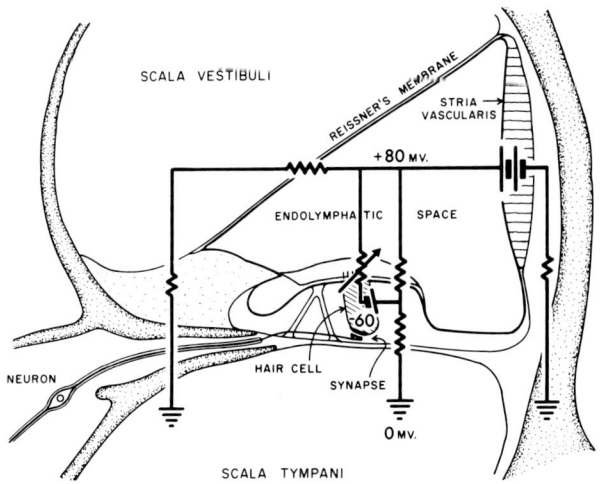

Fig. 2 Model of mechano-electrical excitation in the cochlea. From HEARING AND DEAFNESS, edited by Hallowell Davis and S. Richard Silverman. Copyright 1947, (c) 1960, 1970 by Holt, Rinehart and Winston, Inc. Reprinted by permission of Holt, Rinehart and Winston, Inc.

sound intensity that is accepted by the ear. Well, Dr. Flock may be able to take care of this problem.

The next problem is, what do the efferent auditory nerve fibers really do? The most that is claimed for them is to reduce the sensitivity of the afferent system by perhaps 20 dB when the whole bundle is stimulated at a rate well above its physiological range. I submit that it is biologically ridiculous that such a phylogenetically old and anatomically prominent system has no really significant function. Is this function possibly trophic? Does it provide some missing metabolite that is needed to sustain the function of the external hair cells? And, if so, is this because the meager afferent innervation that Spoendlin has described simply is not a big enough pipeline? Or should I change my question and ask what the outer hair cells really do? Fig. 3 is just to remind you of the efferent system and how impressive all of these great efferent nerve endings are, with the little afferents in between. I submit that one

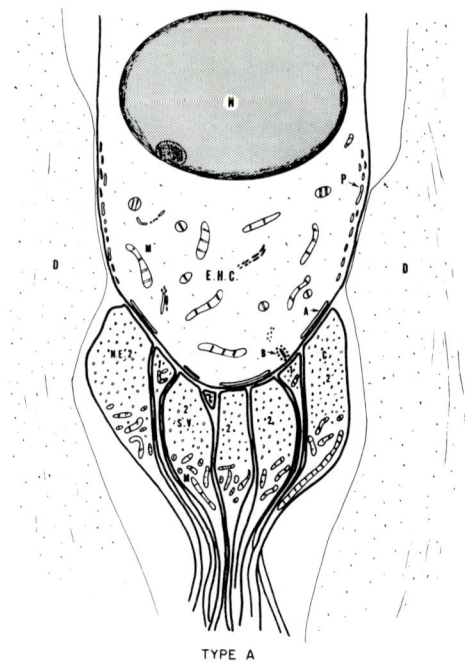

Fig. 3 The efferent system (Smith and Sjöstrand, 1961).

thing that such large structures with many mitochondria can be counted on to have is a high metabolic rate. They ought to be pretty active chemical structures. The efferent system is reported to improve stimulus discrimination in noise (Dewson, 1968). Noise puts a metabolic demand on the hair cells. Perhaps this reveals a sort of trophic action.

Changing the subject completely, what is the basis of temporary threshold shift? We are so familiar with the phenomenon that we are likely to forget that we have no model other than vague speculations about adaptation or fatigue. And, why is its maximum half an octave above the frequency of the exposure tone? Fig. 4 is from our own experiments done about 1942. (It was a war project, heavily classified at the time, and was not published until later, Davis et al., 1950). Notice that at the exposure tone (2,000 Hz), the threshold did not change. Progressively longer

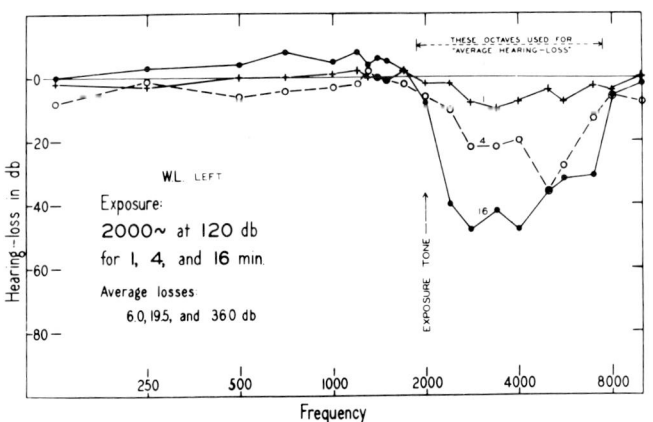

Fig. 4 Temporary threshold shifts. (Davis et al., 1950).

exposures of this particular subject on different occasions gave progressively greater threshold shifts, but always above the frequency of the exposure tone. We discovered this in our first experiment and I still have no explanation that satisfies me as to why there is this displacement. As to mechanisms, perhaps there is more than one process at work in the production of temporary threshold shift, such as metabolic exhaustion and perhaps also a physical effect such as a partial slippage in the attachments of cilia to the tectorial membrane.

The next problem: is the sharpness of tuning of sensory units to be explained as due to a physical tuning, a resonance of the basilar membrane or organ of Corti, which perhaps can only be demonstrated when very small segments are observed separately? The overall Békésy envelope is not sharp enough and simply will not take care of all of the facts as we know them. Are there possibly little resonators which are loosely coupled to the basilar membrane as a whole or to one another that can continue to jingle after a transient stimulus? Were Hartridge and Hallpike correct in interpreting the "phase-change beat" and its electrical counterpart in the action potentials as evidence of such continuing resonant vibration? Hamilton Hartridge was a devoted, aggressive champion of resonance in the ear in the good old Helmholtz style. In this experiment the phase of the stimulating tone, generated by an acoustic siren, was reversed abruptly. The listeners heard a pause, an instant of silence, sometimes accompanied by a click. That was the original phenomenon (Hartridge, 1922). I was not particularly worried about that experiment somehow; Békésy (1960) criticized it rather severely and failed to confirm the presence of the "beat". I found more disturbing the second experiment in which the cochlear microphonics and the action potentials of the mid-brain are compared. Fig. 5, originally by

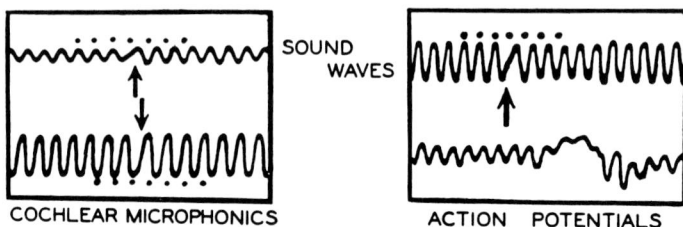

Fig. 5 Oscillographic records of sound-waves, of cochlear microphonics, and of action-potentials from the mid-brain. The phase of the sound-waves is shifted by $180°$ at the points indicated by the arrows. The frequency is 1024 cycles. (After Hallpike et al., 1937). (By permission of The Royal Society of London).

Hallpike et al., (1937), is reprinted from Stevens and Davis in Hearing (1938), and there I presented a possible alternative explanation. Rather brushing off the whole affair, my alternative explanation was vague, in terms of an on-effect and refractory periods. For Hartridge the phase-change beat was the overcoming of the persisting resonance and starting it up again in the opposite phase, which takes a bit of doing. The bit of doing apparently appears in the action potential record, although the cochlear microphonic follows the acoustic stimulus very faithfully. I think I was annoyed because Hallpike and Hartridge deduced from this that the cochlear microphonic must be just an epiphenomenon that did not amount to anything because the action potentials must be right. That was the real pay-off for them. And I said, my conscience is not entirely easy about it. I have had recently some correspondence with Dr. Hallpike who pointed out quite correctly that this experiment has been forgotten and neglected, and I promised that I would raise the question here, in case it turns out that he and his colleagues deserve belated recognition and a degree of priority. The criticism by Békésy of the original experiment cast serious doubt on this later animal experiment, which I think was rather better done.

Finally, how do we reconcile Dr. Kiang's exhaustive exploration of the thresholds of the fibers of the cat's eighth nerve (which has revealed only a single population of very sensitive units (Kiang, 1968)) with the compelling evidence from whole-nerve studies, in guinea pig, in cat and in the human electrocochleogram, which show two sets of receptors in the ear. Fig. 6 is a familiar figure, borrowed from Nelson

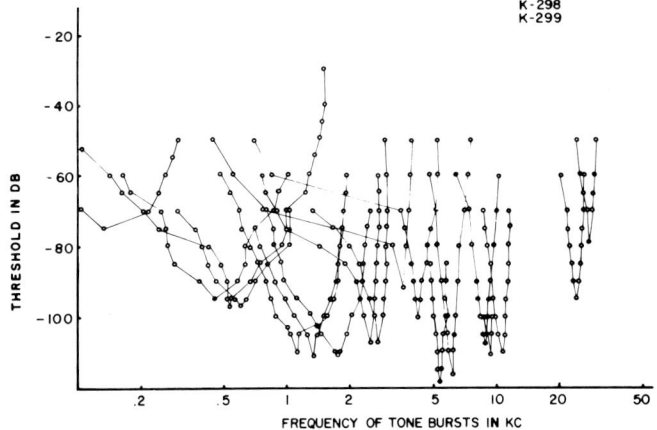

Fig. 6   Tuning curves from two cats combined to show a wide range of characteristic frequencies. (Kiang, 1965).

Kiang (1965), and shows what we mean by the response areas and particularly the high-frequency sharply-tuned narrow response areas. The sensitivities at the best frequencies seem to make a single curve that corresponds well with the overall sensitivity, i.e., a single population. Possibly Dr. Kiang is going to tell us today or tomorrow that he has found another population, but I doubt it. Dr. Spoendlin referred yesterday to the human electrocochleogram. I have just come from the recent XI International Congress of Audiology, in Budapest, in which this was discussed at some length. I shall give you a little more detail about it because I think it is rather relevant. The published reports will appear in due time in Audiology.

In the human there are two sets of neural responses to clicks or to tone pips. (Most of the workers now are using high-frequency tone pips (filtered clicks) and have gotten rid of some of the uncertainties introduced by raw clicks.) The two sets of neural responses have different latencies, different thresholds, and different slopes of their input-output functions. Fig. 7 is copied from a publication by Aran et al.

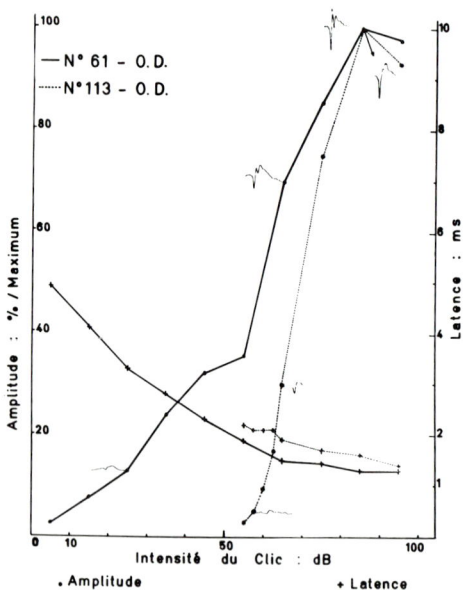

Fig. 7   Comparison of characteristic curves representing the variations in amplitude and the latency of responses as functions of the intensity of the click. Two children: no. 61, normal hearing, threshold at 5 dB. No. 113, threshold at 55 dB, but responses practically normal above this level. (Duration of oscillograms 10 msec., amplification constant.) (Aran et al., 1969).

(1969) of Bordeaux, who are among the very productive and enthusiastic workers in the field. The placement of their active electrode is on the promontory. The electrode is inserted through the tympanic membrane so that it makes contact fairly close to the round window and I think we can accept this as virtually a round-window recording. The reference electrode is on the lobe of the ear. There are two cases illustrated here, both of them children. Look first at the heavy lines. The falling curve shows the latency of the peak of action potential, which first appears here at something over 4 msec. That latency becomes progressively shorter as the intensity of the click is increased. The amplitude follows the trend of the rising solid curve. A fairly clear slope is established at low levels but something happens at about 60 dB: the amplitude suddenly rises quite abruptly over the next increments, while the latency changes very little more and is now of the order of 1.5 msec. I am sorry that the copies of the oscillograms are so small and faint, but in this and many other records that I have seen, the first wave to appear with the weak stimuli is rounded and it is late. In many cases the break in the latency curve is sharper than this, with a clear drop of 0.5 msec or more to the faster curve. What happens is that a new wave appears in front of the early one, grows more rapidly and finally becomes the peak of greatest amplitude. The convention is to measure the tallest peak, which at high intensities is way out in front while the second one is left behind or is absorbed in the falling phase. At the Congress of Audiology everyone seemed to accept this without hesitation as evidence of two sets of receptors, and I find the evidence very compelling myself. Recall also that in cats Peake and Kiang (1962) found evidence for two receptors, on the basis of the whole-nerve action potentials.

It is additionally quite significant that in a certain class of abnormal ears, the kind where we expect to find recruitment, the low-intensity late response is not seen. This is true for Menière's disease and for some of the toxic drugs. Guinea-pig experiments as well as humans tell the same story. In Fig. 7 we have the input-output function of such an ear (light line). It is normalized, which is deceptive because the actual voltage does not necessarily get quite so high as the normal response; but the point is that the threshold is displaced up to about 55 or 60 dB. There we see the high-intensity component, which appears clear and simple in the waveform of the electrocochleogram without the long-latency low-intensity component. If we assume, as many do, that these two sets of receptors are the inner and the outer hair cells, with the low-intensity set represented by the outer cells, the longer latency and lower maximal voltage of the neural responses match qualitatively the longer fibers and the smaller total number of fibers to the outer hair cells that are described by Dr. Spoendlin. Perhaps Kiang <u>et al</u>. (1970) gave a clue when they showed that, in cats treated with kanamycin and showing loss of outer hair cells in the basal turn, the response areas of auditory units with high characteristic frequency had lost their sharply-tuned tails. With your permission, Nelson, here is a figure (Fig. 8) taken from the paper that I have just cited. In

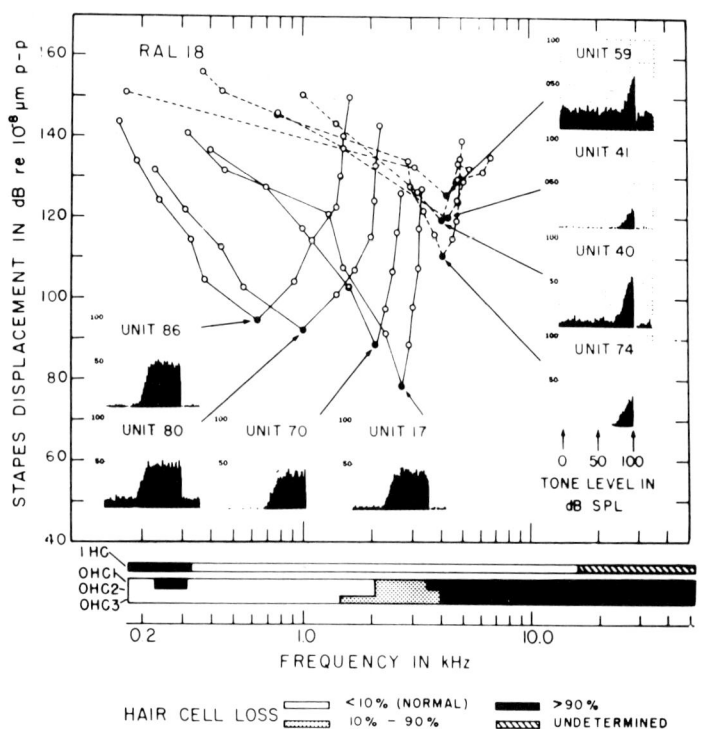

Fig. 8 Tuning curves and histograms of spike rate against SPL for eight units in a kanamycin-treated cat. The shapes of tuning curves denoted by solid lines resemble those of normal cats; the curves denoted   (cont'd)

(Fig. 8, cont'd) by dotted lines are distinctly "abnormal". (Kiang et al., 1970).

the frequency zone corresponding anatomically to the loss of outer hair cells, the response areas have either a small "tail" or practically no "tail" at all.

The obvious inference from all of this is that we must have two sets of receptors on a single unit, on a single neuron! After the low-sensitivity sharply-tuned "tail" is gone, we have a pattern that is compatible with recruitment. The units are there if we use a strong enough stimulus to reach them. They have high thresholds, and as a group of course they have a small dynamic range. Frequency selectivity should be very poor for each unit because the "tails" are lost. Remember that in recruiting ears of Menière's disease the frequency discrimination is so bad that practically it cannot be measured. Tonal quality is gone. (I have verified this proposition by consultation with three audiologists on our staff in St. Louis.) Has each kanamycin-injured neuron lost an <u>anatomical</u> tail that innervated a sharply-tuned resonator? If so, what is the receptor for the remaining high-threshold, unselective part of each response area in these cats, and for the high threshold, short-latency group of nerve responses in human ears?

Does Dr. Dallos have the answer for us in his conclusion that the cilia of inner hair cells do not make contact with the tectorial membrane but are coupled to it by the viscosity of the endolymph? Such coupling should be less efficient and yield higher thresholds. Or is it too fantastic to suggest that in kanamycin poisoning what has been lost is the chemical sensitivity of the nerve endings and that what remains is diffuse electrical stimulation of the nerve fibers? This would correspond to the situation in patients in whom electrodes have been inserted into scala tympani. This has been done and these patients show the same pattern of small dynamic range and no frequency discrimination except for periodicity pitch.

Well, I shall stop here. My imagination is outrunning the facts and I am not sure how much of this to take seriously myself. I ask your help with some answers.

References

Aran, J.M., Portmann, Cl., Delaunay, J., Pelerin, J., and Lenoir, J. (1969). L'électro-cochléogramme: Méthodes et premiers résultats chez l'enfant. Rev. Laryng. (Bordeaux), 90, 615-634.

Békésy, G. von (1960). Experiments in Hearing, pp. 411-414. McGraw-Hill, New York.

Davis, H., Morgan, C.T., Hawkins, J.E. Jr., Galambos, R., and Smith, F.W. (1950). Temporary deafness following exposure to loud tones and noise. Acta Oto-Laryngol. Suppl. 88.

Davis, H. (1961). Some principles of sensory receptor action. Physiol. Rev. 41, 391-416.

Davis, H. (1965). A model for transducer action in the cochlea. Cold Spring Harbor Symp. Quant. Biol. 30, 181-190.

Davis, H., and Silverman, S.R. (1970). Hearing and Deafness. 3rd ed. Holt, Rinehart and Winston, New York.

Dewson, J.H. III (1968). Efferent olivocochlear bundle: Some relationships to stimulus discrimination in noise. J. Neurophysiol. 31, 122-130.

Hallpike, C.S., Hartridge, H., and Rawdon-Smith, A.F. (1937). On the electrical responses of the cochlea and the auditory tract of the cat to a phase reversal produced in a continuous musical tone. Proc. Roy. Soc. London, Ser. B 122, 175-185.

Hartridge, H. (1922). An indication of the resonance hypothesis of audition. Brit. J. Psychol. 12, 362-382.

Kiang, N.Y.S. (1965). Discharge Patterns of Single Fibers in the Cat's Auditory Nerve. Res. Monogr. 35. M.I.T. Press, Cambridge, Mass.

Kiang, N.Y.S. (1968). A survey of recent developments in the study of auditory physiology. Ann. Otol. Rhinol. Laryngol. 77, 656-675.

Kiang, N.Y.S., Moxon, E.C., and Levine, R.A. (1970). Auditory-nerve activity in cats with normal and abnormal cochleas. In: Sensorineural Hearing Loss (G.E.W. Wolstenholme and J. Knight, eds.), pp. 241-273. J. and A. Churchill, London.

Peake, W.T., and Kiang, N.Y.S. (1962). Cochlear responses to condensation and rarefaction clicks. Biophys. J. 2, 23-34.

Smith, C.A., and Sjöstrand, F.S. (1961). Structure of the nerve endings on the external hair cells of the guinea pig cochlea as studied by serial section. J. Ultrastruct. Res. 5, 523-556.

Stevens, S.S., and Davis, H. (1938). Hearing: Its Psychology and Physiology, pp. 411-413. John Wiley and Sons, New York.

Figure 3 reproduced by permission of Journal of Ultrastructure Research.

Figure 4 reproduced by permission of Acta Oto-Laryngologica (Stockholm).

Figure 6 reproduced from DISCHARGE PATTERNS OF SINGLE FIBERS IN THE CAT'S AUDITORY NERVE by N.Y.S. Kiang et al., 1965, by permission of M.I.T. Press.

Figure 7 reproduced by permission of Revue de Laryngologie Otologie-Rhinologie (Bordeaux).

Figure 8 reproduced from SENSORINEURAL HEARING LOSS edited by G.E.W. Wolstenholme and J. Knight, 1970, by permission of J. & A. Churchill, London.

THE PHYSIOLOGY OF INDIVIDUAL HAIR CELLS
AND THEIR SYNAPSES

Åke Flock, Mørup Jørgensen[1], and Ian Russell[2].

King Gustaf V Research Institute
Stockholm, Sweden
and the
Karolinska Hospital
Stockholm, Sweden

1. Introduction

This paper is concerned with peripheral sensory mechanisms at the cellular level. It deals with the passive electrical properties of hair cells and with the hierarchy of electrical events which occur in the hair cell and afferent fibers during transduction. These are the receptor potential, the afferent synaptic transmission, and impulse initiation in the afferent nerve fiber. The paper is also concerned with the way in which the inhibitory efferent fibers interfere with these processes. Finally, the development of hair cells and their dependence on neural connections will be briefly considered.

New techniques have been developed in recent years which now make it possible to probe intracellularly with fine glass microelectrodes and directly measure electrical properties and responses of single hair cells and sensory terminals. It is now also possible to study individual cells in living organs and follow their behavior and development continuously for hours, or on a day to day schedule. It is intended here to give a preview and to document some of the most important results of such work, which are being published elsewhere in original articles.

---

[1]. Zoological Institute, University of Aarhus, Denmark.
[2]. School of Biology, University of Sussex, Falmer, Brighton, England.

2. Electrical properties and responses

The preparation

For several reasons this work has been done on lateral line organs. They develop from the same embryological placode as the sense organs of the inner ear and the ultrastructure of their hair cells is similar to those of the inner ear, and so measurements from them should in general be valid for other acoustico-lateralis organs. Electrical recordings have been made mainly from head canal organs of the fresh water cod fish, the burbot (Lota lota). The ultrastructure of these organs has been studied in detail with transmission electron microscopy as well as scanning electron microscopy and has been described elsewhere (Flock 1965, Flock 1971).

The fish were anaesthetized with 0.025 % tricaine-methane sulphonate (MSS 222, Sandoz), the brain was exposed through the roof of the skull and the forebrain was destroyed by cautery. The spinal cord was pithed from the obex down its length, and the animal was transferred to an experimental tank where it was respired by water flowing through the mouth and over the gills.

Methods of recording and cell identification

Hair cells are small cells, about 8 µ wide and 25-30 µ long. They are constructed to respond to mechanical stimulation. It is, therefore, not surprising that hair cells are easily damaged by microelectrode penetration as is evident from the rapid decline in electrical properties which often shortly follows intracellular penetration. Care was taken to ensure that electrodes were made with sharp tips and that they entered the cell with the minimum of mechanical disturbance to the hair cell.

The size of the electrode tips is illustrated in comparison with an outer hair cell in the organ of Corti in Fig. 1. Their impedance ranges from 20-80 Mohm when filled with 3 M KCL. They were filled by a modification of the capillary method of Tasaki et al. (1968). In this method the electrode tips do not come into contact with the electrolyte. Thus the possibility of blunting the electrodes by electrolytic etching of the glass at the extreme tip is reduced.

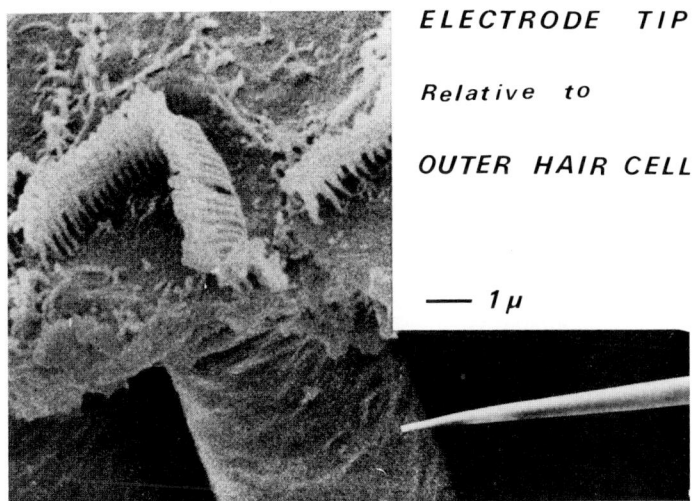

Fig. 1 In order to penetrate hair cells and maintain prolonged recordings the size of the electrode tip has to be small, as illustrated in this montage of two scanning electron microscope pictures taken at the same magnification.

The electrodes were driven into the cell by means of a microdrive driven by a step motor which advanced in 2 μ steps with a rise time of 1 msec (Transvertex). This facilitated penetration and in addition minimized mechanical damage of the cell. Recording was done with a high impedance input amplifier (Mentor) which also provides facilities for resistance measurements by a bridge circuit.

Within the sensory epithelium there are sensory cells, supporting cells and terminal branches of innervating nerve fibers. In order to correlate a particular type of response with a particular type of cell it is necessary to mark the recording site and identify the cellular compartment histologically. This was done by filling the cell electrophoretically with dye from the microelectrode with currents of about 5×10^{-8}A for 10-40 seconds under visual control in the operating microscope. The electrodes were then filled with a 6 % solution of Procion Navy Blue H3RS in distilled water (Stretton and Kravitz, 1968), which also serves as the electrolyte in the electrode.

The resistance of these electrodes was 200-500 Mohm. When a cell had been marked, the organ was fixed in 2 % glutaraldehyde buffered to pH 4 with phosphate buffer (Kaneko and Hashimoto, 1967). The Prociun dye is soluble in water but not in organic solvents, therefore the tissue can be dehydrated, embedded in epon and cut into 4-6 µ sections which are photographed through differential interference contrast (Nomarski, Zeiss. Figs. 4, 5, 6).

3. Membrane potential and resistance

Hair cells may function on principles similar to those in neurons and it is important to determine the electrical properties of the cell under resting conditions (Flock et al., 1973b). In experiments in which membrane potential and resistance were measured in 60 cells within the sensory epithelium, the advancement of the electrode was trigged to occur a short time after the beginning of the oscilloscope

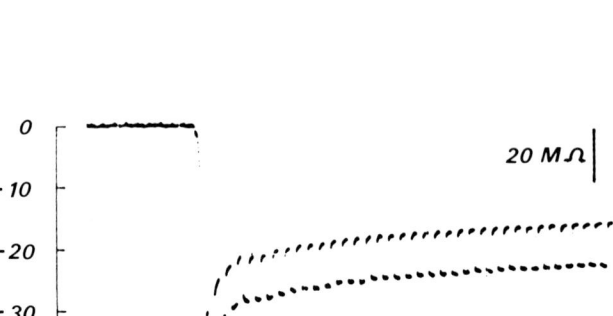

Fig. 2 When the microelectrode penetrates a cell its membrane potential and resistance can be measured in a bridge circuit. Time scale: 10, 50 and 100 msec.

sweep (Fig. 2). Pulses of current are driven through the electrode, and the voltage drop across the electrode resistance was balanced outside the cell with the bridge circuit. When the electrode penetrates the cell there is a voltage drop and an unbalance of the bridge proportional to the resistance of the cell. Withdrawal of the electrode from the cell restores the bridge balance and the voltage goes back to zero. The membrane potential, as measured 300 msec after penetration, varies from one cell to another between 10 and 65 mV and the resistance between 10 and 100 Mohm. There is a clear relationship between membrane potential and resistance, the higher the resistance the higher is the membrane potential. In experiments in which cells were marked with dye, hair cells and supporting cells were not found to have different values; both types of cells were equally likely to have low or high values.

The time span over which an intracellular recording could be maintained varied from one cell to another. Although some cells died within seconds, other recordings could be maintained for periods up to 5-10 min. Some cells maintained their membrane potential quite constantly throughout the recording, while others declined initially and then settled at a lower level. As the membrane potential slowly declined the membrane resistance went down in parallel (Fig. 3). After the initial decline some cells sealed and again increased their resistance and membrane potential (Figs. 3 and 6).

The relationship between membrane resistance and potential for a cell as the two parameters change with time is the same as that measured shortly after penetration from a number of cells with different membrane potentials.

It is probable that cells are damaged to varying extent by the electrode. However, many of them are still viable because the hair cells produce a receptor potential in response to mechanical stimulation and the inhibitory postsynaptic potential generated during efferent stimulation is similar in amplitude to that seen in neurons. Still, the highest membrane potential recorded did not exceed 65 mV. This is lower than the 80 mV claimed for cells within the organ of Corti. However, the origin of the potential recorded in the organ of Corti has not been

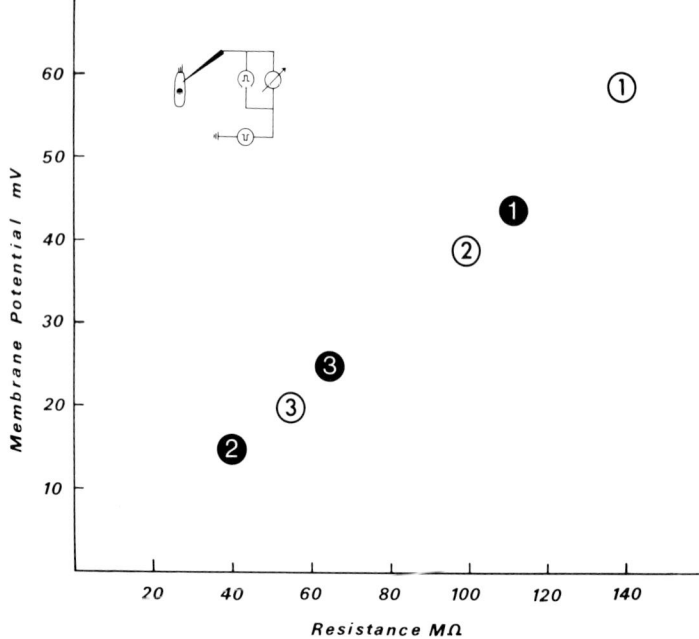

Fig. 3 The resistance of a cell is high when its membrane potential is high. The two parameters are plotted here for two cells at different times, in the sequence 1-2-3, during intracellular recording. One cell (circles) steadily declined, the other cell (filled circles) initially declined but then recovered. Compare with Figs. 5 and 6.

identified by dye marking and is somewhat unclear (Dallos, 1968, Sohmer et al., 1971).

The membrane area of a hair cell in the lateral line canal organ is approximately 1000 µ^2, which gives a specific membrane resistance of about 1000 ohm/cm^2 for a 100 Mohm cell. This is a bit on the low side but still within the order of magnitude of muscle fibers and neurons.

4. Time constant

When a hair cell is mechanically excited, it responds with an oscillation of membrane potential in phase with the stimulus. This is the receptor potential, and the summed receptor potentials from all of the hair cells in an organ give rise to the externally recorded microphonic potential. During the receptor potential, alternating current flows across the apical cell membrane and across the membrane of the cell body. For this current, or the corresponding voltage change, to be effective at the afferent synapse it must reach the base of the hair cell. If depolarizing current enters through the apical membrane then it must exit across the resistances and capacitances which are distributed in parallel throughout the rest of the cell membrane. If the direction of current across the membrane is shifted, the capacitances take some time to charge. The time constant of this process is determined by the values of the resistances and capacitances and if it is large the signal will be attenuated before it reaches the base of the cell. The degree of attenuation depends on the frequency of the signal and so the value of the time constant determines the ability of the cell to transmit high frequency signals.

This has been investigated by injecting current pulses with a fast rise time through the electrode. When the bridge is balanced outside the cell the time constant of the recording system can be determined. The electrode is then advanced into the cell, the bridge is balanced intracellularly, and the time constant is again measured. In no case did the cell prolong the time constant of the recording system which was about 0.2 msec. This means that the cell is capable of conducting signals in the kHz range without attenuation. It is interesting to note that the lateral line canal organ is restricted by its mechanical coupling to the surrounding water to have a natural resonance frequency of about 100 Hz. Thus the hair cells are preadapted to respond to high frequencies of mechanical stimulation for example in the cochlea.

5. Electrical excitability

In many excitable cells signal transmission is by regenerative impulses which develop as a consequence of the electrical excitability of the particular membrane; above a certain threshold the resistance of the membrane decreases with decreasing membrane potential so that all or nothing nerve impulses are generated. Obviously hair cells do not produce such action potentials; they respond in a graded manner to a graded stimulus. There are instances, however, where membranes have a component of electrical excitability which does not produce fully developed spikes but contributes to the amplitude of graded potentials. In order to examine if hair cells are electrically excitable several cells were penetrated and their resistance monitored while the membrane potential was displaced about 15 mV in the depolarizing or in the hyperpolarizing direction. No resistance change could be detected within the limits of sensitivity which was about 6 % of the cell resistance. Since the amplitude of the receptor potential even at maximum stimulation barely exceeds 1-2 mV it is concluded that electrical excitability does not significantly contribute towards its generation.

6. The receptor potential

It is easy to expose lateral line canal organs by cutting off the skin over the roof of the canal. The cupula which rests on the sensory epithelium is then exposed and can be driven mechanically to excite the sensory cells. The sensory area is large, about 1 mm^2. This organ provides an advantage in comparison to vestibular sense organs which are hidden in the temporal bone and where contamination between endolymph and perilymph is difficult to avoid. It has an advantage also compared to epidermal lateral line organs where the sensory area at which the electrode has to be aimed is only about 20 µ wide and 100 µ long; however, epidermal organs do have the advantage, at least in salamanders, in that hair cells are large and measurements from them can be maintained for longer periods of time. Intracellular receptor potentials were obtained for the first time in such organs in Necturus maculosus (Harris et al., 1970). Evidence was obtained that these were true biological potentials and did not result from the mechanical motion of tissue against the electrode tip.

When measurements are made from cells in the lateral line canal organ during mechanical stimulation with a low frequency tone some cells give a response and others do not (Fig. 4). Three types of responses are seen: 1) a signal with the same frequency as the stimulus, 2) a signal of the same type but of opposite phase, and 3) a signal of smaller amplitude which has a frequency twice that of the stimulus. Responses of type 1 and 2 could sometimes be mixed

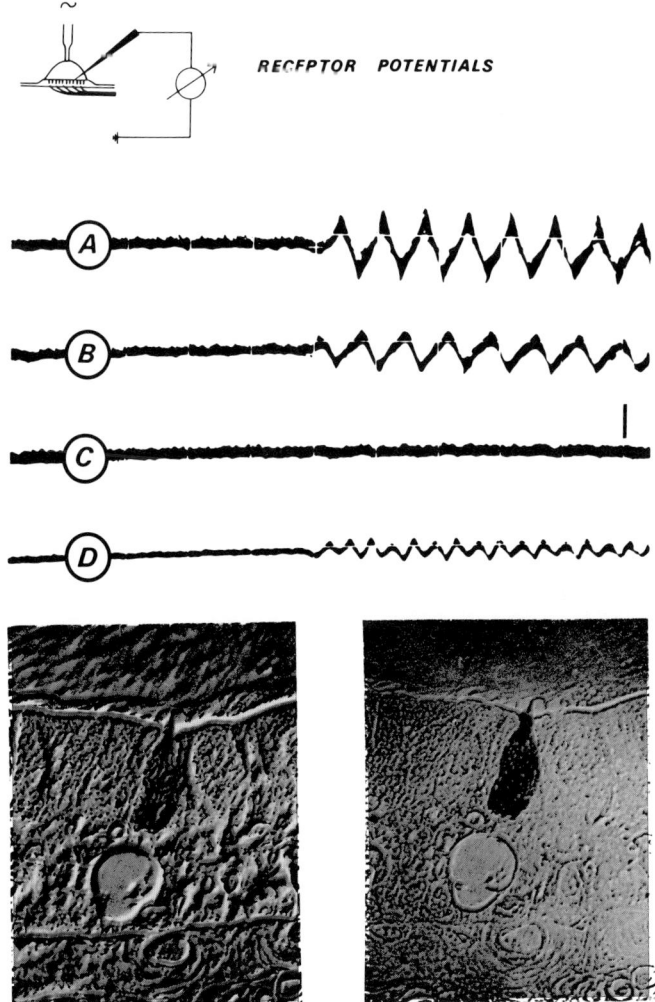

Fig. 4 Hair cells generate a receptor potential when the organ is mechanically stimulated by a 70 Hz tone. Record A was obtained intracellularly from the cell identified below as a hair cell. It was marked by electrophoretic dye injection, and a section through it was photographed, to the left through Nomarski optics, to the right with bright field optics. The next cell to respond (in a new organ) produced record B, which is phase-   (cont'd)

(Fig. 4, cont'd) shifted 180°. Record C was obtained from a supporting cell. In D the external microphonic potential was monitored just before record B. Vertical bar is 500 μV.

with responses of type 3 so that the single frequency response was "notched" by the presence of a second order harmonic component. The external microphonic, which was monitored simultaneously with a second amplifier, is twice the frequency of the stimulus unless the cupula is biased so that one phase of the response dominates.

Out of 30 responding cells which were marked by dye injection 15 were retrieved and identified in sections (Fig. 4). 11 of these were hair cells out of which 8 gave a single frequency response, 2 gave a notched response and 1 gave a small double response, but this cell died rapidly. As the membrane potential (and thus the resistance) of one of the cells which gave a notched response slowly declined the response became smaller and changed gradually into a double frequency response (Fig. 5). This was identified as a hair cell but stain was also found below the base of the cell (Figure 5b). Out of 4 cells identified as supporting cells one gave no response, and one gave a single response but in this case the external microphonic potential had shifted towards single frequency because of biasing. The course of the membrane potential and response of the third cell is illustrated in Fig. 6. It started as a double response, then the cell sealed, the membrane potential increased (and with it its resistance) and the response diminished. One supporting cell gave a single response in spite of the fact that the external microphonic potential was an even double frequency.

We conclude from all this that hair cells generate receptor potentials of the same frequency as the stimulus, with the same or opposite phase depending on their orientation (Fig. 7). The receptor potential can be more or less contaminated by second order harmonics. As the cell deteriorates its resistance decreases and it becomes more and more leaky so that the extracellular microphonic potential is also seen by the electrode; and secondly, in the canal organ of the burbot large areas of neighboring hair cells are in direct opposition without intervening supporting

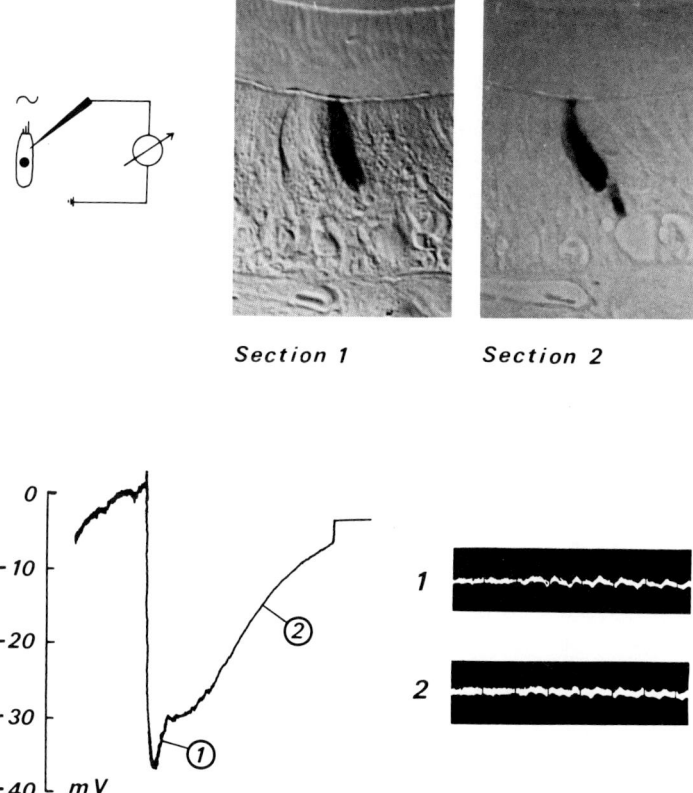

Section 1   Section 2

Fig. 5 These recordings are from a hair cell, identified in section 1 through Nomarski optics and in section 2 with bright field illumination. Below, the decline of membrane potential over a 1 minute period is registered. Records 1 and 2 are obtained at two different times.

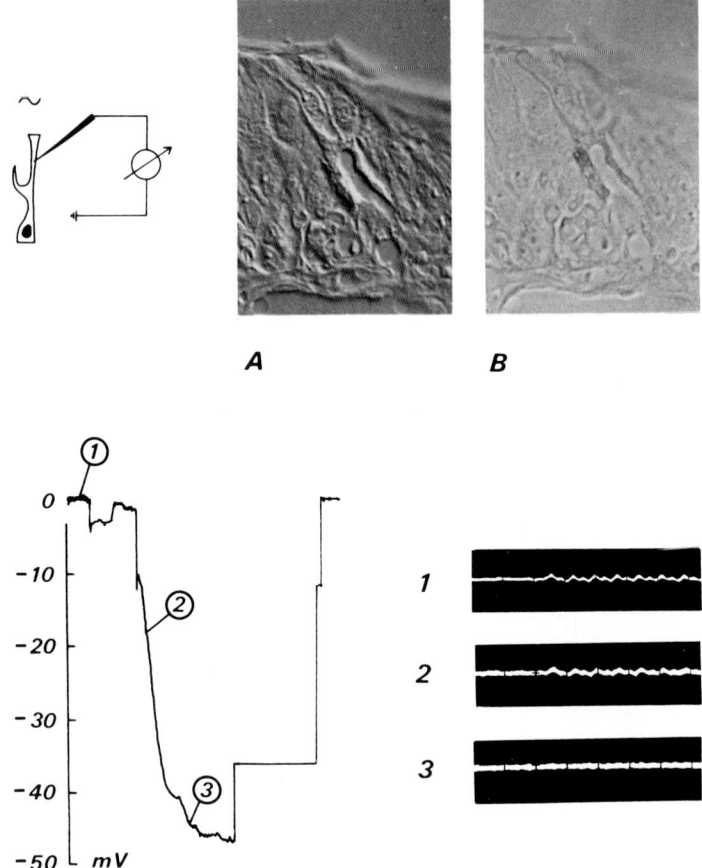

Fig. 6 These recordings are from a supporting cell close to the mantle cell region in the sensory epithelium. In A it is seen through Nomarski optics and in B in bright field. Record 1 is the external microphonic potential, record 2 is just after penetration, record 3 is when the membrane potential has increased.

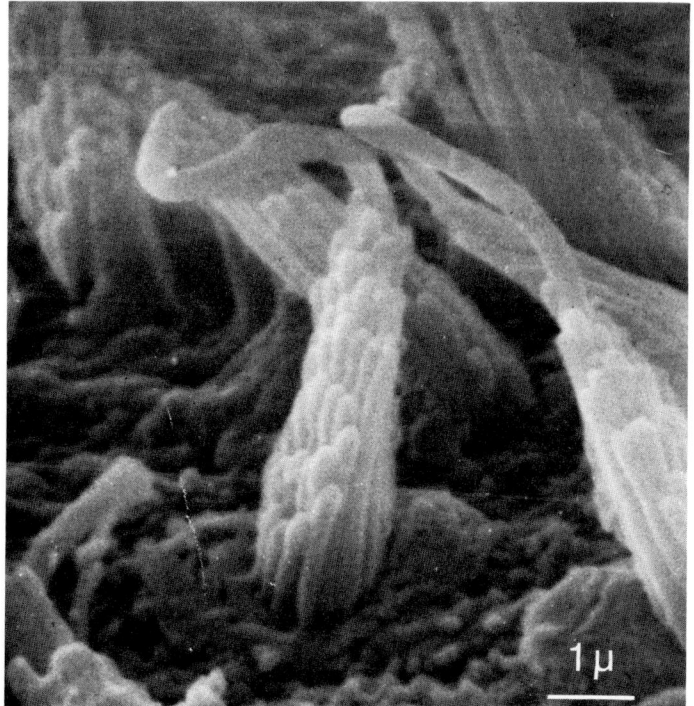

Fig. 7 The stereocilia of the sensory hair bundle increase in length toward the kinocilium which faces opposite directions in neighboring cells.

cells, and cross-talk may well exist. Such passive overhearing does occur between cells with large contact areas (See Katz, 1966) and this does not necessarily imply electrical coupling via low resistance pathways. Gap junctions have never been seen in the lateral line organ (Flock, 1965, Hama, 1965) and procion dye does not pass from an injected cell to neighboring cells as in low resistance gap junctions (Payton et al., 1969).

The external current generated by the hair cells is distributed across the sensory epithelium and the walls of the lateral line canal according to the distribution of trans-epithelial resistances. Part of this current flows through the supporting cells of the sensory epithelium and may give rise to the

small microphonic potentials sometimes recorded in
supporting cells. It may be that a supporting cell
which joins several hair cells which respond in phase
can provide a sink for part of this current and so an
in-phase or mixed potential can be recorded in these
supporting cells. The source and the sink of the receptor current, and the distribution of current between cells in the sensory epithelium, can only be
determined by differential recording between a pair
of electrodes and those measurements have not yet
been performed.

It is fortunate in the lateral line organ that hair
cells are of opposite polarity, because intact sensory cells give a single frequency response whereas
in supporting cells nothing or a small second order
harmonic distortion product is seen. Contamination of
a receptor potential with second order harmonics provides a warning that the external microphonic potential adds to the registered potential because of
damage to the cell. This control will not be present
in organs like the organ of Corti or the crista of
the semicircular canals where all cells have the same
orientation and hair cells and supporting cells give
potential changes of the same phase.

7. Afferent synaptic transmission

Occasionally, recordings have been obtained from the
terminal branches of the afferent sensory neuron
within the sensory epithelium. The terminal dendrites
are myelinated for part of their course in the epithelium but the myelin sheath is lost and the naked
axon travels for some distance before innervating
hair cells. Nerve action potentials are recorded in
these terminals, as is expected from myelinated axons,
but recordings have also been obtained from the non-
myelinated portion. Here, graded potentials are observed which have the characteristics of excitatory
postsynaptic potentials (EPSP's) evoked by release of
a neurochemical transmitter (Fig. 8)(Flock and Russell, 1973a). This is in accordance with observations
in the goldfish sacculus by Furukawa and Ishii (1967).
When dye is injected by electrophoresis very fine
branching strands become visible deep in the sensory
epithelium through the dissecting microscope. The
EPSP's occur spontaneously in these terminals and are
presumably due to the spontaneous release of transmitter at afferent synapses situated at different

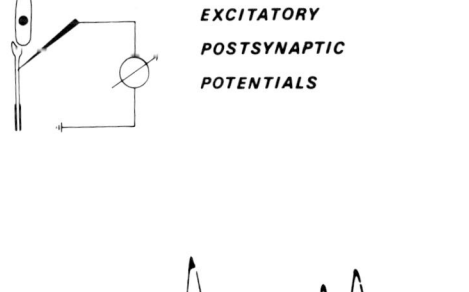

EXCITATORY POSTSYNAPTIC POTENTIALS

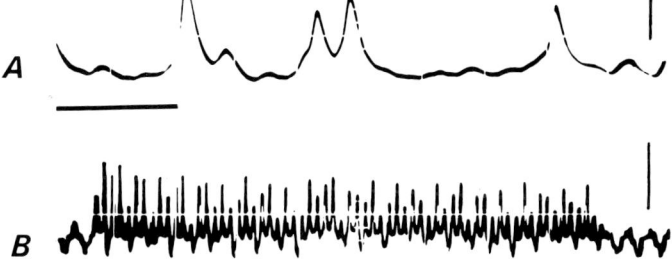

Fig. 8   Excitatory postsynaptic potentials occur spontaneously in the afferent terminal (A). They synchronize in-phase when the organ is mechanically stimulated (B) with a 70 Hz tone (C). Time bar is 10 msec in A, vertical 2 mV.

electrotonic distances from the recording site. When the organ is stimulated mechanically the EPSP's become phase-locked to the stimulus, their amplitude being determined by the intensity of the stimulus (Fig. 8 B). It is assumed that the EPSP's are conducted as graded potentials in the non-myelinated axon and initiate nerve action potentials in the myelinated portion of the terminal when the threshold amplitude is exceeded.

8. Action of efferent fibers

The function of the efferent system is perhaps better known in the vestibular and lateral line organs than it is in the cochlea. It is closely connected to the motor system, and efferent nerve fibers fire prior to and during voluntary movements, inhibiting the activity in the sensory nerve fibers (Russell, 1968 and 1971, Llinàs and Precht, 1969, Klinke and Schmidt, 1970). It is not a feedback system activated by a sensory input, but a control system regulating the sensitivity of the peripheral sense organ during movement.

The canal organs of the burbot are well supplied with efferent fibers which terminate on the base of the hair cells. No contacts have been seen between efferent nerve endings and sensory dentrites. When efferent fibers are selectively stimulated a negative dc-change is recorded extracellularly in the vicinity of the sensory epithelium, the microphonic potential is augmented and afferent nerve impulses are inhibited (Flock and Russell, 1973a). These effects are the same as those caused in the cochlear partition by stimulation of the crossed olivo-cochlear bundle as described by Fex (1962 and 1967). However, efferents in the lateral line organ seem to be more potent than those in the cochlea because these effects are seen when efferent fibers are stimulated at frequencies as low as 10-20 pulses/sec and this is well within the natural firing frequency which may be as high as 60 impulses/sec. At higher frequencies of efferent stimulation the effect is stronger and reaches an optimum at 100-200 pulses/sec.

Direct electrical stimulation of the efferent neurones in the wall of the 4th ventricle is difficult because of their close proximity to the incoming afferent fibers, with the possibility that these may also be excited. Efferent neurones are strongly excited by stimulation of the medial longitudinal fasciculus in the floor of the 4th ventricle. This also causes vigorous movement of the fish. Intramuscular injection of Flaxedil or Curare in low concentrations blocks the efferent synapse within a few minutes (Fig. 9). Therefore, in order to study the effect of selective stimulation of efferents, all the motor nerves had to be sectioned in non-anesthetized fish whose forebrain was destroyed by cautery. The same peripheral effects on DC potential and microphonic potential were produced when the whole nerve to the sense organ was stimulated by pulse trains delivered by bipolar electrodes. This means that efferent fibers are fired ortodromically and afferent fibers

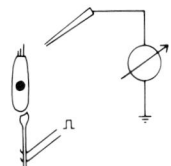

**EXTRACELLULAR
EFFERENT
EFFECTS**

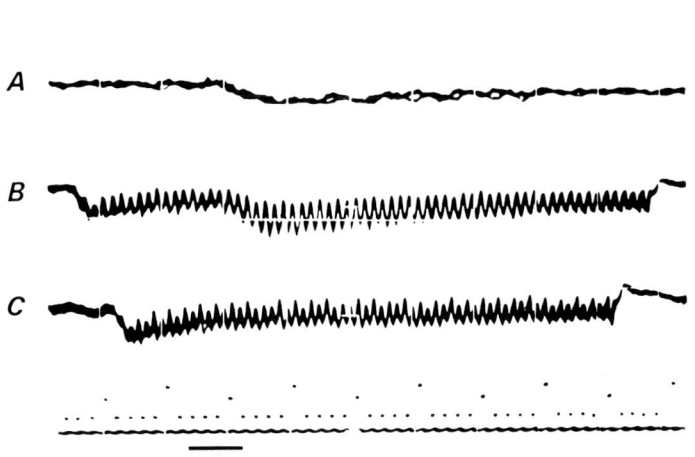

Fig. 9 Repetitive firing of efferent fibers (7 impulses during bar) gives rise to a negative dc potential (A) and an increase in the microphonic potential (B). These effects are blocked by Flaxedil.

are fired antidromically. However, antidromic invasion of afferent terminals has no effect on the hair cell response since the sensory synapse is chemically transmitting. This has been verified by intracellular recordings from hair cells when the efferent synapse has been blocked by Flaxedil during antidromic firing of afferents. For practical purposes this method of stimulating efferent fibers was chosen in a study of the inhibitory mechanism at a cellular level (Flock and Russell, 1973b).

When the efferents are fired by a short pulse train delivered to the nerve, hyperpolarizing inhibitory postsynaptic potentials (IPSP's) develop in some cells but not in others (Fig. 10A). In dye marking experiments responsive cells were identified as hair

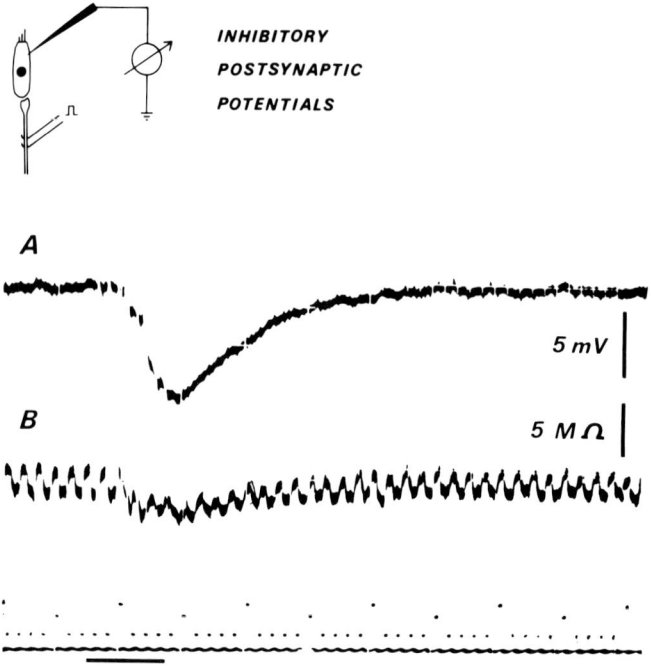

Fig. 10 A hyperpolarizing postsynaptic potential (A) develops in hair cells as a consequence of efferent nerve activity. It is accompanied by a decrease of cell resistance, seen as a reduction in bridge pulse height (B).

cells. During the IPSP the resistance of the cell decreases (Fig. 10B). The receptor potential evoked by a tone is augmented for a period of time equal to that of the IPSP. This provides further evidence that the receptor potential is a true biological potential and no mechanical motion artifact; the activity of a neurochemical synapse would hardly be expected to influence a motion artifact.

In one case EPSP's were recorded in the afferent terminal for more than two hours when efferent fibers could be stimulated at the same time. It was found that efferent stimulation reduces the amplitude of EPSP's for a period of time corresponding to the IPSP (Fig. 11).

In a few cases the size of the IPSP was observed to

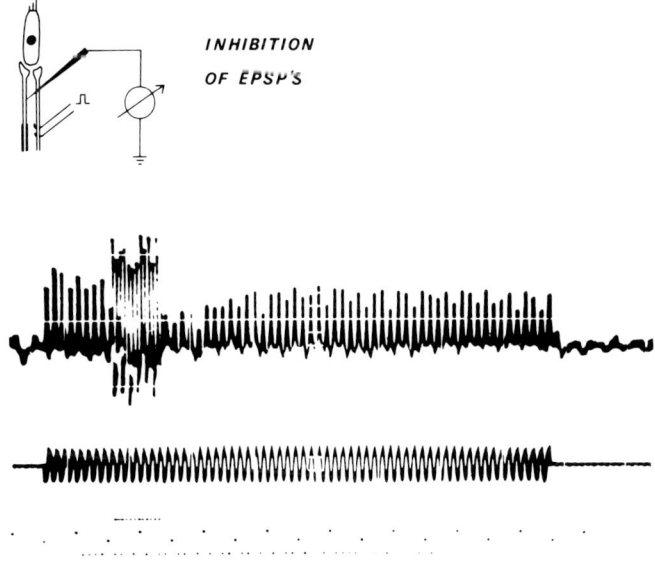

Fig. 11 Excitatory postsynaptic potentials in an afferent terminal are reduced in amplitude by stimulation of efferent nerve fibers. Stimulus pulses are picked up as an artifact by the recording electrode.

vary with the level of membrane potential as seen in Fig. 12. It gets smaller as the resting potential is approached. Although these potential changes developed spontaneously, and not as a consequence of potential displacement by current injection, this may indicate that the reversal potential of the IPSP is close to the resting potential of the cell. In other systems it is known that inhibitory impulses may produce no change in the membrane potential of a cell, or they may produce hyperpolarization or even depolarization depending on the direction in which the membrane potential is displaced (Kuffler and Eyzaguirre, 1955). Inhibition may be seen, with or without a potential change, as a result of shunting of current during the decrease of cell resistance. This implies that in hair cells, the release of a neurochemical transmitter at the sensory synapse is related to current flow across the presynaptic membrane (Fig. 13). The spontaneous afferent discharge can also be inhibited by efferent stimulation and so

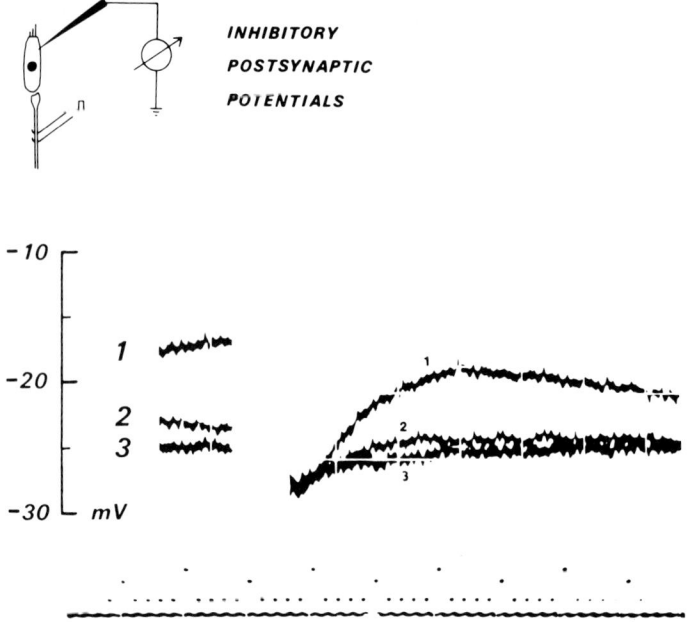

Fig. 12   The size of the inhibitory postsynaptic potential varies with the level of membrane potential.

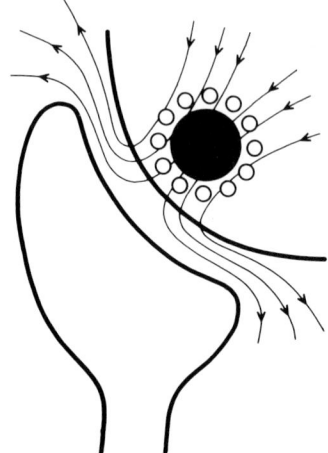

Fig. 13   Quanta of transmitter substance may be released at the afferent synapse as a result of current flow across the presynaptic membrane.

spontaneous activity may be due to a constant flow of current through the hair cell in the nonstimulated state. This is supported by experiments with gentamicin, which has a toxic effect on the membrane of the sensory hairs. When applied to the lumen of the lateral line canal gentamicin blocks spontaneous activity in afferent nerve fibers as well as evoked activity (Flock and Wersäll, 1973).

The shunting action of the efferent synapse appears to cause an increased current flow through the hair cell, because the receptor potential (and the externally recorded microphonic potential) is increased during the IPSP.

It was observed earlier in this paper that membrane potential and specific membrane resistance in hair cells are relatively low. It is possible that the apical membrane of hair cells has a relatively high conductance in the resting state and allows inward flow of current, so that the cell is in a state of partial depolarization, and afferent transmitter is continuously released (Fig. 14). When efferent fibers are active the resistance of the postsynaptic

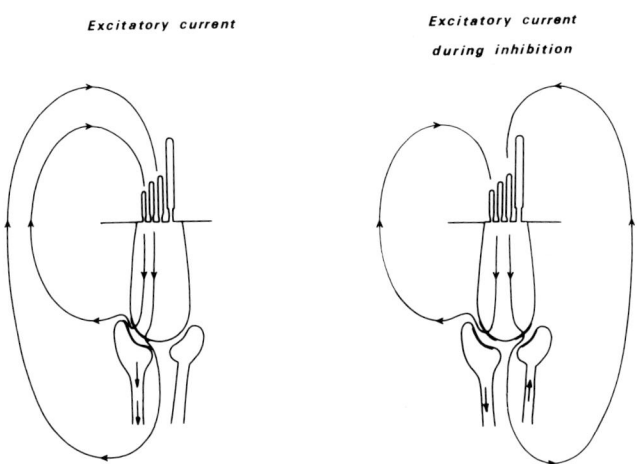

Fig. 14 This diagram illustrates the hypothesis of how efferent nerve fibers cause inhibition of afferent nerve excitation by shunting of excitatory current.

membrane at the efferent synapse is decreased and part of the excitatory current is shunted away from the afferent synapse which is thus inhibited. The mechanism by which efferent fibers exert their inhibitory influence is thus by reducing the release of excitatory transmitter at the afferent synapse.

9. The development of hair cells and nerve connections

The preparation

Tadpoles of the amphibian urodele Ambystoma mexicanum (axolotl) have a translucent tail which contains epidermal lateral line organs. These can be studied in detail in anesthetized living animals in an experimental chamber constructed of a large objective glass with perspex walls. The animals, which are 3-6 cm long, have external gills and are immersed in water containing 0.03 % tricaine methanesulfonate (MS 222, Sandoz). They respire by diffusion and survive without harm for several hours. The tail is held by insect pins connected to pieces of iron which are held by strips of magnetic plastic on either side of the trough. The organs are viewed in transmitted light in a Zeiss photo microscope with differential interference contrast (Nomarski optics). A 40 x water immersion objective with a working distance of 1.6 mm gives high resolution and ample space for manipulation.

In vivo observations

In favorable situations hair cells, supporting cells, and nerve fibers can be studied in considerable detail (Jørgensen and Flock, 1973). When the focus is at the level of the sensory epithelium the sensory hair bundles of individual hair cells can be distinguished (Fig. 15 a). Also, a long and slender kinocilium is seen to extend beyond the bundle of sterocilia. At deeper levels the nucleae are seen (Fig. 15 b), and innervating nerve fibers can be identified (Fig. 15 c).

In the cytoplasm below the hair cell nucleus, round bodies are present just inside the cell membrane (Fig. 15 d). When observed over a period of hours these bodies change their relative positions. They are probably the presynaptic dense bodies which are present at each afferent synapse, but this needs confirmation by electron microscopy.

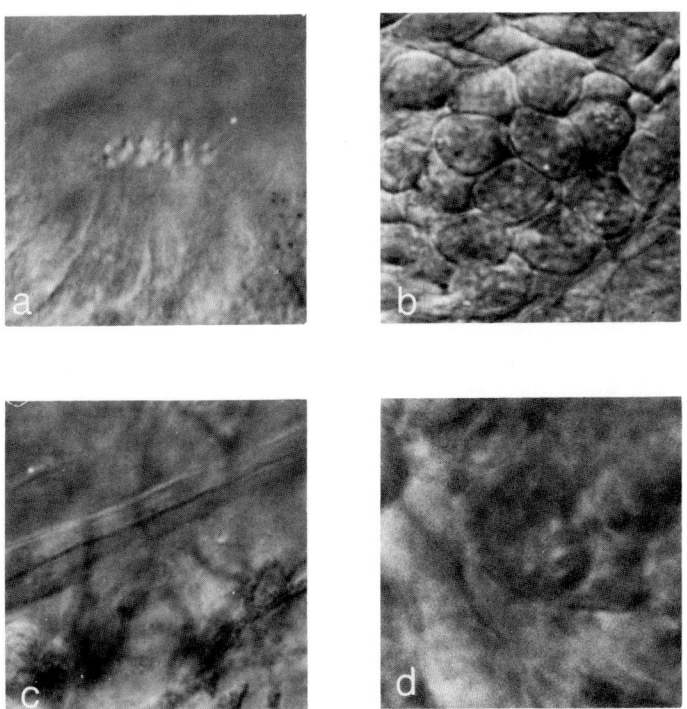

Fig. 15 Hair cells and their innervating nerve fibers can be observed in considerable detail in vivo in epidermal lateral line organs in the translucent tail of salamander tadpoles.

Development of new organs

If the tail is amputated in salamander tadpoles a new tail grows out. During the process of regeneration new lateral line organs develop in the epidermis and after 3-5 weeks a row of organs is seen, all in various stages of development, with the very first stage of development close to the growing tip of the tail and more mature organs close to the point of original sectioning (Speidel, 1947). The progress of development has been studied with the above mentioned technique and organs in various stages of development have been taken for electron microscopy (Flock <u>et al.</u> 1973a). Coincident with the appearance of a nerve growth cone above the basement membrane, cells in the epidermis arrange themselves like cloves in an orange around the point of entrance. Later, synaptic bodies surrounded by vesicles appear in one or a few of these cells, not necessarily in contact with the nerve process but also freely in the cytoplasm.

At the apical ends of these cells a vacuole forms intercellularly, which houses a minute pre-cupula. The centrioles migrate towards the apical end; from one of them a kinocilium develops and behind it primitive stereocilia form, their formation coinciding with the appearance of microtubules in the cytoplasm. Finally, the cupula grows out into the surrounding water when the epidermal cells which overlie it degenerate and are expelled. During continued growth mitosis is frequently seen in peripheral supporting cells but not in hair cells.

The arrival of a nerve growth cone coincides in time with the beginning of differentiation of the epithelial cells. This does not necessarily imply that the development of an organ is induced by the nerve fibers. In fact, Thornhill (1972) has evidence that differentiation of the hair cells in the otocyst of the lamprey precedes the arrival of nerve fibers. However, nerve fibers are in the vicinity, as is the case in the fowl otocyst (Friedmann, 1969) and the developing organ of Corti (Nakai and Hilding, 1968). It has been reported by Speidel (1947) that new organs may develop in regenerating tails where the lateral line nerve is prevented from regrowth by continued sectioning. A number of experiments were performed in an attempt to repeat these results.

In several cases where new organs had been formed, electron microscopy showed that the hair cells were in fact innervated. The lateral line nerve is difficult to localize in small animals and some fibers may have escaped sectioning. However, later experiments have been successful in that new organs have been developed without an innervation. The reason for our continued attempts has been to answer the question of whether normal hair cells can develop in organs which have not had contact with the nervous system, and, if so, whether these cells are able to orient themselves in two opposite directions as in normal organs.

In several tadpoles the tail was amputated and a segment of the lateral line nerve on both sides was taken out through an incision just behind the front limb. Regrowth of the nerve was prevented by repeated operations during the weeks the tail took to regenerate. New organs developed in these tails but they were not as frequent and were spaced at greater intervals than normal organs. Electron microscopy has shown that these organs have completely normal hair cells except in one respect; they completely lack innervating nerve endings (Fig. 16). This has been

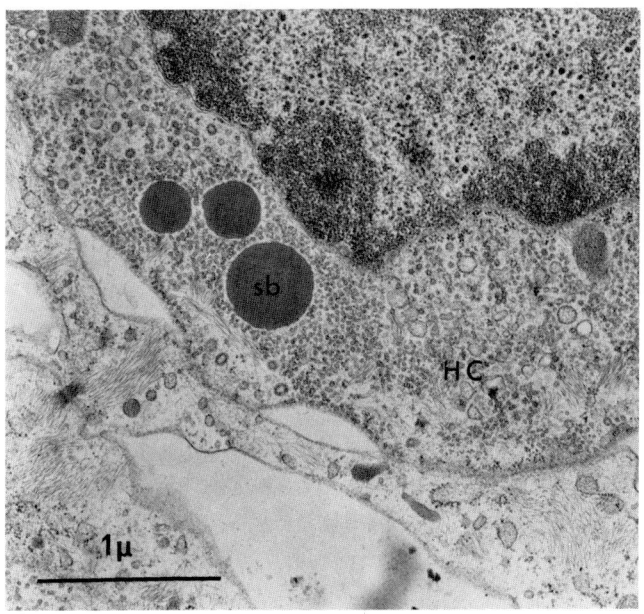

Fig. 16 Hair cells (HC) can develop without contact with innervating nerve fibers. In their basal end are presynaptic bodies (SB) surrounded by synaptic vesicles.

confirmed by sections at different levels in a plane parallel to the surface of the skin. In the basal part of these hair cells a large number of synaptic bodies surrounded by vesicles are freely distributed in the cytoplasm. Cross sections through sensory hair

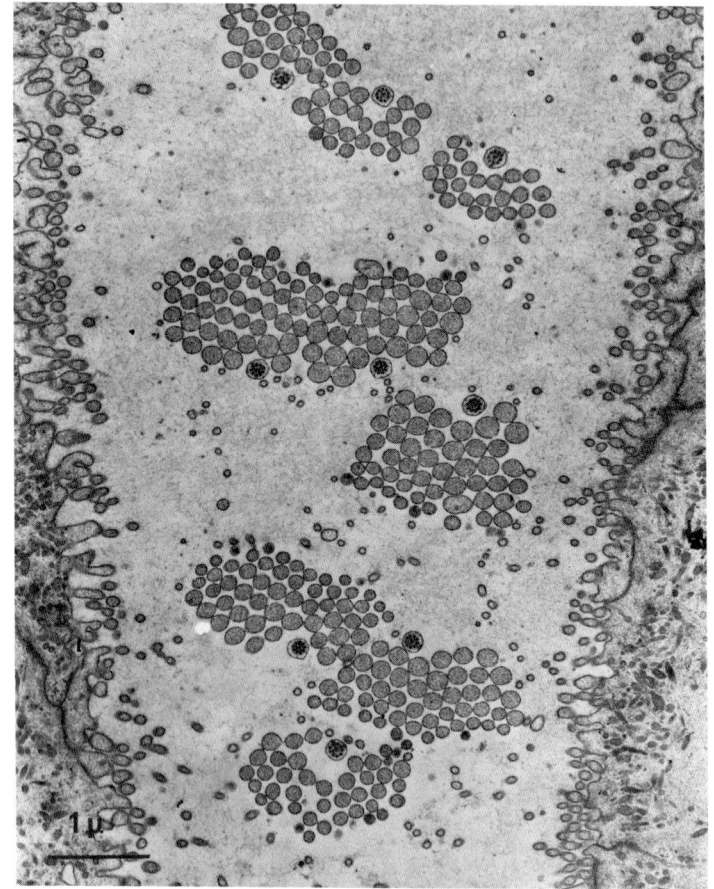

Fig. 17 Hair cells in lateral line organs which develop without contact with the central nervous system are capable of arranging themselves in proper double orientation, as seen here in cross-sections through the sensory hair bundles.

bundles reveal a perfectly normal double orientation (Fig. 17).

It is concluded from these results that the development of normal hair cells in lateral line organs does not depend on the presence of afferent or efferent nerve fibers in the vicinity of the developing organ, which has the capacity of autonomous differentiation and spacial orientation. Inherited deafness and vestibular dysfunction, which includes malformation of receptor cells, are therefore probably not to be blamed on faulty innervation but rather on genetic defects in the hair cells themselves.

Acknowledgements

This work has been supported by grants from the Swedish Medical Research Council (14X-2461), the King Gustaf V Memorial Fund and the Funds of the Karolinska Institute. J. Mørup Jørgensen was supported by the Danish Research Council. Ian J. Russell was supported by a European Program Research Fellowship from the Royal Society and a fellowship from Magdalene College, Cambridge. We thank Mrs. Marie-Louise Spångberg for finding marked cells, Hugo Broström and Tore Engberg for valuable technical assistance.

References

Dallos, P. (1968). On the negative potential within the organ of Corti. J. Acoust. Soc. Amer. 44, 818-819.

Fex, J. (1962). Auditory activity in centrifugal and centripetal cochlear fibres of the cat. Acta Physiol. Scand. Suppl. 189.

Fex, J. (1967). Efferent inhibition in the cochlea related to hair cell D.C. activity: Study of postsynaptic activity of the crossed olivocochlear fibres in the cat. J. Acoust. Soc. Amer. 41, 666-675.

Flock, Å. (1965). Electron microscopic and electrophysiological studies on the lateral line canal organ. Acta Otolaryngol. Suppl. 199, 1-90.

Flock, Å. (1971). The lateral line organ mechanoreceptors. In: Fish Physiology (W.S. Hoar and D.J. Randall, eds.). Vol. V, pp. 241-263. Academic Press, New York.

Flock, Å., and Russell, I.J. (1973a). The postsynaptic action of efferent fibres in the lateral line organ of the burbot Lota lota. (In preparation.)

Flock, Å., and Russell, I.J. (1973b). Efferent nerve fibres: postsynaptic action on hair cells. Science (Submitted).

Flock, Å., and Wersäll, J. (1973). The effect of gentamicin on single unit activity in the lateral line organ. (In preparation).

Flock, Å., Flock, B., and Jörgensen, M. (1973a). The ultrastructure of developing lateral line organs in the salamander Ambystoma mexicanum. (In preparation).

Flock, Å., Jörgensen, M., and Russell, I.J. (1973b). Passive electrical properties of hair cells and supporting cells in the lateral line canal organ. Acta Otolaryngol. (Submitted).

Friedmann, I. (1969). The innervation of the developing fowl embryo otocyst in vivo and in vitro. Acta Otolaryngol. 67, 224-238.

Furukawa, T., and Ishii, Y. (1967). Neurophysiological studies on hearing in gold fish. J. Neurophysiol. 30, 1377-1403.

Hama, K. (1965). Some observations on the fine structure of the lateral line organ of the Japanese sea eel, Lyncozymba nystromi. J. Cell Biol. 24, 193-210.

Harris, G.G., Frishkopf, L., and Flock, Å. (1970). Receptor potentials from hair cells of the lateral line. Science 167, 76-79.

Jörgensen, M., and Flock, Å. (1973). In vivo studies on the development of lateral line sense organs in the regenerating tail of the salamander Ambystoma mexicanum. (In preparation).

Kaneko, A., and Hashimoto, H. (1967). Recording site of the single cone response determined by an electrode marking technique. Vision Res. 7, 847-851.

Katz, B. (1966). Nerve, muscle and synapse (G. Wald, ed). McGraw-Hill, New York and London.

Klinke, R., and Schmidt, C.L. (1970). Efferent influence on the vestibular organ during active movements of the body. Pflügers Arch. ges. Physiol. 318, 352-353.

Kuffler, S.W., and Eyzaguirre, C. (1955). Synaptic inhibition in an isolated nerve cell. J. Gen. Physiol. 39, 155-184.

Llinas, R., and Precht, W. (1969). The inhibitory vestibular efferent system and its relation to the cerebellum in the frog. Exp. Brain Res. 9, 16-29.

Nakai, Y., and Hilding, D. (1968). Cochlear development. Acta Otolaryngol. 66, 369-385.

Payton, B.W., Bennett, M., and Pappas, G. (1969). Permeability and structure of junctional membranes at an electrotonic synapse. Science 166, 1641-1643.

Russell, I.J. (1968). Influence of efferent fibres on a receptor Nature (London) 219, 177-178.

Russell, I.J. (1971). The role of efferent fibres in the lateral line system of Xenopus laevis. J. Exp. Biol. 54, 621-641.

Sohmer, H.S., Peake, W.T., and Weiss, T.F. (1971). Intracochlear potential recorded with micropipets. I. Correlations with micropipet location. J. Acoust. Soc. Amer. 50, 572-586.

Speidel, C.C. (1947). Correlated studies of sense organs and nerves of the lateral line in living frog tadpoles. I. Regeneration of denervated organs. J. Comp. Neurol. 87, 29-55.

Stretton, A.O.W., and Kravitz, E.A. (1968). Neuronal geometry: Determination with a technique of intracellular dye injection. Science 162, 132-134.

Tasaki, K., Tsukahara, Y., Ito, S., Wayner, M.J., and Yu, W.Y. (1968). A simple direct and rapid method for filling microelectrodes. Physiol. Behav. 3, 1009-1010.

Thornhill, R.A. (1972). The development of the
    labyrinth of the lamprey (<u>Lampetra fluviatilis</u>
    Linn. 1758). <u>Proc. Roy. Soc. B.</u> <u>181</u>, 175-198.

DISCUSSION

PFEIFFER: I am curious about the action of the efferent fibers. Some demonstrations of inhibition show no time delay when you look at inhibition in, say, single cochlear nerve fibers under two-tone stimulation. In this type of inhibition there is thus no time delay which would allow the efferent system to work. Is that the inhibition you talk about?

FLOCK: Well, two-tone inhibition could not be due to a neural inhibition.

PFEIFFER: Your data show that the intracellular receptor potential which would originate in the spiral-ganglion dendrites is essentially sinusoidal in shape, and that there is no form of a rectification taking place across that synaptic function. Is that a correct interpretation?

FLOCK: I dare not say anything about linearity or non-linearity on the intracellular recordings. It is quite difficult to maintain cells for a long time and my data so far are qualitative and not quantitative. As a cell is penetrated you see part of the extra cellular current too.

PFEIFFER: Is there any indication that there is a rectification that takes place?

FLOCK: Let me say that we could not detect any impedance change in the experiments on electrical excitability when the membrane potential of the cell is changed. But since in this system fundamentals cancel in the external microphonic potential, and we are still left with a second order harmonic distortion product there is certainly rectification in the input output function of the hair cell.

SPOENDLIN: Do the efferents in a lateral line organ exclusively synapse with the sensory cells or do they also synapse with the dendrites?

FLOCK: In the lateral line canal organ of the burbot, with which I have worked, I have never seen synapses between the efferents and the afferent dendrites. I have looked at hundreds of sections. But in the xenopus toad you do find synapses between the afferent and efferents and we started off by working on the xenopus toad with the efferents. This work, I should mention, is done together with Ian Russell[+]. We could not see any intracellular IPSP in the hair cells, maybe because inhibition often takes place on the afferent dendrite.

FEX: I think you said that the maximum size of the receptor potential was 1-2 millivolts. What was the size of the stimulation and what is the size of natural stimulation?

FLOCK: These experiments were performed with the canal opened and it is not exposed to a natural stimulus. The threshold as determined behaviorally by Cuthers is about 25 Å. I would rather instead of absolute values refer to the threshold for a single afferent unit. The amplitude I have used is about 30 dB above threshold for afferent neurons.

KIANG: Does stimulation of the efferent nerve fibers depress spontaneous activity?

FLOCK: Yes, it does.

BRUGGE: What is the length of the non-myelinated portion of the efferent?

FLOCK: I do not know. When we have been in the nerve

fibers, we have injected a dye into them so we see
the terminal - the stain spread - as the branching
tree. When we then look electronmicroscopically at
the myelin sheath where it passes through the basement membrane we see that it travels for part of the
distance inside the sensory epithelium and then it
loses the myelin sheath so that the terminal part
travels for some distance. For a particular recording
I do not know how long the non-myelinated portion is
because it varies from one terminal to another. What
has to be done now is dye marking for electron microscopy, and this can be done, to really get correlation between neural function and anatomy.

PFALTZ: What was the spike rate in the efferent fibers under normal conditions if the fish was moving?

FLOCK: If you are very careful with your operation
the efferents should be silent. They are silent or
they have a very low spike rate, something like 1 or
2 per second. But if you get a small blood clot on
the cerebellum or in the bottom of the fourth ventricle they increase firing. If you cut the motor nerves, and the sensory input with it, they become tonic
and you get spontaneous activity of up to 60/sec.

MICHELSEN: Do you think that the amplitude of the
microphonics is so large that they can act as receptor potentials? What is the threshold of these
synapses?

FLOCK: Katz and Miledi (1967) and Kusamo, Livengood
and Werman (1967) have shown that they are in the
order of a couple of millivolts and it depends on to
what extent the sensory synapse is exposed to this
voltage or what the resultant current flow is. In
electroreceptors as Dr. Suga has shown you have very
high sensitivity and it takes very little depolarization to produce transmission.

FEX: Do you see spread of stain from one cell to another?

FLOCK: No. Only when the electrode has passed through a cell and it is damaged as you saw, but no gap junctions, no tight junctions.

+) Ian Russell, School of Biology, University of Sussex, Falmer, Brighton, England.

References

Kuiper, J. (1967). Frequency characteristics and functional significance of the lateral line organ. In: Lateral Line Detectors, (P. Cahn, ed.), pp. 105-117. Indiana Univ. Press, Bloomington, Indiana.

Katz, B. and Miledi, R. (1967). Tetrodotoxin and neuromuscular transmission. Proc. Roy. Soc. B. 167, 8-22.

Kusano, K., Livengood, D. and Werman, R. (1967). Correlation of transmitter release with membrane properties of the presynaptic fiber of the squid giant synapse. J. Gen. Physiol. 50, 2579-2601.

Suga, N. (1967). Electrosensitivity of specialized and ordinary lateral line organs of the electric fish, Gymnotus carapo. In: Lateral Line Detectus, (P. Cahn, ed.), pp. 395-409. Indiana Univ. Press, Bloomington, Indiana.

THE IONIC RECEPTIVE MECHANISM IN THE ACOUSTICO-LATERALIS SYSTEM

Yasuji Katsuki

Tsurumi University
Tsurumi, Yokahama
Japan

1. Introduction

Since my electrophysiological studies started on the auditory system more than twenty years ago, there have been two mysteries for me. During the long course of my studies, clues to these mysteries have emerged, and this paper will be mainly concerned with them. One of the mysteries is, why potassium ions play the principal role in the cochlea of higher animals while to most other sense organs sodium ions are known to be indispensable. The other one is why the cochlear nerve fibers are so active spontaneously even in a sound-proofed room. In other systems the peripheral fibers are usually silent in non-stimulus conditions. Later I found that in the acoustico-lateralis system most peripheral nerve fibers are provided with active spontaneous discharges even in the quiet airy or aqueous environment.

I was not able to solve these two questions until quite recently. Someone said that the origin of the spontaneous discharge in the sensory afferent fibers might be the thermal noises at the very endings of the nerve fiber. But there was no direct evidence.

In order to disclose the neural mechanism of hearing I have been accustomed to make experiments from phylogenetical points of view, because such an approach, I believe, is the best way to study the complicated neural mechanism. I began my experimental studies on the lateral-line system of teleosts. At the beginning I planned to record the electrical responses of single fibers of the lateral-line nerve of a bony fish and succeeded in finding the characteristic nature of responses of those nerve fibers to various mechanical stimulations applied on the body surface, that is, water flow or vibratory stimuli with different frequencies applied to the lateral-line pores. The fishes used were marine and fresh water fish such as the eel, the catfish and other teleosts. There was a one to one relationship between the nerve fiber discharges and vibratory stimulation in a relatively low frequency, a different pattern of responses in thick and thin nerve fibers and so on. We found further that the lateral-line canal organs were easily stimulated by direct, alternating and slowly rising electric currents (Katsuki et al., 1950a, 1950b, Katsuki and Yoshino, 1952). Similar features were also observed later in the neural responses of higher animals, cats and monkeys, when I worked on their auditory system with my collaborators, although the frequency range was quite different in aquatic and terrestrial animals. From those experimental results it can be said that from the auditory system of mammals to the lateral-line system of aquatic animals, there may be a straight functional relationship in terms of mechanoreception (Katsuki et al., 1958, 1961).

However when we worked on the lateral-line nerve fibers of a shark in Hawaii with the intention of revealing the receptive mechanism of the lateral-line canal organ, we happened to encounter nerve fibers which did not respond easily to mechanical stimulation, namely mild touches on the end organ with a soft brush. We have had much experience in isolating single lateral-line nerve fibers in various species of teleosts and we know that most of those nerve fibers exhibit active random spontaneous discharges and a typical discharge pattern of responses to soft mechanical stimuli applied to the end organ. From such a change of discharge pattern by an applied stimulation it was confirmed that each single nerve fiber has a very restricted response area of about 1 or 2 cm in length along the lateral-line. By histological studies it has been made clear that between two adjacent lateral-line pores, namely on each body muscle segment, there is a single end-organ, i.e. a single neuromast in the canal (Katsuki et al., 1970, Katsuki and Yoshino, 1952).

In the case of a shark the exposure of the intact lateral-line nerve was not as easy as in the teleosts due to the tough connective tissues surrounding the nerve and the complicated relationship between the nerve and segmental muscles.

We noticed in the shark that many of the lateral-line nerve fibers exposed did not show a typical response to delivered mechanical stimulation. This phenomenon was quite unusual to us. We had not encountered a similar case before that time in any of a variety of teleosts. However we were then notified by Drs. Tester and Kendall (1967) of Hawaii University that in sharks many pit organs, i.e. free neuromasts on the dorsal body surface send afferent fibers to the lateral-line nerve, a branch of the vagus nerve (Fig. 1).

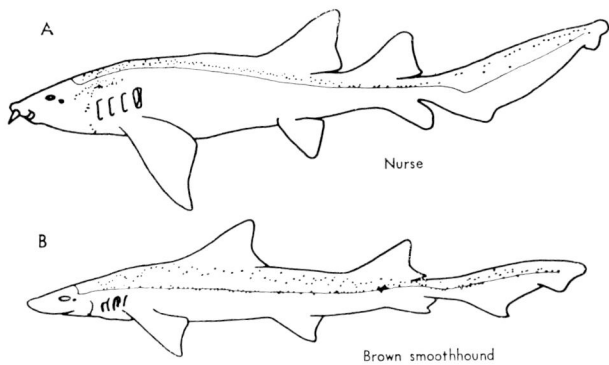

Fig. 1   Lateral distribution of free neuromasts (pit organs) of nurse and brown smoothhound shark. The location of each pit organ is indicated by a dot. Different species have different distributions (Tester and Nelson, 1963).

I tried a chemical stimulation instead of a mechanical stimulation, by pouring a small amount of sea water on the pit organ, the location of which was already identified. This trial was suggested by earlier works of Murray (1962) and also Lowenstein and Ishiko (1962) on Ampulla Lorenzini. Sea water and 1 M NaCl solution were poured over a region innervated by a single nerve fiber from which a recording was being made.

To our surprise a fiber which did not respond beforehand to brief mechanical stimulation did respond readily to chemical stimulation while a fiber which easily responded to mechanical stimulation did not show any response at all to salt solutions. Then we concluded that the lateral-line nerve is composed functionally of two kinds of fibers. One innervating the lateral-line canal neuromasts responds only to mechanical stimulation while the other innervating the pit organs located mostly on the dorsal body surface shows a response to salt solutions, but not much response to mechanical stimuli. By further studies it was found that the pit organ can respond to mechanical stimulation of high intensity, but not to brief stimulation. This kind of chemical response at the lateral-line organs, especially at free neuromasts, has been confirmed not only in sharks, but also in teleosts and in amphibians (Katsuki et al., 1970, 1971, Onoda and Katsuki 1972).

Now we think that this chemical reception at the end-organ, which used to be considered a pure mechanoreceptor, plays a very important role in mechanical reception. The duality of the end-organ function is not mutually independent, but the complementarity of these two functions itself may be the real mechanism at this receptor organ. The following details show the process by which we reached such a conclusion.

2. Materials and Methods

All experiments have been designed from the phylogenetical point of view. Animals used in the serial experiments are seen in table 1.

Animals with gills were usually fixed on a board after being anesthetized lightly with MS 222 (0.03~0.05 gr/liter). The gills were irrigated with aerated sea or fresh water through a mouth piece and the amount of water delivered was carefully controlled. Most parts of the body surface were covered with a wet gauze, kept moist by salt or fresh water. When the lateral-line nerve was exposed by cutting the skin near the operculum where the nerve usually runs just beneath the skin, using a pair of well sharpened tweezers or needles, the distal cut end of the lateral-line nerve was separated under a binocular microscope into very small bundles of a few fibers. If necessary, this small bundle was further divided un-

EXPERIMENTAL ANIMALS

CLASS	COMMON NAME	SCIENTIFIC NAME	HABITAT
Cyclostome	lamprey	*Entosphenus japonicus*	fresh water
Elasmobranchs	sharks	*Ginglymostoma cirratum* *Heterodontus francisci* *Triakis semifasciata* *Mustelus californicus* *Mustelus manazo*	marine
Teleosts	mullet	*Mugil cephalus*	marine
	carp	*Cyprinus carpio*	fresh water
	catfish	*Ictalurus punctatus*	
	eel	*Anguilla japonica*	euryhaline
	mullet	*Mugil cephalus*	
Amphibia	bullfrog (tadpole)	*Rana catesbeiana*	
	African clawed toad	*Xenopus laevis*	fresh water
	mud puppy	*Necturus maculosus*	

Table 1. Animals used in serial experiments.

til one or two fibers were obtained. When those fibers were intact, spontaneous discharges were observed on the oscilloscope through a conventional preamplifier and high gain RC-coupled amplifier. The electrodes used were a chlorinated silver wire, over which a small nerve bundle or individual fibers were looped and a large Ag-AgCl indifferent electrode placed against the side of the fish's wet body.

Most records were registered on a strip chart recorder through an electronic rate meter. By this device the impulse frequency of nerve discharges at a given time interval was registered on a paper, thus making possible observation of change in the impulse rate during experimentation. The advantage of this method is the precise computation of the temporal and sequential change in the discharge rate without delay (Katsuki et al., 1970).

In the case of sharks the lateral-line nerve runs

differently from other fishes. The nerve runs deeply along the vertebral column so that the exposure of the nerve was performed at the tail region (Tester and Kendall, 1967).

In the case of adult Xenopus the lateral-line nerve runs just beneath the skin, so the skin was cut 5≃10 mm from the forelimb and the exposure of the nerve was easily done (Onoda and Katsuki, 1972).

3. Experimental Results

Here I will deal mainly with the neural responses to chemical stimulation. The pit organs of the shark showed responses only to a variety of monovalent cations with different grade, K^+ being the most effective. The order of effectiveness was K^+, $Rb^+ > Na^+$, $NH_4^+ > Cs^+$, Li^+. On the contrary divalent cations, e.g. Ca^{++} produced a suppressive effect. When a diluted Ca^{++} solution was applied with a monovalent cationic solution, e.g. with KCl or NaCl solution, the effect of Ca^{++} was to suppress the excitatory effect of K^+ or Na^+ quickly and drastically. Several minutes after repeated rinsing of the end-organ with sea water, however, the responses to K^+ or Na^+ solution returned completely to the original level (Katsuki et al., 1970); (Fig. 2, Fig. 3).

In the excitable cell membrane Ca^{++} is known to reduce the permeability of Na^+ and K^+. This phenomenon is explained by the supposition that Ca^{++} takes the place of Na^+ and K^+ in the cell membrane. Kusano also reported a similar suppressive Ca^{++} effect on the frog gustatory salt end-organ which is responsive to monovalent cations (Kusano, 1960).

Sr^{++} and Mg^{++} also produced suppressive effects on the end-organ against the stimulating effect of K^+ and Na^+. But their effects were much weaker than that of Ca^{++}. In contrast with other divalent cations Ba^{++} had a completely different effect on the end-organ. Neural discharges increased with diluted Ba^{++} solutions. However this stimulating effect was irreversible and may cause damage in some way to the receptor organ. Anions were found to be almost ineffective (Table 2).

Tetrodotoxin (10^{-6} gr/ml) also produced a suppressive effect on the K^+ or Na^+ or Rb^+ stimulation. Compared

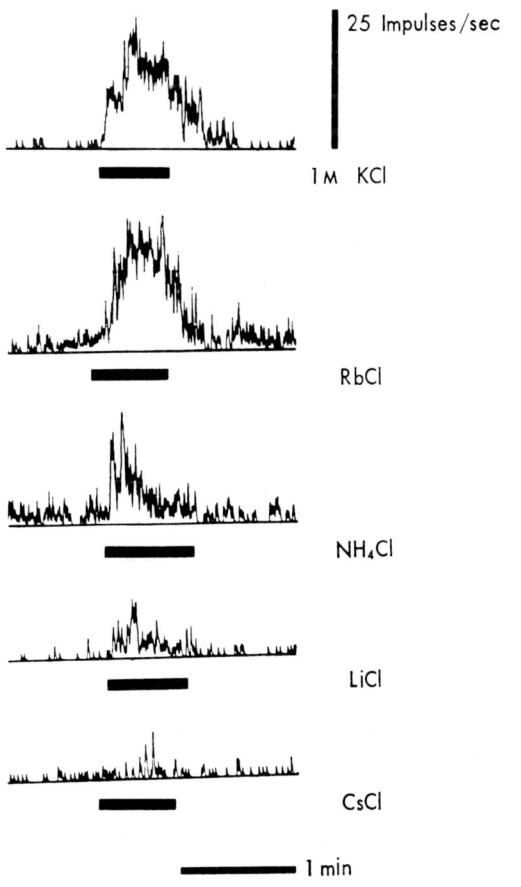

Fig. 2 Salt responses to various monovalent cations. Responses to Na⁺ were almost the same as those to NH$_4$. The ordinate shows the instantaneous average rate of nerve fiber discharges. The abscissa shows the time. A thin black bar indicates 1 minute. The thick black bar below each trace indicates the duration of salt application. At the right end of the bar the end-organ was rinsed thoroughly with sea water. Material: <u>Ginglymostoma cirratum</u> (nurse shark) (Katsuki <u>et al</u>., 1970).

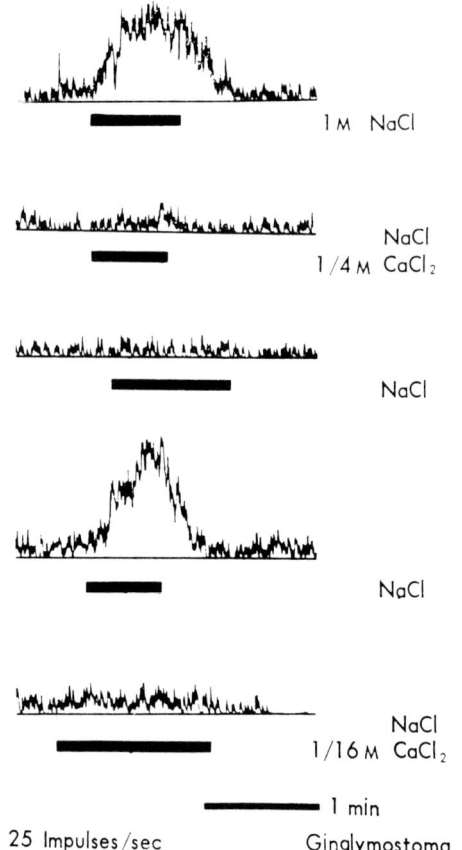

Fig. 3 Inhibitory effect of Ca ions on monovalent cationic responses when they were applied together with or before monovalent cation application. Uppermost trace: the control response to 1 M NaCl solution. Second: the suppressed response with application of the mixed solution of 3/4 M NaCl and 1/4 M $CaCl_2$. Third: the inhibited response to 1 M NaCl solution, 3 minutes after obtaining the second trace. Fourth: the complete recovery of the response. Fifth: reappearance of inhibition with 1/16 M $CaCl_2$ mixture with 15/16 M NaCl solution. Material: Nurse shark (Katsuki et al., 1970).

EFFECTIVENESS OF CHEMICALS

CHEMICALS	EFFECTS	CHEMICALS	EFFECTS
NaCl	++	KCl	+++
$NaNO_3$	++	RbCl	+++
$NaHCO_3$	+	NH_4Cl	++
Na_2SO_4	++	NaCl	++
Na-glutamate	++	LiCl	+
Na-propionate	+	CsCl	+
$NaCH_3SO_4$	+	Choline-Cl	−
$NaC_2H_5SO_4$	+		
Acids	−	$CaCl_2$	− −
Sugar	−	$MgCl_2$	−
Quinine	−	$SrCl_2$	−

Table 2

to the Ca^{++} effect, suppression caused by tetrodotoxin is different in regard to the latency. Both the suppressive and the recovery processes observed were slow.

Cocaine (10^{-3} gr/ml) had no effect. No change was observed in neural discharges with 1 M NaCl solution in which cocaine was dissolved. This is evidence that the salt solution applied to the receptor organ is effective at the receptor cell itself and not at the nerve fiber. Sugar was ineffective and quinine rather suppressive, in 0.005~0.003 M solution of quinine sulphate. H^+ was also found to be suppressive. Distilled water reduced the neural discharge rate and 1 M sucrose solution in distilled water stopped the discharge completely so that sugar or glucose was used to keep the isotonicity of test solutions. Thus the pit organ did not give the response typical of the mammalian taste bud. This organ was considered to be a kind of simple salt detector. The effect of tetraethyl-ammonium chloride (TEA.Cl), which is considered to be a blocking agent of potassium permeability of the cell membrane, was not constant. In this case dissociated $N(C_2H_6)_4^+$ can stimulate the membrane so that this chemical agent may not block potassium permeability of the receptor cell membrane.

Electrical stimulation was also performed. For this experiment a particular region was chosen. At the mandibular region three different lateral-line organs are located: ampullary organs, canal organs and pit organs could be distinguished by mechanical, chemical and electrical stimulation as shown in Table 3. By

RESULTS OF STIMULATION

Organ	Discharges		Threshold (Electrical)
	Mechanical (Touch)	Chemical (KCl)	
Canal	+ + +	—	1000 mV
Pit	+	+ + + **	100
Ampullary	+	+ + + **	10

** Proportional to concentration

Table 3 Responses of the canal, pit, and ampullary organs to three stimulations, mechanical, chemical, and electrical. Electrical threshold values are approximate.

the use of a small bipolar electrode (polar distance being a few mm) distinct differences were found among those three organs in regard to electrical stimulation. One polarity caused an increase of discharge while the opposite polarity its decrease. We were able to determine the threshold value for each end-organ.

During the process of this sort of experiment we occasionally found that many fibers showed burst discharges synchronized with respiratory gill movement. Then we noticed a remarkable increase of burst discharge upon application of a drop of K salt solution on the end-organ which had been known as a pit organ. Changes of impulse number could be counted in a

single burst with different concentrations of K salt
solution. The higher the concentration of K^+, the more
the impulses. A lowering of the electrical threshold
for the end-organ was also observed upon application
of more concentrated K salt solution. In the case of
ampullary or canal organ such a remarkable change was
never observed (Hashimoto and Katsuki, 1972).

This kind of finding may explain the extremely high
mechanosensitivity of the cochlea of a higher animal
by the increase of mechanosensitivity due to the increase of environmental K^+ concentration. The direct
measurement of the increase of mechanosensitivity was
performed in other animals.

Teleosts: In the teleosts similar results were obtained. However the situations were more complicated.
There were some differences between marine and fresh
water fish. We examined the responses of the lateral-
line nerve in several fishes. Generally speaking,
marine fish showed responses similar to the shark
with K^+ and Na^+ stimulation, while the fresh water
fish showed different responses. In marine fish the
effect of K^+ is much stronger than Na^+. The reason
for difference may be the abundance of Na^+ in the environment. On the other hand in the case of fresh
water fish, the differences of the effect between K^+
and Na^+ are not so great, though K^+ is always stronger
than Na^+ (Fig. 4).

Many fishes showed on their lateral-line nerve fibers
chemical responses similar to monovalent cationic
solutions as seen in the shark. However there are
exceptions. Catfish or loaches, which usually live in
muddy water showed **remarkable** differences (Fig. 5).

The effects of divalent cations were found to be not
suppressive but stimulating. The order of effectiveness was $Ca^{++}>Sr^{++}>Mg^{++}$. When Ca^{++} was stimulating,
the monovalent cations were also stimulating, but
less effective. Some fibers showed very high sensitivity to sodium glutamate, which elicited much larger
responses than NaCl solution of the same concentration. Ammonium specific fibers were also found, on
which K^+, Na^+, Rb^+ and TEA-Cl were ineffective. Some
other fibers were responsive to quinine. There were
almost no fibers which responded to sugar solutions.
In the cases described above, the end-organs may be

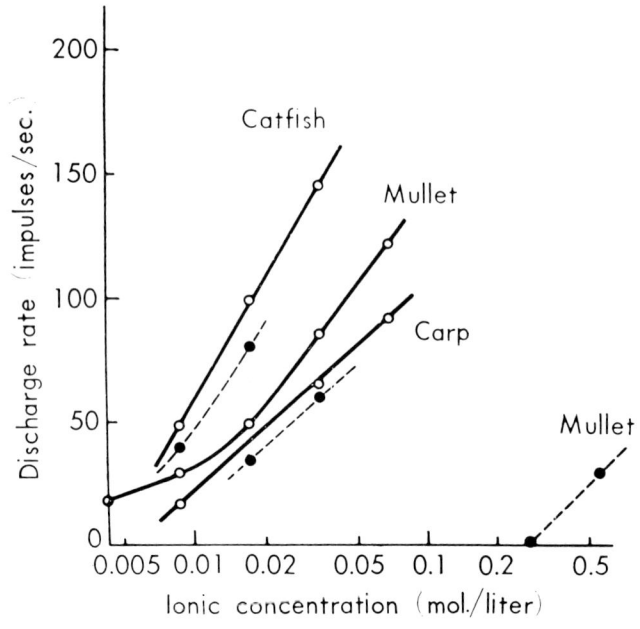

Fig. 4 Neuronal responses of several fishes to various concentrations of the applied salt solution. Ordinate: the impulse frequency of a single unit of the lateral-line nerve. Abscissa: the molar concentration of the applied salt solution (mole/liter). The solid line indicates the response characteristics to KCl solution. The broken line shows the response of the same nerve fiber to NaCl solution. Materials: the catfish (<u>Ictalurus punctatus</u>) and the carp (<u>Cyprinus carpio</u>) are fresh water fishes. The mullet (<u>Mugil cephalus</u>) is an euryhaline fish, which was raised in sea water. ──o── KCl ---o--- NaCl (Katsuki et al., 1971).

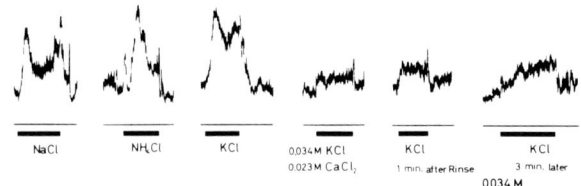

Fig. 5 Single unit responses of the lateral- (cont'd)

(Fig. 5, cont'd) line nerve of carp to monovalent cationic solutions (NaCl, NH$_4$Cl and KCl) and suppressive effects of Ca^{++} to K$^+$ responses, reversible after rinsing with fresh water.

said to be much more differentiated than in other fish (Katsuki et al., 1971); (Fig. 6).

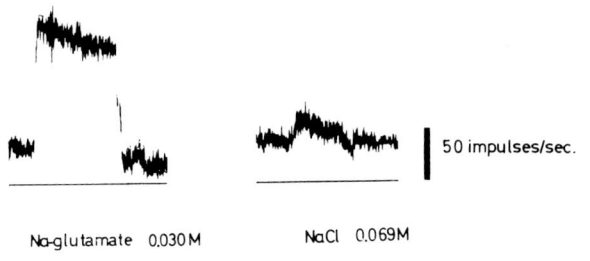

Fig. 6 Response pattern of a glutamate specific fiber in the lateral-line nerve of catfish. Right: the response to 0.069 M sodium chloride solution. Left: the response to 0.03 M sodium glutamate solution of the same endorgan. The concentration of Na$^+$ in the glutamate solution was less than a half of that of the sodium chloride solution, but the response to the former is much larger. (Katsuki et al., 1971).

In teleosts too, the canal neuromasts responded well to mechanical stimulation but not to chemical stimulation, while the free neuromasts and the pit organs responded well to chemical stimulation as well as mechanical stimulation, although there are very little structural differences between the canal and free neuromasts. The only differences so far observed are the amount of polysaccharides covering the surface of hairs (Hama, pers. comm.);(Fig. 7).

Histological studies on the flank skin of catfish showed there were many large and small pit organs and besides them many terminal buds as well. The structure of the terminal bud is extremely similar to that of the taste bud in the oral cavity (Herrick, 1903, Bardach and Atema, 1972). In this sense the variety of responses obtained from the lateral-line nerve fibers of catfish may be designated as the common chem-

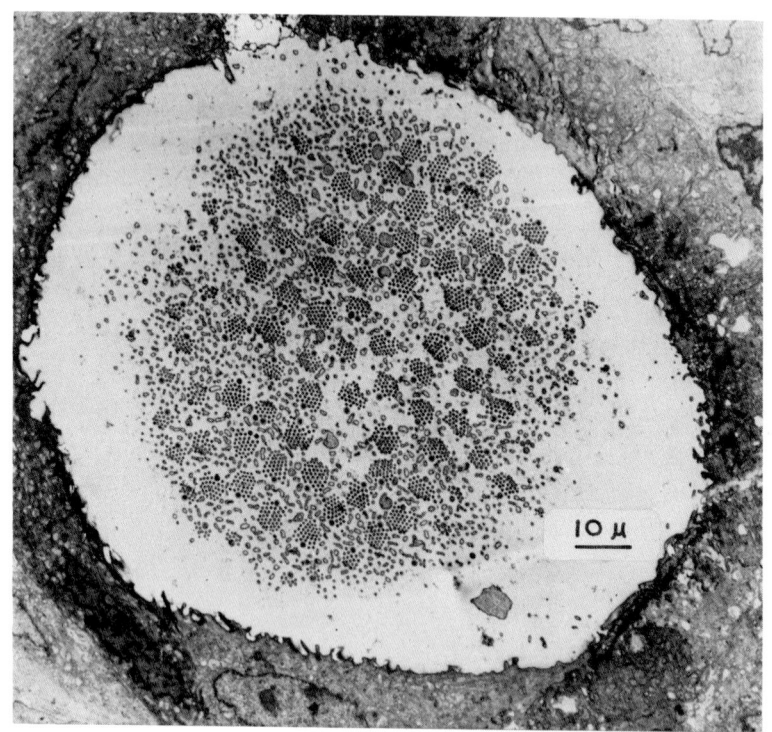

Fig. 7   Electronmicrogram of a pit organ of a sea eel (Astroconger myriaster). This pit organ is located more dorsally along the ordinary lateral-line, less numerous than the lateral-line pores. Arrangements of hair cells, the positional relationship of a kinocilium and stereocilia can be seen clearly. The number of hair cells are also able to be counted. By the courtesy of Prof. K. Hama.

ical sense or the external taste sense. A recent study of the lateral-line nerve showed that it is composed of the main lateral-line nerve and the accessory lateral-line nerve. The latter is composed of 3 branches; the dorsal, ventral and middle branches. They are the branches of the VIIth nerve, the facial nerve (Freihofer, 1963). From these results we concluded that on the flank skin there are two kinds of end-organs distributed diffusely; one is the lateral-line organ (neuromasts including the pit organ described by Hama, pers. comm.) and the other is the taste organ.

Morphologically it has been said that the skin taste organs are innervated by the accessory lateral-line nerve (VIIth nerve) while the canal organs are innervated by the vagal nerve. Several species of teleosts have been known to be provided with terminal buds on the skin surface, especially at the head region. However there are many fishes which have no terminal buds on the skin, but they have many free neuromasts that have been known to be mechanoreceptors. They are also sensitively responsive to chemical stimulation. In those cases only monovalent cations can stimulate the end-organ. The mullet is an example (Table 4).

CLASSIFICATION OF RESPONSES ON LATERAL-LINE NERVE FIBERS

TYPE	STIMULATION		EFFERENT SYSTEM	ENDORGANS
	MECHANICAL	CHEMICAL		
I	+	−	+	CANAL NEUROMASTS
II	+	+	+	FREE NEUROMASTS PIT ORGANS FREE STANDING NEUROMASTS
III	−	+	−	TERMINAL BUDS

Table 4.

Amphibia: Xenopus laevis is an example of an amphibian that has the lateral-line on the body surface for its whole life. The morphological structure of

the lateral-line organs of this animal has been
studied extensively (Flock, 1966). They are called
stitches which are groups of 4-5 end-organs with
cupular formations. Scanning electron microscopy
shows their surface structures very well (Fig. 8).

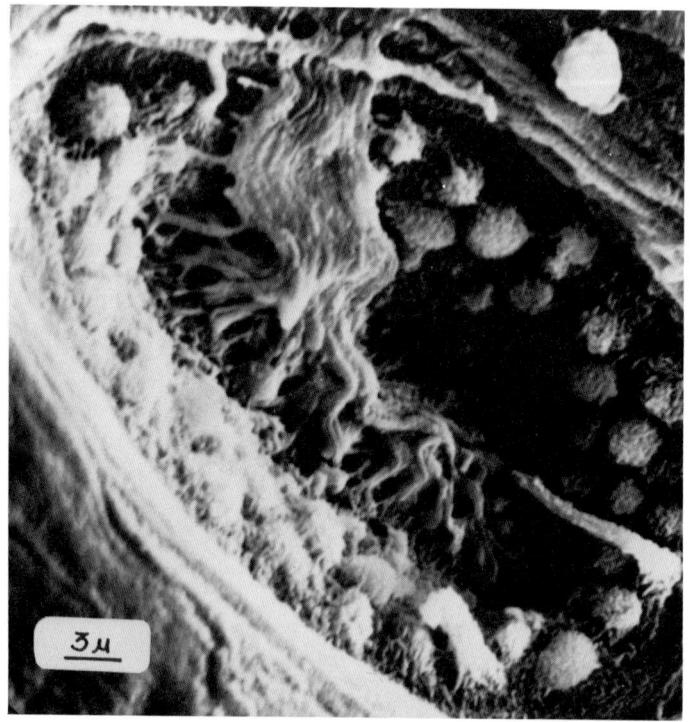

Fig. 8 Scanning electronmicrogram of a lateral-line
organ of <u>Xenopus laevis</u>. Hair cells located
at the center, surrounded by supporting cells,
form a cupola.

Chemical responses were recorded from the lateral-
line nerve fibers. The end-organs were responsive to
mono- and divalent cations. They responded to Na
glutamate most sensitively. In that case the glutamate anions were more effective than the Na cations.
The fact that K^+ produced stronger effects than Na^+
is also worthwhile noting. Sodium ions show very peculiar effects. When they are in diluted solutions,
the effect is rather suppressive. The lateral-line
nerve shows spontaneous discharges to fresh water
(pure water) and a diluted Na^+ solution suppresses

these spontaneous discharges. It is quite striking that the diluted solution (0.001~0.1 M) of NaCl suppressed the discharges. The suppressive effect of 0.05 M solution was the strongest. More concentrated solution than 0.2 M can stimulate the end-organ. In the case of K^+ solution this suppressive effect still exists but is very weak. Even a very diluted solution of K^+, e.g. 0.01 M solution, can stimulate the end-organ. Such a peculiar effect of Na^+ has also been seen on the taste organs of the frog which are innervated by the glossopharyngeal nerve (Fig. 9, Fig. 10).

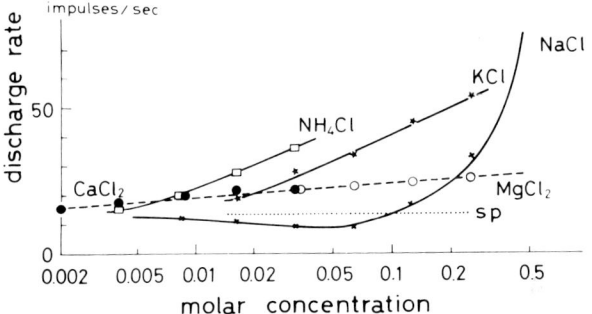

Fig. 9 Relationship between the discharge rate of a single lateral-line nerve fiber of Xenopus and concentrations of various mono- and divalent ionic salt solutions applied on an end-organ. All responses were obtained from the same nerve fiber. The ordinate shows the discharge rate of the nerve fiber and the abscissa gives the molar concentration of a salt solution. The thin dotted line (Sp) indicates the level of the spontaneous discharges. Note that the discharge rate with dilute NaCl solutions was lower than the spontaneous level (Onoda and Katsuki, 1972).

The fact that even in the rat the taste buds on the tongue which are innervated by the glossopharyngeal nerve showed a similar response type, was reported by Pfaffmann et al., (1967). According to their report the response type of the chorda tympani is different. In that case the sensitivity to Na^+ is much better than that to K^+. This means that at the tip of the tongue the sensitivity to Na^+ is much higher than to K^+.

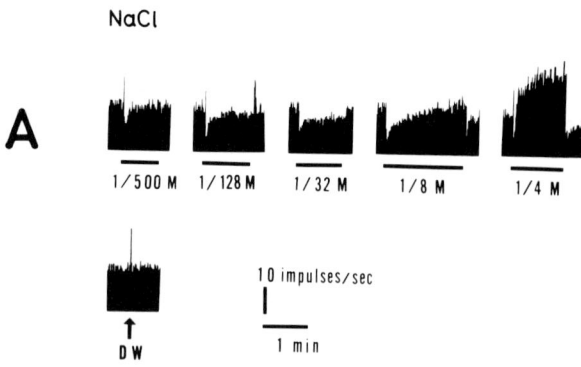

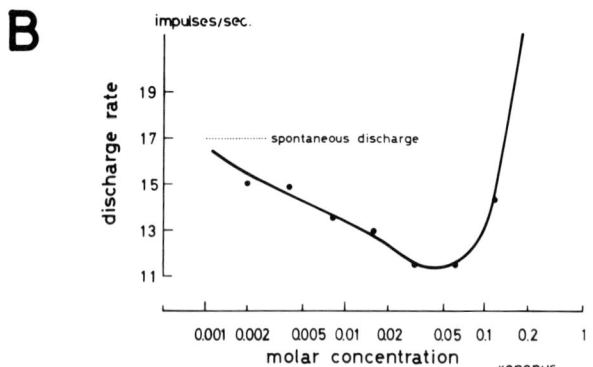

Fig. 10 Suppressive effects of diluted NaCl solutions on the spontaneous discharges of a single lateral-line nerve fiber. A: Rate meter records. Instantaneous discharge rate is shown by a vertical height. A thick horizontal bar below each trace shows the duration of the application of salt solution. The lower record shows the response to distilled water applied at the time indicated by an arrow. There is no tonic increase or decrease in the rate. Results shown in A are plotted in B. B: Rate of impulse discharges per second, averaged for the initial 30 sec. after application of NaCl solutions is shown. The diluted NaCl solution suppresses the spontaneous discharges   (cont'd)

(Fig. 10, cont'd) of the nerve fiber (Onoda and Katsuki, 1972).

In the case of tadpoles (Rana catesboiana and Xenopus laevis) which have lateral-line organs on the flank skin, chemical responses were also observed. In this animal the responses are rather simple, being mostly responses to monovalent cations, and Ca^{++} produced a suppressive effect on the K^+ effect. During the time of metamorphosis the tadpole loses its tail together with the lateral-line organs on it. Then skin taste receptors may disappear and the chemoreception does similarly, while on the other hand the tongue develops newly. The distribution of taste buds in the oral cavity is very similar to those in fish. It can be said that the taste sense on the skin disappears and appears in the oral cavity instead.

We know further that the response type of the glossopharyngeal nerve fiber of the frog is partly similar to those obtained from the free standing organ of Xenopus laevis.

From those experimental results we are of the opinion that the lateral-line organ is, in a sense, the primitive taste organ and in another sense it is a better model of the inner ear of higher animals, because the mechanosensitivity of free neuromasts is increased by the increase of potassium concentration in the environment. The effect of ionic concentration of potassium on the mechanosensitivity was examined by measuring the threshold of the lateral-line nerve response of Xenopus for vibratory stimulations. As shown in the figure, the relation is linear between the concentration of potassium ions and the threshold of the lateral-line organ for the mechanical vibratory stimulation. The more the ionic concentration in the environment, the lower becomes the threshold. The same tendency had already been observed in the pit organ of shark as mentioned before (Katsuki et al., 1970, Hashimoto and Katsuki, 1972);(Fig. 11).

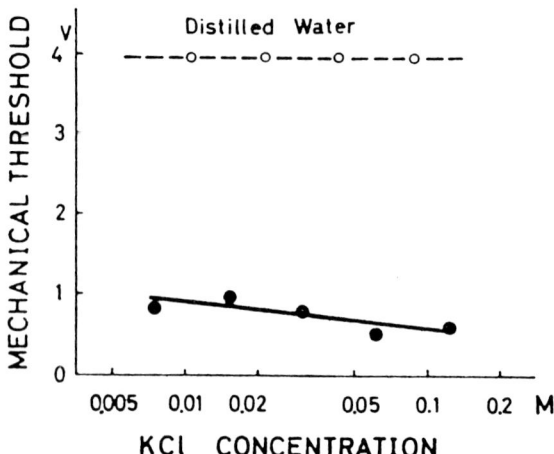

Fig. 11 Effect of potassium chloride solution on the mechanical threshold of the free standing neuromast of Xenopus laevis. The ordinate indicates the threshold of the free neuromast for vibratory stimuli, the magnitude of which is expressed by the voltage driving an electromagnetic vibrator. The abscissa represents the molar concentration of potassium chloride. The open circles represent the threshold in distilled water, which were measured for the control of mechanical sensitivity between the application of potassium chloride solution (Hashimoto and Katsuki, 1972).

4. Discussion

From the phylogenetical point of view the lateral-line nerve of the lamprey (Entosphenus japonicus) was tested. The lamprey is an example of a cyclostome and this primitive animal is still not provided with the lateral-line canal, but only with free neuromasts on the body surface. Recent electron-microscopical studies on this free neuromast have revealed that the sensory cell is not particularly different from that of fish except for the efferent synapses. All synapses at the base of the receptor cell are of the afferent type (Yamada, 1972). In this lateral-line nerve the chemical response to monovalent cations could be seen. The lateral-line nerves of the tadpoles (Rana catesbeiana and Xenopus laevis) were also studied.

They both showed the responses to monovalent cations and the suppressive effect of Ca^{++} on the effect of monovalent cations was observed. The responses observed in tadpoles were very similar to those observed in teleosts.

From all those experimental results the prototype of such chemoreception may be the responses to monovalent cations, K^+, Rb^+, Na^+, NH_4^+, Li^+ and Cs^+. Divalent cations Ca^{++}, Sr^{++} and Mg^{++} suppress the effects of monovalent cations. Quinine and sugar have almost no effect. Distilled water usually stops the spontaneous discharges.

Free neuromasts of cyclostomes, pit organs of sharks, free neuromasts of teleosts and of tadpoles all showed similar responses. In adult amphibians the end-organs can respond much more to chemical stimuli, not only to monovalent cations but also to divalent cations and some anions. They respond particularly to distilled water (Table 5).

In fish and tadpoles the lateral-line organs show active spontaneous discharges. These discharges are stopped, however, by distilled water. They need a minimum amount of cations. River or pond water can activate the end-organ, but distilled water cannot. On the other hand the organ of Xenopus can be stimulated even by distilled water as shown in Fig. 12. Deuterium oxide[1] also can stimulate the end-organ. In this sense, the receptor cells of the Xenopus lateral-line organ are more developed than those of other aquatic animals. In the gustatory cells water responses have often been encountered. Water responses were first discovered by Zotterman (1949). On the other hand Konishi (1967) discovered the DWE (distilled water effect) in the fish gustatory organ. His case was rather different from the former. In the carp gustatory cell remarkable responses to distilled water were raised by application of distilled water successively to a diluted salt solution on the end-organ. Konishi suggested that the mechanism is due to the electrokinetic potential. However the DW-Response observed on the lateral-line organ is different. Diluted salt solutions suppressed the water response.

---

[1] Supplied by Japan Radioactive Isotope Association.

CLASSIFICATION OF CHEMICAL RESPONSES

TYPE	-I-	-II-	-III-
MONOVALENT CATIONS K, Rb, Na, NH_4, Li, Cs	EXCITATORY	EXCITATORY	EXCITATORY
DIVALENT CATIONS Ca, Sr, Mg, EXCEPT Ba	SUPPRESSIVE	EXCITATORY	EXCITATORY
GLUTAMATE (ANION)	—	EXCITATORY	EXCITATORY (SOME FIBERS)
TETRODOTOXIN	SUPPRESSIVE	—	—
QUININE	—	—	EXCITATORY (SOME FIBERS)
SUGAR	—	—	—
STREPTOMYCIN	SUPPRESSIVE	SUPPRESSIVE	—
DISTILLED WATER	—	EXCITATORY	—
ENDORGAN	FREE NEUROMAST PIT ORGAN	FREE STANDING ORGANS	TERMINAL BUDS
ANIMALS	CYCLOSTOMES ELASMOBRANCHII TELEOSTS TADPOLES	AFRICAN TOAD	CATFISH

Table 5

Beidler's hypothesis on the gustatory cell (1965) is that anions have an inhibitory effect on the action of the cations. Certain receptor membranes may differ in their membrane fine structure so that the ratio of anionic to cationic sites on the receptor membrane available for taste stimuli may also vary. If the taste receptor membrane contains a predominance of anionic sites, then the cations of most stimuli presented to the end-organ dominate and the anions play a lesser role. The effects due to the balance between anionic and cationic membrane sites are much more dramatic in the frog, cat and rabbit which exhibit large water responses (Zotterman, 1956). In these animals it may be hypothesized that the cationic membrane sites are more numerous than the anionic and thus the membrane is spontaneously active. When a salt is applied, the anions will be bound to

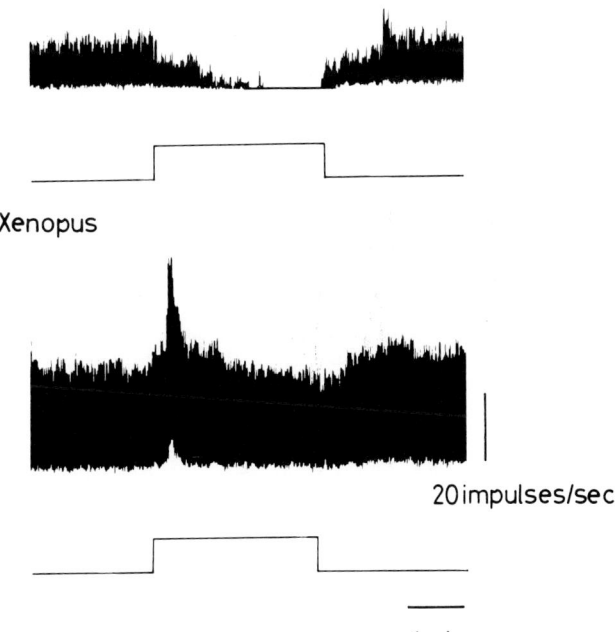

Fig. 12 Responses of a lateral-line nerve fiber to distilled water. A: Tadpole of a bullfrog (Rana catesbeiana). B: African clawed toad (Xenopus laevis). The straight line below each trace represents the duration of distilled water application.

the membrane in greater number and efficiency than the cations, and the magnitude of the spontaneous activity will decrease. As most of the cationic membrane sites are filled, the stimulus cation binds to the anionic membrane sites and a taste response occurs. Thus, there is no fundamental difference between salt and water fibers but only a difference in degree.

At present the meaning of the water response is not clearly understood. However, Xenopus must remain in water, otherwise it cannot be kept alive. The information from the lateral-line organ, therefore is absolutely necessary for that animal. In this sense the active spontaneous discharges at the lateral-line nerve fibers play a very important role in this animal. The spontaneous discharges might lower the threshold for mechanical stimulation.

The responses to various chemicals may also be indispensable for this animal. The location of food in the water may be very important for it. Since Xenopus has no tongue, its lateral-line organ may be requisite for maintaining its life in water. Pfaffmann already showed that there are remarkable differences of salt responses in the glossopharyngeal nerve and the chorda tympani in the rat. The primitive glossopharyngeal nerve shows similar responses to those of the lateral-line nerve.

In order to know the mechanism more precisely, effects of several chemical agents applied to the endorgan were examined by observing the spontaneous discharges of the nerve. Ouabain (10^{-3} gr/ml) gave almost no effect. DNP (dinitrophenol)(10^{-4} gr/ml), Azide (5×10^{-4} gr/ml) and KCN (5×10^{-4} gr/ml) produced slowly a reversibly suppressive effect. On the other hand streptomycin (10^{-4} gr/ml) suppressed within a few seconds the spontaneous discharges which reversibly returned to the original level when the end-organ was flooded with distilled water. From these results the origin of spontaneous discharges in the lateral-line organ of aquatic animals is thought mainly to be the dissolved monovalent cations, particularly K^+, although the anionic effect has been stressed by Beidler. We were able to confirm the change of the sensory cell membrane potential by the change of ionic concentration outside the cell by the use of Nectrus maculosus.

In Xenopus, however, even pure water itself stimulates the end-organ. Adsorption of cations in the receptor site and a certain metabolic mechanism rather than that of a specific ionic pump can be suggested.

In the inner ear of higher animals K^+ has been considered to play the main role in the receptive mechanism (Konishi et al., 1966). In this case too, the chemical origin of the spontaneous discharges observed in the primary afferent fibers and the complementarity between the mechanosensitivity and the K^+ concentration in the endolymph are strongly suggested.

Acknowledgements

This work was collaborated partly with Drs. T. Hashimoto, K. Yanagisawa and N. Onoda, and financially supported by NIH grant NB 06890-02 and NSF grant GB-5768 given to Dr. G. von Békésy of University of Hawaii and by a grant from the Ministry of Education of Japan to the author.

References

Bardach, J.E., and Atema, J. (1972). The sense of taste in fish. In: Handbook of Sensory Physiology (L.M. Beidler, ed.), Vol. IV, pp. 293-336. Springer-Verlag, Berlin.

Beidler, L.M. (1965). Anion influences on taste receptor response. In: Olfaction and Taste (T. Hayashi, ed.), Vol. II, pp. 509-534. Pergamon Press, Oxford.

Flock, A. (1966). Ultrastructure and function in the lateral-line organs. In: Lateral Line Detectors (P.H. Cahn, ed.), pp. 163-197. Indiana Univ. Press, Bloomington, Indiana.

Freihofer, W.C. (1963). Patterns of the ramus lateralis accessorius and their systematic significance in teleostean fishes. Stanford Ichthyol. Bull. 8, 81-189.

Hashimoto, T. and Katsuki, Y. (1972). Enhancement of the mechanosensitivity of hair cells of the lateral-line organs by environmental potassium ions. J. Acoust. Soc. Amer. 52, 553-557.

Herrick, C.J. (1903). The organ and sense of taste in fishes. U.S. Fish Comm. 22, 237-271.

Katsuki, Y., Yoshino, S. and Chen, J. (1950a). Action current of the single lateral-line nerve fiber of fich. I. Jap. J. Physiol. 1, 87-99.

Katsuki, Y., Yoshino, S. and Chen, J. (1950b). Action current of the single lateral-line nerve fiber of fish. II. Jap. J. Physiol. 1, 179-194.

Katsuki, Y., Mizuhira, V. and Yoshino, S. (1951). On the endorgan of the acoustico-lateralis systems of fish. Jap. J. Physiol. 2, 93-102.

Katsuki, Y., and Yoshino, S. (1952). Responses of the single lateral-line nerve fiber to the linearly rising current stimulating the endorgan. Jap. J. Physiol. 2, 219-231.

Katsuki, Y., Sumi, T., Uchiyama, H. and Watanabe, T. (1958). Electric responses of auditory neurons in cat to sound stimulation. J. Neurophysiol. 21, 569-588.

Katsuki, Y., Kanno, Y., Suga, N. and Mannen, H. (1961). Primary auditory neurons of monkey. Jap. J. Physiol. 11, 678-683.

Katsuki, Y., Hashimoto, T. and Yanagisawa, K. (1970). The lateral-line organ of shark as a chemoreceptor. In: Advances in Biophysics (M. Kotani, ed.), Vol. 1, pp. 1-51. Univ. of Tokyo Press, Tokyo.

Katsuki, Y., Hashimoto, T. and Kendall, J.I. (1971). The chemoreception in the lateral-line organs of teleosts. Jap. J. Physiol. 21, 99-118.

Konishi, J. (1967). Studies on the stimulation of chemoreceptors of fresh water fish by dilute solution of electrolytes. In: Olfaction and Taste (T. Hayashi, ed.), Vol. II, pp. 667-692. Pergamon Press, Oxford.

Konishi, T., Kelsey, E. and Singleton, G.T. (1966). Effect of chemical alteration in the endolymph on the cochlear potentials. Acta Oto-laryngol. 62, 393-404.

Kusano, K. (1960). Analysis of the single unit activity of gustatory receptors in the frog tongue. Jap. J. Physiol. 10, 620-633.

Lowenstein, W.R., and Ishiko, N. (1962). Sodium chloride sensitivity and electrochemical effects in a Lorenzinian ampulla. Nature (London) 194, 292-294.

Murray, W. (1962). The response of the ampullae of Lorenzini of elasmobranchs to electrical stimulation. J. Exp. Biol. 39, 119-128.

Onoda, N., and Katsuki, Y. (1972). Chemoreception on the lateral-line organ of an aquatic amphibian, Xenopus laevis. Jap. J. Physiol. 22, 87-102.

Pfaffmann, C., Fisher, G.L. and Frank, M.K. (1967). The sensory and behavioral factors in taste references. In: Olfaction and Taste (T. Hayashi, ed.), Vol. II, pp. 361-382. Pergamon Press, Oxford.

Tester, A.L., and Nelson G.J. (1963). Free neuromasts (pit organs) in sharks. In: Sharks, skates and rays. (Gilbert, ed.), pp. 503-553. Johns Hopkins Press, Baltimore.

Tester, A.L., and Kendall, J.I. (1967). Innervation of free and canal neuromasts in the shark. In: Lateral-line Detectors (P.H. Cahan, ed.), pp. 53-72. Indiana Univ. Press, Bloomington, Indiana.

Yamada, Y. (1972). Evolution of the lateral-line organ. J. Ultrastruct. Res. (in press).

Zotterman, Y. (1949). The response of the frog's taste fibers to the application of pure water. Acta Physiol. Scand. 18, 181-189.

Zotterman, Y. (1956). Species differences in the water taste. Acta Physiol. Scand. 37, 60-70.

Figures 2 and 3 reproduced from ADVANCES IN BIOPHYSICS I edited by M. Kotani, 1970, by permission of University of Tokyo Press.

Figures 4, 6, 9, and 10 reproduced by permission of the Japanese Journal of Physiology.

Figure 11 reproduced by permission of Journal of Acoustical Society of America.

DISCUSSION

BRUGGE: Are these responses sensitive to temperature?

KATSUKI: They are very sensitive to temperature change. We saw this many years ago so (Katsuki et al., 1950) I did not talk about it.

MICHELSEN: I wonder, how fast do these responses adapt? I am thinking about the fishes which are swimming from seawater into freshwater, fishes like the eel and the salmon.

KATSUKI: The response returns to the original level in a few days.

FLOCK: I am a bit worried about the concentrations that you have to use. You used up to 1 molar concentrations. Now, I would not find a strange if cells would react to that high concentration. But maybe you have the control with the canal organ. If you apply these concentrations on the neighboring canal organ, do you not get this chemical response?

KATSUKI: Yes, I could not find the chemical response. This is very funny.

Reference
Katsuki, Y., Yoshino, S., and Chen, J. (1950). Action current of the single lateral-line nerve fiber of fish. Jap. J. Physiol. 1, 87-99.

COCHLEAR POTENTIALS AND COCHLEAR MECHANICS

Peter Dallos

Northwestern University
Evanston, Illinois
U.S.A.

The purpose of this communication is to provide an up-to-date description of the relationships among stimulus-related cochlear potentials and various mechanical events in the inner ear. Of special interest is to consider how well the mechanical tuning characteristics of the basilar membrane are represented in cochlear microphonics (CM) and summating potentials (SP), what important excitatory phenomena are not reflected in these potentials, and what these potentials reveal about the functioning of the two groups of sensory cells of the cochlea; inner and outer hair cells.

The CM and some components of the SP are generally considered to be receptor potentials of the cochlea (Davis, 1961, Dallos, 1971); that is to say, they are the first electrical signs of absorption of stimulus energy by the sensory receptors, but they are not directly responsible for the initiation of neural responses in the fibers of the auditory nerve. It is debatable, and is debated, whether the CM and/or the SP bear a direct causal relation to the process of elicitation of nerve impulses or if they are mere signs of the active functioning of the cochlear transducer. Whatever the outcome of this debate might be, the cochlear potentials provide the investigator with an extremely valuable tool in his quest for unraveling the complex processes that intervene between cochlear output and input. In a sense, a careful study of CM and SP permits one to bring some dim light into the "black box" that needs to be considered. Contempory measurements on basilar membrane motion yield much information about the input, while the wealth of information now available on single 8th nerve unit responses well defines the output of the black box. Knowledge of the behavior of cochlear potentials provides a crack through which one can peer into the box and thus place constraints on its content. When cochlear potentials are studied in a quantitative manner, or when correlations between them and other inner ear phenomena are sought, one must always beware of some pitfalls. The first of these is a consequence of the fact that CM and SP are the gross recordings of the outputs of thousands of spatially distributed generators. As a result of the complex interaction among the elementary constituents of the total response, the latter might have different properties than any of its components. The recording situation is further complicated by the extremely complex electroanatomy of the cochlea, in other words by the arrangement of the sources of electrical potentials in a three-dimensional, nonhomogeneous, conducting medium. Several investigators have addressed themselves to the various problems that stem from these physical properties (Békésy, 1951a, Whitfield and Ross, 1965, Laszlo, 1968, Kohllöffel, 1971, Weiss et al., 1969, Dallos et al., 1971, Cern and Fischler, 1972). A further difficulty lies in the separation of locally and remotely generated electrical responses, particularly when the latter are of greater magnitude. It is now reasonably clear that in the mammalian cochlea the most localized electrical events can be recorded with the aid of the differential electrode technique (Tasaki et al., 1952, Dallos, 1969a, Dallos et al., 1971). Single intracochlear electrodes, whether in scala media or in the perilymphatic scale, or a round window electrode, can not reject remote responses with adequate effectiveness. All results that are presented below were obtained with differential electrodes.

1. Methods

All experiments that are reported in this paper were conducted on guinea pigs. Two types of preparations were used: animals with normal cochleae, and animals in which selective hair cells damage was induced by kanamycin intoxication. We have described details of our preparation in several previous papers (Dallos,

1969a, Dallos et al., 1972a, Wang and Dallos, 1972, and Wang, 1973). Consequently, here a mere outline is given. The animals are anesthetized with intraperitoneal injection of urethane, the auditory bulla on one side is approached and opened, the tensor tympani tendon is cauterized, and after drilling fine holes through the bony cochlear wall electrodes are placed in the scalae tympani and vestibuli of the desired turn. Unless otherwise noted, in all experiments to be described below the bulla is left open. The sound source is directly coupled to the bony external meatus and it is sealed in with vacuum grease, or even cemented in on occasion, to form a closed system. Two types of sound sources are used. In experiments where high frequency sound is not desired, a THD-39 earphone is utilized, while in all others a 1/2 inch condenser microphone driven with a nonlinearity compensating circuit (Molnar et al., 1968) provides the signal. In all cases the sound is monitored near the umbo with appropriate probe tube microphones. These are brought to the vicinity of the eardrum through an enlarged, originally tissue filled, niche on the bulla just ventral to the bony meatus. When the magnitude and phase of high frequency sound are to be monitored, the measuring instrument is a 1/8 inch condensor microphone, attached to a very short (0.2 inch) probe tube. All measurements of ac quantities, sound and CM, are accomplished with a 3 Hz bandwidth wave analyzer, while dc quantities, such as various SP components, are obtained on the basis of computer averaging. In the latter case the stimuli are tone bursts (40 msec ON, 100 msec OFF) in which the carrier is not synchronized to the onset of the burst. With such a stimulus, the CM is averaged out, leaving a true dc response. Our phase measuring scheme was presented in detail in a previous publication (Dallos et al., 1971).

Cochlear lesions are created by subcutaneous injection of kanamycin in a dose of 400 mg/kg/day for 8 to 14 days. A waiting period of at least two weeks is allowed between the last injection and electrophysiological data collection. In these animals after data collection the cochleae are perfused with a solution containing 1% osmium tetroxide; later they are prepared as flat specimens for examination under the phase contrast microscope (Engström et al., 1966). The entire organ, from the apical to the basal end, is examined, and on the basis of accurate hair cell count, a cochleogram is prepared for each cochlea (Wang, 1973). It is our experience, based on examining kanamycin damaged cochleae, that predictable outer hair cell damage can be induced in guinea pig inner ears with the controlled administration of this drug. In Fig. 1, six selected cochleograms are shown to demonstrate the range of damage that can be induced by varying doses of kanamycin injection. The lesions range from very mild to extremely severe. Quantitative descriptions of lesion-dose relations are provided by Wang (1973). For these experiments we endeavored to create damage patterns whereby all outer hair cells are obliterated in the basal half of the cochlea, while over this same region the inner hair cells show minimal or no apparent sign of damage. While we certainly succeeded in obtaining such lesions (cochleograms exemplified by those designated as 17R and 19R in Fig. 1) as defined by the presence or absence of hair cells, we hasten to emphasize that our light microscopic criteria for hair cell normalcy might not be adequate to assure normal hair cell function. In other words, we must entertain the possibility that inner hair cells that appear normal under the phase contrast microscope, might actually be damaged to a degree that interference with normal function could occur. All experiments described below that involved pathologic cochleae are based on animals having damage patterns very similar to those of 17R and 19R (Fig. 1). In these animals the electrodes are situated approximately 16 mm from the apex, in other words, in the center of the region that is denuded of outer hair cells.

2. Results and discussion

One of the most profitable means of studying cochlear mechanisms is to construct frequency response functions for various recording locations. Such functions can be derived for mechanical quantities, such as basilar membrane displacement (Békésy, 1947, B.M. Johnstone and Boyle, 1967; Rhode, 1971; Wilson and J.R. Johnstone, 1972), electrical potentials such as CM and SP (Tasaki et al., 1952, Tonndorf, 1958, Konishi and Yasuno 1963, Honrubia and Ward, 1968, 1969, Engebretson, 1970, Laszlo et al., 1970, Kupperman, 1966) and single unit discharges (Kiang, 1965,

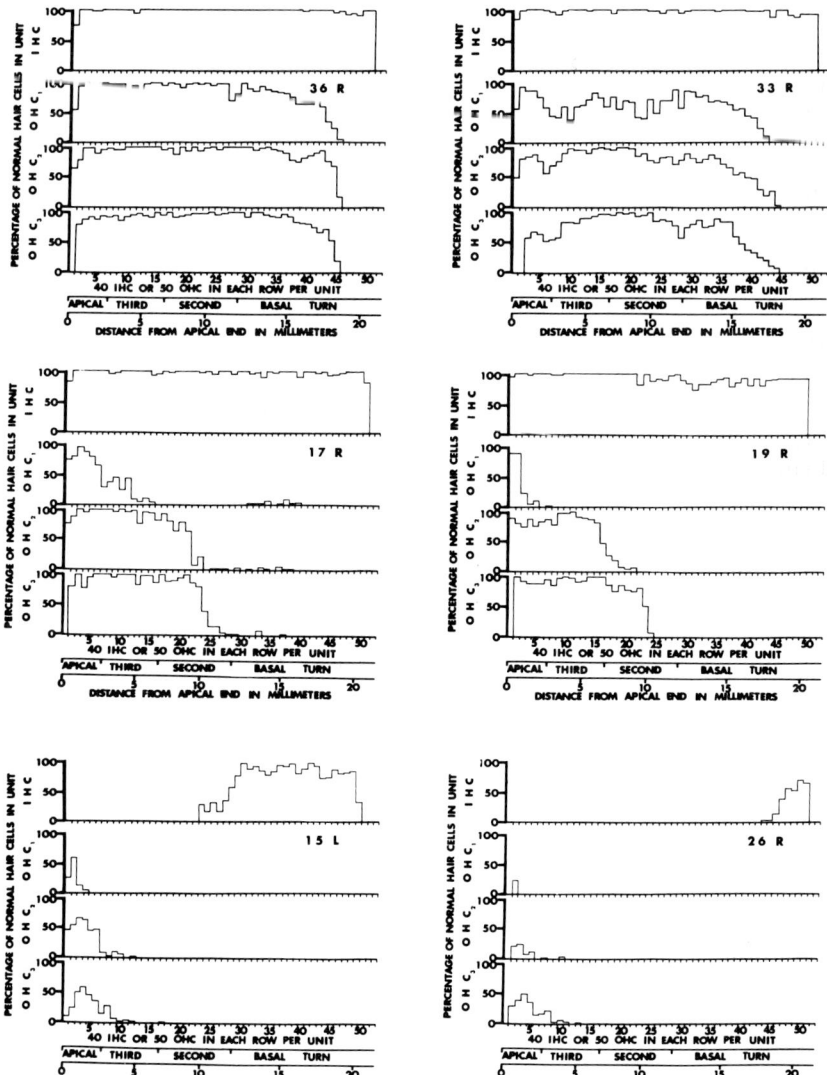

Fig.1 Six cochleograms showing two mild, and two very severe lesions, as well as the pattern of outer hair cell destruction (in 17R and 19R) that is considered ideal for the purposes of the present work (adapted from Wang, 1973).

Hind et al., 1972, Anderson et al., 1971). A frequency response function consists of a pair of plots, one depicting the ratio of output and input quantities, the other showing the phase difference between output and input quantities, both as the function of stimulus frequency. If a system is linear then the frequency response function represents its complete quantitative description, whereas a nonlinear system is only partially described by such functions. Specifically, a frequency response function obtained at a given input level would provide the relations between output and input quantities for harmonic signals of that level only; they could not in general be used to predict responses at other levels or transient properties. Since the auditory system is nonlinear, particularly at high signal levels, it is necessary to obtain frequency response functions for it at relatively low stimulus magnitudes.

The output quantity might be basilar membrane displacement or CM or neural spike rate, depending on the system for which the frequency response function is to be obtained. The input quantity is often chosen as sound pressure at the drum or stapes displacement. Actually, the choice of the input is dictated by the constraints of measurement and the extent of the system to be described. Thus if the middle ear-inner ear combination is the system of interest then sound pressure at the eardrum is the most appropriate input quantity. It is also the easiest to measure. When only cochlear function is to be described, it is advantageous to eliminate the frequency dependent influence of the middle ear (Kiang, 1968). Thus under such conditions stapes displacement might be the input variable of choice, or even more appropriately, stapes velocity. Consider that basilar membrane displacement in the basal end of the cochlea is directly related to sound pressure at the oval window, which in turn is determined by the product of stapes volume velocity and cochlear input impedance. Fortunately, the input impedance of the cochlea is resistive and constant over most of the significant audio frequency range. It does have a significant reactive component in the cat below 100-200 Hz, but in the guinea pig it is purely resistive at least down to 10 Hz (Dallos, 1970a). Consequently, stapes velocity constitutes the best choice for describing the input variable in our frequency response functions. It is usually too cumbersome to measure this quantity, and one is forced to rely on known middle ear transfer characteristics to derive stapes velocity as a function of sound pressure at the eardrum. Such middle ear characteristics have been provided for the cat by Møller (1963) and Guinan and Peake (1967) and for the guinea pig by Zwislocki (1963), B.M. Johnstone and Taylor (1971) and Wilson and J.R. Johnstone (1972).

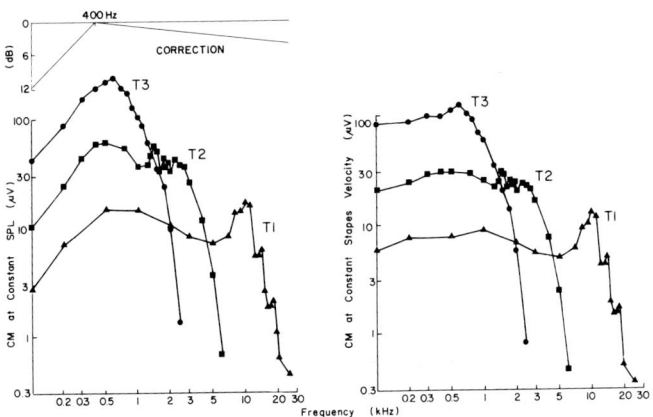

Fig.2 Cochlear microphonic magnitude functions. Left panel: CM magnitude from three cochlear locations at 50 dB sound pressure level at the eardrum. Right panel: CM magnitude at a constant stapes velocity. These curves are obtained from the ones in the left panel by correcting for the middle ear transfer function, and for the displacement-to-velocity transformation. This correction is made according to the plot shown on the top of the picture.

In Figs 2 and 3 CM magnitude and phase functions are presented as recorded with the differential electrode technique from turns one, two, and three of representative guinea pig cochleae. In the left panel of Fig. 2 the rms CM magnitude is shown as a function of stimulus frequency with the sound pressure maintained at a constant value of 50 dB (re 0.0002 dyne/cm^2). In the left panel of Fig. 3 the phase of the CM referred to the phase of the sound field in front

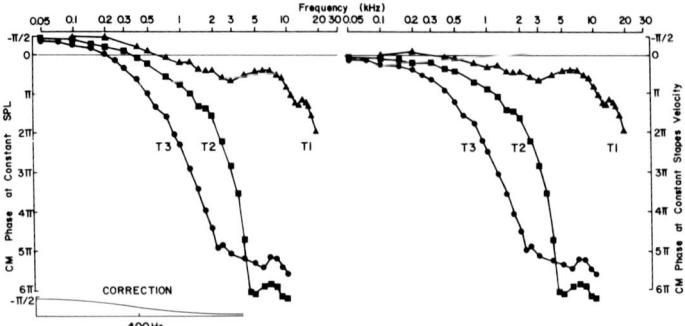

Fig.3 Cochlear microphonic phase functions. Left panel: CM phase referred to the phase of the sound at the eardrum. Measurements are shown from electrode locations in the first three cochlear turns. Right panel: CM phase referred to that of stapes velocity. These curves are derived from the ones in the left panel by correcting them according to the plot shown on the bottom to compensate for middle ear effects and to refer to stapes velocity.

of the eardrum is given. These magnitude and phase plots represent the frequency response functions of the middle ear-inner ear combination, as reflected in the CM as the output quantity. These plots are highly characteristic and their details reveal a great deal about the system. At low frequencies all amplitude plots grow at a rate of 6 dB/octave while the phase plots indicate that at the lowest frequencies the CM leads the sound by 90°. The 6 dB/octave growth is usually terminated at approximately 400 Hz, beyond which the magnitude slowly declines. In the low frequency region there is a systematic increase in CM as the recording point is moved toward the apex of the cochlea. At any recording location there is a fairly distinct frequency beyond which the response shows a drastic decline. Just below this cutoff frequency there usually is a small local maximum. This maximum is very clear, in fact somewhat exaggerated, in the first turn plot. In the region of this peak the phase function usually undergoes a slight but distinct change, a flattening or even reversal, but at higher frequencies it resumes its smooth course. The high frequency slopes of the magnitude functions are approximately -100 dB/decade. The phase functions do not show an ever accumulating phase lag, but level off at about 5 or 6π. The dip in the first turn phase function between 2000 and 5000 Hz is almost certain to be due to middle ear effects.

Since our primary interest is the frequency response function of the inner ear, it is desirable to correct the amplitude and phase plots to eliminate the filter effect of the middle ear. One can deduce from the data of B.M. Johnstone and Taylor (1971) and Wilson and J.R. Johnstone (1972) that at constant sound pressure level the amplitude of the guinea pig's stapes is independent of frequency up to 400 Hz, beyond which it declines at an approximate rate of 8 dB/octave. Consequently, at constant sound pressure level the velocity of the stapes can be assumed to increase at a rate of 6 dB/octave up to 400 Hz and decline at a rate of 2 dB/octave at higher frequencies. This function is sketched in Fig. 2, labeled "correction". If for simplicity we assume that the phase characteristics of the guinea pig middle ear do not significantly depart from that of a simple low-pass filter (that is from a filter whose amplitude response is flat to a corner frequency - in this case 400 Hz - and decreases thereafter at a 6 dB/octave rate) then they should change from zero at low frequencies to 90° lag at high frequencies, with 45° at 400 Hz. Consequently, the stapes velocity phase referred to the phase of the sound should start with a 90° lead at the lowest frequencies and should approach zero at high frequencies, with passing through 45° at 400 Hz. This phase characteristic, again labeled "correction" is included in Fig. 3. If both amplitude and phase plots are corrected so that they should reflect CM magnitude and phase referred to constant stapes velocity, then the right-hand graphs in Fig. 2 and 3 are obtained. These plots then are the frequency response functions (as reflected in CM as the output quantity) of three cochlear locations. These magnitude functions are essentially flat up to a characteristic cutoff frequency beyond which they rapidly decline. The phase functions start from zero at low frequencies, and phase lag rapidly accumulates as frequency is increased. The flatness of the amplitude functions and the zero

low frequency phase clearly indicate that up to a
particular cutoff frequency the CM is proportional
to stapes velocity. This conclusion has been reached
by Weiss et al. (1969) from CM recordings in the
cat's basal turn, and confirmed on the basis of
studying CM transients (Dallos and Durrant, 1972).
A very interesting finding is the small peak in the
amplitude response and the small irregularity in the
phase response that occur just below the cutoff frequency. Together these features suggest the possibility that aside from the traveling wave that establishes the main characteristics of the response,
a secondary resonance might also be present in the
cochlea (Robson, Pers. Comm.).

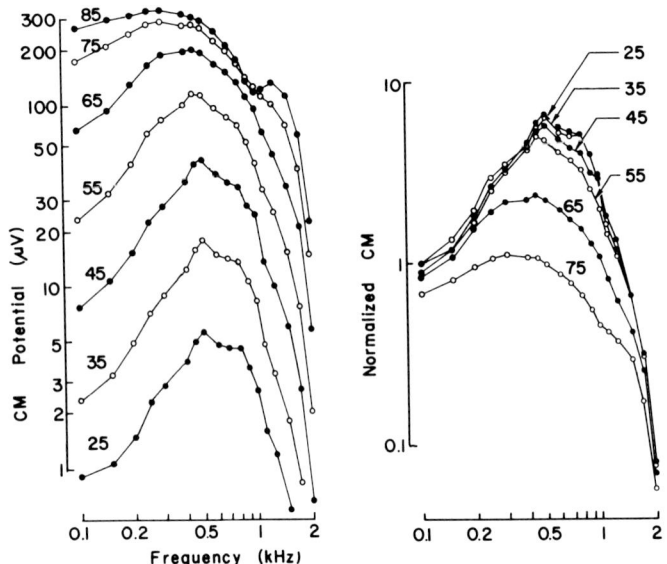

Fig.4 Left panel: CM magnitude plots from the third
       cochlear turn at various sound pressure
       levels. Right panel: Normalized CM magnitude
       plots.

The frequency response function described above provides a fair representation of cochlear processes
over a wide range of low stimulus intensities. In
Fig. 4 CM magnitude functions at various constant
sound pressure levels are shown for one third turn

electrode pair. In the right-hand panel of the figure
some of the same functions are replotted after appropriate vertical shift to linearly compensate for the
magnitude differences. If the CM response were linear
then all plots would superimpose. Departures from
superposition indicate the region and degree of nonlinearity. The 25 and 35 dB sound pressure level
(SPL) functions are completely superimposed, and
there are very minor departures in the 45 dB plot.
These departures occur around the maximum of the
function. As intensity is increased clear violations
of the linearity assumption occur to an ever increasing degree. The most nonlinear region is between
500 and 1200 Hz, while at both lower and higher frequencies the departures from linearity are considerably more moderate. It is demonstrated later
that in the frequency band where the amplitude nonlinearity is most pronounced, nonlinear response
components (e.g. harmonics) are generated in profusion.

Aside from frequency response functions, or tuning
curves, for CM the determination of such functions
for the other receptor potential, the SP, is also of
great interest. We have recently proposed that the
summating potential can best be described as being
composed of two constituents, the DIF and the AVE SP
(Dallos <u>et al</u>., 1970). The former component is simply
the potential difference between scala vestibuli
and scala tympani, and thus it is the gradient across
the cochlear partition. The AVE component is the
common-mode potential of the two perilymphatic scalae. Just as the CM, the two SP components also show
highly systematic changes with frequency and intensity at any given recording location. In Fig. 5 some
of these changes are demonstrated with the aid of
recordings from the second cochlear turn. At low
sound levels the DIF component is negative and the
AVE component is positive in a given frequency band;
in the second turn this band is around 3000-5000 Hz.
Both below and above this band the AVE response
turns negative, while at lower frequencies the DIF
is positive, and it vanishes at higher frequencies.
Thus in both response components there are three
frequency bands in which the response assumes
different character. As intensity increases both
the DIF^- and the AVE^+ bands spread toward the lower
frequencies, while there is negligible upward spread.

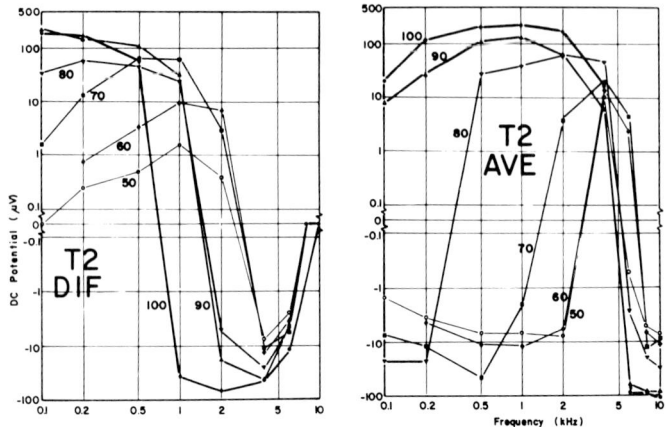

Fig.5 DIF and AVE summating potential components recorded from a second turn electrode pair at a variety of sound pressure levels (from Dallos et al., 1970. Copyright by the American Association for the Advancement of Science).

To demonstrate how the CM and SP tuning curves interrelate, in Fig. 6 recordings from the first cochlear turn are shown. These are plots for CM, AVE, and DIF SP at 50 dB SPL and they are highly characteristic of the common relationship between the three components in the frequency region of greatest interest. In this region the DIF is negative while the AVE is positive. They both peak on the steep high frequency slope of the CM function. To quantify the interdependence of CM, DIF, and AVE SP a so-called frequency map for these components is prepared and presented in Fig. 7. The data included in this plot represent median values obtained from five to ten animals. They represent the frequency at which the given response is 3 dB down from the peak response. The peak in question is not an absolute peak, rather the appropriate local maximum. Thus for example in Fig. 2 the second turn CM has an absolute peak at 500 Hz, but the local peak of interest here occurs at 2250 Hz. It is this latter maximum that is used as reference in establishing the 3 dB - down frequency. The median cutoff frequencies are plotted

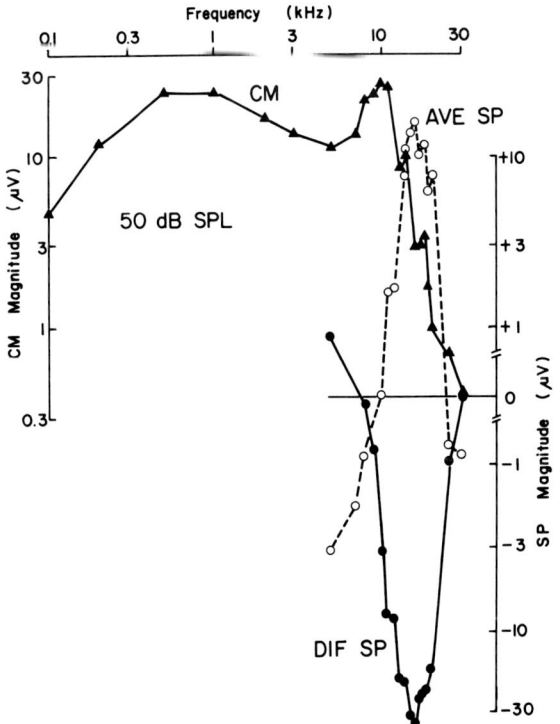

Fig.6 Comparison between CM, DIF SP, and AVE SP recorded from a first turn electrode pair at 50 dB sound pressure level.

as the function of the distance of the recording electrodes from the base. Individual determinations of electrode position were not performed; rather the mean locations of 4, 10 and 14 mm are used on the abscissa. These figures were established for the first and third turn electrode locations on the basis of thirteen actual measurements (courtesy of Dr. G. Bredberg), while the second turn location is interpolated. The median cutoff frequencies for the DIF and AVE responses are virtually superimposed at all three locations, but they are clearly separated from the cutoff frequencies of the CM tuning curves. All data points lie on straight lines in this semi-logarithmic plot, indicating an exponential

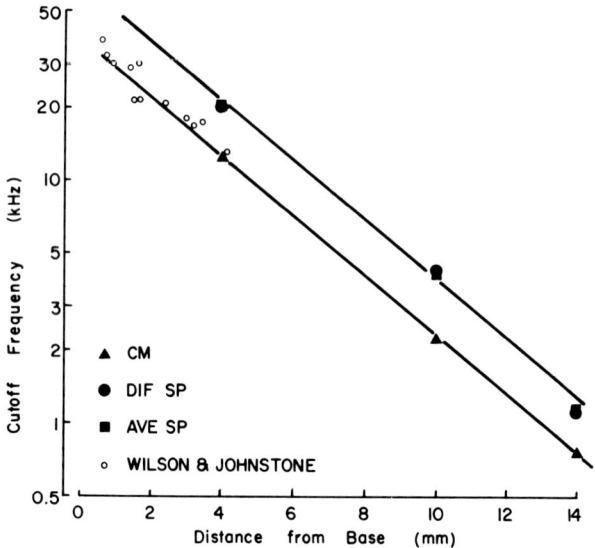

Fig.7 Median cut-off frequencies in turns one, two, and three for CM, DIF SP, and AVE SP. Cutoff frequency is defined as the frequency at the magnitude that is 3 dB below the high frequency local maximum. For comparison the mechanical cutoff frequencies obtained in individual animals by Wilson and Johnstone (1972) are also shown.

relation between cutoff frequencies and place along the basilar membrane. To obtain a comparison between these data and the displacement characteristics of the cochlear partition, recently obtained results from Wilson and J.R. Johnstone (1972) are also included in the plot. These points represent the "highest frequency before the response starts to drop rapidly" and thus are quite commensurate with our 3 dB-down frequency. The agreement between CM data and basilar membrane displacement data is impressive. This agreement tends to indicate that the CM does reflect the displacement pattern of the cochlear partition to a better degree than has been thought recently. The separation between CM and SP reponses is about 2/3 octave. The fact that the CM and mechanical data agree with one another suggests that the difference in location between CM and SP peaks is not simply due to the spatial filtering effect operating detrimentally on the CM (Whitfield and Ross, 1965, Kohllöffel, 1971) but that the dc responses do actually peak on the steeply falling skirt of the traveling wave.

One further consideration involves the phase of the CM at the cutoff frequency. Our data indicate that the phase difference between CM and stapes velocity ranges between 0.7π and 1.27π at the 3 dB-down frequency. From the capacitive probe measurements of basilar membrane motion (Wilson and J.R. Johnstone, 1972) one can deduce that the corresponding phase difference is between 0.93π and 1.35π. This agreement is again quite excellent. In contrast, other available phase measurements of basilar membrane motion do not correlate well with the CM data, or with each other for that matter. Thus the corresponding phase difference obtained by B.M. Johnstone and Taylor (1970) is about 0.25π, while Rhode's (1971) data yield approximately 4.5π.

Inner versus outer hair cell mechanics

It has been known for some time (e.g. Davis et al., 1958, Hawkins, 1959) that outer hair cells produce more CM than inner ones. Today it is possible to quantify the differences between the two groups of cells thanks to a more effective control over means of destroying one cell group, and due to better methods of evaluating such destruction. Better control is achieved by using kanamycin as an ototoxic agent to destroy portions of the outer hair cell population, while the surface preparation technique (Engström et al., 1966) enables the investigator to obtain actual numerical counts of cells present and absent. The discussion that follows is based on data obtained from cochleae in which the outer hair cells are obliterated over the basal half of the cochlea, while the inner hair cells over this same region remain present and in good condition as ascertained by light microscopy. The two cochleograms designated 17R and 19R in Fig. 1 can serve as the prototype for the ears from which the data are derived. It is recalled that the recording electrodes are located approximately 16 mm from the apex. Thus they are in a region where there are virtually no outer hair cells around them over an extent of about ±4mm.

The best means of testing the difference in CM production between inner and outer hair cells is to compare the CM that can be measured at high frequencies from a normal cochlea with that obtainable from an animal like 17R or 19R. High frequency test signals are chosen because the corresponding traveling wave is confined within the region of the cochlea from where the outer hair cells are removed.

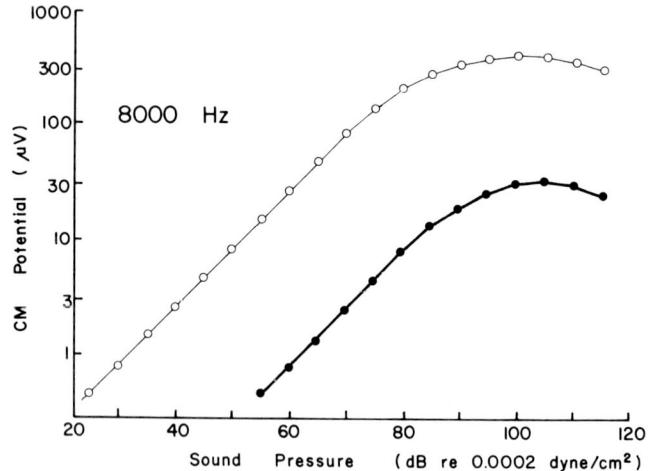

Fig.8   Median normal CM input-output function from the first cochlear turn at 8000 Hz compared with such a function obtained from a kanamycin treated animal.

In Fig. 8 the representative normal CM input-output function is compared with that of animal 17R. The stimulus is 8000 Hz, and the recording is performed with the differential electrode technique. The linear segments of the two functions are separated by a constant 30 dB, indicating that the inner hair cells alone are this much less sensitive than the normal organism. If the function representing the output of the inner hair cells is subtracted from the normal one, then the remainder can be expected to approximately represent the output of the outer hair cells.

Since the CM output of the inner hair cells is less than one-tenth of the normal CM at any intensity, it follows that when the former is subtracted from the latter a function is obtained that is at most 1 dB below the normal CM input-output curve. It is thus quite apparent that the statement that the normal CM is overwhelmingly determined by the outer hair cells is a reasonable one. Thus whatever CM one records from a normal cochlea is produced by the outer hair cells, while the inner hair cells contribute negligibly to this potential. From other animals having the desired pattern of outer hair cell damage one can usually obtain inner hair cell CM between 30 and 40 dB below the normal level. It is this difference (30 to 40 dB) that we consider to represent the sensitivity differential between outer and inner hair cells. Note finally, that both input-output functions in Fig. 8 reach their maximum at about the same sound pressure level. Consequently, saturation and bendover of these functions is unlikely to depend on the magnitude of the potential itself; instead the determining factor might be sought in mechanical events prior to CM production.

A study of the apparent structural differences between inner and outer hair cells suggests that the two groups might differ not only in sensitivity but in dynamic characteristics as well (Billone, 1972). Electronmicrographic investigations of the organ of Corti reveal that aside from important morphological differences between the cells themselves, the relation between their stereocilia and the tectorial membrane is significantly different (Kimura, 1965, Lim, 1971, and pers. comm.). While the tallest row of cilia of the outer hair cells apparently makes a quite intimate contact with the bottom of the tectorial membrane, no such contact is demonstrable for any inner hair cell cilia. Since it is generally assumed that the most likely means of stimulating the hair cells is by the bending or lever action of their cilia, it is apparent that the relation between the hairs and the tectorial membrane could have a profound influence upon the mechanism of hair cell stimulation. Cilia that attach to the tectorial membrane can be bent in proportion to the relative shear-displacement between the reticular lamina and the tectorial membrane. Cilia that are not attached, however, should be displaced (bent) by the movement of endolymph around them. In other words, free standing cilia would be moved by viscous fluid drag, exerted by the streaming of the surrounding fluid. As a consequence, the displacement of a free standing cilium is ultimately proportional not to the displacement of the basilar membrane, but to its velocity (Billone, 1972).

Cochlear microphonic potentials produced by normal hair cells and by inner hair cells alone offer the means to investigate the dynamic differences proposed in the previous paragraph. If the inner hair cells are indeed velocity detectors then a derivative relationship should be demonstrable between their CM and the CM obtained from the normal cochlea. This is the case, since as we have shown previously, in the normal animal the recorded CM reflects the output of the outer hair cells. When measured in the steady-state condition, in other words with pure tones, the derivative operation should manifest itself by decreasing the response magnitude at a rate of 6 dB/octave as frequency is reduced, and by increasing the phase lead toward $\pi/2$ as frequency is lowered. Thus when compared to the normal responses, the inner hair cell derived CM sensitivity curves should show not only the already discussed sensitivity difference but in addition they should have an added 6 dB/octave tilt toward the low frequencies. Furthermore, the phase curves (CM phase versus phase of the sound at the eardrum) should start at very low frequencies at π radian lead instead of the $\pi/2$ radian that was shown in Fig. 3. As Fig. 9 illustrates, these predictions are generally proven correct. In the figure the sensitivity (SPL at 1 µV CM) difference between the first turn CM output of three kanamycin treated animals and the corresponding median normal measure is shown in the top panel, while the difference in phase (CM phase minus phase of sound at the drum) between the three preparations and the normal median is plotted in the bottom panel. The interrupted line is drawn with a slope of 6 dB/octave. It is apparent that the sensitivity of all three kanamycin poisoned animals decreases toward the low frequencies when compared to the median normal sensitivity. The overall rate of change below 5000 Hz is approximately 6 dB/octave, even though there are absolute sensitivity differences among the three impaired ears. The three phase curves show remarkably good agreement, and, bearing out the prediction, below 5000 Hz the phase lead increases toward π/2 as frequency drops. The high frequency behavior, while consistent from animal to animal, is not predicted by the simple displacement-to-velocity transformation, and we do not yet have an explanation for the rapid increase in phase lag shown by the ototoxic ears.

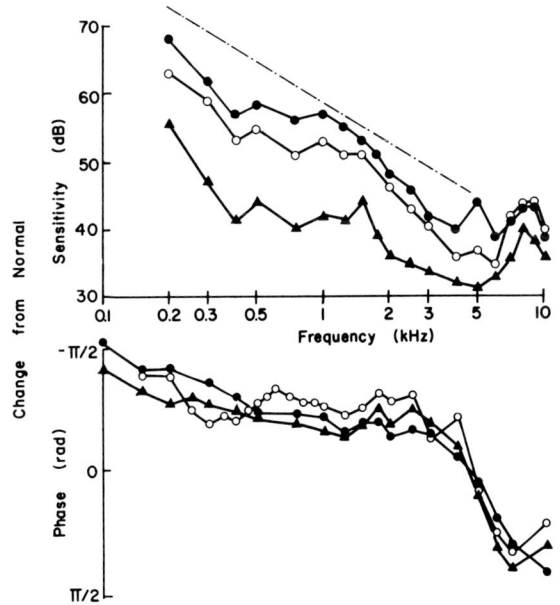

Fig.9 Difference between sensitivity and phase functions obtained from three kanamycin treated animals and the normal median. The sensitivity functions are the sound pressure as a function of frequency that is required to produce 1μV CM response from the first turn electrodes. The phase functions are obtained by measuring the difference between CM phase and the phase of the sound at the eardrum.

The difference in response characteristics between the two types of hair cells can also be demonstrated by utilizing stimuli that are more complex than the sinusoidal input. One especially suitable test signal is a low frequency triangular displacement of the stapes. With such an input the stapes velocity alternates between a certain positive and an equal negative value, resulting in a square-wave change in the pressure at the oval window. We have shown (Dallos and Durrant, 1972) that with this stimulus pattern the resulting CM also approximates a square-wave at all points in the cochlea. In the left-hand panel of Fig. 10 such responses are shown from a normal animal with the recording electrodes being in the first and third cochlear turns. The CM in the first

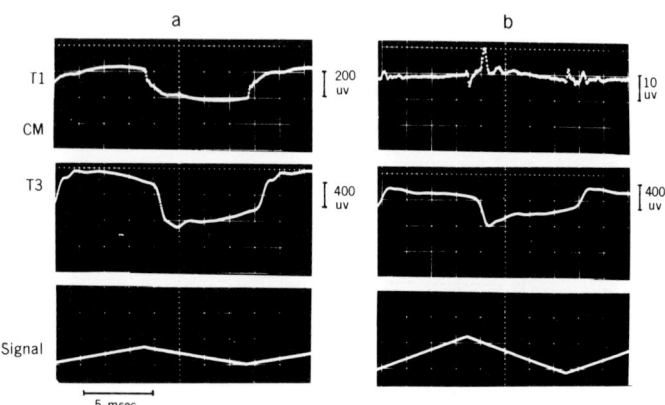

Fig.10 Average CM responses from (a) a normal guinea pig and (b) a guinea pig treated with kanamycin. The two top traces show the averaged CM response obtained from electrodes in the first (T1) and third (T3) cochlear turn. The bottom traces show the stimulus waveform (electrical signal across the transducer). The stimulus is applied to the manubrium of the malleus with a piezoelectric driver. It has been demonstrated (Dallos and Durrant, 1972) that the displacement pattern of the malleus and the electrical driving signal are identical. Furthermore, since the transmission characteristic of the guinea pig's middle ear is flat at low frequencies, the bottom traces represent the motion pattern of the stapes as well as that of the malleus. Stimulus frequency is 73 Hz and stimulus amplitude is measured as 0.3 μm, p-p (from Dallos, et al., 1972b, copyright by the American Association for the Advancement of Science).

turn is in time registration with the triangular stimulus, while the third turn response lags the stimulus with the appropriate traveling wave delay of about 0.9 msec. Remembering that in the normal animal the recorded CM reflects the output of the outer hair cells, one can state that the CM produced by this hair cell group in responce to a triangular stapes displacement approximates a square-wave. If in the region of the recording electrodes the outer hair cells are destroyed, and if our contention about the derivative relationship between inner and outer hair cells stimulation is correct, then the resulting CM (the output of the remaining inner hair cells) should approximate the derivative of a square-wave. That time function of course consists of impulses of alternate polarity. In the right-hand panel of Fig. 10 the results of such an experiment are shown. The recording from the third turn is a square-wave, rather like that obtained from a normal ear. Note again that this response clearly shows a traveling wave delay of the right magnitude. This result is not surprsing, since a glance at cochleograms 17R and 19R in Fig. 1 indicates that in the third turn (approximately 6 mm from the apex) the majority of outer hair cells are present and thus they generate an essentially normal response. In contrast, the first turn response is decidedly different. In time registration with the peaks of the stimulus triangle one sees small pulses of alternating polarity. There are also some response peaks occurring later, but these are apparently uncancelled remote microphonics from more intact regions of the ear. The fact that the first pulse occurs in coincidence[1] with the peak of the stimulus indicates that it is a local response and thus that it is a product of the inner hair cells. This conceptually very simple experiment

---

[1] From measurement of CM phase difference between the customary first turn electrode location and the round window it can be estimated that the traveling wave delay at the site of the first turn electrodes is 20 μsec. The time resolution in Fig. 10 is insufficient to display this small delay, hence it is reasonable to refer to the time relation between stimulus and first turn response as coincident.

provides a relatively clear verification of the hypothesis that, at least as an approximation, the dynamic properties of the two types of hair cells are related by a derivative transformation. Thus if the normal CM (the output of outer hair cells) is proportional to the displacement of the basilar membrane as Békésy has shown (1951b) then the CM generated by inner hair cells is proportional to the velocity of the basilar membrane.

Distortion processes

Some of the most provocative experiments of recent years have dealt with various distortion phenomena in the ear. The distortion components $(n+1)f_1 - nf_2$ and particularly $2f_1 - f_2$ (where f_1 and f_2 are the lower and higher frequency primaries in the two-tone stimulus complex) have generated the most interest. These components have a number of distinctive properties that do not need to be catalogued here; suffice it to say that the psychophysical experience that these components evoke is essentially the same as would be expected if a tone of frequency $2f_1 - f_2$ would have been added to the f_1, f_2 stimulus (Goldstein, 1967, Smoorenburg, 1972). Of course $2f_1 - f_2$ is not present in the stimulus; it is generated in the cochlea in some process of nonlinear distortion. What makes $2f_1 - f_2$ so significant is not some of its undoubtedly fascinating properties, but the implications that one can draw from its behavior about cochlear mechanics and transduction. All evidence now available indicates that $2f_1 - f_2$ is transduced in the cochlea at its "appropriate" place; that is to say if $2f_1 - f_2$ is 3000 Hz, then it is transduced at a place where a 3000 Hz pure tone would be. Evidence for this comes from cancellation, masking, and neurophysiological experiments (Goldstein, 1967, Greenwood, 1971, Smoorenburg, 1972, Goldstein and Kiang, 1968). In addition, it is highly unlikely that $2f_1 - f_2$ would be originated in the actual spike generation process of the 8th nerve fibers; instead it is most probably present at the input of the hair cell - neural junction (Goldstein, 1972). In contrast with these "stimulus like" properties of the $2f_1 - f_2$ component studied either psychoacoustically or in the discharge pattern of the 8th nerve, is our observation that the properties of the $2f_1 - f_2$ components that can be measured in the CM are rather undistinguished (Dallos, 1969b; 1970b). All indices of description that we have been able to amass on the $2f_1-f_2$ CM component support the notion that this component behaves as all other nonlinear CM products. Their behavior could simply be described by stating that these components are apparently not mediated by individual traveling waves, that they all seem to be localized in the region of their primaries, that their generation could be explained by assuming that a polynomial nonlinearity operates in the cochlea, and that the source of the nonlinearity is apparently central to the hydrodynamic processes of the inner ear (Sweetman and Dallos, 1969, Dallos et al., 1969, Dallos 1969b, Worthington and Dallos, 1971). Virtually all of these properties of the CM distortion are in direct contrast to those of the psychoacoustically (or neurophysiologically) measured $2f_1-f_2$. An additional important observation is that of Wilson and J.R. Johnstone (1972) who searched in vain for a significant $2f_1-f_2$ component in the displacement pattern of the basilar membrane. One can summarize by stating that $2f_1-f_2$ is not present in the basilar membrane motion; that is, there is no traveling wave corresponding to it, and it is also absent from the CM. It is, however, very much present in the activity of the nerve fibers that are tuned to the pure tone frequency of $2f_1-f_2$. Clearly, this set of observations can contain the key to our understanding of cochlear transducer processes. In the following few paragraphs some new CM data, pertaining to $2f_1-f_2$, are presented, and then a tentative attempt is made to reconcile, at least to a degree, the seemingly conflicting observations.

We have stated before that as much as one can ascertain on the basis of CM data, at low and moderate sound levels no distortion component in the cochlea appears with maximal strength at the place that is tuned to the frequency of the distortion component (Sweetman and Dallos, 1969, Dallos and Sweetman, 1969, Dallos, 1969b, Worthington and Dallos, 1971). Instead of being determined by the frequency of the distortion component, the spatial locus of prominence is governed by the frequency of the fundamental or frequencies of the primaries. Thus all distortion components that are elicited with a given stimulus complex appear in the same region of the cochlea. To underscore these contentions in Fig. 11 a family

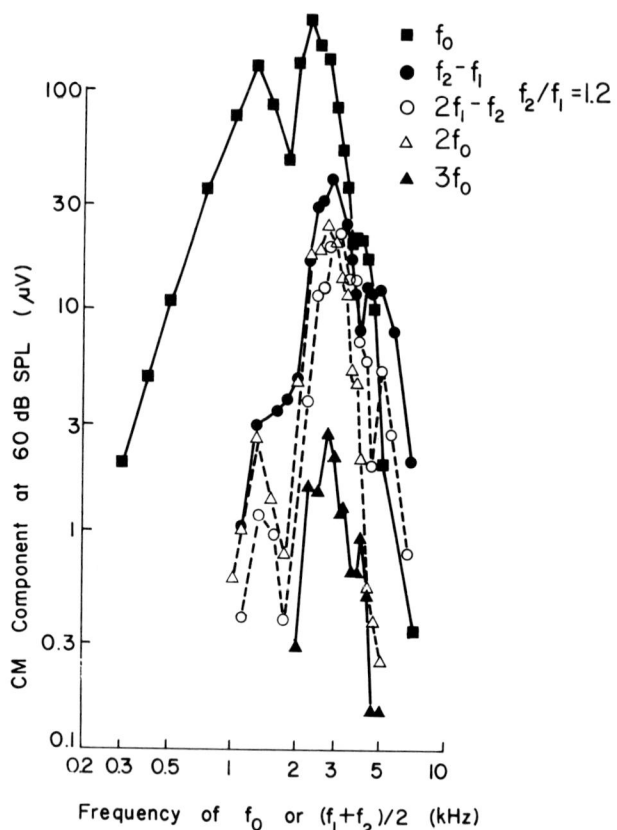

Fig. 11 Frequency response function (■) of a second turn electrode location (closed bulla) and various distortion components measured at 60 dB sound pressure level. Harmonic magnitudes are plotted at the frequency of their fundamental, while combination tone magnitudes are shown at the intertone $((f_1+f_2)/2)$ frequency.

of CM magnitude versus frequency functions are shown, all obtained at a constant 60 dB sound pressure level from a pair of differential electrodes in the second turn of the cochlea. In this particular animal the auditory bulla was closed. The filled squares represent the magnitude of the fundamental primaries of 4000 and 5600 Hz. In both cases the f_2/f_1 ratio is 1.4. It is quite apparent that it is when the primaries are centered around the peak frequency of the recording location (case A) and not when the distortion component frequency is in that vicinity (case B) that the $2f_1-f_2$ achieves its largest magnitude. The difference between plots A and B in the sound pressure level where $2f_1-f_2$ can first be detected is a very impressive 36 dB.

When the various pieces of information on the $2f_1-f_2$ content of the normal CM are gathered together, one is tempted to conclude that at the level of CM-generation the $2f_1-f_2$ component is not any more significant than any other nonlinear distortion product in the cochlea. Such a conclusion would lead to several possible suggestions about the origin of $2f_1-f_2$. The first possibility is that a nonlinearity in the organ of Corti yields $2f_1-f_2$ and that this nonlinearity would produce such a hair cell deformation that appropriate transmitter release could be affected but no CM production would occur. This scheme implies that CM is not a causal agent in initiating neural responses. It also implies that the mechanical input at the hair cell that is responsible for the CM-producing deformation is not necessarily the same as the one which is the precursor of transduction. Presumably with a traveling wave input both types of deformation would be produced, but an intra-organ of Corti source might yield one type.

A second possibility is that $2f_1-f_2$ arises beyond the process of CM generation. This would imply that the nonlinearity is associated with the hair cell-neural junction (J.R. Johnstone, pers.comm.) or even with the dendritic region of the 8th nerve. Clearly, with a nonlinearity of this type one would not expect the distortion components to manifest themselves in either basilar membrane vibrations or in the CM.

A final suggestion about the origin of $2f_1-f_2$, and one that we find appealing, emerges from the realization that the adequate stimulus to, and the possible role of, the inner and outer hair cells are quite different. As was discussed in the previous section, in a normal animal the production of CM is dominated by the outer hair cells. In contrast, the vast majority of 8th nerve fibers innervate the inner hair cells (Spoendlin, 1966) allowing for the distinct possibility that both neurophysiological and psychoacoustical manifestations of $2f_1-f_2$ are mediated by fibers that originate on inner hair cells. If this would be the case then the lack of correlation between CM experiments and single unit experiments on $2f_1-f_2$ would not be unexpected. What needs to be considered, however, is that no matter which hair cell group transduces this distortion component it must arise after the gross mechanical vibration of the basilar membrane. If the two hair cell groups would be stimulated by similar mechanisms then it would be hard to conceive why one would be more prone to respond to $2f_1-f_2$ than the other. In the previous section of this paper it was demonstrated, however, that the adequate stimulus to the two types of hair cell is different, and thus the possibility remains open that the distortion production is somehow tied in with these differences. Consider specifically that the stimulation of the outer hair cells is in a sense much simpler than that of the inner hair cells. The former group receives its input from the bending of the cilia that are anchored between the tectorial membrane and the reticular surface. From the consideration of the organ of Corti geometry by Rhode and Geisler (1967) one can conclude that the linear motion of the basilar membrane results in a linear displacement of the cilia. Consequently, if the $2f_1-f_2$ distortion component is not present in the basilar membrane vibration, it is not expected to be present in the stimulus of the outer hair cells either. From the work of Wilson and J.R. Johnstone (1972) it is known that the basilar membrane displacement is linear, and our normal (outer hair cell) CM results also indicate a lack of distinctive $2f_1-f_2$ content. These results are consistent with one another. Since the inner hair cells do not receive the stimulus directly from the mechanical displacement differential between reticular lamina and tectorial membrane, but via an additional hydrodynamic step, the streaming of fluid between these two surfaces, it is conceivable that a strong nonlinear input component might arise in association with this more complex stimulation process. If this would be the case, then one would expect that the CM produced by inner hair cells would have distortion properties unlike those measured from outer hair cell CM. In fact one might expect the inner hair cell generated CM to reflect the $2f_1-f_2$ behavior seen in single unit discharges. These possibilities are now being investigated in our laboratory with the use of kanamycin intoxicated preparations.

No matter which of the possible schemes one might propose, it is necessary to consider that the production of $2f_1-f_2$ would need to occur in the cochlea at the place that is tuned to that frequency, and since there is no traveling wave present that corresponds to $2f_1-f_2$, it is the primary energy at that location which must act as the input to the nonlinearity. This energy is small since the primary vibration amplitude decreases from the $(f_1+f_2)/2$ site to the $2f_1-f_2$ site at a rather rapid rate corresponding to the apical slope of the intertone's traveling wave. It is conceivable, however, that particularly at the lower primary frequencies this remaining energy is sufficient to stimulate the source of $2f_1-f_2$ (J.R. Johnstone, pers.comm.). It still needs to be explained why the distortion would be prominent at the location of the distortion component instead of that of the primaries. A possible explanation relies on the presence of a second cochlear filter that would accentuate the distortion component at the appropriate location (J.R. Johnstone, pers.comm.). It is proper to point out that the "two-filter" hypothesis of cochlear function is gaining some ground on the basis of considering various experimental evidence. Among these are the discrepancies between mechanical and neural tuning, two-tone suppression, and the $2f_1-f_2$ phenomenon (Pfeiffer, 1970, Evans and Wilson, 1971, Evans, 1972, J.R. Johnstone, pers.comm.).

3. Summary

Ever since their discovery the cochlear microphonic and summating potentials have actively been studied, and their role and relation to other cochlear phenomena have been the subject of much controversy and debate. Opinion is divided about the importance of these potentials. Some feel that they are indispensible intermediate links in the peripheral tranducer process and attempt to seek one-to-one correlations between them and more central events. Others contend that the source of these potentials is too diffuse and that their measurement is too imprecise to warrant serious consideration, and indeed even the investigation, of gross electrical responses from the cochlea. It appears that neither of these extreme positions is warranted. Thus, it is almost certain that the gross electrical potentials under most conditions do not accurately reflect the outputs of individual hair cells. It is also unknown whether even the potential of a singular generator is causally involved in the transducer process. Furthermore, the normal CM is determined by the outer hair cells while central events are likely to be dominated by the output of inner hair cells. Consequently, it is probably not fruitful to assume that gross CM or SP actually would mediate more central auditory responses. On the other hand, even though possibly indirectly, both CM and SP are involved in the tranducer process; they are a sign of it and they can be a measure of it. They are apparently a good index of simple hydromechanical events as well, as the agreement between mechanical and CM cutoff frequencies (Fig. 7) suggests. Thus the investigation of CM and SP can yield extremely valuable results, provided that these are interpreted within the constraints of the complexity of the recording situation and the nature of these gross receptor potentials.

In this report some selected problems of cochlear biophysics are treated in relation to their gross potential correlates. One of these problems pertains to the frequency response characteristics of specific cochlear locations. It is apparent that at a given recording site as a function of frequency, the normal CM magnitude is proportional to stapes velocity up to a characteristic cutoff frequency beyond which it rapidly declines. A small maximum is often seen below the cutoff frequency. The CM phase referred to that of stapes velocity is zero at low frequencies and it accumulates up to 5π to 6π and then levels off at approximately two octaves above the cutoff frequency. Most of the CM measures of frequency response agree qualitatively and even quantitatively with descriptions of basilar membrane vibrations. Where discrepancies are evident, such as in some aspects of phase characteristics, the various available measures of mechanical performance are not in agreement with one another. One important difference between CM and mechanical tuning is in the steepness of the high frequency slope. The electrical tuning curves have high frequency slopes between 30 and 40 dB/octave, not systematically dependent on recording location, while the corresponding slopes of mechanical tuning curves can be estimated to range between 35 and 90 dB/octave with systematic increase toward the base (Evans, 1972). This difference is likely to be the consequence of the more localized nature of the mechanical recordings. While at low stimulus levels the CM is linear, it becomes markedly nonlinear as intensity increases. This familiar nonlinearity is in contrast with the majority of the mechanical data on basilar membrane displacement. Due to this discrepancy, it is virtually imperative to make CM measurements below 40-50 dB SPL when their correlation with mechanical events is sought.

Both summating potential components, DIF and AVE, are shown to be tuned about 2/3 octave higher than the CM. At low intensities they are also more localized than the ac receptor potential. The magnitude of the SP is quite commensurate with that of the CM, and its properties are just as well-defined and quantifiable. It is probably not appropriate to dismiss the importance of the dc receptor potential components, or to a priori attribute less significance or a lesser potential role to them than to the CM.

One new development in cochlear biophysics, the study of which is made possible by appropriate CM measurements, is proposed difference in dynamic properties between inner and outer hair cells. The properties of the CM produced by inner hair cells, recorded from cochlear regions from where all outer hair cells are removed by kanamycin poisoning, are such that one can deduce that inner hair cells respond to the derivative of the stimulus that excites the outer hair cells. Since normal CM (overwhelmingly the product of outer hair cells) is proportional to basilar membrane displacement (Békésy, 1951b), the CM produced by inner hair cells is proportional to basilar membrane velocity. These dynamic differences also imply differences in the frequency response of the two hair cell groups. One of the most important manifestations of these is the steeper (by 6 dB/

octave) low frequency slope of inner hair cell tuning curves. Since the most striking discrepancy between mechanical and neural tuning is in the steepness of their low frequency slopes, it is comforting that the inner hair cells that innervate most of the afferent 8th nerve fibers do provide some small measure of sharpening over the mechanical response.

The difference in stimulation of the two hair cell groups is also invoked as a conceivable explanation for the apparent discrepancies between mechanical and CM measures on the one hand, and single unit data and psychoacoustic information on the other hand, as these pertain to the peculiar distortion component $2f_1-f_2$. This most prominent of all subjective distortion components, the $2f_1-f_2$, is apparently not present in the vibration pattern of the basilar membrane or in the normal CM. It is, however, clearly demonstrable in the discharge properties of the neurons tuned to the frequency $2f_1-f_2$. If this distortion arises in a nonlinearity that is peculiar to inner hair cell stimulation, that is one which resides in a hydrodynamic process central to basilar membrane displacement, then $2f_1-f_2$ would not be seen either in the gross mechanical measure of basilar membrane vibration or in normal CM. It would, however, be present in the discharges of those 8th nerve fibers that innervate inner hair cells.

Acknowledgements

This work is supported by grants from the National Institute of Neurological Diseases and Stroke, NIH, US Public Health Service. Several of my associates, W. Ballad, M.A. Cheatham, J.D. Durrant, and C.Y. Wang, contributed to this work.

References

Anderson, D.J., Rose, J.E., Hind, J.E., and Brugge, J.F. (1971). Temporal position of discharges in single auditory nerve fibers within the cycle of a sine-wave stimulus: Frequency and intensity effects. J. Acoust. Soc. Amer. 49, 1131-1139.

Békésy, G. von (1947). The variation of phase along the basilar membrane with sinusoidal vibrations. J. Acoust. Soc. Amer. 19, 452-460.

Békésy, G. von (1949). The vibration of the cochlear partition in anatomical preparations and in models of the inner ear. J. Acoust. Soc. Amer. 21, 233-245.

Békésy, G. von (1951a). The coarse pattern of electrical resistance in the cochlea of the guinea pig (electro-anatomy of the cochlea). J. Acoust. Soc. Amer. 23, 18-28.

Békésy, G. von (1951b). Microphonics produced by touching the cochlear partition with a vibrating electrode. J. Acoust. Soc. Amer. 23, 29-35.

Billone, M.C. (1972). Mechanical stimulation of cochlear hair cells. Thesis. Northwestern Univ., Evanston.

Cern, Y., and Fischler, H. (1972). Significance of resistance measurements in the scala media. J. Acoust. Soc. Amer. 51, 2057-2059.

Dallos, P. (1969a). Comments on the differential electrode recording technique. J. Acoust. Soc. Amer. 45, 999-1007.

Dallos, P. (1969b). Combination tone $2f_1-f_h$ in microphonic potentials. J. Acoust. Soc. Amer. 46, 1437-1444.

Dallos, P. (1970a). Low frequency auditory characteristics: Species dependence. J. Acoust. Soc. Amer. 48, 489-499.

Dallos, P. (1970b). Combination tones in cochlear microphonic potentials. In: Frequency Analysis and Periodicity Detection in Hearing (R. Plomp and G. Smoorenburg, eds.), pp. 218-226. Sijthoff, Leiden, The Netherlands.

Dallos, P. (1972). Cochlear potentials: A status report. Int. Audiol. 11, 29-41.

Dallos, P., and Durrant, J.D. (1972). On the derivative relationship between stapes movement and cochlear microphonic. J. Acoust. Soc. Amer. 52, 1263-1265.

Dallos, P., and Sweetman, D.H. (1969). Distribution pattern of cochlear harmonics. J. Acoust. Soc. Amer. 45, 37-46.

Dallos, P., Schoeny, Z.G., Worthington, D.W., and Cheatham, M.A. (1969). Cochlear distortion. Effect of direct current polarization. Science 164, 449-451.

Dallos, P., Schoeny, Z.G., and Cheatham, M.A. (1970). Cochlear summating potentials: Composition. Science 170, 641-644.

Dallos, P., Schoeny, Z.G., and Cheatham, M.A. (1971). On the limitations of cochlear microphonic recording. J. Acoust. Soc. Amer. 49, 1144-1154.

Dallos, P., Schoeny, Z.G., and Cheatham, M.A. (1972a). Cochlear summating potentials: Descriptive aspects. Acta oto-laryngol. Suppl. 302, 46.

Dallos, P., Billone, M.C., Durrant, J.D., Wang, C-y., and Raynor, S. (1972b). Cochlear inner and outer hair cells: Functional differences. Science 177, 356-358.

Davis, H. (1961). Some principles of sensory receptor action. Physiol. Rev. 41, 391-416.

Davis, H., Deatherage, G.H., Rosenblut, B., Fernández, C., Kimura, R., and Smith, C.A. (1958). Modification of cochlear potentials produced by streptomycin poisoning and by extensive venous obstruction. Laryngoscope 68, 596-627.

Engebretson, A.M. (1970). A study of the linear and nonlinear characteristics of microphonic voltage in the cochlea. Thesis. Washington Univ. St. Louis.

Engström, H., Ades, H.W., and Andersson, A. (1966). Structural Pattern of the Organ of Corti. Almquist & Wiksell, Stockholm.

Evans, E.F. (1972). Does frequency sharpening occur in the cochlea? Symposium on Hearing Theory 1972, pp. 27-34. IPO Eindhoven, Holland.

Evans, E.F., and Wilson, J.P. (1971). Frequency sharpening of the cochlea. The effective bandwidth of cochlear nerve fibers. Proc. Int. Congr. Acoust. 7th, Vol. 3, pp. 453-456. Akademiai Kiado, Budapest.

Goldstein, J.L. (1967). Auditory nonlinearity. J. Acoust. Soc. Amer. 41, 676-689.

Goldstein, J.L. (1972). Evidence from aural combination tones and musical tones against classical temporal periodicity theory. Symposium on Hearing Theory 1972, pp. 186-208. IPO Eindhoven, Holland.

Goldstein, J.L., and Kiang, N.Y.S. (1968). Neural correlates of the aural combination tone $2f_1-f_2$. Proc. IEEE 56, 981-992.

Greenwood, D.D. (1971). Aural combination tones and auditory masking. J. Acoust. Soc. Amer. 50, 502-543.

Guinan, J., and Peake, W.T. (1967). Middle ear characteristics of anesthetized cats. J. Acoust. Soc. Amer. 41, 1237-1261.

Hawkins, J. (1959). The ototoxicity of kanamycin. Ann. Otol. Rhinol. Laryngol. 68, 698-715.

Hind, J.E., Rose, J.E., Brugge, J.F., and Anderson, D.J. (1972). Some effects of intensity on the discharge of auditory nerve fibers. In: Physiology of the Auditory System (M.B. Sachs, ed.), pp. 101-111. National Educational Consultants, Inc. Baltimore.

Honrubia, V., and Ward, P.H. (1958). Longitudinal distribution of the cochlear microphonics inside the cochlear duct (guinea pig). J. Acoust. Soc. Amer. 44, 951-958.

Honrubia, V., and Ward, P.H. (1969). Properties of the summating potential of the guinea pig's cochlea. J. Acoust. Soc. Amer. 45, 1443-1450.

Johnstone, B.M., and Boyle, A.J.T. (1967). Basilar membrane vibrations examined with the Mössbauer technique. Science 158, 389-390.

Johnstone, B.M., and Taylor, K.J. (1970). Mechanical
aspects of cochlear function. In: Frequency
Analysis and Periodicity Detection in Hearing
(R. Plomp and G. Smoorenburg, eds.), pp. 81-93.
Sijthoff, Leiden, The Netherlands.

Johnstone, B.M., and Taylor, K.J. (1971). Physiology
of the middle ear transmission system. Otolaryngol. Soc. Aust. 3, 226-228.

Kiang, N.Y.S. (1965). Discharge Patterns of Single
Fibers in the Cat's Auditory Nerve. Res. Monogr.
35. M.I.T. Press, Cambridge, Mass.

Kiang, N.Y.S. (1968). A survey of recent developments
in the study of auditory physiology. Ann. Otol.
Rhinol. Laryngol. 77, 656-672.

Kimura, R. (1965). Hairs of the cochlear sensory
cells and their attachment to the tectorial
membrane. Acta oto-laryngol. 61, 55-72.

Kohllöffel, L.U.E. (1971). Studies of the distribution of cochlear potentials along the basilar
membrane. Acta oto-laryngol. Suppl. 288.

Konishi, T., and Yasuno, T. (1963). Summating potential of the cochlea of the guinea pig. J. Acoust.
Soc. Amer. 35, 1448-1452.

Kupperman, R. (1966). The dynamic dc potential in the
cochlea of the guinea pig (summating potential).
Acta oto-laryngol. 62, 465-480.

Laszlo, C.A. (1968). Measurement, modeling and simulation of the cochlear potentials. Thesis.
McGill Univ. Montreal.

Laszlo, C.A., Gannon, R.P., and Milsum, J.H. (1970).
Measurement of the cochlear potentials of the
guinea pig at constant sound-pressure level at
the eardrum: I. Cochlear microphonic amplitude
and phase. J. Acoust. Soc. Amer. 47, 1063-1070.

Lim, D. (1971). Morphological relationship between
the tectorial membrane and the organ of Corti-
Scanning and transmission electron microscopy.
J. Acoust. Soc. Amer. 50, 92(A).

Møller, A. (1963). Transfer function of the middle ear. J. Acoust. Soc. Amer. 35, 1526-1534.

Molnar, C.E., Loeffel, R.G., and Pfeiffer, R.R. (1968). Distortion compensating, condenser-earphone driver for physiological studies. J. Acoust. Soc. Amer. 43, 1177-1178.

Pfeiffer, R.R. (1970). A model for two-tone inhibition of single cochlear nerve fibers. J. Acoust. Soc. Amer. 48, 1373-1378.

Rhode, W.S. (1971). Observations of the vibration of the basilar membrane in squirrel monkeys using the Mössbauer technique. J. Acoust. Soc. Amer. 49, 1218-1231.

Rhode, W.S., and Geisler, C.D. (1967). Model of displacement between opposing points on tectorial membrane and reticular lamina. J. Acoust. Soc. Amer. 42, 185-190.

Smoorenburg, G. (1972). Combination tones and their origin. J. Acoust. Soc. Amer. 52, 615-632.

Spoendlin, H. (1966). The Organization of the Cochlear Receptor. Karger, Basel-New York.

Sweetman, R.H., and Dallos, P. (1969). Distribution pattern of cochlear combination tones. J. Acoust. Soc. Amer. 45, 59-71.

Tasaki, I., Davis, H., and Legouix, J.-P. (1952). The space-time pattern of the cochlear microphonics (guinea pig) as recorded by differential electrodes. J. Acoust. Soc. Amer. 24, 502-518.

Tonndorf, J. (1958). Localization of aural harmonics along the basilar membrane of guinea pigs. J. Acoust. Soc. Amer. 30, 938-943.

Wang, C-y. (1973). Cochlear damage by kanamycin: A quantitative analysis of histopathological findings. Ann. Otol. Rhinol. Laryngol. (In press).

Wang, C-y., and Dallos, P. (1972). Latency of whole nerve action potentials: Influence of hair cell normalcy. J. Acoust. Soc. Amer. 52, 1678-1686.

Weiss, T.F., Peake, W.T., and Sohmer, H. (1969). Intracochlear responses to tones. M.I.T. Quart. Progr. Rep. 94, 305-316.

Whitfield, I.C., and Ross, D.A. (1965). Cochlear microphonic and summating potentials and the outputs of individual hair cell generators. J. Acoust. Soc. Amer. 38, 126-131.

Wilson, J.P., and Johnstone, J.R. (1972). Capacitive probe measures of basilar membrane vibration. Symposium on Hearing Theory 1972, pp. 172-181. IPO Eindhoven, Holland.

Worthington, D.W., and Dallos, P. (1971). Spatial patterns of cochlear difference tones. J. Acoust. Soc. Amer. 49, 1818-1830.

Zwislocki, J. (1963). Analysis of middle ear function Part II: Guinea pig ear. J. Acoust. Soc. Amer. 35, 1034-1040.

DISCUSSION

ZWISLOCKI: I have one comment and several questions. Let me start with the comment. I notice in your phase curves that, past a 6 π angle, the phase stops changing, as in Rhode's experiments. I am very happy about this because it agrees with the theoretical prediction that, past the resonance point of the cochlear duct, the phase should not change, since there is no wave propagation there. However, it seems to me that some other experiments do not show this phase plateau, which has to be considered.

One of my questions is: I think, it was stated in the literature not so long ago that even differential recordings of cochlear microphonics represented events that were integrated over a certain portion of the cochlea. From the recordings you showed today, it seems that they really agree quite well with an assumption of an extremely small area of integration.

DALLOS: I would not go that far. One measure of the differences between mechanical and microphonic data is in the high frequency slope of the tuning curves. We obtain a high frequency slope of about 100 dB/decade and of course the people who record mechanical events get about 100 dB/octave. There is thus a significant difference which most likely is due to the fact that the microphonic measurements are integrated over a wide spatial segment.

ZWISLOCKI: We are dealing with what you hypothesize to be inner hair cells. You show a phase difference of half a π relative to the normal up to, I think about 5 kHz. Then, the phase difference suddenly drops. Would you comment on that?

DALLOS: The inner hair cell phase behavior at high frequencies is of course a question that puzzles us a great deal and we have no explanation for it at the present time. My colleague Mike Billone actually presented a very complete model (Billone 1972) that predicts our amplitude and phase results rather well at low frequencies but not at the high frequencies.

STEELE: Well, I am happy to see from the results that you have presented, that several things fit together.

My question is: Did you record the summating potential for the kanamycin treated animal?

DALLOS: Yes. I have an illustration of that (Fig. 1).

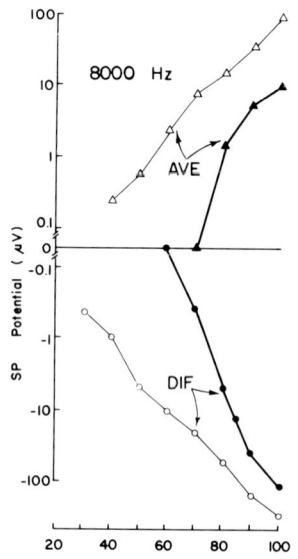

Fig. 1 Summating potential input-output functions in response to 8 kHz tone bursts from representative normal (open symbols) and from kanamycin-treated (closed symbols) cochleas. Recording is from the basal turn, where there were no outer hair cells remaining in the ototoxicated ear.

In the kanamycin-treated animal in which there are only inner hair cells intact in the basal region, the summating potential at low intensities also declines approximately by the same amount as the cochlear microphonic. As you see in the figure, as intensity is increased both the DIF^- and the AVE^+ components rise at approximately twice the rate as they do in a normal animal. Thus, in a normal animal at low sound levels, the outer hair cells produce all or virtually all the recordable summating potential. As sound pressure level is increased beyond 100 dB, the inner hair cells start to contribute significantly. This is well above the intensity range where we like to collect our data. In order not to have nonlinear effects interfere with the measurements, levels below 60 dB SPL should be used. There the outer hair cells produce the overwhelming amount of summating potential just as they produce the overwhelming amount of cochlear microphonic.

KOHLLÖFFEL: I would like to make a comment on your phase plateau. As you said mechanical measurements and cochlear microphonic measurements show the strongest deviation on the high frequency side. If this holds for amplitude it would be surprising if it did not hold for phase. Furthermore, it is quite possible to record a flat cochlear microphonic phase curve provided the wavelength along the basilar membrane is sufficiently short for the electrodes not to resolve the phase difference. Thus the cochlear microphonic phase plateau can either indicate a mechanical phase plateau, i.e. an extremely long wavelength, or just the opposite, an extremely short wavelength. One cannot compare the phase plateau in the cochlear microphonic directly with the mechanically measured phase plateau, I think.

DALLOS: Well, the striking feature is that we get quite similar results which at least one group obtained with the mechanical measurement.

KOHLLÖFFEL: Did you get it at the same frequency?

DALLOS: Yes, I did. This is exactly the point. At the cut-off frequency we get exactly the same phase as they do.

KOHLLÖFFEL: As regards the phase plateau, Wilson and Johnstone (1972) obtained it at about 2π phase lag in the basal turn of the guinea pig; you show it around 6π, presumably in a higher turn.

DALLOS: Yes, there is a difference in the total accumulated phase at the plateau, but the agreement up to and at the cut-off frequency is good.

References

Billone, M. (1972). Mechanical stimulation of cochlear hair cells. Thesis. Northwestern Univ., Evanston.

Wilson, J.P., and Johnstone, J.R. (1972). Capacitive probe measure of basilar membrane vibration. Symposium on Hearing Theory 1972, pp. 172-181, IPO Eindhoven, Holland.

NEUROPHARMACOLOGY AND POTENTIALS
OF THE INNER EAR

Jörgen Fex

Center for Neural Sciences
Indiana University
Bloomington, Indiana
USA

This report is concerned with the recording of potentials in the organ of Corti as a basis for neuropharmacological experiments and with the olivocochlear inhibition. Excitation in the cochlea is discussed elsewhere (Fex, 1972).

1. First Series, 1967. Intracellular and Extracellular Recording from the Organ of Corti

1.1 Technique

Many of the details concerning preparation, electrical stimulation, acoustic stimulation and recording technique have been presented before (Fex, 1967) and will be only summarized here.

The experiments were carried out in 1967 on 28 cats, weighing between 2.0-3.0 kg and anesthetized with intraperitoneal pentobarbital, 36-42 mg/kg b.w. They were paralyzed with gallamine triethiodide and artificially respirated. Most of the outer ear, the bulla, and the septum, were removed. In some of the animals the whole middle ear was also removed so that it would be easier to move the microelectrode in parallel with the rows of outer hair cells. In the other animals this could be done with the tympanic membrane and the bonelets in position, and these structures were then left intact. The round window membrane was removed and care was being taken to stop all the bleeding in this region.

Two or three electrodes for electrical stimulation of the crossed olivocochlear fibers were implanted in the floor of the fourth ventricle.

Capillary microelectrodes filled with 3M KCl and having a resistance in perilymph of 2.5-25 Megohm were used. The electrodes were connected by a switch with an Ag - AgCl wire to a cathode follower amplifier with capacity neutralization. The reference electrode, an Ag - AgCl wire embedded in gauze soaked in saline or artificial perilymph, was placed in the open left bulla or between intact neck muscles. A low-resistance voltage calibrator and a low-resistance dc balance circuit were between the reference electrode and the room ground.

Tip potentials (Adrian, 1956) were not measured but must often have been large, since most of the microelectrodes were stored for a long time in a refrigerator before they were used.

1.2 Experimental Procedure

As much perilymph as possible was sucked away from the basilar membrane of the basal turn. The shaft of the microelectrode was approximately aligned with the optical axis of the binocular operating microscope. The tip of the microelectrode was aimed so that in the organ of Corti it would move towards the apex in a direction parallel to that of the rows of hair cells. Also, the electrode was aimed to penetrate the basilar membrane at rather an acute angle, so that the electrode might penetrate the one hair cell after the other, in the same row but at different heights, while coming deeper and deeper into the organ of Corti.

The touching of the perilymph with the tip of the microelectrode was signalled by the monitoring loudspeaker. The ink-writer for dc recording was then started. It was set to zero reading by the dc balance circuit. The olivocochlear nerve fibers were electrically stimulated with single shocks, 3-10 shocks/sec. The master trigger and the other triggers were set so that single sweeps appeared on the screen of the oscilloscope synchronously with the single shocks (Fig. 1).

The tip of the electrode was then advanced; generally after 50-100 μm the lower, ac high gain beam of the oscilloscope started to swing up and down. This swinging sometimes stopped if the electrode was stopped, sometimes only if the electrode was withdrawn

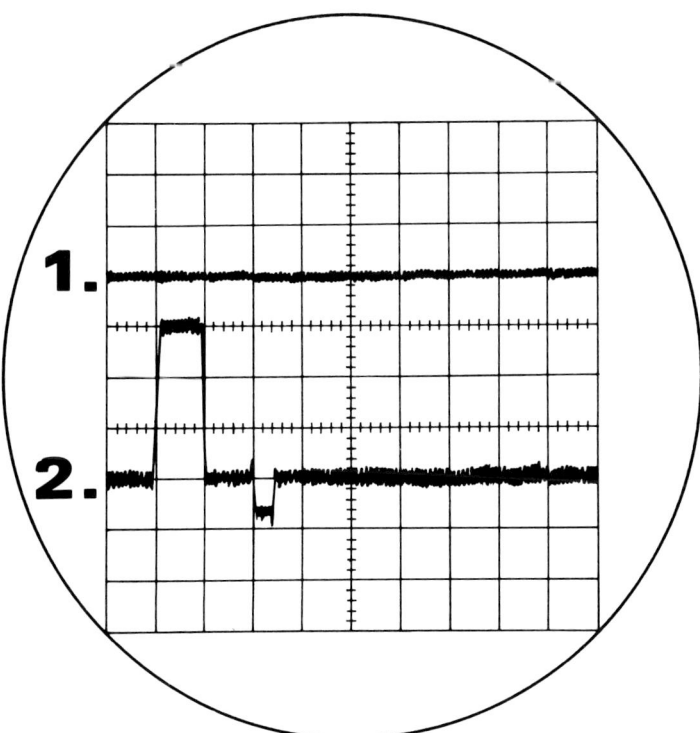

Fig. 1   Diagram illustrating the procedures.

A single sweep of the monitoring oscilloscope is represented. Beam 1 was used to monitor the dc potential at low gain, 50 mV/unit. Beam 2 was used to monitor ac potentials at high gain, 0.2-2.0 mV/unit, with a time resolution of 1 msec/unit, sometimes 2 msec/unit. The first potential on beam 2 represented the electrode resistance and the amount of capacity neutralization; the second potential represented the timing of the single shock for olivocochlear activation. It was particularly important to notice even small changes of the electrode resistance and of the stability of the ac base line.

1 - 2 - 5 µm. The electrode was then again advanced by 1 - 2 - 5 µm, the swinging of the beam would start again, and the electrode was advanced further, only

a few microns at a time (Fig. 2 A). It often happened

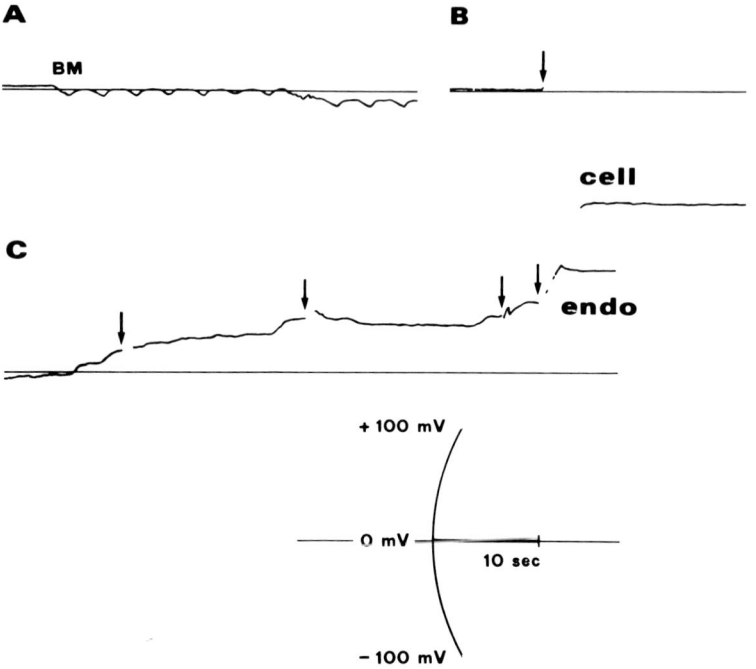

Fig. 2   Records illustrating typical intracochlear potentials.

A. Corresponding to the tracing to the left of BM the electrode tip was in scala tympani and was moved 5 μm forwards, towards the basilar membrane. This caused a small negative dc shift, on which was superimposed a negative potential that was synchronized with the respiratory movements. BM was taken to represent the contact between the electrode tip and the basilar membrane, in time and space. Slightly more than 20 sec after BM the electrode was again moved, 8 μm forwards. This typically increased the negative dc shift.

B. The electrode tip had passed through three stages of relatively small negative dc shifts after BM and the potential had then returned to approximately   (cont'd)

(Fig. 2, cont'd) 0 mV. Just before the arrow the electrode tip had been moved forwards in a region of 0 mV, and this has caused the electrode resistance to increase from 13 Megohm to 17 Megohm. At the arrow, current was passed through the electrode. Immediately after this (cell), a potential of -100 mV was recorded and the electrode resistance had returned to 13 Megohm. This lasted for more than 4 minutes; then the electrode was moved purposely.

C. The electrode tip had passed through several regions with negative potentials and with potentials close to 0 mV and the beginning of this record was reached. Before each arrow the electrode tip had been moved forwards a few microns; at each arrow current was passed through the electrode. In this way it was possible to record a relatively stable potential at almost any level between 0 mV and the EP (endo).

In each record, the straight horizontal line represents approximately 0 mV (relative to scala tympani). The calibration of voltage and time is common to all the records. NOTE: all dc potentials are larger by 10 % than is indicated by the calibration.

after the penetration of the basilar membrane that there was a region for which the ink-writer registered a potential of about zero mV, while the ac beam on the oscilloscope showed that the electrode resistance was the same as it had been in scala tympani. Then, often, there was an increase of the electrode resistance when the electrode was advanced, sometimes with only a few Megohms; the ac beam showed added fluctuations and the monitoring loudspeaker sounded more noisy. Current was then passed through the micropipette by overcompensating for the resistance change with the feed back circuit for capacity neutralization. This often caused the electrode resistance to go back to its initial value, while the recorded dc potential became negative and large (Fig. 2B) and stable. On the other hand, if current was not applied to the pipette as a means for getting the negative potential, and if the pipette was simply advanced in a situation as the one just described, any negative potential that then might appear would as a rule be unstable, disappearing after a few seconds.

The electrode was advanced until the endolymphatic potential could be recorded. The olivocochlear fibers were then stimulated also by trains of shocks and the evoked potential (COC-; see Fex, 1967; Fex, 1968) was recorded with the ink-writer set at a high gain for dc recording. The corresponding evoked potential was often also recorded in the organ of Corti, both in regions of zero dc potential and of large negativity. Different methods were tried to get a stable base line for the recordings. Often the baseline was good when the electrode tip was in the endolymph, but sometimes not. Much experimental time was used to find out how stopping the artificial respiration might change the different potentials. Stopping the pump shortly for stable recordings was, of course, quite safe and often useful. Stopping the pump for longer periods caused the centrifugally evoked potentials to increase during and immediately after the asphyxia.

1.3 Results

In the 28 cats, 82 penetrations of the organ of Corti were carried out and large negative potentials were recorded 110 times. In all, 23 of these potentials were held unchanged during 4 minutes or more, in twelve of the animals. Thus five potentials were held for 4 minutes, thirteen potentials for 5-8 minutes, two potentials for 10-13 minutes, two potentials for 20 minutes, and one potential for 31 minutes. In thirteen of the animals the endolymphatic potential was +90 mV or larger with a mean amplitude of +101 mV and a range of +90 - +108 mV. Five out of these thirteen cats with seemingly normal endolymphatic potentials (cf. Sohmer et al., 1971) had between them eleven longlasting negative potentials with a mean amplitude of -93 mV and a range of -78 - -105 mV. Much the same mean amplitude and range of both shortlasting and longlasting large negative potentials were found in some of the experiments in which the endolymphatic potential was abnormally low, +60 mV or lower.

To note is, that out of all the 23 longlasting large negative potentials only one was lost by some uncontrolled movement of the electrode tip. In all the other 22 cases the electrode tip was moved purposely relative to the stationary parts of the micromanipulator before the negativity disappeared.

In all experiments potentials close the zero mV were found and could be kept indefinitely, before, between and after recordings of large negativities, short-lasting and longlasting, during the passage of the electrode tip through the organ of Corti.

The centrifugally evoked potential was larger when superimposed upon a large negativity than when recorded in a region with zero dc potential.

2.   Second, Third and Fourth Series.
Intracellular and Extracellular Recording from the
Organ of Corti - Pharmacological Studies

2.1   Auxiliary Studies

2.1.1 The Use of Methylene Blue Chloride for Improving the Precision of Electrode Placement

Békésy (1960) used methylene blue in vivo in order to make hair cells stain selectively. Richardson (1968) found that toxic effects of methylene blue chloride at a concentration of 2 mg/100 cc could be seen under the electron microscope. Richardson stressed that methylene blue chloride rather specifically stained structures that also stain for acetylcholinesterase (AChE).

In five full experiments I used methylene blue chloride in order to try to visualize the hair cells of the organ of Corti. This was done also at the end of several other experiments. Whether actually the inner and outer hair cells, or the inner spiral fibers under the inner hair cells and the large efferent endings on the outer hair cells were stained, was immaterial to my purpose. I found two stained regions, running like ribbons along the organ of Corti. Between the ribbons was an unstained region along which an artery was running. I took the inner, thinner ribbon that was running extremely close to the modial bony lip to represent the inner hair cells. The unstained region outside the inner hair cells was taken to represent the tunnel of Corti. It had a width of about 25 microns, while the stained structure further to the periphery was estimated to be about 30 microns wide, probably corresponding to the outer hair cells.

The basilar membrane was approximately 100 microns wide between the bony lips in the region inside the round window that was penetrated with microelectrodes.

Training precision placement of the microelectrode tip I found it easy to penetrate the organ of Corti peripheral to all hair cells and possible to cause the blue color to disappear from localized spots on the outer stained ribbon. I could also with some confidence place the tip inside the outer hair cells without breaking the electrode tip against the bony, medial, lip. This was when the electrode shaft was placed so that the tip traveled approximately in a plane tangent to a hair cell row at right angles to the basilar membrane. The precision was not good enough to enable me to aim at the row of inner hair cells with any confidence. The precision radially, across the organ of Corti, was understandably much better than that along the organ. It was found that the layer of fluid on the basilar membrane had to be very thin or thick not to spoil the precision. In practice it became important to work with a thin layer of fluid and fast refill of perilymph could therefore become a serious problem. A considerable source of error was bending of the electrode tip.

2.1.2 Latency Measurements of Crossed Olivocochlear Nerve Impulses, 1965

One cat, weighing 2.5 kg, was anesthetized with pentobarbital, paralyzed with gallamine triethiodide and prepared for recording from single crossed olivocochlear nerve fibers in the vestibulo-cochlear anastomosis as described earlier (Fex, 1962). Particular care was taken to keep the posterior fossa and the vestibulo-cochlear anastomosis at normal temperature. A microelectrode filled with 3 M KCl and with a resistance of 35 Megohm was used for probing the anastomosis. Seven nerve fibers were identified as belonging to the crossed olivocochlear bundle by responding to single shocks from two electrodes in the floor of the fourth ventricle.

The evoked resonses from five out of these seven nerve fibers were displayed on the oscilloscope screen and photographed (Fig. 3 A). The latencies from the beginning of the shock to the inflection point of the initial positive phase of the potentials were, in msec: 0.7, 0.7, 1.2, 1.2 and 1.4. Corresponding am-

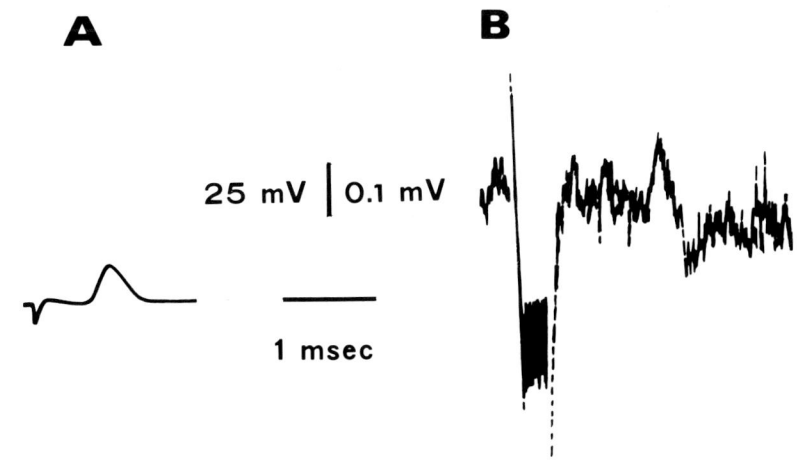

Fig. 3   Records illustrating potentials evoked by single shocks applied to the crossed olivo-cochlear fibers in the midline of the floor of the fourth ventricle.

A. Potential recorded from a single crossed olivocochlear fiber in the vestibulo-cochlear anastomosis, approximately 12 mm from the site of stimulation.

B. Potential recorded extracellularly with the microelectrode tip in the organ of Corti.

The initial deflection, on both traces, is the shock artifact.

plitudes of the monophasic positive spikes were, in mV: 4, 20, 2, 8, and 7. The two additional nerve fibers were lost before film could be taken: one of these had an estimated latency of 0.8 msec. The impulses had a rather poorly defined duration of the order of 0.6-0.7 msec. The distance between the sites of stimulation and recording was approximately 12 mm.

2.2   Technique

The technique was much the same as described above, (Section 1.1) except for details in the preparation of the animal.

Experiments were carried out on a series of 39 cats

during 1968, weighing 1.7-2.8 kg and anesthetized with intraperitoneal pentobarbital, 36-46 mg/kg b.w., paralyzed with gallamine triethiodide and artificially respirated. In 1969, 23 cats were used for these experiments, weighing 1.9-2.8 kg, decerebrated and decerebellated under anesthesia with Fluothane and then paralyzed with gallamine triethiodide and artificially respirated. In 1970 and 1971, 17 cats were used for these experiments, weighing 1.8-2.5 kg; 6 cats were anesthetized with pentobarbital and 11 cats with Fluothane and prepared as the cats of 1968, respectively of 1969.

In many of the cats the round window region of the cochlea was made as accessible as was possible. Thus, most of the bulla and of the septum was removed. The incudo-stapedial joint was dislocated, the incus was removed and the outer ear with the tympanic membrane was deflected forwards. The tendon of the stapedius muscle was cut to prevent dislocation of the stapes during the opening of the canal of the facial nerve; the nerve was cut. Part of the temporal bone above the round window was removed with forceps and fine rongeurs. Drills were never used. It often happened that a semicircular canal was opened; this seemed to cause problems only the first few times. It should be noted that there were animals in the series in which all the structures were left intact that were necessary for inner ear responses to be normal; Evans (1970) has shown that single auditory nerve fibers respond normally to sound also when the round window membrane and the perilymph in the basal turn have been removed.

Stimulation and recording were carried out as described above in section 1; in some of the 1969, 1970, and 1971 experiments a signal averager was used for recording. For many of the experiments microelectrodes more than one year old were used. Again, tip potentials were tolerated and not measured.

A 30 % solution of urea in invert sugar was found not only to combat edema of the brain (cf. Fex, 1962, also for references), but also to help to slow down the refill of perilymph in the scala tympani. Therefore, urea was used in many of the experiments. Fast refill was detrimental to the precision of electrode placement and often to the stability of the preparation.

2.3 Experimental Procedure

2.3.1 The 1968 Series

The experimental procedure except for the two last experiments was much the same as during the 1967 experiments. However, more care than before was taken to supply scala tympani with freshly oxygenated artificial perilymph at regular intervals, each 20-30 minutes. The technique for doing this has been described before (Fex, 1967); this technique was used also now for the pharmacological experiments.

2.3.2 The 1969 Series

During these experiments, and during the two last experiments of the 1968 series, electrodes were pushed through the organ of Corti faster than before and the technique of passing current through the microelectrode was used less.

2.3.3 The 1970 - 1971 Series

Microelectrodes were pushed quickly through the organ of Corti, peripheral to the tectorial membrane in order to cause the smallest possible lesion. Electrically and acoustically evoked potentials were recorded with the microelectrode tip sitting stationary in the scala media. The fluid in the basal part of the scala tympani was exchanged with the electrode in this position.

2.4 Results

2.4.1 1968 Series, Recording of Potentials

Out of the 39 cats, one was used only for pharmacological experiments and the two last cats of the series were used for relatively rapid penetration of the organ of Corti. The results of potential recording from the remaining 36 cats were:

a) The organ of Corti was penetrated 116 times and the electrode tip seemed to have been well aimed in 66 of these penetrations.

b) In 30 animals, in 99 instances, a large negative stable potential was recorded that did not disappear until the electrode had been moved on purpose. A larger, uncounted, number of large, unstable, negative potentials were also recorded.

c) In the first 19 cats of the series the electrode was occasionally aimed for cells much peripheral to outer hair cells. Twenty-two negativities, stable or instable, from the periphery had a mean potential of -96 mV. The mean potential was -97 mV of thirty-eight, respectively twenty-one, potentials when the electrode had been aimed at outer hair cells, respectively at the tunnel of Corti or at inner hair cells, in these 19 cats.

d) In seven cats, altogether 15 penetrations of the organ of Corti were made much peripheral to the outer hair cells. Out of these penetrations, the full endolymphatic potential (EP) was reached immediately after a large negativity 5 times and after about zero mV 5 times; the EP was reached via intermediate positive values 4 times from a large negative potential and once from about zero mV. In twenty cats, altogether 33 penetrations were made of the organ of Corti with a good aim for outer hair cells. The EP was reached immediately after a large negativity 10 times and after a stable zero mV 5 times; the EP was reached via intermediate positive values 13 times from a large negative potential and 5 times from about zero mV. In six cats, 6 penetrations were made with a good aim for the tunnel of Corti. The potential changed directly from about zero mV to EP 5 times and once via intermediate positive values. In three cats, 12 penetrations were made with the aim for the inner hair cells. The potential went directly to the EP from a large negativity 4 times and from about zero mV twice; the EP was reached via intermediate values twice from a large negative potential and 4 times from about zero mV.

e) During two penetrations in one cat and one penetration in one cat electrical stimulation of crossed olivocochlear nerve fibers by single shocks evoked large negative potentials that were superimposed on potentials of -66 mV, -33 mV, and -62 mV, respectively. It was estimated from direct observation of the evoked potentials on the high gain ac beam on the screen of the oscilloscope that they had the following characteristics, all figures being approximate: latency, between 2 msec and 4 msec; amplitude, between 5 mV and 10 mV; duration, several msec, perhaps

10 msec. These evoked potentials and the negative potentials on which they were superimposed disappeared simultaneously, after 1.5 sec, 1.0 sec, and 2.5 sec, respectively. Such evoked potentials were never seen superimposed on stable negative potentials.

f) In five cats, during 9 penetrations, single shocks that were applied to crossed efferent fibers evoked an extracellular potential (pre-COC potential; Fig. 3 B) that could be recorded over an indefinite period of time and over a large part of the distance between the basilar membrane and the endolymph.

2.4.2 1969 Series, Recording of Potentials

a) In twenty out of the twenty-three cats of this series 39 penetrations were made in attempts to record the pre-COC potential. This succeeded in eight cats, in 12 penetrations; in ten cats, only one penetration was made, 4 of these were successful. The characteristics of the 21 pre-COC potentials from the two series together were the following: latency from beginning of shock to beginning of potential was generally estimated to be of the order of 1.5 msec and measured values were, in msec, 1.2, 1.3, 1.4, 1.4, 1.6, 2.0, and 2.5; duration, less than 1 msec; amplitude, generally between 50-200 µV. A potential corresponding to the pre-COC potential was never seen intracellularly or in the endolymph. On the other hand, a pre-COC potential could be found on both sides of a region of cells. A pre-COC potential could also be seen when the microelectrode recorded an intermediate positive value on its way between zero mV and the EP. 13 of the pre-COC potentials were seen both before the electrode tip had entered the endolymph and when the tip had been drawn back into the organ of Corti from the endolymph.

b) Only very few stable large negativities were recorded.

c) In none of the 39 penetrations, out of which at least 29 were aimed for outer hair cells, tunnel of Corti, or inner hair cells, was a large negative potential found that was evoked by a single shock to the efferent fibers.

d) One penetration was aimed much peripheral to the outer hair cells; the potential went directly from about zero mV to the EP. Out of 29 penetrations that were aimed for outer hair cells, tunnel of Corti or inner hair cells, one showed a direct jump from a large negative potential to the EP, 7 showed a direct jump from about zero mV to the EP, and 21 showed that the EP was reached from about zero mV via intermediate values (on one occasion via -30 mV, once via -45 mV)(see Fig. 2 C).

2.4.3   Pharmacological Experiments: 1968 - 1971

2.4.3.1 The pre-COC Potential in Pharmacological Experiments

In one experiment, strychnine hydrochloride was given intravenously, 0.2 mg/kg b.w.; the pre-COC potential was unchanged both 3 min and 63 min after the injection. In two experiments, d-tubocurarine chloride (dTC), at a concentration of 3.5×10^{-5} g/ml, was applied in 0.2 ml artificial perilymph to scala tympani in the basal turn of the cochlea, without seeming to change the pre-COC potential, while the COC-disappeared. In one experiment, applying 0.2 ml artificial perilymph with dTC, 1.4×10^{-5} g/ml, caused the pre-COC potential, as recorded through a signal averager, to decrease in amplitude by 10 %. Later, in the same animal, 0.01 ml of perilymph with tetrodotoxin (TTX) (Kao, 1972; Narahashi, 1972), 10^{-7} g/ml, was applied to scala tympani; the pre-COC potential decreased to a third of its original amplitude in less than 60 sec.

In a second experiment with TTX, 0.01 ml of TTX, 10^{-7} g/ml, reduced the amplitude of the pre-COC potential to half its value, as recorded through the signal averager, within 2 min. Later, applying 0.2 ml of the TTX solution did not further reduce the pre-COC potential.

2.4.3.2 The COC- Potential in Pharmacological Experiments

Strychnine hydrochloride in 0.2 ml at a concentration of 5×10^{-7} g/ml quickly blocked the COC-, in four animals (cf. Fig. 4). In three similar experiments, strychnine hydrochloride, 10^{-7} g/ml, partially blocked the COC-, In thirteen cats, depending on the rate of spontaneous refill of scala tympani, presumably through the cochlear aqueduct, 0.01-0.2 ml of dTC, 10^{-5} g/ml, was needed to block the COC- totally or subtotally within few minutes.

0.01 ml of TTX in artificial perilymph, 10^{-7} g/ml,

totally or subtotally blocked the COC- in four experiments. In one of these experiments, with little spontaneous refill of scala tympani, the block was total within 30 sec. In another of these experiments, with fast spontaneous refill of scala tympani, there was still some COC- after 6 min; when the COC had been restored to its original value through repeated applications of artificial perilymph, 0.2 ml of the TTX solution totally blocked the COC- within 45 sec. In a fifth experiment, 0.2 ml of TTX, 2×10^{-8} g/ml, totally blocked the COC-, leaving a click-evoked AP seemingly intact. Hemicholinium (HC-3)(Schueler, 1960) was used in eight animals; 0.03-0.05 ml of HC-3, 2×10^{-5} g/ml, caused relatively slowly a subtotal or total block of the COC- (Fig. 4, top). The block re-

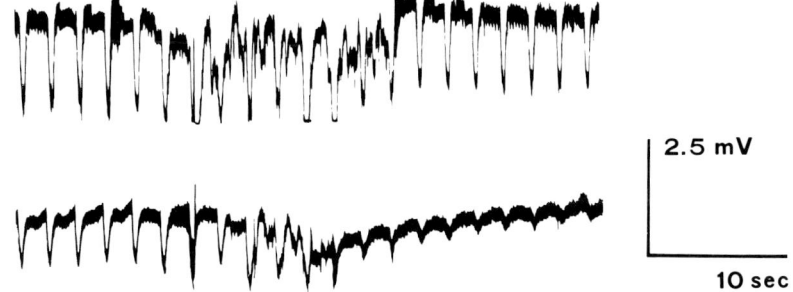

Fig. 4   Records illustrating the initial time course of the action of HC-3, respectively of strychnine, on the COC- potential.

Top record. Corresponding to 10 sec after the beginning of this record, HC-3 in 0.04 ml of artificial perilymph, 2×10^{-5} g/ml, was applied to the basal turn of scala tympani. At the end of the record, i.e. more than 20 sec after the application of the HC-3, the COC- had declined only slightly.

Bottom record. Corresponding to 17 sec after the beginning of this record, strychnine chloride in 0.03 ml of artificial perilymph, 2×10^{-6} g/ml, was applied to the basal turn of scala tympani. Eight seconds later, the COC- was much reduced in amplitude.

The calibration of voltage and time is common to both records. The COC- was in both cases evoked by trains of electrical (cont'd)

(Fig. 4, cont'd) shocks applied to the crossed olivocochlear fibers in the midline of the fourth ventricle: each shock 0.3 msec in duration at a current strength of 100 μA; each train of shocks lasted for 300 msec; 300 shocks/sec.

versed very slowly, and not fully, when only artificial perilymph was used in order to wash out the HC-3 from the cochlea. When choline chloride, 10^{-4} g/ml was added to the artificial perilymph for washing out the HC-3, the COC-potential was fully restored (Fig.5).

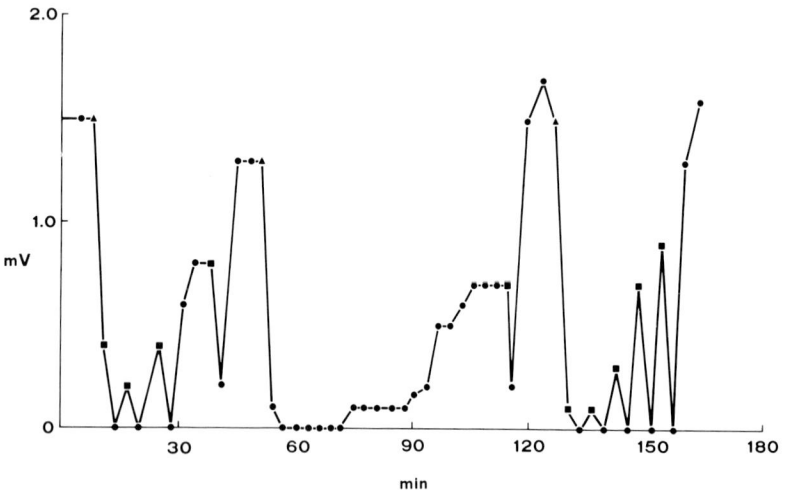

Fig. 5   Diagram illustrating that the action of HC-3 on the COC-potential was reversed with choline.

COC- potentials were evoked and recorded as illustrated in Fig. 4. Approximately every third minute the fluid in the basal turn of scala tympani was sucked out and 0.05 ml of artificial perilymph (circle), of artificial perilymph with HC-3 (triangle), 2×10^{-5} g/ml, or of artificial perilymph with choline chloride (square), 10^{-4} g/ml, was applied.

In one animal for each of the three substances, 0.2 ml with, respectively, glycine chloride (10^{-4} g/ml), γ-aminobutyric acid (GABA)(10^{-4} g/ml), and bicuculline (10^{-6}, 3×10^{-6}, and 3×10^{-5} g/ml), did not change the COC-.

Gallamine thriethiodide (Flaxedil) in 0.2 ml, 10^{-5} g/ml, respectively 2 × 10^{-5} g/ml, was applied to scala tympani in two experiments. The COC- declined by approximately 30 %, respectively by 50 %. The Flaxedil was, as it were, superimposed on the 4-5 mg/kg b.w. of Flaxedil that had been injected intravenously each 30-60 min. On the other hand, during and after such routine injections of Flaxedil, the COC never seemed to change as a result of the injection. Also, in two experiments, 22.3 mg/kg b.w., respectively 40 mg/kg b.w. of Flaxedil was injected, with no change of the COC-. This indicated that Flaxedil had no untoward effects in my experiments (cf. Galley et al., 1971).

2.4.3.3 AP in Pharmacological Experiments

In one experiment, strychnine hydrochloride in 0.01 ml, 10^{-5} g/ml, caused no change of the AP evoked by a click; the COC- went down to less than one fourth of its original value. In another experiment, 0.05 ml of the strychnine solution, 10^{-5} g/ml, was used and the AP remained unchanged while the COC- quickly disappeared. In four animals, dTC, 1 × 10^{-5} g/ml, in 0.05 ml caused the AP to decrease in amplitude by an amount that corresponded to a decrease of sound pressure of 2-10 dB. 0.2 ml artificial perilymph with glycine chloride, 10^{-3} g/ml, applied to scala tympani in one animal left the AP and the olivocochlear inhibition of AP unchanged. In a similar experiment, in another cat, the AP was unchanged when 0.2 ml of artificial perilymph was used with TTX, 2 × 10^{-8} g/ml, while the COC- disappeared.

2.4.3.4 Olivocochlear Inhibition of AP in Pharmacological Experiments

In one animal strychnine hydrochloride, 10^{-5} g/ml, in 0.01 ml artificial perilymph took the COC- down from -2.0 mV to -0.5 mV while the efferent inhibition of the AP seemed to change little, if any. Conditions were restored, and the experiment was repeated, giving the same result. The AP was not changed by strychnine. In another cat, 0.2 ml of the strychnine solution caused the COC- to vanish during the first few seconds. The efferent inhibition of the AP was little changed after 100 sec and even after 400 sec there was still some inhibition. The AP was not changed by the strychnine. Also, in one cat, dTC, 10^{-5} g/ml, in artificial perilymph in scala tympani caused the COC- to disappear completely while there was still some inhibition of the AP. Glycine chloride, 10^{-3} g/ml, in 0.2 ml of artificial perilymph left the olivocochlear inhibition of AP unchanged, in one experiment.

3. Fifth Series, 1970-1. dTC and Efferent Inhibition of Activity in Single Auditory Neurons

3.1 Technique

The experiments were carried out on 6 cats, weighing 1.7-2.5 kg. Five cats were anesthetized with Fluothane and decerebrated; one cat was anesthetized with pentobarbital i.p., 38 mg/kg b.w. The preparation of the cats for recording from single nerve fibers of the auditory nerve and for stimulation of the crossed olivocochlear fibers has been described before (Fex, 1962). The application of dTC to the basal turn of scala tympani, inside the round window of the cochlea, has also been described (cf. above; also Fex, 1967).

The microelectrodes for recording were filled with 3M KCl and had a resistance of 9-20 Megohm.

3.2 Experimental Procedure

The tip of the microelectrode was pushed from inside the open skull of the cat through the internal auditory meatus out into the modiolus of the cochlea. Whenever a single auditory nerve fiber gave a stable recording, its response to sound stimulation with and without simultaneous efferent inhibition was monitored through the screen of a slave oscilloscope inside the quiet room. A camera outside the quiet room photographed single sweeps from a master oscilloscope in several series of twenty sweeps: in each series, ten sweeps displayed the response to sound and ten sweeps showed the efferent inhibition of the sound response. With the camera still running, dTC in 0.05-0.20 ml of artificial perilymph at a concentration of 10^{-5} g/ml was then applied to scala tympani. Several or many additional series of twenty sweeps were photographed and the dTC was then washed out with artificial perilymph.

No attempts were made to calibrate the sound stimuli:

50 msec tone bursts. Pulses for electrical stimulation of the efferent fibers were delivered in trains of 100 msec, 300 pulses/sec, with a pulse length of 0.3 msec and a current strength of 50-200 µA. The pulse trains were synchronized with the sweep trigger and with the sound stimulus at a frequency of one train every other second. The negative potential at the beginning of each photographed sweep in the second and fourth column of Fig. 6 is the artifact from the last pulse in a train. This also corresponds to the time, for all sweeps, at which the tone burst started.

3.3 Results

Nine single auditory nerve fibers were studied with dTC; one fiber was studied with glycine chloride.

In three nerve fibers, the acoustically evoked activity seemed unchanged by 0.2 ml, respectively 0.05 ml of the dTC solution, while the efferent inhibition was blocked (Fig. 6). In one experiment, 0.05

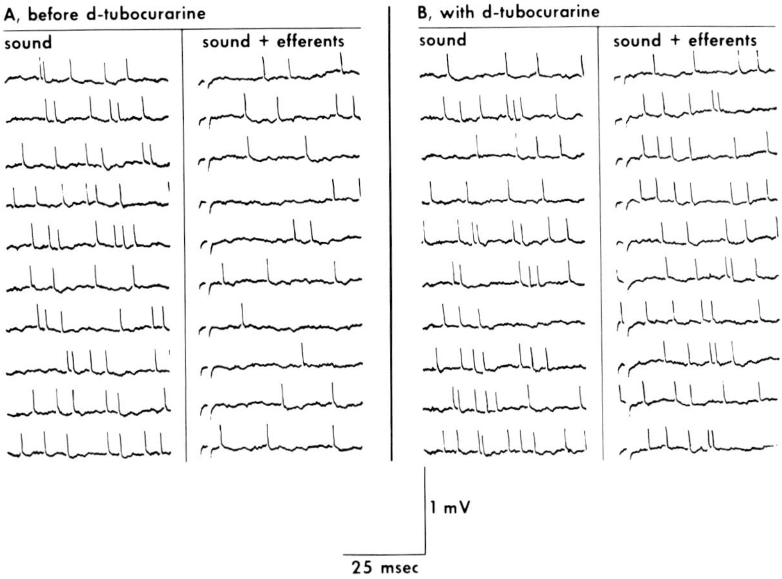

Fig. 6 Records illustrating that dTC in the cochlea can block efferent inhibition, seemingly with no change of sound-evoked auditory activity.   (cont'd)

(Fig. 6, cont'd)
A. Records to the left show nerve impulses in a single auditory nerve fiber in response to sound and, to the right, in response to the same sound during efferent inhibition.

B. Between A and B dTC had been applied to scala tympani. Otherwise stimulating conditions were unchanged.

Note that while the efferent inhibition was clear-cut in A, no inhibition can be seen in B.

ml of dTC solution was applied four times, during seven minutes, which finally resulted in a block of the efferent inhibition and a slight decrease in the number of impulses in response to the sound stimulus. Similar results, but after only one application of dTC were seen with another nerve fiber. One fiber showed an increase of threshold to sound by 20 dB ($\pm$ 5 dB) after dTC and another fiber needed a stronger sound, by 20 dB ($\pm$ 5 dB), to give the same response as before the application of dTC, as monitored by counting impulses. In two additional nerve fibers, dTC seemed to cause no decrease in the response to the tone burst.

Glycine chloride, 10^{-3} g/ml, in 0.05 ml of artificial perilymph caused no change in the response of one nerve fiber to sound, or in the efferent inhibition of the response to sound.

4. Sixth Series, 1968. Is ACh Released by Olivocochlear Nerve Fibers?

Perilymph from the cat's cochlea was assayed for the possible presence of ACh with a thin strip of the longitudinal muscle of the terminal ileum of the guinea pig, before and after electrical stimulation of the crossed olivocochlear fibers.

4.1 Technique

Guinea pigs were selected, fed, and prepared according to guide lines given by Paton (1957), Blaber and Cuthbert(1961), and Dawson et al. (1965), except that fine strips of the longitudinal muscle of the terminal ileum were used, instead of segments of the ileum.

Thus, the end-product of the preparation was the following. The thin muscle strip was stretched with two loops of silk between a hook on a strain gage and a hook on the bottom of a vertical glass chamber that could hold 1.2 ml of fluid before overflowing. The muscle was submerged in 1 ml of Tyrode solution containing 5 mg/ml of morphine sulfate and 2 g dextrose/l. During the first two hours the Tyrode solution contained also the anti-cholinesterase diisopropyl fluorophosphate (DFP) at a concentration of 2 mg/l.

The strain gage was connected to a differential transformer, the output of which was amplified and fed into an ink-writer, giving a continuous record of the tension of the muscle. The resting tension of the muscle was usually kept between 20-60 mg. As a rule, the muscle strip was prepared late in the evening and left overnight for 8-12 hours in the 1.2 ml chamber which had a circular, uncovered, opening, 8 mm in diameter. It was also left without change of fluid during successive nights. Out of 23 muscle strips prepared in succession, 5 gave good responses during 4 days, 13 during 3 days and one during 2 days. Two muscle strips failed and two gave good responses only during the day after the preparation.

Cats were prepared for electrical stimulation of the crossed olivocochlear fibers through Fluothane anesthesia and decerebration, immobilization with gallamine triethiodide, and artificial respiration; and for application of DFP through surgical removal of the outer and middle ear and removal of the round window membrane. Often, a 30 % urea solution with 10 % inert sugar was used to reduce the rate of spontaneous refill of scala tympani; hourly doses of up to 1 cc/kg b.w. were used.

Twenty-three cats were used for preliminary experiments until the above technique could be used to carry out experiments on 18 cats.

4.2 Experimental Procedure

Every 10 minutes during one hour the basal turn of scala tympani was emptied by suction and refilled with artificial perilymph containing DFP at a concentration of 2×10^{-5} g/ml. Then, continuing the application of DFP, the artificial perilymph that was sucked out was mixed with Tyrode to a volume of 0.2

ml and applied to the test-chamber containing the
muscle strip. The response was recorded and the chamber was emptied twice and washed out twice with 5 ml
of Tyrode. This control test was sometimes repeated,
sometimes electrical stimulation of the crossed efferent fibers was started immediately after the first
control test. At the end of ten minutes of electrical
stimulation the perilymph in the basal turn of scala
tympani was again sucked out and applied to the testchamber. Sometimes the time intervals varied, sometimes the basal turn of scala tympani was emptied and
filled several times in succession in attempts to
collect for testing as much as possible of any substance that might have diffused into the scala tympani during rest or electrical stimulation.

4.3 Results

In 2 out of the 18 cats, the first batch of perilymph
tested for ACh after electrical stimulation of the
crossed olivocochlear nerve fibers caused a stronger
contraction of the muscle strip than did the perilymph before the olivocochlear stimulation (Fig. 7).

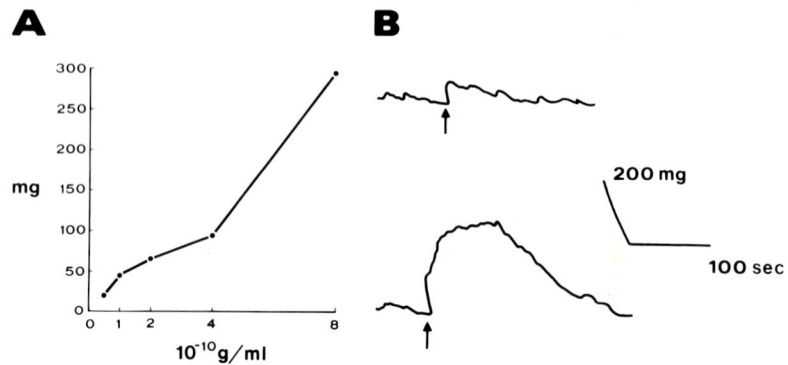

Fig. 7 Records illustrating that activation of the
crossed olivocochlear fibers may cause an
increase of ACh in the perilymph.

A. Response (mg) of muscle strip to ACh
(10^{-10} g/ml) in increasing doses.

B. Top record shows response of muscle strip
to perilymph before electrical stimulation
of crossed olivocochlear fibers. (cont'd)

(Fig. 7, cont'd)
Bottom record shows response of muscle strip to 0.007 ml of perilymph in 0.2 ml of Tyrode; the perilymph was removed after the crossed olivocochlear fibers had been electrically stimulated during 10 min. 30 sec; 20 shocks/sec; 400 µA.

Two other experiments gave similar findings but with the important difference that a second batch of perilymph, from ten - twenty minutes after finishing stimulating the olivocochlear fibers electrically, caused a stronger contraction of the muscle than did the first post-stimulatory batch. In the remaining 14 experiments there was no difference between responses to perilymph before and after electrical stimulation of the cochlear efferents.

In the 4 experiments with positive findings there was little if any blood in scala tympani during the olivocochlear stimulation and little if any spontaneous refill of scala tympani with perilymph. In 11 out of the 14 remaining experiments there was relatively much blood in scala tympani and also more spontaneous refill than in the other experiments. In the remaining 3 cats, and in two others with negative findings, there was an edema of the brain stem with displacements of the stimulating electrodes.

5. Discussion

5.1 Intracochlear Potentials

Sohmer et al. (1971) concluded on the basis of strong experimental evidence that large negative dc potentials that are recorded inside the organ of Corti correspond to cellular membrane potentials. My results confirm this and show that intracellular potentials in the organ of Corti can give longlasting and stable records if an adequate technique is used.

In the present study (section 2.4.1.e) three evoked potentials were found that probably represented intracellularly recorded inhibitory postsynaptic potentials (IPSPs) of outer hair cells, evoked by crossed olivocochlear stimulation; it is unlikely that evoked potentials recorded from inside the large efferent endings would be negative. Also, out of all the cochlear structures that may permit intracellular recording, only outer hair cells are likely to receive crossed efferent innervation. There may be at least three reasons why only three potentials of this kind were found. It is conceivable i) that it was particularly difficult to penetrate outer hair cells successfully with my techniques; ii) that synaptic bombardment from crossed efferent fibers generally causes little change of the outer hair cell membrane potential; iii), but unlikely, that only relatively few crossed efferent fibers were successfully stimulated in my experiments.

Logically, the next step in this field of research is to combine my recording technique with a technique for intracellular marking (Potter et al., 1966, Stretton and Kravitz, 1968, Pitman et al., 1972); new exciting knowledge about cochlear intracellular activity seems close at hand.

Lawrence's (1967) statement that there is a "negative potential of the organ of Corti -- controlled by the basilar membrane" implies that the basilar membrane is a diffusion barrier between scala tympani and the organ of Corti. However, there are many experimental results (e.g. Tasaki, 1957, Misrahy et al., 1960) that show that the organ of Corti is easily accessible to solutions that are applied to scala tympani. The present new results, often showing strong effects of small amounts of substances in small volumes of artificial perilymph shortly after application (cf. Fig. 4, strychnine), seem inexplicable under the assumption that these substances cannot diffuse through the basilar membrane.

When in the present study the electrode had been aimed for the tunnel of Corti the EP was preceded by a potential of about zero mV, which had been recorded along most of the electrode track. In other penetrations the technique seemed to decide whether the EP would be preceded by a large negativity, by approximately zero mV, or by a series of values between zero mV and the EP. Also, with the adequate technique, during a single penetration a long series of potentials was often recorded before the EP was reached, zero mV alternating with large negativities. Furthermore, the pre-COC potential was always recorded superimposed on a potential close to zero mV, often between negativities and often just before the EP was reached and immediately after the withdrawal of the electrode tip from the region of the EP. The only exooption was that the pre-COC could also be seen when an intermediate value between zero mV and the EP was recorded. All these potentials close to zero mV are interpreted as representing extracellular spaces in the organ of Corti. In particular, I have no reason for believing that any of the many stable zero mV records of this study represent the tectorial membrane. The possibility exists, of course, that an electrode tip in the tectorial membrane would record not the EP but a different potential, perhaps because of the suspension effect (cf. Tasaki and Singer, 1968, Fig. 1). However, because of both theoretical and practical considerations (Tasaki and Singer, 1968) it may be both difficult and not very meaningful to let a specific potential represent the tectorial membrane. Also, any claims that such a potential has been defined (Lawrence and Nuttall, 1970) cannot be well defended unless it can be said (to repeat recommendations by Sohmer et al., 1971) i) that microelectrodes without tip potentials were used; ii) that the electrode resistance was monitored during the experiment; iii) that the electrode tip was in the tectorial membrane as determined by other means than the recording of dc potentials.

This is a good place to stress that in the present study the problem with tip potentials was disregarded. Therefore I cannot safely claim to have shown that the intracellular potential of most cells in the organ of Corti lies between -90 mV and -100 mV, relative to scala tympani. However, the results permit the conclusion that cells from several different regions of the organ of Corti have about the same membrane potential. Again, there are no results, here or elsewhere, that permit the specific assumption that the intracellular potentials of inner hair cells are the same as those of the outer hair cells, or that hair cell membrane potentials are the same as membrane potentials of other cells of the organ of Corti.

Recording from single nerve fibers in the vestibulocochlear anastomosis I found that impulses needed 0.7-1.4 msec to travel approximately 12 mm. Since the fiber diameter is 5 µm or less (Rasmussen, 1946, Fex, 1962) these results agree with other results on conduction velocity (Wagner and Buchthal, 1972). The pre-COC potentials had a latency of 1.2-2.5 msec, were quickly suppressed by small quantities of TTX but not by strychnine or dTC. It is concluded that the pre-COC potential corresponded to activity in olivocochlear fibers in the organ of Corti and in the habenula perforata but not to postsynaptic activity. Note that i) some pre-COC potentials were evoked at a current strength of only 50 µA, ruling out antidromic stimulation of fibers of the auditory nerve; ii) potentials evoked by electrical stimulation and conducted through thin unmyelinated efferent nerve fibers (cf. Terayama and Yamamoto, 1971) from the midline of the brain stem to the habenula, or further, would in all probability have a latency much longer than 2.5 msec.

5.2 Sites of Action of Cochlear Efferent Inhibition

Often referred to in discussions about inhibitory cochlear synaptic sites is the finding that a single shock, applied to the midline of the brain stem of a cat with degenerated cochlear hair cells, caused an evoked potential at the round window (Desmedt, 1965). Desmedt suggested that this potential corresponded to postsynaptic activity of cochlear dendrites, but his illustration (Desmedt, 1965, Fig. 1) indicates that the potential had a latency of 0.2 msec or less with strong shocks. It is highly unlikely that 0.2 msec would be enough for both conduction and synaptic delay; Desmedt's (1965) potential in all probability corresponded to intracranial activity. It is well-known that intracranial activity may be recorded with an electrode at the round window, since the auditory nerve can serve as an extension of the recording electrode (Davis et al., 1950, Mikaelian, 1967). Therefore, it is often advisable to use intracochlear application of pharmacological agents if problems are to be solved about the origin of a potential recorded from the cochlea.

Desmedt et al. (1971) reported that crossed olivocochlear inhibition did not change the latency from the click to the peak of the AP. They stated i) that this absence of latency change is readily explained if the crossed efferents produce a postsynaptic inhibition on auditory dendrites; ii) that Fatt and Katz (1953) and Eccles (1964) have documented in other preparations the absence of latency shift in postsynaptically inhibited responses. However, Galambos (1956, Fig. 4) and Wiederhold and Peake (1966, Fig. 2) illustrated an increase of latency of AP with crossed olivocochlear inhibition; Wiederhold stated (1963): "At higher click intensities the latency of N_1 has been seen to decrease with increasing OCB stimulation.", (OCB = olivocochlear bundle); and both Sohmer (1966) and Dayal (1968) stressed that olivocochlear inhibition increases the AP latency. Both Sohmer (1966, Fig. 2) and Dayal (1968, Fig. 1) recorded increase of CM amplitude simultaneously with increase of AP latency and Sohmer (1966, Fig. 5) stimulated the nuclei of origin of the crossed olivocochlear fibers in some experiments with positive findings. It is therefore most unlikely that unintended activation of the facial nerve caused the increase of the AP latency in these two studies. Furthermore, and unfortunately, there is no such simple test as measuring latency for deciding whether a particular inhibition is postsynaptic or presynaptic (cf. Euler et al., 1968). There is no instance in Eccles' book of 1964 of postsynaptic inhibition without change of latency of postsynaptic nerve impulses; to the contrary, Eccles illustrates an instance in which inhibition delays the onset of spikes (Eccles, 1964, Fig. 83). Also, Eccles (1964, Fig. 40) illustrates that changes of amplitude and of rise time of excitatory postsynaptic potentials (EPSPs) can give changes of latency of the nerve impulse, when the latency of the EPSP is unchanged. Therefore, the absence of latency shift of the postsynaptically inhibited, non-propagated potential of the crustacean muscle in the study of Fatt and Katz (1953), which in this discussion corresponds to a neuronal, non-propagated EPSP, is not evidence that the latency of propagated spikes in auditory nerve fibers should be unchanged under efferent inhibition, if this inhibition were postsynaptic.

For a full discussion of problems that concern the sites of action and the pharmacology of the cochlear efferent inhibition it is necessary to mention recent advances in cochlear innervation. Fig. 8 illustrates the main features of the most recent concept of the efferent innervation of the cochlea of the cat as clarified by Spoendlin (cf. Spoendlin, this volume). On the basis of these features and of the findings by Kiang et al. (1965) it has been hypothesized (Lynn, 1969, Lynn and Sayers, 1970) that activity in the

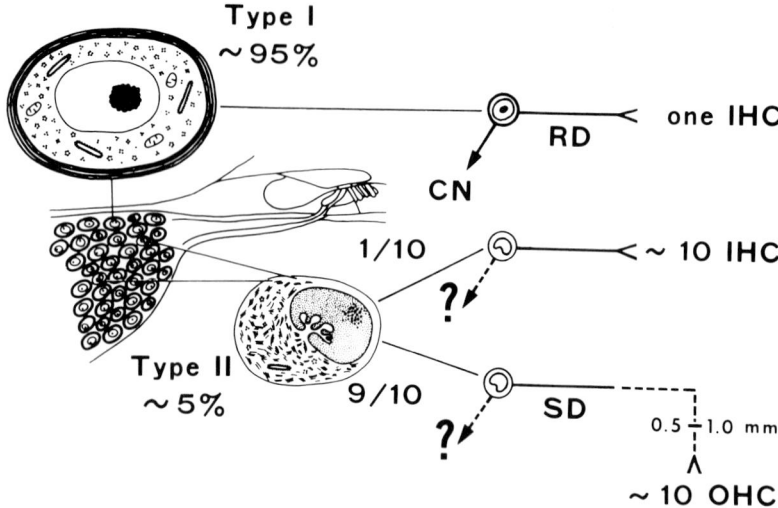

Fig. 8 Diagram of the afferent innervation of the cochlea of cat. CN, cochlear nucleus; IHC, inner hair cell; OHC, outer hair cell; RD, radial dendrite; SD, spiral dendrite.

To the left are illustrated cells of the spiral ganglion. Approximately 95 % are the Type I cells. These cells are myelinated and each cell sends an axon to the cochlear nucleus and a dendrite to one inner hair cell. The remaining ganglion cells, Type II, are unmyelinated and may or may not send axons centrally. Approximately one in ten of the Type II cells innervates approximately 10 inner hair cells. Each of the remaining Type II cells sends a spiral dendrite that runs 0.5-1.0 mm to innervate approximately 10 outer hair cells.

(The left half of the figure is redrawn from Fig. 10 of Spoendlin, 1971).

spiral dendrites, coming from outer hair cells, regulates activity in the radial dendrites, coming from inner hair cells. The hypothesis is attractive, not the least because it helps to focus attention on specific questions about basic mechanisms of hearing. One problem is that there is no morphological evi-

dence for an interaction between the different kinds
of cochlear dendrites (see Fig. 9), or between different groups of hair cells. Fig. 10 illustrates how the

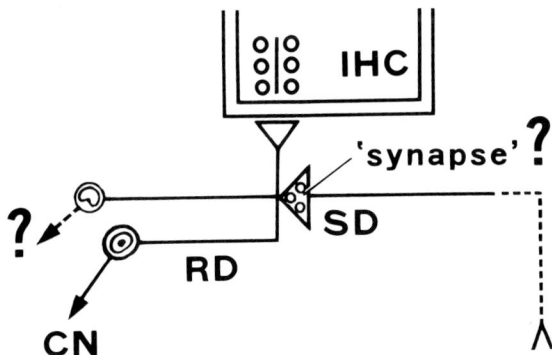

Fig. 9   Diagram to illustrate the problem posed by
the Lynn-Sayers concept that spiral dendrites
regulate activity in radial dendrites. CN,
cochlear nucleus; IHC, inner hair cell; RD,
radial dendrite; SD, spiral dendrite.

It is indicated by "?" that there are no
known synapses between spiral dendrites and
radial dendrites. Also, "?" at the symbol for
the unmyelinated ganglion cell, corresponding
to the spiral dendrites, again stresses that
this cell type may send no axons centrally.

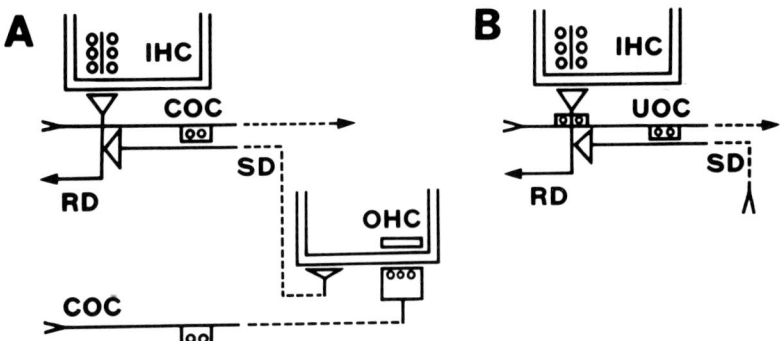

Fig. 10 Diagram illustrating how the efferent synapses may be distributed in the cochlea of the
cat. COC, crossed olivocochlear nerve fiber;
IHC, inner hair cell; OHC, outer hair cell;
RD, radial dendrite; SD, spiral   (cont'd)

(Fig. 10, cont'd) dendrite; UOC, uncrossed olivocochlear fiber.

A. Note that it has not yet been shown conclusively that COC synapses with RD (cf. text).

B. Note that UOC synapses also with OHC although this is not indicated here.

efferent synapses perhaps are distributed in the cochlea of the cat. The crossed olivocochlear fibers synapse extensively with outer hair cells but synapse little if at all with afferent spiral dendrites or their endings under outer hair cells, and there are in all probability no efferent synapses with inner hair cells, or very few (Sponedlin, 1970). There are perhaps no synapses between crossed efferents and radial dendrites in the chinchilla (Iurato et al., 1968, Iurato, 1972). The finding by Spoendlin (1970) that cutting the crossed cochlear efferents reduces the amount of AChE of the inner spiral fibers (medial to the tunnel of Corti) in the cat is evidence that the crossed efferents of this species form synapses with radial dendrites; however, this evidence is not conclusive.

Almost all or all primary auditory neurons may be inhibited by crossed olivocochlear activity (Fex, 1962, Wiederhold and Kiang, 1970). Also, very likely, almost all or all primary auditory neuronal axons, from which recordings have been carried out with microelectrodes, have come from Type I spiral ganglion cells with radial dendrites to inner hair cells (cf. Lynn and Sayers, 1970). Thus, all the crossed cochlear efferent inhibition can be carried out through efferent endings on cochlear hair cells and spiral dendrites, if and only if radial dendritic activity is regulated through activity from outer hair cells. And, if activity in radial dendrites is not regulated by spiral dendritic activity or outer hair cell activity, then it seems necessary to assume that crossed olivocochlear fibers synapse with radial dendrites. A detailed discussion of experiments that bear on this concept of interaction between afferents is presented elsewhere (Fex, 1972). It should be added here that Wiederhold (1970) found a decrease from a maximum of the crossed olivocochlear inhibition of activity in single fibers of the auditory nerve, that according to Wiederhold appeared to correspond qualitatively to a decrease from a maximum of the longitudinal distribution of AChE stain near outer hair cells as described by Ishii and Balogh (1968); no such variation of AChE stain was found near the inner hair cells (Ishii and Balogh, 1968).

My new findings, that the COC- potential can be suppressed before the inhibition of the AP has become blocked, cannot be evaluated quantitatively. The findings may seem to indicate that the efferent endings on outer hair cells are of minor importance, if the COC- potential truly mirrors all activity of outer hair cells that corresponds to inhibition. However, valid conclusions about how functionally important the efferent synapses are on outer hair cells can probably only be based on results of intracellular recording from these cells and on studies of the activity of single auditory nerve fibers, with perfect control of the acoustic stimuli.

5.3 ACh as Candidate for Efferent Transmitter Substance

It is well-known that the olivocochlear neurons contain acetylcholinesterase (AChE) and also that the presence of AChE in a neuron need neither affirm nor

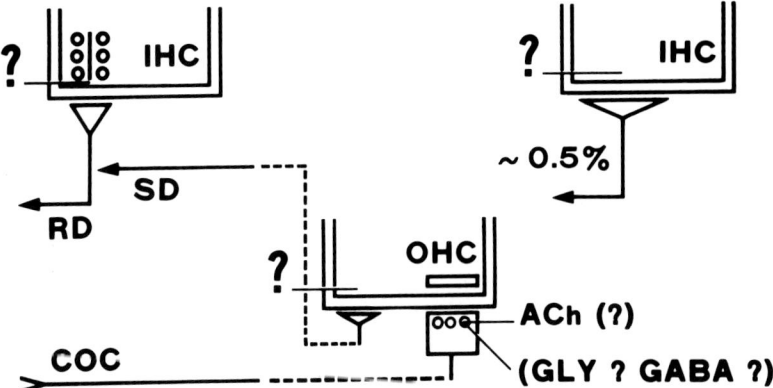

Fig. 11 Diagram to stress that we know very little about transmitter substances in the cochlea. ACh, acetylcholine; COC, crossed olivocochlear nerve fiber; GABA, γ-aminobutyric acid; GLY, glycine; IHC, inner hair cell; (cont'd)

(Fig. 11, cont'd) OHC, outer hair cell; RD, radial dendrite; SD, spiral dendrite.

The "?"s are to stress that nothing is known about the nature of any chemical transmitter substance that may be active at the afferent synapses of the three different kinds of dendrites. There may, for instance, be three different kinds of excitatory transmitter substances.

The efferent synapse in the diagram, between COC and OHC, is probably cholinergic, as indicated by "ACh(?)", but glycine or γ-aminobutyric acid may conceivably also be an inhibitory transmitter substance, as indicated by "(GLY?GABA?).

deny the hypothesis that the neuron is cholinergic ("cholinergic" is used as identical with "using ACh as a transmitter substance or synthesizing ACh or both")(see Fex, 1972, section IV A 2, for references). In particular, it may not be necessary for AChE to be a structural component of the postsynaptic membrane at a cholinergic synapse (Hall and Kelly, 1971).

It has not been shown that olivocochlear fibers contain also choline acetyltransferase (ChAc). However, findings (section 2.4.3.2) that HC-3 suppression of the COC- is fully reversed if choline is used, indicate that ACh may be synthesized during olivocochlear stimulation, since HC-3 blocks ACh synthesis (Schueler, 1960). Of course, by blocking the uptake of choline, HC-3 may interfere also with metabolic processes in which ACh is not involved (cf. Diamond and Milfay, 1972).

It also remains to prove the hypothesis that ACh is released during olivocochlear activity. My new results (section 4.3) are not more than consistent with the hypothesis, while Guth *et al.* (1972) seem to claim that they have proof; I hope that the claim will prove valid in the eventual full paper. My results indicate that, if necessary, these kinds of experiments may be extended to give a conclusive series of positive findings in the cat if i) the cochlear aqueduct is closed to prevent blood and cerebrospinal fluid from bringing an excess of AChE into scala tympani; ii) the olivocochlear stimulation is monitored so that relatively weak currents may be used, in order that poststimulatory "spontaneous" efferent activity may be avoided.

dTC has since long been used to block transmission postsynaptically at cholinergic synapses. My new findings on single auditory neurons (section 3.3) indicate that dTC can block the efferent cochlear inhibition without changing the afferent activity. However, dTC can also influence the response of auditory neurons to sound, to judge from an illustration by Tanaka and Katsuki (1966, Fig. 8) and from my results (section 2.4.3.3; 3.3). It is conceivable that dTC competes with ACh for efferent postsynaptic sites on outer hair cells; this could change conditions for afferent synaptic transmission (cf. Kosay et al., 1972, also for references). It is also conceivable that dTC directly interferes with afferent synaptic transmission but then perhaps not by blocking ACh receptors, since Bobbin and Konishi (1971) found that ACh mixed with eserine can, as a late effect, block efferent inhibition of the AP, without blocking the AP itself. There may be several other possible explanations for this observed action of dTC. Again, only studies of the hair cell synapses through intracellular recording are likely to tell what the exact action of dTC at these synapses is. It may be useful to keep in mind that dTC can block certain receptors for 5-hydroxytryptamine (5-HT)(Stefani and Gerschenfeld, 1969) and dopamine (Ascher, 1972), and is thus no specific blocker of ACh.

It is likely that the efferents of some of the different acoustico-lateralis organs have the same transmitter substance(s). Russell's studies (1968, 1971) indicate that the efferent synapses in the lateral-line system of Xenopus laevis release ACh. Whether it is easier to define transmitter substances of the cochlea or of other acoustico-lateralis organs is hard to tell, but Russell has already shown that the Xenopus may be very useful also for auditory neuropharmacological research.

Strychnine in a nonconvulsive dose blocks the olivocochlear inhibition (Desmedt and Monaco, 1960) which need not imply that the cochlear efferents are noncholinergic. A study by Alving (1961) on the actions of strychnine on the neuromuscular junction of the frog showed that strychnine block resembles that produced by curare. Furthermore, there may be a cholinergic inhibition in the cortex of cat that is blocked by strychnine as well as by cholinergic antagonists (Phillis and York, 1968). Also, two out of the three different kinds of ACh-sensitive receptors on certain Aplysia neurons can be blocked by strychnine (Kehoe, 1972b)

5.4 Other Candidates than ACh for Efferent Cochlear Transmission

Since strychnine blocks the efferent cochlear inhibition (Desmedt and Monaco, 1960), the action on cochlear synapses of glycine (Werman and Aprison, 1968), GABA, and blockers of these substances should be studied. Strychnine rather specifically blocks glycine (Curtis et al., 1971), while bicuculline specifically blocks GABA (Curtis et al., 1970).

I found (see above) that glycine chloride in one cat did not change the COC-; in one cat did not change the AP or the efferent inhibition of the AP; and in one cat did not change the response of a nerve fiber to sound or the efferent inhibition of this response. These new findings indicate that glycine is not a cochlear inhibitory transmitter substance. However, I would like to see the experiments repeated. with increasing doses of glycine until there eventually is an effect at cochlear synapses. Then strychnine would be used in an attempt to show whether or not the eventual glycine effect is specifically mimicking the olivocochlear inhibition.

In one cat GABA did not change the COC-, neither did bicuculline in another experiment. In both instances, dTC reduced the COC-, as usual. This indicates that GABA is not a cochlear inhibitory transmitter substance, but also these observations need to be extended. Bobbin and Guth (1970) believed that their findings of a decrease of AP through intracochlear infusion of GABA, in three guinea pigs, was an unspecific effect. However, their results do not rule out the possibility that GABA is an efferent cochlear transmitter.

It should be noted that primary catecholamines and 5-HT in all probability are ruled out as candidates for efferent cochlear transmission (Fex et al., 1965).

5.5 Mechanisms of the Cochlear Efferent Inhibition

Since the cochlear efferents may release ACh it is of interest that "ACh can open ionic gates to Na and Cl on the same neurone" (Levitan and Tauc, 1972), while another type of cell membrane will react to ACh by changing its permeability to potassium and chloride (Kehoe, 1972a). It has also been shown that differences in ion contents of cells can cause differences in the cell response to ACh (Kerkut and Meech, 1966). To speculate on what the ionic mechanism of the olivocochlear inhibition may be seems meaningless; the publications referred to here tell what kind of experiments need to be done and that intracellular recordings at the synapses are indispensable, if synaptic mechanisms are to be defined.

It would be interesting to learn whether the efferents that bend off from the olivocochlear bundle to innervate cells in the cochlear nucleus (Rasmussen, 1960) are axonal collaterals of cochlear efferents. If they are, it would be of value to find out whether they are excitatory or inhibitory, in view of the claim that there are no known cells in the mammalian brain that can excite by one set of synapses and inhibit by another set (Eccles, 1970).

6. Summary and Conclusions

New results concerning the pharmacology of the efferent inhibition in the cochlea are described and discussed. It was found

a) in section 2.4.3.2, that the centrifugally evoked potential COC- is suppressed by hemicholinium (HC-3) as if acetylcholine (ACh) is synthesized during crossed efferent activity in the cochlea;

b) in section 4.3 and by Guth et al. (1972), that after activation of the crossed cochlear efferents the perilymph can cause contraction of the longitudinal muscle of the guinea pig ileum as if ACh had been released during efferent activity;

c) by Bobbin and Konishi (1971), that ACh mixed with eserine first mimics the actions of the crossed efferents by suppressing the AP and increasing the CM and, later, keeps the efferent inhibition blocked while the AP returns to its original value;

d) in section 3.3, that d-tubocurarine (dTC) can suppress the efferent cochlear inhibition;

e) in section 5.3, that the fact that strychnine blocks the crossed efferent cochlear inhibition need not imply that ACh is not an inhibitory transmitter substance in the cochlea.

The evidence seems strong that ACh is a transmitter substance of the crossed efferent nerve fibers in the cochlea. However, the evidence that corresponds to items a), b), and d) immediately above is not conclusive (see section 5); the evidence in c) above that ACh mimics efferent actions needs to be strengthened through intracellular recording.

In conclusion, ACh probably causes efferent inhibition in the cochlea, but conclusive evidence for this is still lacking.

It may be useful to try to show conclusively that glycine and γ-aminobutyric acid (GABA) are not inhibitory transmitter substances in the cochlea (cf. section 5.4); primary catecholamines and 5-hydroxytryptamine (5-HT) in all probability are already ruled out (Fex *et al.*, 1965).

Statements concerning the sites of action of the crossed cochlear efferents are discussed. To be noted is that *if* activity from outer hair cells does not regulate activity in radial dendrites, *then* crossed efferents most likely have synapses on radial dendrites. Histological findings (Spoendlin, 1970) show that there may be such synapses, but the evidence is not conclusive.

Publications are mentioned that may provide useful guidance for future studies on the cochlear efferent mechanisms in terms of ionic gates.

Findings (Tanaka and Katsuki, 1966, Fig. 8; above, sections 2.4.3.3 and 3.3) that dTC may suppress sound-evoked activity in the auditory nerve need not be taken to imply that ACh is a transmitter substance for excitation in the inner ear (cf. section 5). It is useful to state here that there is no good candidate for a substance that may transmit excitation from hair cell to auditory nerve fiber. Neural excitatory processes of the inner ear are discussed in detail elsewhere (Fex, 1972).

Techniques and procedures are described (Sections 1 and 2) that led to longlasting recordings from inside cells from different regions of the organ of Corti. Activity of outer hair cells probably was recorded on three occasions. Extracellular potentials were found that in all probability corresponded to activity of crossed efferent nerve fibers in the organ of Corti and in the habenula perforata.

The present new findings lead also to the following statements that agree with similar, earlier, statements by Sohmer et al. (1971).

a) Many regions in the organ of Corti have a potential of about 0 mV (relative to scala tympani); the tunnel of Corti is one such region.

b) In all probability, no extracellular region in the organ of Corti has a large negative potential.

c) It has not yet been shown that the tectorial membrane may be assigned a well defined potential.

Also, the basilar membrane in all probability permits free diffusion of electrolytes and of pharmacological agents in general (cf. Tasaki, 1957, Misrahy et al., 1960).

Acknowledgements

The experiments of 1967, 1968 and 1969 were carried out while the author was a Visiting Scientist at the Laboratory of Neurobiology, National Institute of Mental Health, Department of Health, Education and Welfare; Bethesda, Maryland, U.S.A. The friendly encouragement of Dr. Ichiji Tasaki made that work even more pleasant than it would otherwise have been.

The experiments of 1970 and 1971 and the manuscript of this paper were completed at the Center for Neural Sciences, Indiana University; Bloomington, Indiana, U.S.A. During this time, grant NASA NGL 15-003-077 contributed to making this study possible.

Discussions with Dr. William D. Neff concerning this study have been encouraging, stimulating and most enjoyable.

The technical advice and assistance of Mr. Merrill Gater has been invaluable as have the friendliness and excellent typing of Ms. Rebecca Mattix.

References

Adrian, R.H. (1956). The effect of internal and external potassium concentration on the membrane potential of frog muscle. J. Physiol. 133, 631-658.

Alving, B.O. (1961). The action of strychnine at cholinergic junctions. Arch. Int. Pharmacodyn. 131, 123-150,

Ascher, P. (1972). Inhibitory and excitatory effects of dopamine on Aplysia neurones. J. Physiol. 225, 173-209.

Békésy, G. von (1960). Experiments in hearing. p. 488ff. McGraw-Hill, New York.

Blaber, L.C., and Cuthbert, A.W. (1961). A sensitive method for the assay of acetylcholine. J. Pharm. Pharmacol. 13, 445-446.

Bobbin, R.P., and Guth, P.S. (1970). Evidence that gamma-aminobutyric acid is not the inhibitory transmitter at the crossed olivocochlear nerve-hair cell junction. Neuropharmacol. 9, 567-574.

Bobbin, R.P., and Konishi, T. (1971). Acetylcholine mimics crossed olivocochlear bundle stimulation. Nature, New Biol. (London) 231, 222-223.

Curtis, D.R., Duggan, A.W., Felix, D., and Johnston, G.A.R. (1970). GABA, bicuculline and central inhibition. Nature (London) 226, 1222-1224.

Curtis, D.R., Duggan, A.W., and Johnston, G.A.R. (1971). The specificity of strychnine as a glycine antagonist in the mammalian spinal cord. Exp. Brain Res. 12, 547-565.

Davis, H., Gernandt, B.E., and Riesco-MacClure, J.S., (1950). Threshold of action potentials in ear of guinea pig. J. Neurophysiol. 13, 73-87.

Dawson, W., Hemsworth, B.A., and Stockham, M.A. (1965), Influence of ascorbic acid on the sensitivity of guinea-pig ileum. J. Pharm. Pharmacol. 17, 183.

Dayal, V.S. (1968). The effects of olivocochlear bundle stimulation on latency of action potential. Laryngoscope 78, 1590-1596.

Desmedt, J.E. (1965). Discussion. Acta Oto-laryngol. 59, 168-170.

Desmedt, J.E., and Monaco, P. (1960). Suppression par la strychnine de l'effet inhibiteur centrifuge exercé par le faisceau olivocochléaire. Arch. Int. Pharmacodyn. 129, 244-248.

Desmedt, J.E., La Grutta, V., and La Grutta, G. (1971). Contrasting effects of centrifugal olivo-cochlear inhibition and of middle ear muscle contraction on the response characteristics of the cat's auditory nerve. Brain Res. 30, 375-384.

Diamond, I., and Milfay, D. (1972). Uptake of (^{3}H-methyl)choline by microsomal, synaptosomal, mitochondrial and synaptic vesicle fractions of the rat brain. The effects of hemicholinium. J. Neurochem. 19, 1899-1909.

Eccles, J.C. (1964). The physiology of synapses. Springer-Verlag, Berlin.

Eccles, J.C. (1970). Facing reality. Philosophical adventures by a brain scientist. p. 15ff. Springer-Verlag, New York.

Euler, C. von, Skoglund, S., and Söderberg, U. (eds.) (1968). Structure and function of inhibitory neuronal mechanisms. Wenner-Gren Center Int. Symp. Ser. Vol. 10. Pergamon Press, Oxford.

Evans, E.F. (1970). Narrow "tuning" of the responses of cochlear nerve fibers emanating from the exposed basilar membrane. J. Physiol. 208, 75P-76P.

Fatt, P., and Katz, B. (1953). The effect of inhibitory nerve impulses on a crustacean muscle fiber. J. Physiol. 121, 374-389.

Fex, J. (1962). Auditory activity in centrifugal and centripetal fibers in cat. A study of a feedback system. Acta Physiol. Scand. 55, Suppl. 189.

Fex, J. (1967). Efferent inhibition in the cochlea related to hair cell DC activity of the crossed olivocochlear fibers in the cat. J. Acoust. Soc. Amer. 41, 666-675.

Fex, J. (1968). Efferent inhibition in the cochlea by the olivocochlear bundle. In: Hearing Mechanisms in Vertebrates, Ciba Symp. pp. 169-181. J. & A. Churchill, Ltd., London.

Fex, J. (1972). Neural excitatory processes of the inner ear. In: Handbook of Sensory Physiology, Vol. V: Auditory System. Springer-Verlag, Berlin.

Fex, J., Fuxe, K., and Lennerstrand, G. (1965). Absence of monoamines in olivocochlear fibers in cat. Acta Physiol. Scand. 64, 259.

Galambos, R. (1956). Suppression of auditory nerve activity by stimulation of efferent fibers to cochlea. J. Neurophysiol. 19, 427-437.

Galley, N., Klinke, R., Pause, M., and Storch, W.-H. (1971). The effect of flaxedil (gallamine triethiodide) on the efferent endings in the cochlea. Pflügers Arch. 330, 1-4.

Guth, P.S., Burton, M., and Norris, C.H. (1972). Release of acetylcholine by the olivocochlear bundles. J. Acoust. Soc. Amer. 52, 144.

Hall, Z.W., and Kelly, R.B. (1971). Enzymatic detachment of endplate acetylcholinesterase from muscle. Nature, New Biol. (London) 232, 62-63.

Ishii, D., and Balogh, K., Jr. (1968). Distribution of efferent nerve endings in the organ of Corti. Acta Oto-laryngol. 66, 282-288.

Iurato, S. (1972). Efferent innervation. In: Handbook of Sensory Physiology. Vol. V: Auditory System. Springer-Verlag, Berlin.

Iurato, S., Smith, C.A., Eldredge, D.H., and Henderson, D. (1968). Electron microscopic observations and cochlear potentials after section of the crossed olivo-cochlear tract in the chinchilla. Electron Microsc. Proc. Eur. Reg. Conf., 4th, Rome, pp. 561-562.

Kao, C.Y. (1972). Pharmacology of tetrodotoxin and saxitoxin. Fed. Proc. 31, 1117-1123.

Kehoe, J. (1972a). Ionic mechanisms of a two-component cholinergic inhibition in Aplysia neurones. J. Physiol. 225, 85-114.

Kehoe, J. (1972b). Three acetylcholine receptors in Aplysia neurones. J. Physiol. 225, 115-146.

Kerkut, G.A., and Meech, R.W. (1966). Microelectrode determination of the intracellular chloride concentration in nerve cells. Life Sci. 5, 453-456.

Kiang, N.Y.S. (1965). Discharge Patterns of Single Fibers in the Cat's Auditory Nerve. Res Monogr. 35. M.I.T. Press, Cambridge, Mass.

Kosay, S., Riker, W.K., and Guerrero, S. (1972). Effects of d-tubocurarine on the frog sympathetic ganglion cell and on synaptic function. J. Pharmacol. Exp. Ther. 180, 255-264.

Lawrence, M. (1967). Electric polarization of the tectorial membrane. Ann. Otol. Rhinol. Laryngol. 76, 287-312.

Lawrence, M., and Nuttall, A.L. (1970). Electrophysiology of the organ of Corti. In: Biochemical Mechanisms in Hearing and Deafness, pp. 83-96. C.C. Thomas, Springfield, Ill.

Levitan, H., and Tauc, L. (1972). Acetylcholine receptors: topographic distribution and pharmacological properties of two receptor types on a single molluscan neurone. J. Physiol. 222, 537-558.

Lynn, P.A. (1969). Processing of signals in the peripheral auditory system in relation to aural perception. Thesis. University of London.

Lynn, P.A., and Sayers, B.McA. (1970). Cochlear innervation, signal processing, and their relation to auditory time-intensity effects. J. Acoust. Soc. Amer. 47, 525-533.

Mikaelian, D.O. (1967). Experiments with VIII nerve section and the cochleo-cochlear mechanisms. Ann. Otol. Rhinol. Laryngol. 76, 1033-1039.

Misrahy, G.A., Spradley, J.F., Beran, A.V., and Garwood, V.P. (1960). Permeability of cochlear partitions: Comparison with blood-brain barrier. Acta Oto-laryngol. 52, 525-534.

Narahashi, T. (1972). Mechanism of action of tetrodotoxin and saxitoxin on excitable membranes. Fed. Proc. 31, 1124-1132.

Paton, W.D.M. (1957). The action of morphine and related substances on contraction and on acetylcholine output of coaxially stimulated guinea pig ileum. Brit. J. Pharmacol. Chemother. 12, 119-127.

Phillis, J.W., and York, D.H. (1968). Pharmacological studies on a cholinergic inhibition in the cerebral cortex. Brain Res. 10, 297-306.

Pitman, R.M., Tweedle, C.D., and Cohen, M.J. (1972). Branching of central neurons: intracellular cobalt injection for light and electron microscopy. Science 176, 412-414.

Potter, D.D., Furshpan, E.J., and Lennox, E.S. (1966). Connections between cells of the developing squid as revealed by electrophysiological methods. Proc. Nat. Acad. Sci. 55, 328-336.

Rasmussen, G.L. (1946). The olivary peduncle and other fiber projections of the superior olivary complex. J. Comp. Neurol. 84, 141-219.

Rasmussen, G.L. (1960). Efferent fibers of the cochlea nerve and cochlea nucleus. In: Neural mechanisms of the Auditory and Vestibular Systems, pp. 105-115. C.C. Thomas, Springfield, Ill.

Richardson, K.C. (1968). Cholinergic and adrenergic axons in methylene blue-stained rat iris: an electronmicroscopical study. Life Sci. 7, 599-604.

Russell, I.J. (1968). Influence of efferent fibers on a receptor. Nature (London) 219, 177-178.

Russell, I.J. (1971). The pharmacology of efferent synapses in the lateral-line system of Xenopus laevis. J. Exp. Biol. 54, 643-658.

Schueler, F.W. (1960). The mechanism of action of the hemicholiniums. Int. Rev. Neurobiol. 2, 77-97.

Sohmer, H.S. (1966). A comparison of the efferent effects of the homolateral and contralateral olivocochlear bundles. Acta Oto-laryngol. 62, 74-87.

Sohmer, H.S., Peake, W.T., and Weiss, T.F. (1971). Intracochlear potential recorded with micropipets. I. Correlations with micropipet location. J. Acoust. Soc. Amer. 50, 572-586.

Spoendlin, H. (1970). Structural basis of peripheral frequency analysis. In: Frequency Analysis and Periodicity Detection in Hearing. pp. 2-40. A.W. Sijthoff, Leiden, The Netherlands.

Spoendlin, H. (1971). Degeneration behaviour of the cochlear nerve. Arch. Klin. Exp. Ohr-Nas, Kehlk-Heilk 200, 275-291.

Stefani, E., and Gerschenfeld, H.M. (1969). Comparative study of acetylcholine and 5-hydroxytryptamine receptors on single snail neurons. J. Neurophysiol. 32, 64-74.

Stretton, A.O.W., and Kravitz, E.A. (1968). Neuronal geometry: determination with a technique of intracellular dye injection. Science 162, 132-134.

Tanaka, Y., and Katsuki, Y. (1966). Pharmacological

investigations of cochlear responses and of olivocochlear inhibition. J. Neurophysiol. 29, 94-108.

Tasaki, I. (1957). Hearing. Ann. Rev. Physiol. 19, 417-438.

Tasaki, I., and Singer, I. (1968). Some problems involved in electrical measurements of biological systems. Ann. N.Y. Acad. Sci. 148, 36-53.

Terayama, Y., and Yamamoto, K. (1971). Olivo-cochlear bundle in the guinea pig cochlea after central transection of the crossed bundle. Acta Otolaryngol. 72, 385-396.

Wagner, A.L., and Buchthal, F. (1972). Motor and sensory conduction in infancy and childhood: reappraisal. Develop. Med. Child Neurol. 14, 189-216.

Werman, R., and Aprison, M.H. (1968). Glycine: the search for a spinal cord inhibitory transmitter. In: Structure and Function of Inhibitory Neuronal Mechanisms, Proc. Int. Meet. Neurobiol., 4th, pp. 473-486. Pergamon Press, Oxford.

Wiederhold, M.L. (1963). Effects of efferent pathways on acoustic evoked responses in the auditory nervous system. Thesis. M.I.T., Cambridge, Mass.

Wiederhold, M.L. (1970). Variations in the effects of electric stimulation of the crossed olivocochlear bundle on cat single auditory-nerve fibers responses to tone bursts. J. Acoust. Soc. Amer. 48, 966-977.

Wiederhold, M.L., and Kiang, N.Y.-S. (1970). Effects of electric stimulation of the crossed olivocochlear bundle on single auditory-nerve fibers in the cat. J. Acoust. Soc. Amer. 48, 950-965.

Wiederhold, M.L., and Peake, W.T. (1966). Efferent inhibition of auditory-nerve responses: Dependence on acoustic-stimulus parameters. J. Acoust. Soc. Amer. 40, 1427-1430.

DISCUSSION

EVANS: You showed in your last slide a very interesting connection running from the outer hair cells by fibers labeled FD to end on the inner hair cells. Would you like to comment on this?

FEX: Well, actually, they did not end on the inner hair cells. They ended on the radial dendrites (see Figs. 9 and 10, above). If there are no crossed-efferent synapses on the radial dendrites or on the inner hair cells, then there must be some interactions between the outer hair cell afferent system and the inner hair cell afferent system, between cells or between dendrites, or there would not be inhibition in practically all afferent fibers when the efferents are stimulated electrically (cf. Wiederhold and Kiang, 1970). Now, on the other hand, Dr. Spoendlin has shown that if you cut the crossed efferent fibers in cat only about half the inner spiral bundle will stain for acetylcholinesterase, while the whole bundle takes stain in the normal cat. Dr. Spoendlin seems to feel fairly sure, although he does not feel that this evidence is conclusive I think, that the fibers in the inner spiral bundle that come from the crossed efferent fibers do not go to outer hair cells. If they do not, then they end somewhere under the inner hair cells and where would they end if not on radial fibers? With crossed efferents ending on radial fibers one does not need any regulation of radial fiber activity by spiral fibers to explain the findings by Wiederhold and Kiang.

Reference

Wiederhold, M.L., and Kiang, N. Y.-S. (1970). Effects of electric stimulation of the crossed olivo-cochlear bundle on single auditory-nerve fibers in the cat. J. Acoust. Soc. Amer. 48, 950-965.

INNER EAR POTENTIALS IN LOWER VERTEBRATES:
DEPENDENCE ON METABOLISM

J. Schwartzkopff

Ruhr-Universität Bochum
463 Bochum-Querenburg
Germany

1. Introduction of the problems

The vertebrates can be characterized by the labyrinth organ as well as by the vertebrae. Both are common to all groups. The former organ is closely related to the lateral line system of the Anamnia (i.e. fish and amphibians). Like the lateral line system, the labyrinth organ comprises hair cells as receptors. During phylogentic development these receptors in the labyrinth, above all, became adapted to serve hearing functions. While the morphological transformations of the inner ear are known satisfactorily, this is not true of the physiological mechanisms. The Sauropsida (a group including both birds and reptiles), with a basilar membrane extending between scala tympani and scala media, holds an interesting intermediate position in respect to morphology. A sound probably sets up a traveling wave and the location of the maximal vibration amplitude along the membrane depends on the frequency of the sound. In addition, there is a polarization of the hair cells, in which, however, a kinocilium is maintained up to the adult state. With its perpendicular orientation to the long axis of the basilar membrane, and "outward", this kinocilium corresponds with that of the Mammalia. On the other hand the well developed lagena resembles the appendage of the Anamnia. The lagena apparently serves the perception of low frequency tones and the sense of equilibrium. Most significant, however, is the formation of a homogeneous sensory epithelium (papilla basilaris) in contrast to the organ of Corti, of which 20-40 hair cells with interconnecting supporting cells are lying side by side in one transversal section. A gradient of differentiation between the hair cells is shown only by the length/width relation, decreasing steadily from "inner" to "outer" cells (Retzius, 1884, Takasaka and Smith, 1971).

The afferent nervous supply of the papilla basilaris also resembles the simpler interrelations in the lowest vertebrates. The transformation of the major part of the cochlear duct to become the tegmentum vasculosum is a <u>peculiar differentiation</u> in sauropsids. The tegmentum appears hypertrophic in birds, but it is well developed also in caimans (tropical American crocodilian). The richly folded, single-layered epithelium is formed by adjacent "light" and "dark" cells of the same substructure as found within the stria vascularis (marginal cells) and the transitional zone of the cristae ampullares (Dohlman <u>et al.</u>, 1959, Jahnke <u>et al.</u>, 1969, Ishiyama <u>et al.</u>, 1970, Hládky <u>et al.</u>, <u>1971</u>). Outside the tegmentum vasculosum, only a slender scala vestibuli has developed. It communicates with the ample scala tympani apically through the helicotrema, as well as basally through the ductis brevis (de Burlet, 1934, Schwartzkopff and Winter, 1960).

The inner ears of birds and reptiles appear less uniform in their physiology than in their morphology which scarcely differ at least in birds and caimans. The birds, being homoiothermic, have the same high intensity of life functions as that of the mammals. Especially known is the excellent hearing performance of birds (Schwartzkopff, 1960a,b, 1962). Crocodiles and alligators, among other poikilothermic reptiles, show a rather indolent acoustic behavior. At first therefore the question arises, as to whether the excitatory mechanisms of the various sauropsid cochleae have developed similarly, according to the morphological conformity, or divergingly, corresponding to the differences in general physiology and behavior.

Finally, we have concentrated our efforts in studying the dependence of cochlear potentials on metabolism, aiming at the enzymatic predisposition of the auditory excitatory processes.

2. Methods

2.1 Experimental procedure

The principles of the technique used have been published by Schwartzkopff and Bremond (1963), and by Necker (1970a). The details of the surgery on the reptile are to be published elsewhere (Kauffmann, in preparation). The bony cochlea with round and oval window was exposed under pernocton or nembutal anesthesia without affecting the middle ear. Ag-AgCl-electrodes were brought into contact with the round window or introduced into the scala tympani or into the crevices of scala vestibuli. An indifferent electrode was placed underneath the skin of the frontal region, within a Ringer-pool. In the course of another experimental procedure, capillary microelectrodes were advanced through the tegmentum vasculosum up to the basilar membrane. The experimental animal received artificial respiration through a tracheal cannula, providing air, N_2 or air-N_2-mixtures. The biochemical predispositions of electrogenesis within the cochlea were altered by infusion or perfusion of metabolic inhibitors (cyanide, ouabain) into scala tympani. For a similar purpose, the inner ear was cooled or warmed up, locally under thermocouple control.

The effects of inner ear manipulations upon the receptor processes were tested by recording the cochlear potentials in response to submaximal auditory stimulation (by click and pure tone signals). Controlled outward and inward displacements of the tympanum were generated by positive or negative dc-pulses applied to the loudspeaker or the earphone. The leading and the trailing edge of a 10 msec rectangular pulse applied to the loudspeaker induces movements of the tympanic membrane of opposite directions. Correspondingly the generated cochlear microphonic potentials become independent of each other and of opposite polarity (Schwartzkopff, 1958). In addition, short time after-oscillations can be seen. These are electrically superimposed upon the immediately following discharges of the auditory nerve. They are, however, sufficiently damped so as not to interfere with the second microphonic potential, which appears 10 msec later (Fig. 1).

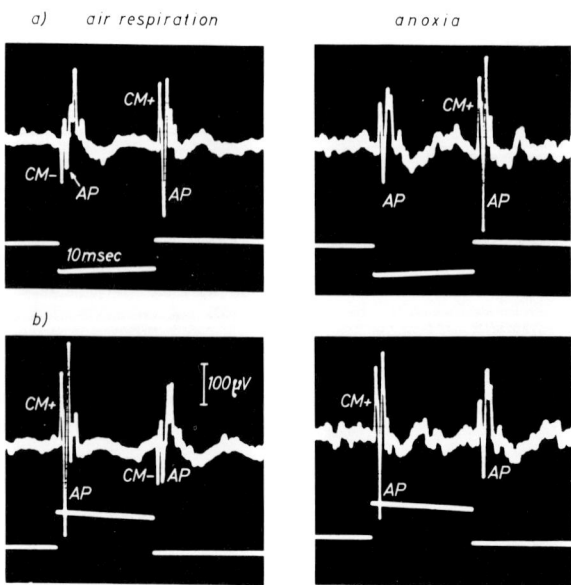

Fig. 1 Pigeon (Columba livia dom.); cochlear potentials evoked by "rectangular" stimuli of alternating polarity a) Condensation-click, b) rarefaction-click at the beginning. CM- appears as first event after condensation-, CM+ after rarefaction-click, respectively. AP is distorted by superimposed CM. Notice the reversible, selective abolishment of CM- by short-time anoxia. (After Necker, 1970a).

2.2 Terminology

Shearing of the hairs towards the kinocilium (or outward shift of the tympanum and upward displacement of the basilar membrane) causes depolarization of the receptor membrane. Shearing into the opposite direction produces hyperpolarization in the cochlea of sauropsids as well as in the other organs developed from the lateral line organ (Flock, 1967, 1971). The cochlear potentials are usually recorded from the round window with the indifferent electrode placed at the body of the animal. In that way a depolarization of the hair cells appears as a positive deflection (endolymph-negative), while a hyperpolarization

results in a negative potential (endolymph-positive).
Accordingly, the cochlear microphonic which is the
result of a depolarization is called CM+ while a hyperpolarization is called CM-, irrespective of the
fact that the polarity depends on the actual position
of the electrode (Necker and Schwartzkopff, 1969).

3. Results

3.1 Qualitative differentiation of cochlear potentials

A peculiar, reversible differentiation of CM+ and CM-
was revealed during the experiments, by which the influence of metabolic alteration upon the inner ear
of birds was compared with the better known situation
in mammals. Ensuing studies on the caiman showed general conformity with birds (Kauffmann and Schwartzkopff, 1971). The other components of the cochlear
potentials (EP, SP and AP) in the sauropsids did not
differ essentially from the findings in the other
vertebrates. But the metabolic control of the latter
components appears to be linked more or less closely
with the differentiation of CM+ and CM-, on which
the following presentation is therefore based.

Cochlear microphonics submitted to oxygen shortage

The stimulus used in the experiments, shown in Fig.
1 a, first caused the eardrum to shift inward and
then after 10 msec outward with the same amplitude.
Fig. 1 b shows the results obtained using a reversed
stimulus sequence. In the recordings in the animal
breathing normally shown in Fig. 1 a - b the CM-
resp. CM+ can be recognized as the earliest event
after stimulation. The action potential of the auditory nerve (AP) appears about 0.5 msec after the
corresponding CM. The AP is distorted by the damped
oscillations of the CM.

Short time deprivation of O_2 (anoxia) causes CM- to
disappear reversibly within 40 - 80 sec in the bird,
while CM+ remains more or less unchanged (see Fig.
1). This reaction does not depend on the sequence of
the two phases of tympanic displacement. The same
differential effect on CM as a result of N_2-respira-
tion is seen in the caiman (Fig. 2). In this animal

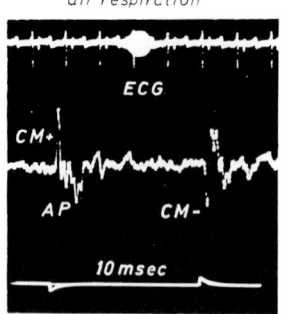 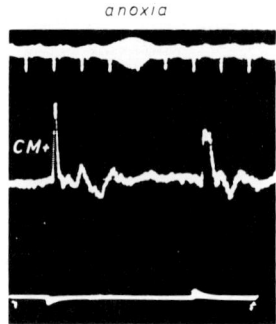

Fig. 2 Caiman (Caiman crocodilus); cochlear potentials evoked by "rectangular" stimuli, as in Fig. 1 b), ECG electrocardiogram, accelerated under anoxia. Notice the depression of CM- by anoxia of 30 min. (Kauffmann, in preparation).

however, it takes about 50 times as long N_2 respiration as in the bird before the influence of O_2-shortage appears. The possible reasons for the delayed reaction are discussed later. Otherwise the AP of Fig. 2 is comparatively small, probably a corollary to the anatomical situation in the caiman.

The selective sensitivity of CM- to O_2-shortage is not related to the special shape of a click-stimulus used in the experiment described above. The choice of this type of stimulus was made because the CM generated can be easily referred to the phase of the vibration and the two components can be separated from the following AP. Such a discrimination is difficult to make in response to high frequency tones. The sinusoid CM in responses to low frequency tones, however, shows only negligible contamination by AP. Fig. 3 demonstrates that one half wave of the microphonics in a pigeon, corresponding to CM-, has disappeared after N_2-respiration. In principle, this kind of distortion during anoxia was also found in response to medium frequency stimulation. This has even been mentioned by Riesco-McClure et al. studying CM postmortally in the guinea pig as early as 1949. A quantitative analysis of the distortion at higher frequencies becomes more difficult since a

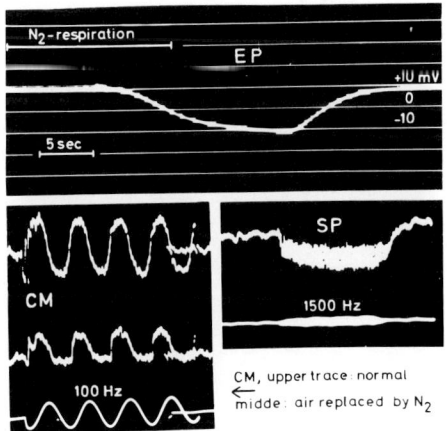

Fig. 3 Components of cochlear potentials in birds; upper part showing EP of the sparrow (Passer domesticus) responding reversibly to short-time anoxia. Left side: combined cochlear potentials of the pigeon, stimulated by a 100 Hz tone pip; notice the rectification (cutting off CM-) by short-time anoxia. At the right: SP of the starling (Sturnus vulgaris) under normal respiration (After Necker, 1970a).

summating potential (SP) is generated above 500 Hz. Its amplitude increases up to the optimal range of hearing sensitivity (1500 Hz in birds), and reacts to anoxia in a specific way (Necker, 1969, 1970a).

3.2 Time course of the anoxia effects on the cochlear potentials

It is well known from numerous earlier studies on mammals that interruption of the O_2-supply to the cochlea impairs electrogenesis partially, at short notice and reversibly. This is also true for a component of CM formerly called "physiological", while a "physical" component remains visible postmortally, even after considerable time (cf. Schwartzkopff, 1960a, 1962, Necker, 1970a). CM+, in our experiments on birds, can be recorded up to about 30 min after the heart has stopped beating, though we prefer not

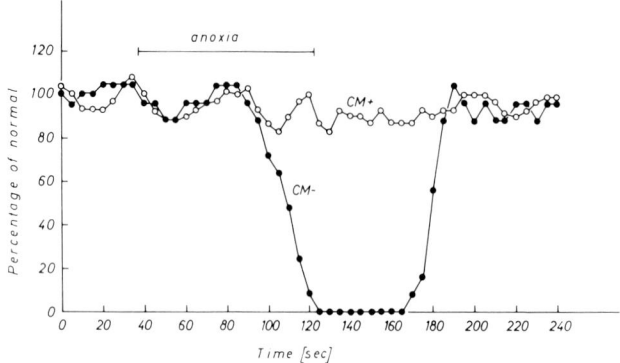

Fig. 4 Pigeon; reversible differentiation of CM+ and CM- by 85 sec anoxia (After Necker, 1970a).

to characterize it as a "physical" event. Further information about the differentiating effects of N_2-respiration upon the other components of the cochlear potentials was obtained by watching the short time variations in CM more precisely.

3.2.1 Cochlear microphonics (CM, CM+, CM-)

The cochlear potentials in birds usually do not change before 30-40 sec after the onset of N_2-respiration. It seems reasonable to assume that O_2-stores within the respiratory tract and within the blood and the tissues are used down to a critical O_2-tension during this period. The blood O_2-tension was not measured directly in our experiments, but was in those of Misrahy et al. (1958) on the guinea pig. The time course reported by these authors corroborates our hypothesis. After the latency period, CM- decreases very regularly within the following 40-80 sec until it disappears (Fig. 4). Shortly afterwards the heart may stop fatally and the impairment of CM- becomes irreversible. After resumption of the normal respiratory support recovery begins with a short latency. The full height of the initial potential is usually obtained more rapidly after resumption of O_2-respiration than was the decay after termination of O_2.

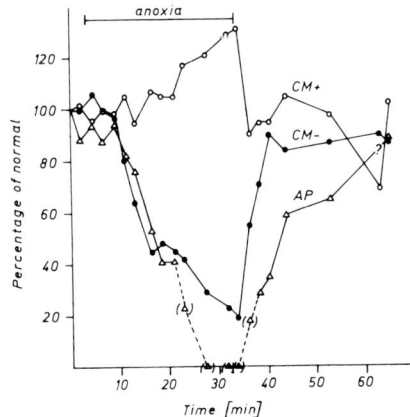

Fig. 5 Caiman; time course of CM+, CM- and AP under reversible anoxia; notice the overshoot of CM+ and the slowing down of the reactions, compared with birds (Kauffmann, in preparation).

CM+ differs from CM- in its reaction to O_2-shortage also by a considerable interexperimental variation. Besides experiments, like the one presented in Fig. 4, in which CM+ is nearly not influenced at all by short-time anoxia, a modest initial depression is observed more frequently, followed by a substantial overshoot. The recovering CM+ returns to normal at about the same time CM- does (Fig. 7). If the animal dies because of prolonged anoxia CM+ at first returns quickly to its initial value, thus behaving differently from CM- which never reappears. Later CM+ decreases slowly and fades away within about 30 min.

The comparison of the reactions in cold- and in warm-blooded sauropsids shows conformance in principle (Fig. 5), though the time course is retarded significantly. The latency after N_2-respirations runs up to several min and the waning of CM- proceeds about 23 times more slowly in the caiman than in the bird. CM- does not reach its (reversible) minimum until 30 min after the onset of N_2-respiration. The recovering course is distinctly steeper than the drop, in the caiman as well as in the bird. The mean ascending rate in Fig. 5 is 7.1 %/min against 2.7 % in the descent. CM- of the caiman differs furthermore from

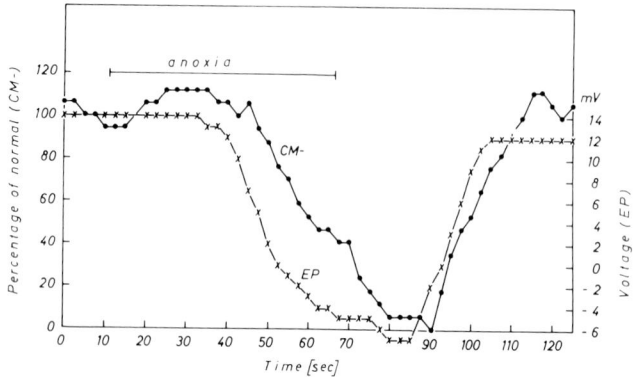

Fig. 6 Starling; time course of EP and CM- under reversible anoxia; notice the phase shift between the components while the general shape of the responses corresponds closely (After Necker, 1970a).

that of the bird since it cannot be abolished by O_2-shortage completely, and at the same time reversibly. On the contrary, 20 % to 40 % of the initial value of CM- was preserved in all experiments in which permanent damages by prolonged metabolic shortage were avoided. This may be indicative of anaerobic processes of energy utilization in the caiman, corresponding with diving.

3.2.2 Endocochlear DC potential (EP)

The maximum values obtained with the unimpaired EP in 5 species of birds barely reach +20 mV (Schmidt and Fernández, 1962, Necker, 1970a). Even this voltage is not equalized in most experiments because of leak currents through lesions of the tegmentum vasculosum caused by the penetrating microcapillary. Thereby the normal EP of birds achieves less than 1/4 the strength known from the mammals.

The time course of EP, changing under metabolic stress, resembles closest that of CM-, among the other components of cochlear potentials. This finding is illustrated by Fig. 6, which shows results of an experiment in a sparrow. EP parallels the course

of CM-, however preceding it by some (5-10) sec in
the experiment demonstrated, as it did in all comparable experiments in pigeons, starlings and thrushes.
This seems to be correlated with the direct blood
supply to the tegmentum vasculosum, which is most
reasonably the generator of EP. The papilla basilaris, generator of CM, has no blood vessels of its own
(cf. Schwartzkopff and Winter, 1960, Schmidt, 1964)
and receives the O_2 required through diffusion from
the tegmentum.

Also the EP of birds (+20 mV normally) becomes negative (-20 to more than -30 mV) after a short period
of anoxia. The corresponding "inversion-value" of
mammals amounts to about -50 mV. Thus the EP's in
mammals and birds are clearly in closer relation with
each other during anoxia than under normal physiological conditions (Necker, 1970a). The negative EP's of
birds and mammals can therefore both be interpreted
as diffusion potentials, corresponding to the similar K- (and Na-) concentration gradients within the
inner ear of both groups (Johnstone et al., 1963).
EP of the caiman does not surpass +5 to +6 mV, as
Schmidt and Fernández (1962) have found earlier, and
as we confirmed. We did not succeed because of methodological difficulties in following the changes of
this potential over larger periods of time than 30
min., as required here. Qualitatively, there exists
consistency with the EP of birds.

3.2.3 Summation potential (SP)

SP is produced by stimulating the ear with tone pips
of 10 msec duration (1000 or 1500 Hz in birds), alternating with click signals. The SP of caimans had
too low an amplitude to allow a thorough investigation. In the birds, SP has its highest amplitude
when recorded from the scala media. SP shows the
same polarity as CM+ does (i.e. endolymph-negative)
and changes sign as soon as the recording microelectrode penetrates the hair cell surface (simultaneously with polarity changes of CM+ and CM-; Necker and
Schwartzkopff, 1969). When the electrode is kept in
place no change of polarity occurs in the SP of birds
in response to prolonged or supramaximal auditory
stimuli. This is in contrast to the finding in mammals (Honrubia, 1969, 1970, Honrubia and Ward, 1969a,
Honrubia et al., 1964). Furthermore, the SP of birds

is not extinguished by short-time anoxia. Because
the mammalian SP is related to the spatial position
of the electrode in respect to the coiled cochlea
(Honrubia and Ward, 1969b, Dallos et al., 1970), the
divergency might be explained at least partially by
the stretched shape of the inner ear and the homogeneous composition of the papilla basilaris in the
bird.

The SP shows a general relationship with the behavior
of CM+ when the bird undergoes N_2-respiration and
other metabolic loads (Fig. 7). Certain differences
can be explained by methodological difficulties and
consecutive inaccuracies in measuring SP. In most
cases, SP and CM+ both show correlations with general
heart functions, measured as pulse rate. A causal
linking by the way of the blood pressure is supposed,
which however was not measured during our experiments.
But it is reasonable to assume that it parallels
heart frequency. The blood pressure could become effective through the arteria cochlearis, running freely with several loops at the bottom of the recessus
scalae tympani (Schwartzkopff and Winter, 1960). Increasing volume of this artery would force the perilymph of the scalae tympani to displace the basilary
membrane "upward".

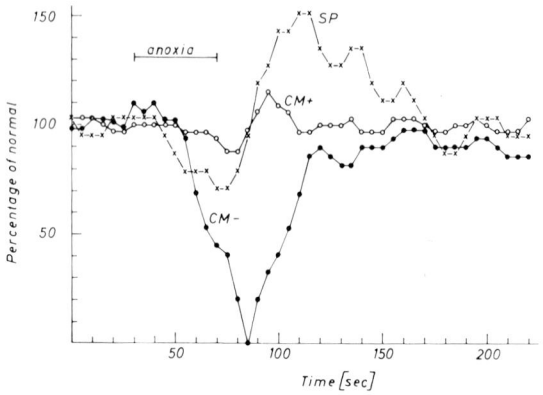

Fig. 7 Starling; response of CM+, CM- and SP to
anoxia; notice the initial depression and the
following overshoot of CM+ and SP, thus showing parallel variation while CM- changes
independently (After Necker, 1969).

3.2.4 Action potential (AP)

The AP of birds and caimans (Fig. 5) reacts sensitively when O_2 supply is disturbed in accordance with the AP of mammals. That is, it behaves in general similarly to CM-. This is surprising at first, since the latter indicates a hyperpolarization of the hair cells to which an inhibition of the synaptic spike-generator process corresponds. However, the explanation, close at hand, is that the O_2-shortage controls metabolic processes of the same kind, but as parts of the generators of CM- or AP, independently. The concept of independent interfering with identical biochemical events is corroborated also by the finding that AP shows frequently a passing by "recovery" after its descent has been initiated by continuing metabolic impair. Such intercalated maxima are sufficiently clearly correlated with the overshoot of CM+, generated at the same time of the experiment (Fig. 9). An indication of a rather loose coupling between CM- and AP is further offered by the finding that AP in the caiman disappears under reversible anoxia while CM- stays at a residual value.

3.3 Temperature dependence of cochlear potentials

The differentiation of the various inner ear potentials by short-time O_2-deprivation proves the interference of diverse metabolic mechanisms. For further elucidation, the general influence of the intensity of metabolism was tested by varying the temperature. A significant increase above normal body temperature (40°C) or cooling beyond 20°C was not possible in the pigeon without damage. In the caiman however, the adaption temperature (25°C) could be exceeded reversibly (up to ca. 30°C). The lower limit of compatibility in this animal was not attained by cooling until 10°C. Methodological difficulties arose in both experimental animals from considerable counterreactions of the whole body to temperature manipulations, and from the time needed to achieve a satisfactory homogeneity of body temperature. The preferred method was a localized cooling (or warming) of the tissues surrounding the inner ear. But even then, sensoric reflex actions as well as temperature convection through the circulating blood produced side effects which could not be controlled completely. Only an approximation results from measuring the temperature of the tissue adjacent to the cochlea.

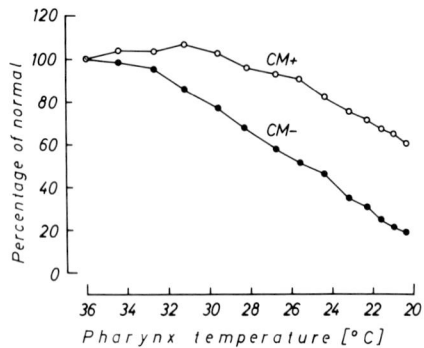

Fig. 8 Pigeon; differentiation of CM+ and CM- by cooling the head (After Necker, 1970b).

This, however, is close enough to the temperature inside the cochlea, considering the general accuracy of our finding (Necker, 1970a).

The various inner ear potentials are differentiated in a similar way by temperature manipulation as found under anoxia; there is general agreement also with the situation in mammals (Butler et al., 1960) if the discrimination of CM+ and CM- is disregarded. Lowering the temperature induces the most accurately reproducible changes in CM- of the bird, as was found similarly for N_2-respiration. The relations are close enough to utilize the readings of CM- for measuring the temperature inside the cochlea (Fig. 8). The Q_{10} of CM- was found to be 2.0 as an average of our experiments. CM+ behaves more complexly under changing temperature, though no serious overshoot is induced by decreasing temperature in birds as seen frequently with N_2-respiration. Sometimes CM+ reacts weakly when cooling starts, but then decreases more steeply than CM- does, beyond a critical point of temperature. The gradient of CM+ is less steep than that of CM- in experiments with a rather continual course; here a Q_{10} (for CM+) of 1.54 results. It is true also for CM- and CM+ of the caiman that the first decreases between 30 and $10°C$ more steeply than the second.

The reactions of SP to cooling are rather variable, but resemble in general that of CM+, comparable with the behavior under anoxia. Correspondingly, Butler et al. (1960) have found in the guinea pig that SP depends on temperature only in a rather loose and occasionally paradoxical way. AP too is influenced by temperature changes, similarly to CM+, thus diverging from its anoxia behavior. The amplitude of AP in the bird is nearly constant for temperatures between 40° and 25° similar to the situation in the mammal. If cooling is continued beyond 25°C the AP decreases rather abruptly. In contrast, the latency changes steadily increasing with decreasing temperature in agreement with what is known generally from nervous processes (Necker, 1970a).

3.4 Biochemical interference with cochlear potentials

Various studies of the cochlear potentials in mammals show that short-time metabolic manipulations impair the oxidative phosphorylation and energy utilization within the cells of the inner ear. The obvious assumption is that the rapid changes of CM- (and EP) in birds depend also directly on changes in oxidative energetic processes while the latter are not responsible for CM+ in the same direct way.

3.4.1 Cyanide-poisoning

CN-ions contaminate the cytochromoxidase abundantly found within the hair cells and elsewhere (Gerhardt, 1962). Tsunoo and Perlman (1969) and other authors succeeded in cautiously perfusing the scala tympani of the guinea pig with cyanide and depressing CM reversibly. The effects reported resemble those produced by hypoxia. Applied simultaneously, an additive impairment is produced by CN and hypoxia. Infusion of KCN into the scala tympani of birds depresses immediately CM-, while CM+ decreases with considerable retardation. The time course of the potential variations under anoxia including the postmortal waning of CM can be completely reproduced by carefully dosing the cyanide (Necker, 1970a, 1970b). A reversible contamination of CM- and CM+ can also be achieved in the caiman by infusion of a small amount of KCN (40 μl, 4×10^{-7}M). The time course of the potential corresponds with the anoxic effects (Fig. 9). Here it can be assumed that the cyanide was diluted up to inefficiency by the blood circulation, which remained untouched. It is interesting to note that AP was reduced irreversibly to 30 % of its initial value

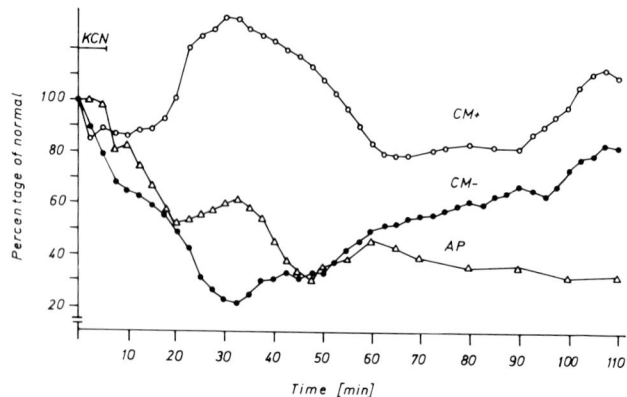

Fig. 9 Caiman; response of CM+, CM- and AP to infusion of KCN (40 µl, 4×10^{-7}M) into scala tympani. Notice the differentiation of CM+ and CM-, both depressed almost reversibly, while AP does not recover (After Kauffmann and Schwartzkopff, 1971).

during the experiment described in Fig. 9. This underlines the idea that AP depends on the same biochemic process as CM+ does, but that both potentials can be manipulated independently.

3.4.2 Effects of ouabain

The energy activated through the intracellular metabolism is utilized for the synthesis of ATP and for the active transport of ions and charges across membranes. A Na-, K-sensitive ATP-ase participates in the transport and can be disengaged selectively by ouabain (Glynn, 1964, Konishi and Mendelsohn, 1970). It has been shown that ouabain-sensitive mechanism is involved in the generation of CM by the macula sacculi of the goldfish, where the enzyme blocking agent becomes effective only when administered upon the basal surface of the hair cells (Matsuura et al., 1971). Also in the mammal the influence of ouabain is much stronger when applied through scala tympani than through scala media (Konishi and Mendelsohn, 1970). ATP-ase activity has been demonstrated within the hair cells and the supporting cells of the mammalian organ of Corti, at a very high level, within

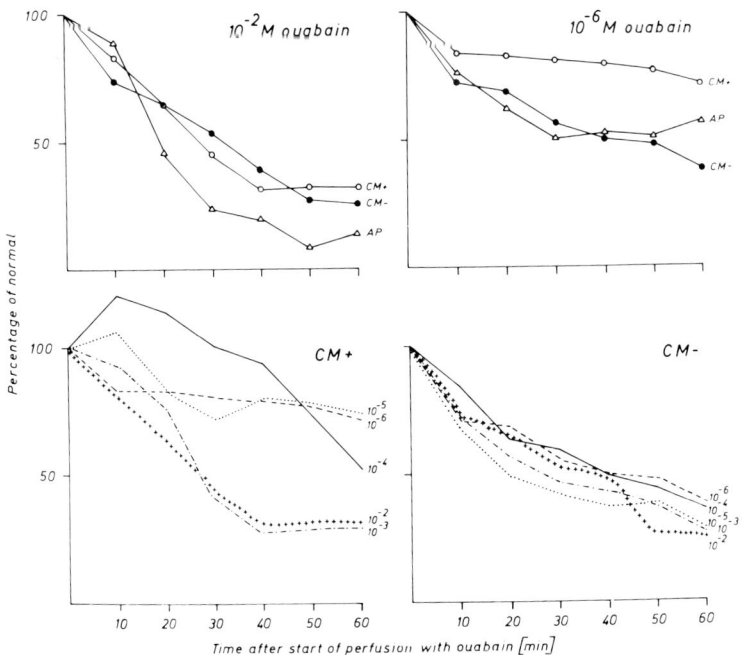

Fig. 10 Caiman; response of cochlear potentials to perfusion of scala tympani by various concentrations of ouabain. Notice the initially positive response of CM+ to intermediate concentrations of the drug, while CM- and AP are depressed in close relation to the strength of the ouabain administered (Kauffmann, in preparation).

the stria vascularis and also within the avian tegmentum vasculosum. The contamination of the K-transport through the walls of the cochlear duct as well as the corresponding detriment of EP and CM has been proved by various studies in mammals and, generally speaking, in the birds too (Nakai and Hilding, 1967, Kuijpers, 1969, Kuijpers and Bonting, 1970a, 1970b, Kuijpers et al. 1970, Chou, 1970).

In the caiman, it was found by continuous perfusion of scala tympani that a concentration of 10^{-6}M ouabain is close to threshold for AP and CM (Kauffmann, in preparation). The saturation value of the ouabain effect on the cochlear potentials is surpassed at 10^{-2}M (Fig. 10). This working range of ouabain is in agreement with the data reported by Chou (1970) and by Kuijpers and Bonting (1970) in the guinea pig, and by Kuijpers et al., (1970) in the chicken.

CM+ and CM- of the caiman both decrease in amplitude almost identically when 10^{-2}M ouabain is administered. Both components are reduced to approximately 25 % of the initial value, while AP is affected even more. The effects of ouabain are lessened generally when the concentration is reduced. However, a differentiation between CM+ and CM- is the most remarkable outcome. CM- behaves "orthodoxly", showing at all concentrations of ouabain an impairment which starts at the onset of the perfusion and continues in an approximately exponential way (Fig. 10). CM+, on the other hand, reacts by an initial overshoot to intermediate concentrations of ouabain, followed by an eventual descent. Maximal overshoot is obtained by 10^{-4}M ouabain. This finding resembles observations in the guinea pig (Kuijpers and Bonting, 1970a), according to which very low concentrations of ouabain induce an activation of the Na-, K-sensitive ATP-ase.

But it must be admitted that these authors did not find a corresponding variation of EP or CM. Prázma (1969), however, describes a distinct increase of CM at ouabain concentrations of 10^{-4}M during analogous experiments with the mammal. The reaction resembles that of CM+ in the caiman (Fig. 10).

Considering all ambiguities of interpretation, ouabain does certainly create a differentiation of CM+ and CM- within the caiman cochlea, in the course of which CM- is injured generally more than CM+ by low and medium concentrations. The latter is enhanced during the initial phase or perfusion by intermediate doses.

4. Discussion

The comparative exploration of the receptor cells in the vertebrate acoustico-lateralis system has been pushed forward by studies on various representative animals (Schmidt and Fernández, 1962) and has been reviewed repeatedly (Schwartzkopff, 1960a, 1962, Grinnell, 1969, Flock, 1971). This discussion may justifiably concentrate on placing the findings presented here into a framework already at hand.

4.1 Comparison of homoiothermic with poikilothermic sauropsids

While the inner ear of the caiman is anatomically very close to that of the bird, these sauropsids differ physiologically. This is true generally for the metabolic level and for the time course of the cochlear potentials under stress. Following up details of CM-, the reaction to metabolic shortage is remarkably slower in caimans than in birds, by far surpassing the expected influence of the differences in body temperature. It can be assumed so far only that additional adaptations to the diving behavior of the rapacious saurian are involved, e.g. increased energy storage and oxygen-independent metabolism. A hint in this direction is that we did not succeed in suppressing CM-completely by reversible N_2-respiration or cyanide infusion. The possibility of a more pronounced contribution of glycolytic energy-utilization must be taken into consideration.

The dependency of the cochlear potentials of mammals on temperature changes (Butler et al., 1960) is found also in the warm- as well as in the cold-blooded sauropsid. Furthermore a temperature-controlled differentiation of CM+ and CM- was discovered in birds, and in reptiles correspondingly.

4.2 Comparison of cochlear potentials within the Vertebrates

4.2.1 The endolymphatic DC-potential (EP)

EP is generated by the stria vascularis in the mammal, reaching more than +80 mV. In birds and probably in caimans it originates from the tegmentum vasculosum and it does not surpass +20 mV (bird) or reaches little more than +5 mV (caiman), though the volume and the surface of the tegmentum seem to exceed relatively those of the stria. EP is either lacking or poorly developed within the lateral line organ, the inner ear of the Anamnia and around the cristae.

The difference in size of the mammalian and avian EP cannot be explained by the degree of activity of the

ATP-ase, which is responsible for generation of EP, since this is practically equal in both classes (Kuijpers et al., 1970). Nor does there seem to exist an interrelation with the cation concentration in the scala media (Johnstone et al., 1963). The divergent structure of the stria vascularis (multi-layered epithelium, only the external layer with the enzyme-active marginal cells) may offer an explanation when compared with the tegmentum vasculosum (single-layered, though richly folded epithelium). Furthermore, the backside of the tegmentum borders the perilymphatic space of scala vestibuli, similar to the position of Reissner's membrane. It is conceivable that the electric isolation by the walls of the cochlear duct is sufficient only in the mammal for maintaining the high level of endolymphatic potential. This idea is supported indirectly by the finding (Bosher and Warren, 1971) that the full enzymatic mechanism of cation transport is present already at the 8th postnatal day in the young rat. Also the endolymphatic ion concentration nearly reaches the final values at early developmental stages. The EP however is built up essentially between the 13th and 14th day. These authors assume that the membrane resistance is insufficient before this time.

In any case, certain cellular elements of the membraneous labyrinth generate EP by active transport of ions according to the findings of various authors (Bosher and Warren, 1968, Konishi and Mendelsohn, 1970, Ishiyama et al., 1970, Kuijpers et al., 1970). The recent observation that metabolic manipulation interferes with CM-, producing a short but distinct delay to EP, but otherwise depressing it in the same way, leads us to the conclusion that a fraction of the ATP-ase activity, responsible for the generation of CM-, is localized within the papilla basilaris itself (within the hair cells or the surrounding supporting cells).

4.2.2 Summating potentials (SP)

SP - and microphonics - are generated at the endolymphatic surface of the sensory epithelium, in mammals as well as in birds. This has been proved by the abrupt turnover of polarity when a microelectrode penetrates the respective region of the cochlea (Necker and Schwartzkopff, 1969). In the birds, SP is found regularly to be endolymph-negative. Divergencies in morphology cannot explain satisfactorily the observation that the mammalian SP decreases or even changes polarity under metabolic stress, while the same conditions frequently enhance SP in birds.

No special difficulties in interpretation arise when the reactions of SP to certain mechanical stimuli are compared, if the particular ascription to the inner hair cells of mammals is disregarded (Davis et al., 1958, Stopp and Whitfield, 1964). Static displacement of the basilar membrane in the mammal or of the sacculus-otolith in the goldfish (Furukawa and Ishii, 1967) can be compared with mechanical influences in the cochlea of birds, e.g. of infusion or of the changing heart activity as a counter-reaction to metabolic stress. Thereby the assumption is made that an increasing pulse rate results in a variation of the blood pressure and produces a pressure gradient across the basilar membrane.

4.2.3 The cochlear microphonics (CM)

The general properties of the cochlear microphonics show good agreement in the various vertebrates. It has been suggested (Flock, 1971) that CM is part of the mechanism of sensory transduction, based upon active ion transport, and followed by synaptic transfer of (afferent) excitation. The differentiation of CM into a depolarizing and a hyperpolarizing component (CM+ and CM-) as found in our experiments by alteration of the metabolic conditions, however, is not supported directly by previous studies. As a matter of fact, Riesco-McClure et al. (1949) have mentioned a rectification in the CM of the guinea pig after death, comparable to Fig. 3 of this paper. But apparently this observation has not been followed up.

It seems to the author that the morphological and physiological polarization of hair cells, indicated by the asymmetric kinocilium, could be correlated with the differentiation of CM+ and CM- (cf. Flock, 1967, 1971). It is well known that the input/output functions of the lateral-line receptors, revealed by bending the sensory hairs into hyper- or depolarizing direction, are asymmetric. This is at least compatible with the decomposition of CM into two physiological components, if there is not a closer correlation to be assumed.

4.3 General biochemical predispositions for the generation of cochlear potentials

Older observations are confirmed by the findings presented here showing a sensitive reaction of EP to disturbances of the oxidative phosphorylation or of the activity of the Na-, K-sensitive ATP-ase. The avian EP is turned to a negativity of about -30 mV by a short-time anoxia, i.e. it approaches the mammalian EP under anoxia (-40 to -50 mV), as Necker (1970a) has underlined. This backs the hypothesis that the comparatively low value of EP in the normal ear of the bird is to be linked with the conductance of the cochlear walls, rather than with enzyme activity. This concept is in agreement with the conclusion of Kuijpers and Bonting (1970b) that the EP of the guinea pig depends on two components. The one is built up by an ouabain-sensitive electrogeneous K-pump; the other is based upon a negative K-diffusion potential. Their conclusions were made on the basis of results from experiments in which the metabolic stress and the perilymphatic ion composition were varied.

The two-component concept seems to be useful not only for a better understanding of EP, but also for an interpretation of the differential behavior of CM+ and CM-. The various experimental conditions induce the hyperpolarizing component CM- to change by the same function that EP does. The parallelism between the course of these two potentials proves that the same mechanism is responsible for the generation of CM-, which produces the ouabain-sensitive component of EP. The site of generation is, however, different. The electrogeneous ion pump, which hyperpolarizes the hair cell receptor membrane, is also responsible for the generation of EP. CM+ and SP, on the other hand, are thought to represent a diffusion potential which is generated by depolarization (of the receptor membrane). A general confirmation of this concept is offered by the temperature coefficients. The Q_{10} of ouabain-sensitive, hyperpolarizing membrane activities is in general found to surpass that of depolarizing processes (Lüttgau, 1963, Glynn, 1964). This corresponds with the difference between CM- and CM+ reported here (Necker, 1970a). According to our hypothesis, the physiological asymmetry of the membrane polarization in hair cells, stimulated mechanically, from opposite directions (Flock, 1967, 1971, Harris et al., and earlier authors) is connected with the different mechanisms of potential generation. A conductance change is indicated by CM+, caused by shifting of the stereocilia towards the kinocilium. The normal CM-, on the other hand, is based upon an instantaneous enhancement of the active ion transport, induced by the opposite displacement. CM- therefore is coupled directly with the activity of the Na-, K-sensitive ATP-ase, while the latter produces indirectly the predisposition for CM+ by providing an ionic concentration gradient.

The question as to how the mechanoelectric transducer processes at the endolymphatic hair cell surface may control the synaptic transfer of excitation is not touched here by the observations and interpretations presented. Of course, we assume that the functions are comparable throughout all vertebrate phyla, also in this respect. This means a disagreement with the classic theory (Davis, 1965) that a detector mechanism of sensitive resistors alone controls essentially the excitatory current from the energy storage of the endolymph to the synaptic region of the organ of Corti. The findings in the sauropsids, and in the Anamnia as well, corroborate the idea that processes of "active" inhibition are involved in hair cell physiology together with excitation by depolarization. The high level of frequency and time pattern analysis by the auditory system is achieved only by the alternating cooperation of both mechanisms and is not found generally in neurosensoric systems.

Acknowledgement

This work is supported by the Deutsche Forschungsgemeinschaft; part of the program of SFB 114 (Bionach).

References

Bosher, S.K., and Warren, R.L. (1968). Observations on the electrochemistry of the cochlear endolymph of the rat: a quantitative study of its electrical potential and ionic composition as determined by means of flame spectrophotometry. Proc. Roy. Soc. London, Ser. B. 171, 227-247.

Bosher, S.K., and Warren, R.L. (1971). A study of the electrochemistry and osmotic relationships of the cochlear fluids in the neonatal rat at the time of the development of the endocochlear potential. J. Physiol. 212, 739-761.

de Burlet, H.M. (1934). Vergleichende Anatomie des statoakustischen Organs a) Die innere Ohrsphäre. In: Handbuch der vergleichenden Anatomie der Wirbeltiere. (Bolk, Göppert, Kallius, Lubosch, eds.), 2/2, pp. 1293-1380, Urban and Schwarzenberg, Berlin and Vienna.

Butler, R.A., Konishi, T., and Fernández, C. (1960). Temperature coefficients of cochlear potentials. Amer.J. Physiol. 199, 688-692.

Chou, J.T.-Y. (1970). The effect of cardiac glycoside on microphonic potential. Arch. Klin. Exp. Ohr.- Nas.- Kehlk. Heilk. 195, 246-256.

Dallos, P., Schoeny, Z.G., and Cheatham, M.A. (1970). Cochlear summating potentials: composition. Science 170, 641-644.

Davis, H. (1965). A model for transducer action in the cochlea. Cold Spring Harbor Symp. Quant. Biol. 30, 181-190.

Davis, H., Deatherage, B.H., Eldredge, D.H., and Smith, C.A. (1958). Summating potentials of the cochlea. Amer. J. Physiol. 195, 251-261.

Dohlman, G., Ormerod, F.C., and McLay, K. (1959). The secretory epithelium of the internal ear. Acta Oto- Laryngol. 50, 243-249.

Flock, Å. (1966). Ultrastructure and function in the lateral-line organs. In: Lateral Line Detectors (P.H. Cahn, ed.), pp. 163-197. Indiana Univ. Press, Bloomington, Indiana.

Flock, Å. (1971). Sensory transduction in hair cells. In: Handbook of Sensory Physiology I. Principles of Receptor Physiology (Loewenstein, ed.), pp. 361-441. Springer, Berlin.

Furukawa, T., and Ishii, Y. (1967). Effects of static bending of sensory hairs on sound reception in the goldfish. Jap. J. Physiol. 17, 572-588.

Gerhardt, H.J. (1962). Die Cytochromoxydasereaktion in der Meerschweinchenschnecke. Arch. Klin. Exp. Ohr.- Nas.- Kehlk. Heilk. 179, 283-289.

Glynn, J.M. (1964). The action of cardiac glycosides on ion movements. Pharmacol. Rev. 16, 381-407.

Grinnell, A.D. (1969). Comparative physiology of hearing. Ann. Rev. Physiol. 31, 545-580.

Harris, G.G., Frishkopf, L.S., and Flock, Å. (1970). Receptor potentials from hair cells of the lateral line. Science 167, 76-79.

Hladký, R., Dvorák, M., and Cada, K. (1971). Elektronenmikroskopische Untersuchungen zur funktionellen Morphologie der Stria vascularis. Z. Mikrosk. Anat. Forsch. 83, 166-176.

Honrubia, V. (1970). Temporal and spatial distribution of the CM and SP of the cochlea. In: Frequency Analysis and Periodicity Detection in Hearing (R. Plomp and G.F. Smoorenburg, eds.), pp. 94-105, Sijthoff, Leiden, The Netherlands.

Honrubia, V., and Ward, P.H. (1969a). Properties of the summating potential of the guinea pig's cochlea. J. Acoust. Soc. Amer. 45, 1443-1450.

Honrubia, V., and Ward, P.H. (1969b). Cochlear potentials inside the cochlear duct at the level of the round window. Ann. Otol. Rhinol. Laryngol. 78, 1189-1200.

Honrubia, V., Johnstone, B.M., and Butler, R.A. (1964). Maintenance of cochlear potentials during asphyxia. Acta Oto-Laryngol. 60, 105-112.

Ishiyama, E., Cutt, R.A., and Karls, E.W. (1970). Ultrastructure of the tegmentum vasculosum and transitional zone. Ann. Otol. Rhinol. Laryngol. 79, 998-1009.

Jahnke, V., Lundquist, P.-G., and Wersäll, J. (1969). Some morphological aspects of sound perception in birds. Acta Oto-Laryngol. 67, 583-601.

Johnstone, C.G., Schmidt, R.S., and Johnstone, B.M. (1963). Sodium and potassium in vertebrate cochlear endolymph as determined by flame microspectrophotometry. Comp. Biochem. Physiol. 9, 335-341.

Kauffmann, G., and Schwartzkopff, J. (1971). On the dependence on metabolim of the cochlear potentials in Caiman (Caiman crocodilus). Z. Vergl. Physiol. 75, 105-107.

Konishi, T., and Mendelsohn, M. (1970). Effect of ouabain on cochlear potentials and endolymph composition in guinea pigs. Acta Oto-Laryngol. 69, 192-199.

Kuijpers, W. (1969). Cation transport and cochlear function. Acta Oto-Laryngol. 67, 200-205.

Kuijpers, W., and Bonting, S.L. (1970a). The cochlear potentials. I. The effect of ouabain on the cochlear potentials of the guinea pig. Pflügers Arch. 320, 348-358.

Kuijpers, W. and Bonting, S.L. (1970b). The cochlear potentials II. The nature of the cochlear endolymphatic resting potential. Pflügers Arch. 320, 359-372.

Kuijpers, W., Houben, N.M.D., and Bonting, S.L. (1970). Distribution and properties of ATPase activities in the cochlea of the chicken. Comp. Biochem. Physiol. 36, 669-676.

Lüttgau, H.C. (1963). Nervenphysiologie (einschl. Electrophysiolgie des Muskels). Fortschr. Zool. 15, 92-124.

Matsuura, S., Ikeda, K., and Furukawa, T. (1971). Effects of Na^+, K^+, and ouabain on microphonic potentials of the goldfish inner ear. Jap. J. Physiol. 21, 563-578.

Misrahy, G.A., Shinabarger, E.W., and Arnold, J.E. (1958). Changes in cochlear endolymphatic oxygen availability action potential, and microphonics during and following asphyxia, hypoxia, and exposure to loud sounds. J. Acoust. Soc. Amer. 30, 701-704.

Nakai, Y., and Hilding, D. (1967). Adenosine triphosphatase distribution in the organ of Corti. Acta Oto-Laryngol. 64, 477-491.

Necker, R. (1969). Mikrophon- und Summationspotentiale des Vogelohres bei N_2-Beatmung. Naturwiss. 56, 143-144.

Necker, R. (1970a). Zur Entstehung der Cochleapotentiale von Vögeln: Verhalten bei O_2-Mangel, Cyanidvergiftung und Unterkühlung sowie Beobachtungen über die räumliche Verteilung. Z. Vergl. Physiol. 69, 367-425.

Necker, R. (1970b). Physiologische Differenzierung der Mikrophonpotentiale im Innenohr von Vögeln in De- und Hyperpolarisation. Verh. Deut. Zool. Ges. Köln, pp. 178-182.

Necker, R., and Schwartzkopff, J. (1969). Entstehungsort und räumliche Verteilung der Mikrophon- und Summationspotentiale im Vogelohr. Naturwiss. 56, 92.

Prazma, J. (1969). Active ion transport from scala vestibuli into scala media. Acta Oto-Laryngol. 67, 631-638.

Retzius, G. (1884). Das Gehörorgan der Wirbeltiere II. Das Gehörorgan der Reptilien, der Vögel und der Säugetiere. Samson and Wallin, Stockholm.

Riesco-McClure, J.S., Davis, H., Gernandt, B.E., and Covell, W.P. (1949). Ante-mortem failure of the aural microphonic in the guinea pig. Proc. Soc. Exp. Biol. Med. 71, 158-160.

Schmidt, R.S. (1964). Blood supply of pigeon inner ear. J. Comp. Neurol. 123, 187-203.

Schmidt, R.S., and Fernández, C. (1962). Labyrinthine dc potentials in representative vertebrates. J. Cell. Comp. Physiol. 59, 311-322.

Schwartzkopff, J. (1958). Über den Einfluß der Bewegungsrichtung der Basilarmembran auf die Ausbildung der Cochlea-Potentiale von Strix varia und Melopsittacus undulatus. Z. Vergl. Physiol. 41, 35-48.

Schwartzkopff, J. (1960a). Vergleichende Physiologie des Gehörs. Fortschr. Zool. 12, 206-264

Schwartzkopff, J. (1960b). Der Einfluß der Impuls-Folge-Frequenz auf die Komponenten des Cochlea-Potentials von Vögeln. Verh. Deut. Zool. Ges. Bonn, pp. 416-424.

Schwartzkopff, J. (1962). Vergleichende Physiologie des Gehörs und der Lautäußerungen. Fortschr. Zool. 15, 213-336.

Schwartzkopff, J., and Brémond, J.C. (1963). Méthode de dérivation des potentiels cochléaires chez l'oiseau. J. Physiol. 55, 495-518.

Schwartzkopff, J., and Winter, P. (1960). Zur Anatomie der Vogel-Cochlea unter natürlichen Bedingungen. Biol. Zentralbl. 79, 607-625.

Stopp, P.E., and Whitfield, J.C. (1964). Summating potentials in the avian cochlea. J. Physiol. 175, 45P-46P.

Takasaka, T., and Smith, C.A. (1971). The structure and innervation of the pigeon's basilar papilla. J. Ultrastruct. Res. 35, 20-65.

Tsunoo, M., and Perlman, H.B. (1969). Respiration of the cochlea and function. Acta Oto-Laryngol. 67, 17-27.

Figures 1, 3, 4, 6, 8, and 9 reproduced by permission of Zeitschrift für Vergleichende Physiologie.

Figure 7 reproduced by permission of Naturwissenschaften.

DISCUSSION

DAVIS: Dr. Schwartzkopff has given us some further insight with this distinction between the hyperpolarizing and the depolarizing cochlear microphonics. This will bear much thinking about.

KATSUKI: As I said before we used the ouabain from the top of the cells and ouabain did not work. Matsuura et al. (1971) studied the ear of the fish. They also found that the ouabain from the top surface did not work but at the base the ouabain was effective.

SCHWARTZKOPFF: Well, we applied it from the base. We knew these papers and have therefore not done experiments from the endolymphatic side. I think that somebody (Kuijpers and Bonting, 1970) has done it in the mammal and has repeated the experience of Matsuura et al. (1971). It takes a couple of minutes for ouabain to work in the mammal and according to our results, almost the same time in the crocodile.

KATSUKI: We use the concentration 10^{-3} mol. without any effect. But you used 10^{-2} mol. That is a very, very concentrated solution which might damage the cell.

SCHWARTZKOPFF: This is completely true. The experiment in which we used 10^{-2} mol. was a little bit different from the other. It gives a supermaximal effect. It was only a short-time perfusion; otherwise it would have damaged the cell. All the other experiments in which we used concentrations of 10^{-3} to 10^{-6} mol. could be done with continuing perfusion.

DALLOS: There could be one component among the cochlear potentials in the mammalian cochlea that might very well correspond or be similar to your CM^-. This is one of the summating potential components that I call AVE^- which can be recorded at frequencies below the best frequency of the electrode location. This potential has the same polarity in both scalae, vestibuli and tympani, and it immediately disappears upon death. It is much more oxygen dependent than the other summating potential components.

SCHWARTZKOPFF: We have certainly recorded this CM^- potential from scala vestibuli or from scala media at the opposite sign. I have only shown the one.

SUGA: When a high frequency sound is delivered, the electrogenic pump should be turned on and off very quickly to produce the negative component of the cochlear microphonic according to your illustration. I wonder if such a fast change in the activity of the electrogenic pump is possible.

SCHWARTZKOPFF: We can see the effects only up to 1000 Hz.

References

Kuijpers, W., and Bonting, S.L. (1970). The cochlear potentials I. The effect of ouabain on the cochlear potentials of the guinea pig. Pflügers Arch. 320, 348-358.

Matsuura, S., Ikeda, K., and Furukawa, T. (1971). Effects of Na^+, K^+, and ouabain in microphonic potentials of the goldfish inner ear. Jap. J. Physiol. 21, 563-578.

IV
NEURAL CODING AT LOWER LEVELS

STIMULUS CODING AT CAUDAL LEVELS OF THE CAT'S
AUDITORY NERVOUS SYSTEM: I. RESPONSE
CHARACTERISTICS OF SINGLE UNITS

N.Y.S. Kiang
D.K. Morest[1]
D.A. Godfrey[1]
J.J. Guinan, Jr.[2]
E.C. Kane[3]

1. Introduction

The primary purpose of these papers is to present some ideas based on combined physiological and anatomical studies of stimulus coding in the mammalian auditory nervous system. The papers are presented together to emphasize the unity of the approach. The general approach is to show how single units in selected regions of the cat's auditory system respond to simple acoustic stimuli and to correlate the responses with structural features in each region. The regions selected were the auditory nerve (AN), the cochlear nucleus (CN), and the superior olivary complex (SOC). Each region was studied independently, and more complete reports will be published elsewhere. The present paper will examine a few results significant for describing the processing of signals

---

From the Center for Communication Sciences, Research Laboratory of Electronics, Massachusetts Institute of Technology; Department of Anatomy, Harvard Medical School; and the Eaton-Peabody Laboratory of Auditory Physiology, Massachusetts Eye and Ear Infirmary.

[1] Presently at Washington University School of Medicine, Dept. of Pharmacology, St. Louis, Missouri

[2] Presently at University College London, Dept. of Biophysics, London

[3] Presently at Harvard Medical School, Dept. of Pathology, Boston, Massachusetts

at these levels of the auditory system. It appears that the main characteristics of the system at these levels are very similar for most mammals with the possible exception of animals with special abilities such as echolocation. The cat was chosen as the experimental animal, because descriptions of the anatomy are more available than for other species.

The scope of this report is indicated roughly by Fig. 1, which summarizes some of the known relationships between nuclei and fiber tracts in the auditory parts of the caudal brain stem of the cat (Ramón y Cajal, 1909, Lorente de Nó, 1933, Stotler, 1953, Rasmussen, 1960, 1964, 1967, Warr, 1966, 1969, 1972, Morest, 1968, van Noort, 1969, Osen, 1970, 1972, Cohen, 1972, Cohen et al., 1972). This simplified diagram ignores a number of unresolved complications that do not appear to be crucial for the immediate issues. For instance, the auditory nerve is represented by a single channel, because the possible existence of auditory-nerve fibers with different peripheral innervation patterns is not critical here (Lorente de Nó, 1937, Polyak et al., 1946, Spoendlin, 1972).

On entering the brain stem, each auditory-nerve fiber bifurcates into an ascending branch that projects to the anteroventral cochlear nucleus (AVCN) and a descending branch that projects to the posteroventral cochlear nucleus (PVCN) and dorsal cochlear nucleus (DCN). In addition, there are cells in the interstitial region of the nerve that receive endings from the auditory-nerve fibers either before or just after their bifurcations. Thus the auditory nerve projects to many groups of cells in the CN in parallel. The general response characteristics of auditory-nerve units in cats have been described (Kiang et al., 1965b). If the nerve signals, recorded in the internal auditory canal, are transmitted faithfully to the terminals, the specification of response characteristics of the postsynaptic cells (Kiang, 1968) would give input-output relations for these cells. Knowledge of the projections of these cells in the CN to other regions would then facilitate the detailed physiological study of signal transmission at the next level.

The idea of signal transmission in the nervous system implies activity transmitted in specific sequences by interrelated cells. A wiring diagram, such as Fig. 1, shows only that connections are known to exist for certain regions. Since most regions contain more than one type of cell, the idea of tracing signals through pathways is feasible in only a few special cases at this time. A brief review of some of the relevant anatomical features of certain regions in the cat will serve to indicate why those regions were chosen for discussion here. In this paper, the name of a region may sometimes be used to identify the location of specific units. In these situations it should be clear that there is no implication that all units in that region behave similarly.

The anteroventral cochlear nucleus (AVCN) of cats contains cells that project to the ipsilateral lateral superior olive (LSO) and the medial superior olive (MSO) of both sides (Warr, 1966). Probably at least some of these cells, particularly in the rostral pole of the AVCN, receive large endings (endbulbs of Held) from the AN (Ramón y Cajal, 1909, Lorente de Nó, 1933, Lenn and Reese, 1966).

The region of the interstitial nucleus (IN) contains cells that project via the trapezoid body (TB) to the medial nucleus of the trapezoid body (MNTB) of the contralateral side (Warr, 1972). These cells receive many small endings from the AN, but their projections in the MNTB terminate in very large endings, the calyces of Held (Held, 1893, Ramón y Cajal, 1909, Morest, 1968). The posterior part of AVCN (PAVCN) and the anterior part of PVCN (APVCN) contain a mixture of cell types, the projections of which are not yet completely defined.

The PPVCN contains large cells that Osen (1969) called octopus cells. These cells project via the intermediate acoustic stria (IAS) to the dorsomedial periolivary nucleus (DMPO) and the dorsolateral periolivary nucleus (DLPO) (Warr, 1969). The DMPO and the DLPO are especially interesting, in that the cells of origin of the olivocochlear bundles are located in or around these regions (Fig. 1).

The anatomy of the DCN is extremely complex (Ramón y Cajal, 1909, Lorente de Nó, 1933, Osen, 1969, Cohen, 1972). At least one group of cells, called the fusiform cells, receives endings from the auditory nerve

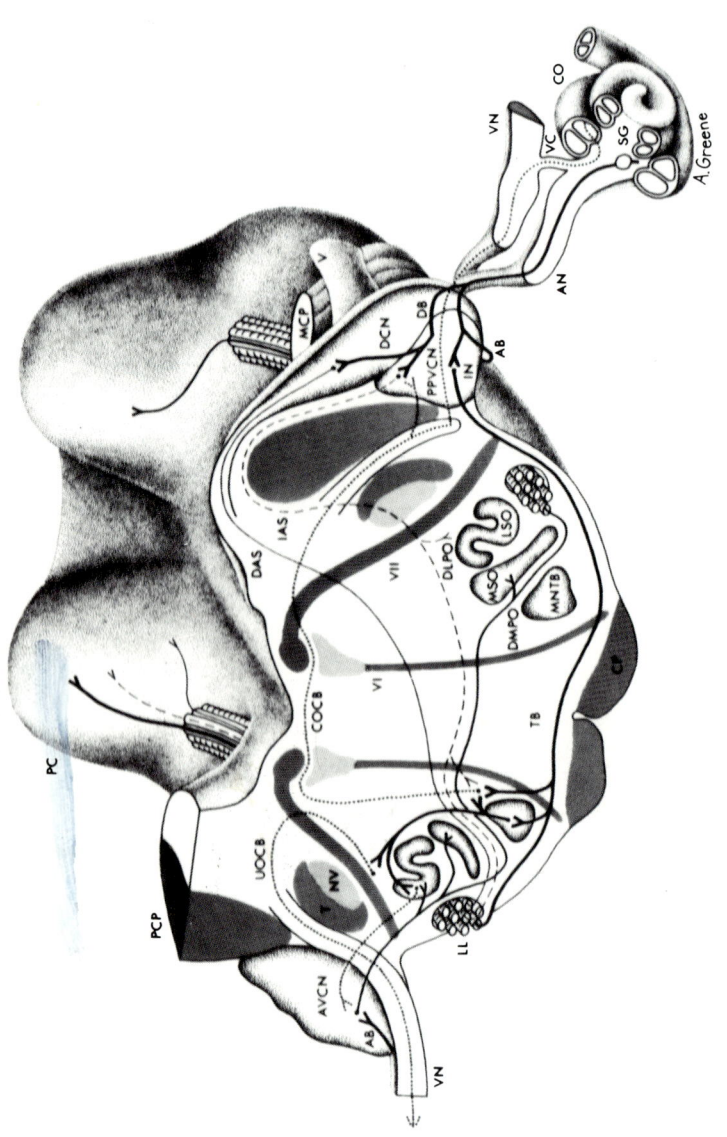

Fig. 1

Fig. 1 Schematic representation of the principal auditory nuclei and pathways of the cat treated in the present papers. List of abbreviations of anatomic terms used in the text and figures follows:

AB	ascending branch of AN	MNTB	medial nucleus of TB
AN	auditory nerve	MSO	medial superior olivary nucleus
APVCN	anterior part of PVCN	NV	(see TNV)
AVCN	anteroventral CN	PAVCN	posterior part of AVCN
CN	cochlear nucleus	PC	posterior colliculus
CO	cochlea	PCP	posterior cerebellar peduncle
COCB	crossed olivocochlear bundle	PPVCN	posterior part of PVCN
CP	cerebral peduncle	PVCN	posteroventral CN
DAS	dorsal acoustic stria	SG	spiral ganglion
DB	descending branch of AN	SOC	superior olivary complex
DCN	dorsal CN	TB	trapezoid body
DLPO	dorsolateral periolivary nucleus	TNV	descending tract and nucleus of V
DMPO	dorsomedial periolivary nucleus		
IAS	intermediate acoustic stria	UOCB	uncrossed olivocochlear bundle
IN	interstitial CN	VC	vestibulo-cochlear anastomosis (Oort)
LL	lateral lemniscus		
LSO	lateral superior olivary nucleus	VCN	ventral cochlear nucleus
MCP	middle cerebellar peduncle	VN	vestibular nerve
		V	trigeminal nerve
		VI	abducens nerve root and nucleus
		VII	facial nerve root

(Cohen et al., 1972) and sends projections via the DAS that bypass the SOC to reach the pons and midbrain (van Noort, 1969, Osen, 1972). Also receiving AN projections are many intrinsic neurons with axons that form a complicated pattern of connections within the DCN without projecting from the CN (Cohen, 1972, Cohen et al., 1972). It should always be remembered that throughout much of the CN are cells, including intrinsic neurons, the morphology and projections of which remain to be clarified.

2. Methods

For the physiological experiments, adult cats were anesthetized by intraperitoneal injections of sodium pentobarbital (37 mg/kg) or diallyl barbituric acid in urethane solution (75 mg/kg). After the appropriate surgical exposure, each animal was placed in a "sound-proofed," vibration-isolated, electrically-shielded chamber. A closed acoustic system (Kiang et al., 1965b) with a 1" Brüel & Kjaer microphone as a sound source was sealed into one or both external auditory canals. Stimulus levels in this paper are expressed in sound-pressure levels after correcting for the properties of the acoustic system. The electrodes, used in recording activity from fiber tracts, were micropipets, filled with 2M KCl. The electrodes, used in recording from nuclei, were indium-filled pipets with platinum tips (Dowben and Rose, 1953, Kiang, 1965); the metal electrodes showed less tendency to record from fibers than the fluid-filled micropipets. Electrophysiological data were processed by computers either during the experiments or from taped recordings. Localization of electrodes required histological reconstruction of electrode tracks. In critical cases locations were more closely specified by placing a radiofrequency lesion at the site of recording. An atlas of the nuclear boundaries was prepared from series of Nissl- and Protargol-stained sections, cut in the three standard planes. In the case of the cochlear nucleus a block model (with blocks 80 µm to a side) was generated and the location of units denoted by block numbers. The locations of superior olivary units were plotted on atlas sections. More detailed accounts of methods and results appear elsewhere (Godfrey, 1971, Guinan et al., 1972a, 1972b).

3. Results

Of the myriad response characteristics that can be used to describe the behavior of single units, three will be discussed here. These are latency, frequency selectivity, and time pattern of responses to short tone bursts.

3.1 Latencies of responses to clicks

A basic characteristic of most systems is the time taken for a response to occur following a stimulus. The time of occurrence of the stimulus is most sharply defined for an impulsive stimulus such as a click. Fig. 2 shows latencies of responses to standard clicks for auditory-nerve fibers and single units in certain parts of the cochlear nucleus and superior olivary complex. With a few exceptions, single units at the medullary level respond to clicks, although units with very high characteristic frequency (CF) might not respond to the clicks, unless the stimulus level were increased. In the cochlear nucleus, the shortest latencies are found in the ventral cochlear nucleus (VCN), and the longest latencies in the dorsal cochlear nucleus (DCN). In Fig. 2 only data for certain units in each region were used. For instance, the AVCN units are restricted to those with a complex waveform that has a positive component, appearing approximately 0.5 msec before a negative spike (Kiang et al., 1965a, Pfeiffer, 1966a). Within the cochlear nucleus this complex waveform is seen only in the AVCN and tends to become more common in the rostral part of the AVCN. Other units in the AVCN, not associated with complex waveforms, have a greater range of latencies and are not represented in Fig. 2. Some of these other units in the AVCN exhibit a particular time pattern of response (chopper pattern) to tone bursts, and still others have a prominent peak at the onset of the tone bursts. These same patterns are seen in the APVCN. The APVCN units in this paper show "chopper" patterns in response to tone bursts. IN units and PPVCN units have been selected to represent the preponderant type of unit in these regions. The DCN units selected were localized in the fusiform-cell layer. A greater range of latencies would be represented if data for units in the deep DCN were included.

The latency of responses in the SOC is shortest in the MNTB, where the units respond only to stimulation

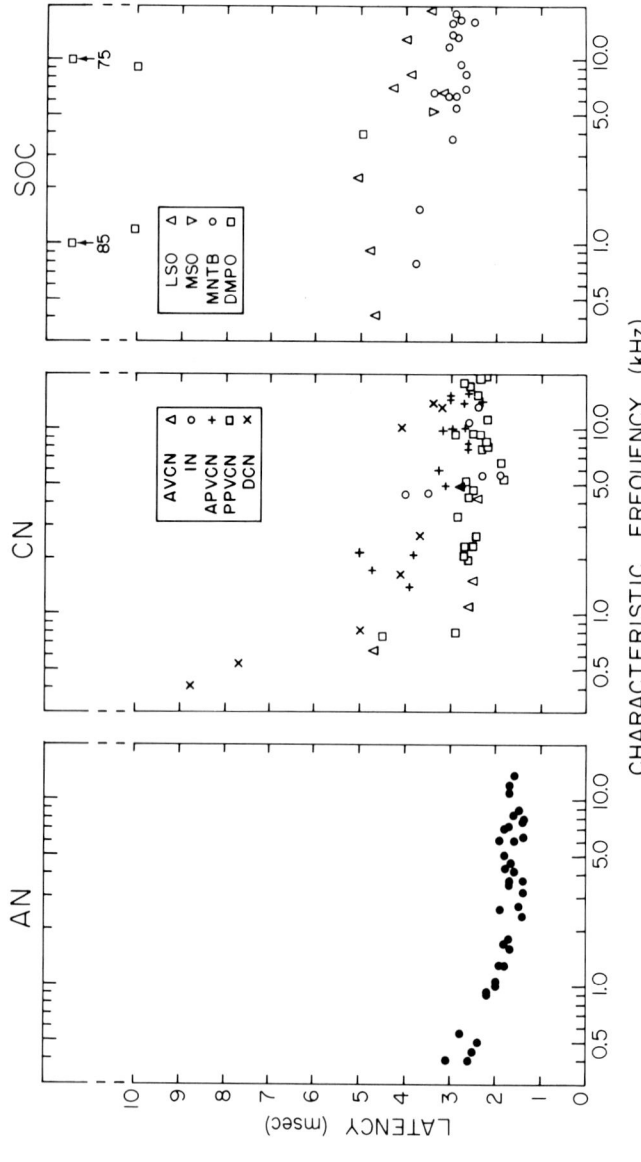

Fig. 2

Fig. 2 Latency of responses to clicks for single units at three levels of the auditory nervous system:

Auditory Nerve (AN), Cochlear Nucleus (CN), and the Superior Olivary Complex (SOC).

Rarefaction clicks were used in the AN and CN units. Condensation clicks were used in the SOC units. This difference would be unimportant at high frequency but might be significant for the lower frequencies (< 2 kHz). The repetition rate was 10/sec except in the DMPO units, where it was 2-5/sec, because the units would not respond to 10/sec clicks. Each point represents the latency of the first peak in a poststimulus time (PST) histogram. Zero time is the time at which a 100-μsec electric pulse is delivered to the earphone. Acoustic travel time from the earphone to the tympanic membrane with this sound system is less than 0.1 msec. In all except a few instances, the pulse was -50 dB re 100 V into the earphone; the click level was approximately 1 μbar peak at the tympanic membrane. In the few exceptional instances the level was 5-10 dB lower. Since latency of responses in auditory units is a function of characteristic frequency (CF), the latency of each unit is plotted versus its CF. The different symbols in the plots for CN and SOC units indicate the anatomical locations that are specified by the abbreviations in the insets. The auditory-nerve units were in a single animal; the other units were taken from many different animals. Note that two units in the DMPO had such long latencies (85 and 75 msec) that they could not be accommodated by the chosen vertical scale without a break in the vertical axis.

of the contralateral ear. These units are almost all associated with complex waveforms (similar to those found in the AVCN) and are found nowhere else in the SOC. Many SOC units are binaural, in the sense that responses are elicited by stimuli to either ear and the responses cannot be attributed to acoustic cross-talk. Data are virtually unavailable for the MSO, not only because of the paucity of units recorded there with present techniques, but also because the gross field potential is large in response to clicks and tends to obscure the unit responses. The responses of LSO units are for ipsilateral stimulation, since the effect of contralateral stimulation is to inhibit activity. The latency of responses of units in the DMPO shows a very broad range, including some of the longest latencies yet recorded in the SOC. In general, the latencies of click responses show considerable overlap for CN and SOC units.

3.2 Tuning curves

A second response characteristic is frequency selectivity. Typical tuning curves for single units at three levels of the system are shown in Fig. 3. Here the intention is to show the tuning curves in a context that indicates possible lines of signal transmission. Auditory-nerve activity is presumably the exclusive peripheral input to the cochlear nucleus. The tuning curves of AN units are sharp and show a single characteristic frequency, or CF, at which the unit is most sensitive to tonal stimuli. The cells in the ACVN all show sharp tuning curves. Unit PH 19-9, the tuning curve of which is shown in Fig. 3, had responses with complex waveforms and presumably represents a cell that receives large endings from the AN. The AVCN is known to send projections to the ipsilateral LSO and to the MSO of both sides. The tuning curves in the LSO have been studied extensively by Boudreau and Tsuchitani (1970) and need not be described in detail here. The LSO appears to be represented predominantly by units with high CF, whereas the MSO appears to be represented predominantly by units with low CF (Guinan et al., 1972b). Both regions contain units with sharp tuning curves that do not differ greatly from those of AN or AVCN units. If Osen (1970) is correct in stating that the cells in the rostral pole of the AVCN receive mainly AN fibers from the more apical turns of the cochlea, then there could be a separation of AVCN units into those that project to LSO and those that project to MSO with perhaps some overlap. However, the structure of this region has not been fully analyzed, and one should proceed with some care in attempting to force correlations solely on the basis of presently available descriptions.

Units in the interstitial region of the CN (IN) have tuning curves that resemble those of AN units. Since the projections of cells in the region of the IN form the large endings in the MNTB, it is not entirely surprising that the tuning curves for units in the MNTB with complex waveforms are like those of primary units in the AN. However, the MNTB also contains other units that characteristically respond to the turning off of a tone. Some of these units also respond during the presence of a tone, but this response is represented by a separate tuning curve (dotted curve in Fig. 3).

Sharp tuning curves are found for all units in the PAVCN and the APVCN. The particular example chosen here was for a unit with a "chopper" pattern in response to short tone bursts (Fig. 4).

The PPVCN contains many units that have broad tuning curves, sometimes with a very sharp tip. These units usually respond best to the onset of stimuli, but they will respond in a phase-locked manner to individual cycles of low-frequency stimuli. The frequency range, where the "on" pattern and the phase-locked pattern merge, is usually marked by an indentation of the tuning curve (near 4 kHz for unit 54-24). One of the few places where broad tuning curves are found in the CN is the PPVCN, in the region of the octopus cells. Broad tuning curves are also found in the DMPO, the region of the SOC to which the octopus cells of the PPVCN are said to project.

The tuning curves of units in the DCN fusiform-cell layer resemble those of AN units. Some of the units in the deep DCN may show somewhat broader tuning curves, but the response patterns change drastically in different frequency ranges. Some units respond only by showing a decrease in discharge rate.

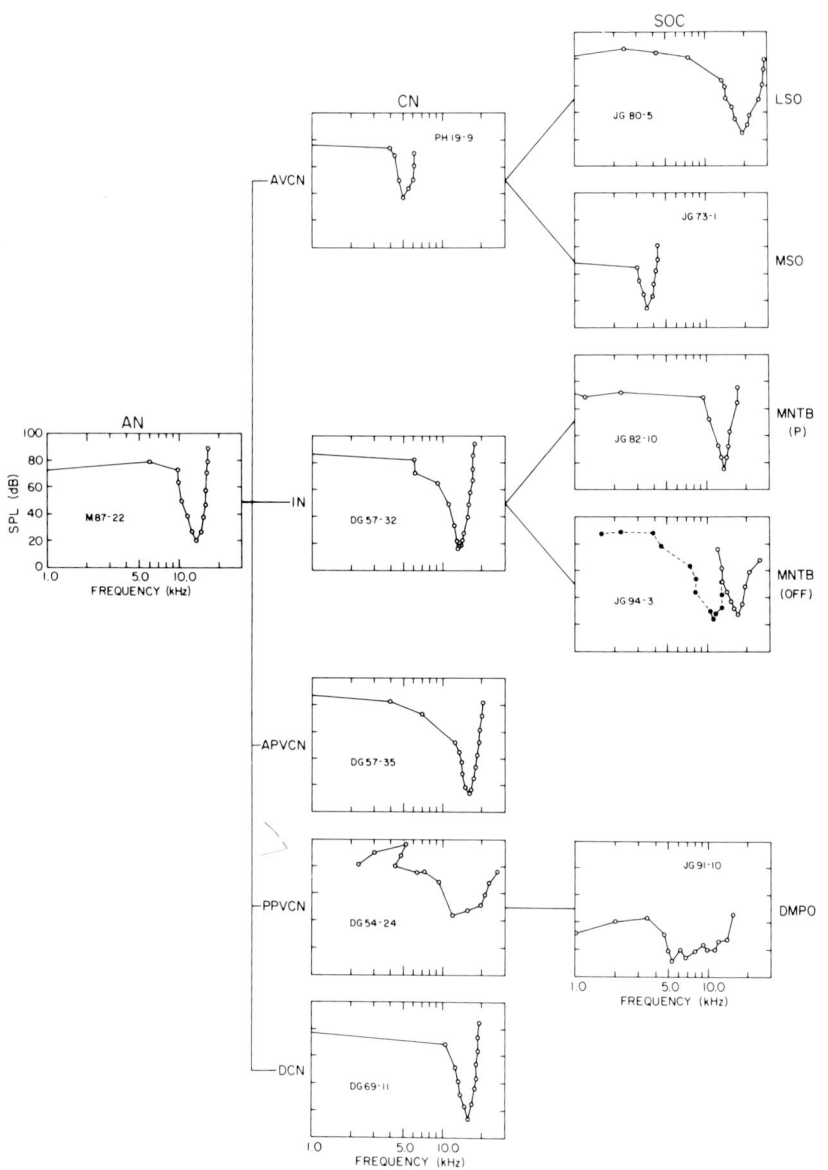

Fig. 3 Tuning curves for single units at three levels of the auditory nervous system (AN, CN, and SOC). Abbreviations for locations are as in Fig. 2. Each column of graphs represents units found at one of the three levels. The lines, cross-connecting columns, represent the existence of demonstrated anatomical projections between the regions indicated (see Fig. 1). Each point on a tuning curve repre-

(Fig. 3 cont'd) sents the "threshold" level for responses to short tone bursts at that frequency. The data points are connected by straight lines. A line, interrupted by the vertical axis, indicates that a data point exists for a lower frequency. The vertical scale is in sound-pressure level re 0.0002 dynes/cm^2 and is the same for all graphs. Note that the MNTB is represented by two units. The graph labeled "P" represents a unit with complex waveshape that had a response pattern resembling that of units in the AN. The graph labeled "OFF" represents a unit that responded when the tone burst was turned off (see Fig. 4). The identifying code, supplied for each graph, gives the experimental series, the cat number, and the unit number. The rate of spontaneous discharge in spikes per second is given in parentheses for each unit: M 87-22 (66.4), PH 19-9 (83.4), DG 57-32 (78.4), DG 57-35 (92.5), DG 54-24 (0.0), DG 69-11 (44.6), JG 80-5 (0.0), JG 73-1 (not available), JG 82-10 (not available), JG 94-3 (0.0), and JG 91-10 (not available).

3.3 Time patterns of responses to short tone bursts

The most useful single criterion thus far defined for classifying units is the appearance of the post-stimulus time (PST) histogram for short (25-msec) tone-burst stimuli at the CF (STBCF) (Kiang et al., 1965b, Pfeiffer, 1966b). Fig. 4 shows such histograms for selected units.

The response patterns of all auditory-nerve fibers are essentially the same. There is a sharp increase in response rate, when the tone is turned on. After reaching a peak, there is a gradual decrease to a sustained level. After the tone is turned off, there is a sharp decrease below the level of spontaneous activity, followed by a gradual increase to the spontaneous rate. For low-frequency stimuli there is time-locking to individual cycles of the tone. The response pattern of units with complex waveforms in the AVCN (PH 19-9 in Fig. 4, for example) is almost indistinguishable from that of AN units. The PST histograms of units in the LSO to ipsilateral stimula-

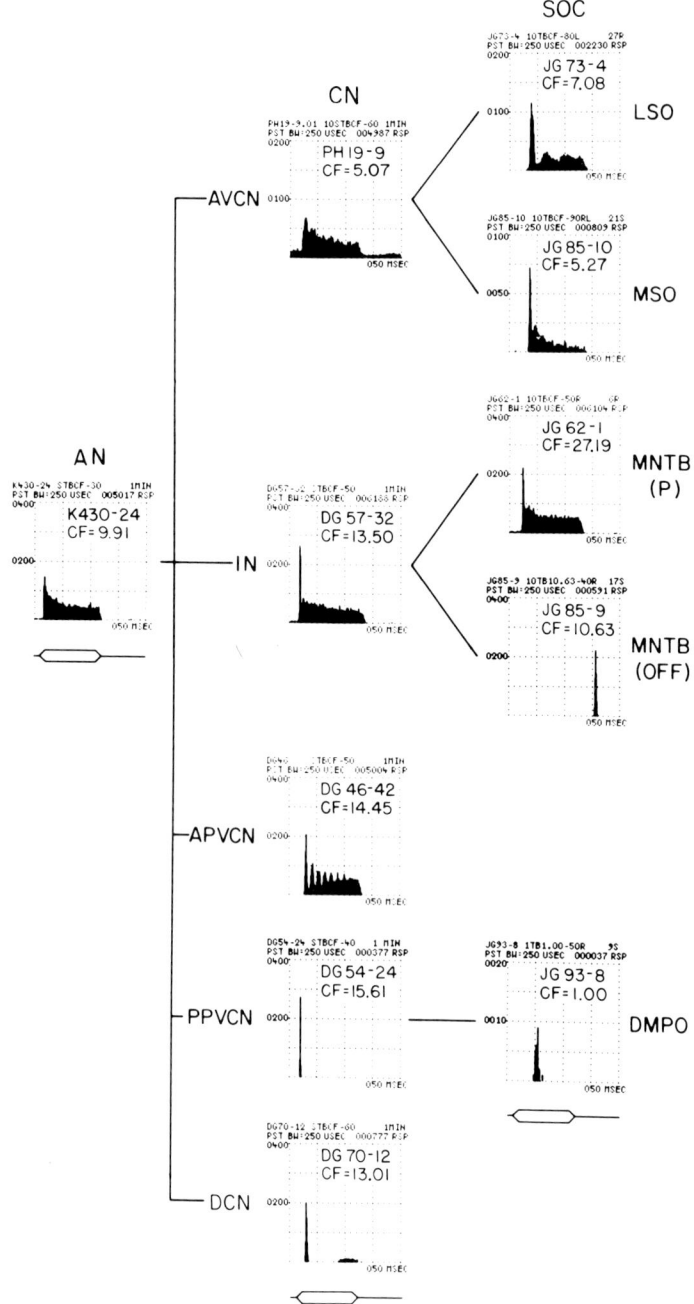

Fig. 4 Time patterns of response to short tone bursts at the CF (STBCF) for units at three levels of the auditory nervous system (AN, CN and SOC). The organization of this figure is as in Fig. 3, except that the PST histo-

(Fig. 4 cont'd) grams are presented instead of tuning curves. The histograms have time (50 msec full scale) as the abscissa, and number of spikes as the ordinate. All histograms shown in this paper have 200 bins and are based on one-minute samples of data. The symbol at the base of each column of histograms in this figure shows the envelope of the stimulus waveform (25-msec duration tone burst with a 2.5-msec rise-fall time). Zero time in each histogram is 2.5 msec before the onset of the electric signal to the earphone. The insets within each histogram give the identifying code for the unit (see Fig. 3) and the "uncorrected" CF of the unit, as obtained during the experiment. This CF can be "corrected" by considering the properties of the acoustic system and the middle ear (Kiang et al., 1967). The stimulus level in dB SPL for each unit is: K 430-24, 100; PH 19-9, 44; DG 57-32, 54; DG 46-42, 63; DG 54-24, 63; DG 70-12, 35; JG 73-4, 35; JG 85-10, 22 (both ears); JG 62-1, 53; JG 85-9, 66; JG 93-8, 69.

tion show a sharp initial peak, followed by an undulating pattern that resembles some "chopper" units in the cochlear nucleus. Most units in the MSO are excited by stimulation to both ears; the patterns seen in the few PST histograms available resemble the patterns for AN units, except that the initial peak is more prominent and is followed by a notch or dip in the histogram. This latter pattern is also found for many AVCN and IN units that do not have complex waveforms, and for MNTB units with complex waveforms. This pattern is seen more clearly on an expanded time scale in Fig. 5. Many of the cells in the AVCN and IN receive numerous terminal boutons from the AN. One effect of convergence of many AN endings on a single cell could be to increase the probability of response to the onset of the tone to the point that the refractory periods of the units become noticeable as a notch. This notch usually lasts less than 2 msec and can thus be distinguished from the "pause" pattern.

The response patterns of many units in regions near the IN (the posterior part of the AVCN and the an-

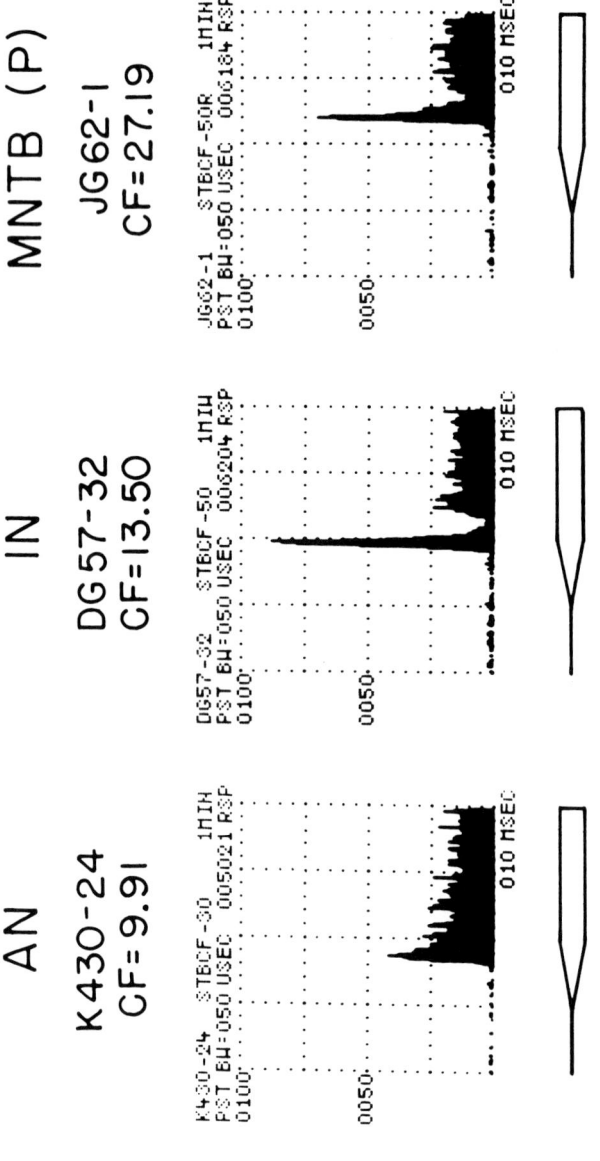

Fig. 5 Three of the histograms of Fig. 4, displayed on a total time base of 10 msec, to show the presence of a notch or dip after the initial peak in the response of the units in the IN and MNTB.

terior part of the PVCN) and in the DCN show patterns characterized by a series of peaks ("chopper" pattern). The envelopes of these histograms resemble those of AN units. At the level of the SOC, such "chopper" patterns are found, predominantly for units in the DLPO and possibly in the LSO, where a weak "chopper" pattern is observed. Perhaps there is a functional connection between these locations but the patterns could just as well be independently generated. For this reason, a sample of the patterns seen in the CN is shown in Fig. 4 without a corresponding pattern in the SOC (see Fig. 6 for response patterns of a unit in the DPLO).

The predominant pattern seen in the posterior part of the PVCN is a single sharp peak in response to the onset of the tone. Following this peak there is a low level or no response, as long as the tone is left on. In the octopus-cell region, which occupies most of the PPVCN, the units almost all show such "on" patterns. Although some "on" patterns are seen in other parts of the CN, "on" patterns with no activity following the single initial peak are not seen for units outside the PPVCN. Although data are sparse for the DPMO, it is one of the few places in the SOC, where "on" response patterns have been seen. The response patterns of units in the present sample of the DMPO and the DLPO are so different from those described by Fex (1962, 1965) for the olivocochlear bundle, that one must entertain doubts that the present units correspond to the cells of origin for the efferent fibers to the cochlea.

The PST histograms for activity of units in the fusiform-cell layer of DCN almost all show either a "pauser" or a "buildup" pattern. A "pauser" pattern has a single initial peak at the onset, followed by a pause, lasting longer than the notch seen in Fig. 5, followed by resumption of activity. A "buildup" pattern resembles "pauser" patterns but without the initial peak. The "pauser" and "buildup" patterns have not been seen for SOC units in the present study. This is an especially significant point, since the DAS fibers from the DCN are thought to bypass the SOC (Fig. 1). Units with pauser patterns have been reported to be in the LSO by Clark and Dunlop (1969), but the evidence is not entirely convincing. As shown in Fig. 6, a unit in the superior olivary complex

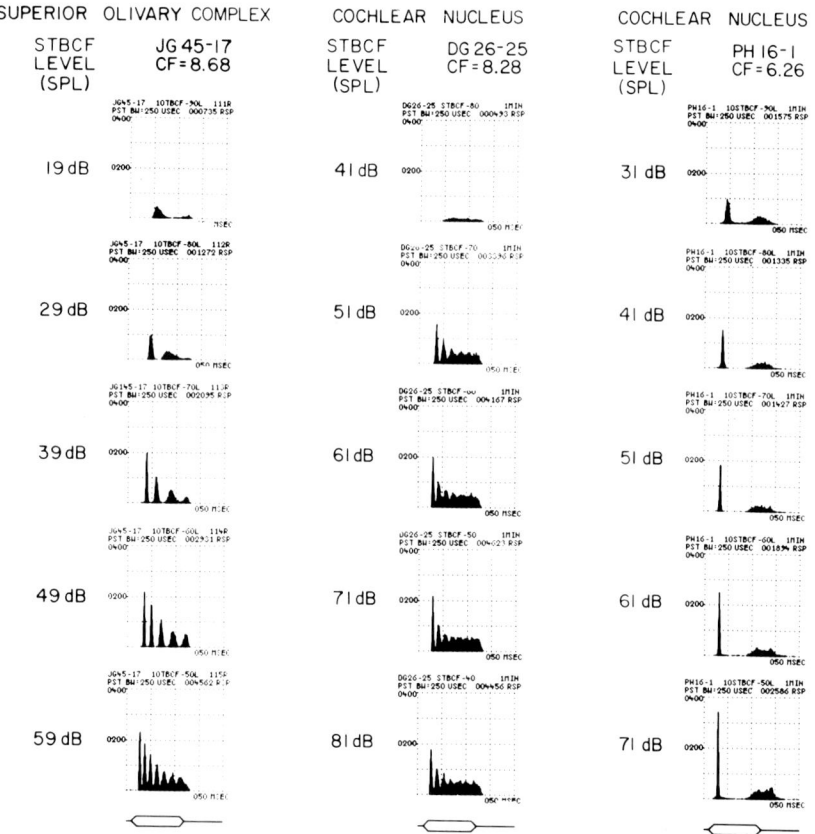

Fig. 6 Response patterns of three single units to STBCF as a function of stimulus level. Unit JG 45-17 (left column) was located in the dorsolateral periolivary nucleus (DLPO). Unit DG 26-25 (middle column) was located in the anterior PVCN. Unit PH 16-1 (right column) was located in the DCN. The envelope of the stimulus waveform is shown at the bottom of each column. The rate of spontaneous discharge was zero for unit DG 26-25, 1 spike per sec for PH 16-1, and fluctuated between zero and a few spikes/sec for unit JG 45-17.

(DLPO) can have a PST histogram that resembles a "pauser" pattern at low stimulus levels. However, as the stimulus level is increased, the pattern becomes clearly a "chopper" pattern. Since the period of chopping for the lowest stimulus levels is so long that only two peaks are present for a 25-msec tone burst, the unit does not show the typical behavior of a "pauser" type unit. Fig. 6 also shows response patterns of two units from the cochlear nucleus for comparison. The unit (DG 26-25) from the APVCN was a typical "chopper" type, while the unit (PH 16-1) from the DCN was a typical "pauser" type. Clearly a single histogram is insufficient to distinguish "chopper" units from "pauser" units. A series of histograms for many stimulus levels provides a better basis for classification.

The observation that "pauser" units are not found in the SOC raises the issue of whether the activity of "pauser" units in the DCN might fail to be relayed out of the cochlear nucleus. A similar question could be asked of each type of activity seen in the nucleus. Fig. 7 shows sample histograms of the responses recorded in the three major fiber output tracts of the CN in some preliminary experiments. Out of 10 units presumed to be fibers in the DAS, seven had "pauser" patterns, two had "buildup" patterns, and one had a "chopper" pattern, in response to short tone bursts. As the recording micropipet passed into the region where the fibers of the IAS are presumably located, the patterns of activity encountered were almost all "on" in character. Out of 45 fibers encountered in this region, 28 responded to acoustic stimuli with a large initial peak at the onset of a short tone- or noise-burst. This peak was followed by no activity or a very low, steady level of activity. These patterns are the predominant ones found in the octopus-cell region of the PPVCN. The remaining units in the IAS region either did not respond to acoustic stimuli or were not classifiable with the data obtained. Fibers from the restiform body and elsewhere also travel in this region and might account for these remaining units. The trapezoid body is so large a tract that no adequate sample of unit activity is available. A few recordings with micropipets have been made in the lateral trapezoid body, where most of the fibers from the VCN presumably course. Activity of some of the fibers (perhaps the large fibers) appears to be recordable with the platinum-indium electrodes, used also in the SOC. With either type of electrode, many units with response patterns resembling those of units in the AN or the IN have been found, but not units with "chopper" patterns. As mentioned before,

Fig. 7

Response patterns of single units in the fiber output tracts of the cochlear nucleus. The recordings were made by inserting fluid-filled micropipets into the dorsal acoustic stria (DAS), the intermediate acoustic stria (IAS), or the lateral part of the trapezoid body (TB). As shown at the bottom of the figure, the stimuli were short tone bursts at the CF (STBCF). In all three cases the stimulus was at least 30 dB above the unit's threshold at CF.

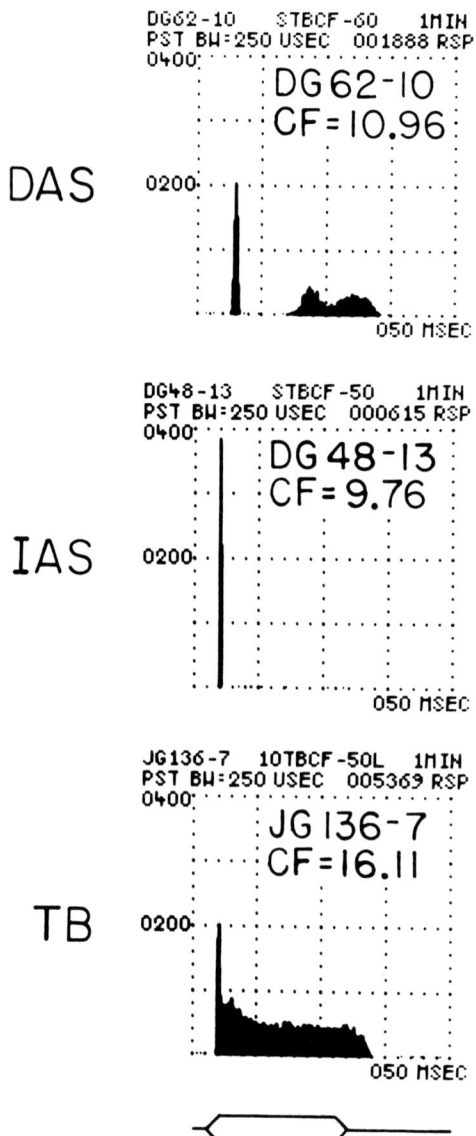

the only places in the SOC, where "chopper" patterns were seen, are the DLPO and possibly the LSO. It is not known whether these "chopper" patterns are generated locally in the SOC or whether they reflect "chopper" patterns of activity relayed from the CN.

4. Discussion

The present study shows that anatomical "wiring" diagrams, such as Fig. 1, can be useful in organizing data on response characteristics of single cells. However, representation of the tuning curves and time patterns of auditory units in the apparent form of a wiring diagram in Figs. 3 and 4 must not be misconstrued. It is not yet possible to relate types of units in a given part of the cochlear nucleus to particular units in the superior olivary complex. Nor is it possible to state which types of neurons participate in a particular pathway, since most nuclear regions contain a variety of cells. Present techniques do not permit routine physiological studies on the input-output functions of a particular cell in the mammalian brain. A possible exception occurs in the case of units with complex waveforms. These units are located only in regions where large endings are found. In the auditory system, two such regions are the AVCN with the end-bulbs of Held and the MNTB with the calyces of Held. Here the indications favor the interpretation of one component of the response as being presynaptic in origin and another component as being postsynaptic. However, it is not yet possible to relate the presynaptic component to a particular cell of origin in the preceding stage of the system. In some invertebrate preparations it is feasible to record from individually identified neurons that are synaptically linked (Gardner and Kandel, 1972). In mammals, many cells have consistently recognizable morphological characteristics, including their connections. Consequently, one can treat particular single units as representatives of specific groups of well defined cells.

If one chooses to adopt this approach, one soon encounters conceptual difficulties in classifying units. The physiologist could occupy himself endlessly with the accumulation of case histories for individual units. The burden of organizing these data can become overwhelming.

Other disciplines, such as anatomy or psychology, can help by providing an independent set of organizing principles. The introduction of anatomical considerations permits interesting new formulations of data. For example, the following statements are now possible: "on" units with no background activity are found only in the octopus-cell region of the PPVCN; units in the fusiform-cell layer of the DCN almost all show "pauser" or "buildup" patterns; or, "pauser" units are not obtained in data from the SOC. Such classifications of response patterns must have significance beyond being merely descriptive labels. In paper II (Patterns of Synaptic Organization), the morphology of selected regions will be examined more closely with this point in mind.

Because of the paucity of reliable physiological data that permit comparison of single unit responses at different levels of the system, it would be advantageous to pool results from many different laboratories. Attempts to do so are frequently frustrated by the variety of methods, criteria, and standards. Serious problems often occur in connection with species, anesthesia, stimulus control, choice of recording electrodes, and procedures for classifying units.

With the present limited comparative data it is not possible to assess with confidence the generality of the results for different species. Similarly, anesthesia is important in most central nervous system work, but no means for comparing results obtained under different states has yet proved satisfactory.

It is axiomatic that a signal-transmission approach requires careful specification of the stimulus. Effects of extraneous sounds, such as background acoustic noise, switching transients, harmonics, and acoustic cross-talk are widely recognized but still appear inadvertently from time to time. For instance, few workers have paid sufficient attention to acoustic cross-talk in binaural experiments, where one seldom sees calibration for cross-talk as a function of frequency. Even in monaural work, deficiencies in stimulus control can lead to faulty conclusions on major issues (e.g. see Katsuki et al., 1962, Kiang et al., 1967, Price, 1972, Weiss and Peake, 1973).

No less important for a signal-transmission approach is the ability to define the part of the system from which responses are recorded. In practice, the procedure is to establish the location of the electrode tip. The locations, established in this way, are imprecise with regard to specific cells, except perhaps in intracellular recordings, combined with dye injection (Caspary, 1971). Recording the extracellular potentials with large microelectrodes could conceivably give spurious unit locations, if the fields were extensive. However, the use of micropipets and sharpened wires as electrodes presents an even more serious problem. Such electrodes can record activity of incoming fibers, outgoing fibers, or fibers of passage, as well as cell bodies and dendrites. For example, the electrode tip could be in the MSO but record a fiber, projecting from somewhere else. The electrode may be recording the activity of single units in the MSO, but such results could lead to confusion over the conceptual stages at which signal processing takes place. For this reason, interpretations, based on such data (Katsuki et al., 1958, Moushegian et al., 1964, Clark and Dunlop, 1969, Caspary, 1971), should be examined cautiously. Actually it is desirable to use many different kinds of electrodes, in order to check whether a particular type of electrode has an unusual bias in the recording situation. However, lack of appreciation of how different types of electrodes sample activity has understandably generated misinterpretations.

While it is always useful, and frequently a boon, to have a physiological criterion for electrode location (Rose, 1960), many criteria (Hall, 1965, Rupert et al., 1968) are not so firmly established as to remove the need for careful histological verification of electrode locations.

Perhaps a more subtle type of methodological pitfall lies in the procedure for classifying units. An example was given in the results to show how a single histogram is, in general, insufficient for classification by the scheme used here. Because this scheme has been stated only qualitatively, some misunderstandings have arisen. For example, a study, based on marked cells in the cochlear nucleus, contains several statements that apparently contradict some of the present findings but which appear to be based on different usage of the terms for classification (Caspary, 1971).

There is no attempt in this paper to speculate on the functional significance of the findings. The present state of our knowledge of central mechanisms is far too sketchy to permit any but the most obvious conclusions. Much current interest has been focused on correlating binaural effects in single unit recordings with behavioral functions, but this seems to be based on as much guesswork as evidence. The introduction of behavioral considerations certainly places new perspectives on both the morphological and physiological studies, but how effective psychology can be in organizing the present data can only be answered by the test of time.

"Feature detection" in single units has become a popular concept in recent years. At first sight this seems to provide a useful way for behavioral work to interact with physiology. However, it seems questionable whether a specific function can be isolated and defined for a single unit without reference to the framework in which the unit operates. For example, what purpose would be served by identifying an "on" unit in the DMPO as a detector of stimulus onsets, if the inputs to these units from the PPVCN already showed an "on" pattern? Or what sense would it make to identify an "on" unit in the PPVCN as a detector of stimulus onsets, if the units to which it projects showed a different pattern on the next level? One cannot answer these questions in the absence of systematic analyses of the response characteristics and synaptic organization at each stage of the system. One could argue that a bold plunge into unknown territory could result in new ways of thinking about the system. Ideally this approach can provide clues for further, more systematic work. However, such an approach should not disguise poorly executed experiments, inadequate sampling, or superficial thinking. While there is little question that the game of assigning roles for specific cells, nuclei, and pathways is a fascinating one, good science, systematically pursued, can be as stimulating as the most ingenious speculations.

Acknowledgments and references: entered collectively at the end of paper II (Morest et al.)

STIMULUS CODING AT CAUDAL LEVELS OF THE CAT'S
AUDITORY NERVOUS SYSTEM: II. PATTERNS
OF SYNAPTIC ORGANIZATION

D.K. Morest
N.Y.S. Kiang
E.C. Kane
J.J. Guinan, Jr.
D.A. Godfrey

1. Introduction

The physiological results demonstrate that changes occur in neural signals between the auditory nerve and more central locations in the auditory system. While wiring diagrams can help to elucidate the paths of signal transmission, they are insufficient to clarify the mechanisms by which the signals are modified. To examine this question, one needs to know in detail the nature of the relationships between the pre- and postsynaptic cells. The distinct morphological arrangements of the afferent axons and of the neuronal structures, contacted by the synaptic endings, impose certain constraints on the activity of the neurons, involved in signal transmission. Some structural features would tend to preserve the original signal patterns, others to transform them. Certain morphological data give promise of some insights into the mechanisms, involved in stimulus coding in the auditory system. The geometrical aspects of the morphological basis for tonotopic organization in the auditory system have been treated elsewhere (Morest, 1965a, 1968).

2. Methods

The morphological results in this paper have been based on Nissl and reduced silver techniques, Golgi methods, electron microscopy, and experimental degeneration methods (Morest, 1965b, 1968, 1971, Morest and Morest, 1966, Cohen, 1972).

3. Results

<u>In the region of ACVN and IN</u> several types of neurons have been recognized in rapid Golgi preparations from the cat. Two of the principal types are the bushy cell and the stellate cell. These cells are quite different with respect to the major morphological and geometrical features that provide for their synaptic organization (see description of Fig. 1). These cell types are not taken into account in the available parcellations and descriptions of the cochlear nucleus with the traditional cytoarchitectonic approach, using Nissl and Protargol stains (e.g. Osen, 1969, Harrison and Feldman, 1970). For example, it is not clear whether the spherical cells, multipolar cells, or globular cells (Osen, 1969) correspond to either bushy cells or stellate cells, or to a combination of both. It does not seem safe to assume that parcellations, resulting from the cytoarchitectonic approach, necessarily provide a useful frame of reference for studies of neural connections and functions. An example of this danger occurs in studies of the neuronal architecture of the medial geniculate body, where a strict adherence to the tenets of Nissl-body cytoarchitectonics has limited the meaningful correlation of structural and physiological data (Morest, 1964).

Although some information on the connections of the AVCN and IN region in the cat is available (Warr, 1966, van Noort, 1969), it is not certain which types of neurons give rise to these projections. It seems probable that the units, exhibiting complex waveforms, short latencies, narrow tuning curves, and time-patterns similar to those of AN units, would correspond to cells, receiving end-bulbs of Held (Fig. 1). However, it is not clear which types of postsynaptic cells are involved. In particular, it is not yet known if the stellate neuron may receive end-bulbs of Held, or if there may be varieties of bushy cells that differ in the sizes and numbers of the end-bulbs received. Furthermore, the units in this region have not been adequately sampled. Finally, the available electron microscopic studies (DeRobertis, 1956, Lenn and Reese, 1966, Bruner, 1970, McDonald and Rasmussen, 1971) cannot be used to relate cytological structure to function, since they do not distinguish the neuronal types. For these reasons it would be risky to speculate on the precise nature of the signal transformations in the region of the ACVN-IN and its projection sites. Nor can one as yet surmise the possible relationships between the synaptic organization in this region and the time-pattern of auditory activity recorded.

In the PPVCN it has been possible to localize in rapid Golgi preparations (Cohen, 1972) a region that is occupied by a distinct type of stellate neuron, the octopus cell, so-named by Osen (1969) because of its fancied shape in the Nissl-stained sections. In a way the cell looks more like an ostrich (Fig. 2). The region, occupied by this cell type in Golgi preparations, does correspond to the octopus-cell area, delineated on cytoarchitectonic grounds by Osen (1969). Except for a few small, intrinsic neurons, the octopus cell appears to be the only neuronal type in this area. The anatomical analyses of this cell have uncovered a number of morphological features of its synaptic organization that may be related to its response characteristics (Fig. 2).

One of the most striking features of the octopus cell is the intense concentration of synaptic endings on the cell body. Over 50% of the surface area of the cell body is covered by the large AN endings alone. This compares with lower values for all of the axosomatic inputs of 23% for pyramidal cells of the rat's visual cortex (Kaiserman-Abramof and Peters, 1972) and of 47% for motor neurons of the cat's spinal cord (Conradi, 1969). Most of the primary afferent endings on the octopus cell are quite large (3 to 8 μm in diameter) and arise from thick fibers, presumably with rapid conduction times. Also, more than 70% of the surface area of the proximal dendritic trunks is covered by large primary afferent endings. These features, no doubt, provide a basis for secure, short-latency responses.

The long dendrites of octopus cells usually extend perpendicularly across a large number of the descending AN branches. It might be predicted that these cells would have much broader tuning curves than spiral ganglion cells or than stellate cells in the AVCN with dendrites arranged parallel to the "isofrequency plane" or bushy cells without dendrites. Osen (1969) in the cat and Harrison and Feldman (1970) in the rat made similar suggestions, although they did not fully demonstrate the branching affer-

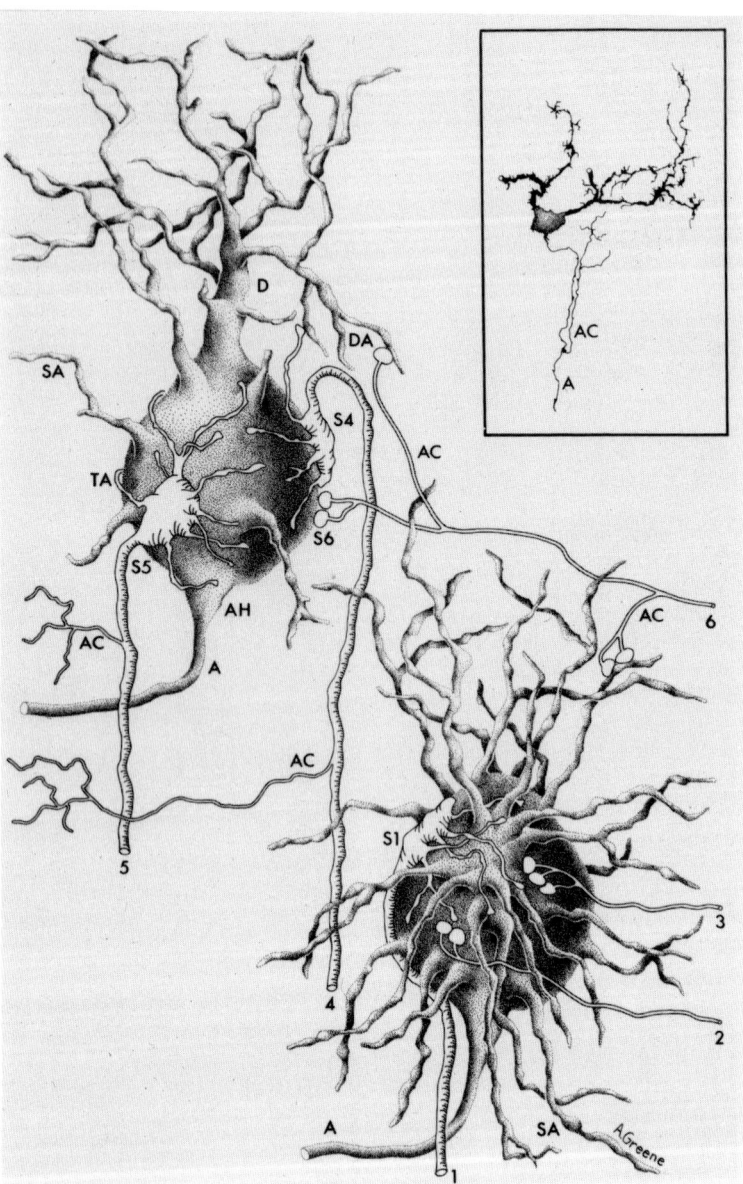

Fig. 1

Fig. 1 Neurons from the region of the interstitial and anteroventral cochlear nuclei of the cat. The drawing is based on an interpretation of the literature (Ramón y Cajal, 1909, Lorente de Nó, 1933, Vincenzi, 1900) and unpublished observations of Golgi preparations. At the lower right, the bushy neuron has a cell body, about 30 μm in diameter, with long, thin somatic appendages (SA). The bushy neuron at the upper left has a similar arrangement, but a dendrite (D) bears most of the appendages (DA). These neurons contact the synaptic endings of thick and thin afferent axons. The thick axons (e.g., nos. 1,4,5), from the ascending branch of the auditory nerve, form the large end-bulbs of Held (e.g. S1, S4, S5). One to three of these endings may contact a single cell (Ramón y Cajal, 1909). These terminals also contact the cell body and its appendages by means of thready extensions, the terminal appendages (TA). The thin afferent axons (e.g., nos. 2, 3, 6) form small synaptic endings on the cell bodies (e.g., S6) and on the somatic and dendritic appendages, often by means of collaterals (AC). The cell body and the appendages are encrusted with a large number of the small endings. Many of the thin axons probably project from the lateral superior olive (Rasmussen, 1967, McDonald and Rasmussen, 1971), and the posterior colliculus (Rasmussen, 1964), but there may be other sources, too, e.g., the collaterals of ascending auditory-nerve branches (6-AC, 4-AC) or recurrent collaterals (inset:AC) of the efferent axons. Inset: A stellate neuron, shown at a lower magnification than the bushy cells, has a cell body of about the same size. In this example the main dendrites extend in a plane parallel to the ascending branches of the auditory nerve. The kinds of endings associated with the stellate cell remain to be elucidated.
Abbreviations: A, axon initial segment; AC, axonal collaterals; AH, axon hillock; D, dendrite; DA, dendritic appendage; SA, somatic appendages; S1,S4,S5, synaptic terminals; TA, terminal appendages; 1--6, afferent axons, including branches of auditory-nerve fibers.

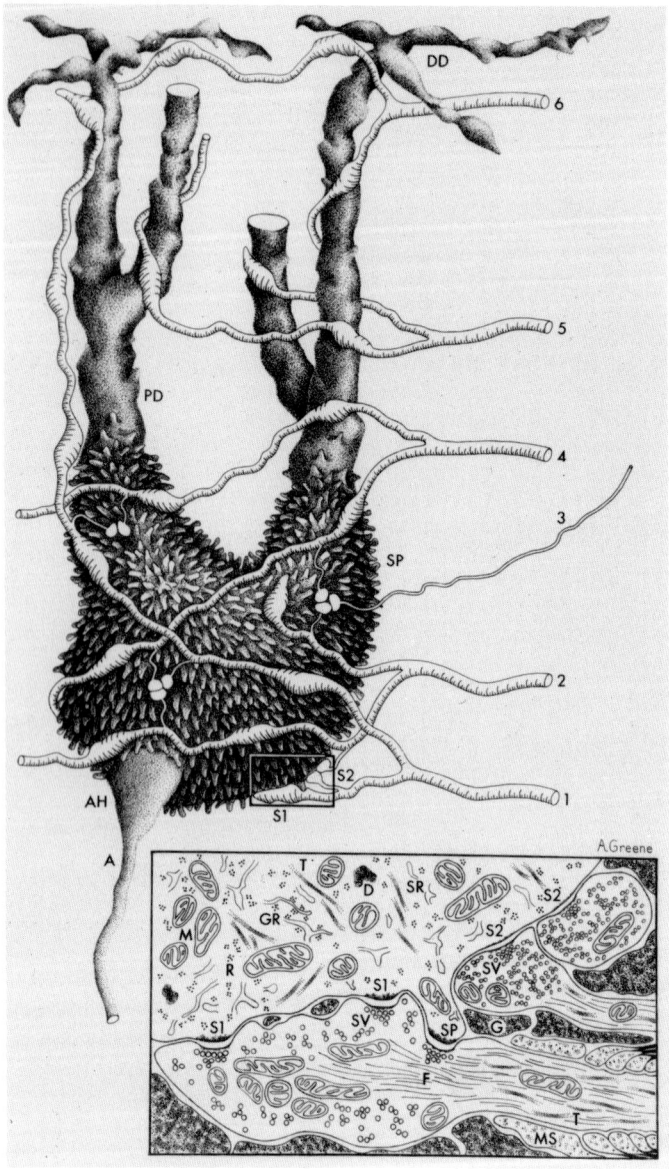

Fig. 2

Fig. 2 An octopus neuron, as seen in an interpretative drawing, based on observations of Golgi preparations and electron micrographs (Cohen, 1972) from the posteroventral cochlear nucleus. The cell body, over 35 µm in diameter, is cloaked with short stubby appendages, the somatic spicules (SP), which greatly increase the surface area involved in axosomatic synapses. Synaptic endings cover approximately 70% of the surface area in electron micrographs of the cell body and proximal dendrites (PD). In these regions there are several varieties of axonal endings. Shown here are large endings (e.g., S1) from the thick, descending branches of the auditory nerve (e.g., 1,2,4,5,6) and small endings (e.g., S2). The small endings are formed secondarily by thin collaterals of the large descending branches or primarily by thin axons (e.g., 3) of undetermined origin. The large synaptic endings occur as isolated, elongated enlargements, either terminal or in passage. Each auditory-nerve fiber contacts a number of octopus cells. Each octopus cell receives many auditory-nerve endings on the cell body and dendrites.

Abbreviations: A, axon initial segment; AH, axon hillock; DD, distal dendrites; PD, proximal dendrite; SP, somatic spicules; S1, S2, axosomatic endings; 1--6, afferent axons, including auditory-nerve fibers.

Inset: The large axonal endings are readily identified by their characteristic size, shape, and locations in electron micrographs, where they cover about 50% of the perikaryal surface. These synaptic endings (Type 1 of Cohen, 1972) are characterized by a moderate collection of neurofilaments (F) and microtubules (T) in the center, surrounded by an accumulation of mitochondria and clear spherical synaptic vesicles (SV), about 0.064 µm in diameter. The synaptic vesicles gather in multiple synaptic complexes (S1), characterized by widened intercellular clefts, post synaptic elevations, and prominent postsynap-

(Fig. 2 cont'd) tic membrane densities. Each large ending is insulated by glial processes (G), some of which also insinuate between the axonal ending and the perikaryal surface. Synaptic complexes of the same type also involve the somatic spicules (SP), which, however, do not synapse with the small endings. The latter (S2, type 2 of Cohen, 1972) are characterized by a lack of neurofilaments and by smaller synaptic vesicles, about 0.058 µm in diameter. These vesicles are pleomorphic and flatter or more oval than those of the large endings. The synaptic complex is marked by a narrower cleft, flatter postsynaptic surface, and much less conspicuous postsynaptic density than in the large synapse. The small endings, which cover about 13% of the perikaryal surface in electron micrographs, are often packed together in contiguity within small clusters, surrounded by glial processes. Since these small endings are often found in clusters in electron micrographs, they can be identified in Golgi impregnations with the small endings of the same size and shape that occur in clusters on the cell body and proximal dendrites. Thus it can be inferred that at least some of the thin collaterals of the thick auditory nerve branches have cytological features similar to the S2 synapses. To be sure, it has not been possible to demonstrate such a collateral in its entirety in the ultrathin sections, used for electron microscopy. Also, it is possible that some of the small collateral endings of the auditory-nerve fibers do not occur in clusters and have the features of S1 synapses. In any case, many of the small (S2) endings must arise from central or indigenous neurons, since a number of the small synapses do not degenerate after cochlear ablations that do result in the disappearance of all of the large endings (Rasmussen, 1967, Cohen, 1972). Junctions, resembling those associated with electrical synapses elsewhere, have not been found.

<u>Abbreviations for inset:</u> D, dense body (lysosome); F, neurofilaments; G, glial process (astrocyte); GR, granular endoplasmic reticulum; M, mitochondria; MS, myelin sheath; R, ribosomes; SP, somatic spicule; SR, smooth endoplasmic reticulum; SV, synaptic vesicles; S1, synaptic complex of large endings; S2, synaptic complex of small endings; T, microtubules.

(end of legend for Fig. 2).

ent axons and octopus-cell dendrites or the arrangement of the synaptic endings. The present results show that the dendrites of the octopus cells along their entire lengths do in fact associate with the AN endings. However, individual axons quite often turn out of their "iso-frequency planes" to ascend or descend along the dendrites and bodies, which they contact repeatedly by means of synapses in passage (e.g. Fiber no. 1 in Fig. 2). Moreover, the secondary dendritic branches often extend within particular "iso-frequency planes." It is possible that these last two morphological features could affect the tuning properties of octopus cells. Furthermore, the dendrites extend predominantly in the dorsal direction, and the octopus-cell area extends across only part of the low-frequency region of the PPVCN. Thus, units with low CF could be fewer than those with high CF. This is consistent with the observation that low-frequency "on" units are relatively rare. Directional sensitivity to sweeping frequencies of tone might be another interesting consequence of the axonal and dendritic arrangements of these cells. In a few preliminary experiments, some units in the PPVCN have shown asymmetric sensitivity to tones swept in frequency.

Perhaps the most intriguing electrophysiological property of the octopus cell is its "on" response pattern. In order to account for this modification of the input activity, it seems likely that inhibitory events in the cochlear nucleus need to be invoked. One possibility is the existence of inhibitory interneurons, projecting to the octopus cells from other sites, that have short-latency responses, time-locked to the onset of the stimulus. Such cells have not been demonstrated. The extreme rapidity with which these units stop firing (frequently after a single spike) argues in favor of a local inhibitory mechanism. One may speculate that the small ($\simeq 2$ μm diameter) synaptic endings, clustered on the cell body and proximal dendrites (Fig. 2), might be involved in inhibitory activity. Many of these small endings arise from AN fibers, often by means of thin collaterals (less than 0.5 μm in diameter) of the descending branches; by contrast, the large afferent endings arise from thick collaterals (0.7 to 1.5 μm in diameter). If the small endings formed inhibitory synapses, they could provide the basis for the cessation of firing shortly after the arrival of excitatory inputs from the AN. The required delay for inhibition might be a consequence of the more slowly conducting thin collaterals and a considerable degree of convergence at the small endings. The cytological appearance of the small AN terminals (Fig. 2: inset) is at least consistent with the fine structure of synaptic profiles that many neurocytologists choose to regard as inhibitory in other parts of the brain (see Gray, 1969). Of course, other hypotheses can be advanced. Perhaps some of the thin afferents arise directly from branches derived from one of the two types of spiral ganglion cells described by Spoendlin (1972). For that matter, not all of the small endings need be inhibitory in action. Nor can the possibility be excluded that some of the large endings might be inhibitory or that an excitatory ending might fail.

In the MNTB, three types of neurons have been recognized: the principal cell, the stellate cell, and the elongate cell (Morest, 1968). Of these, only the principal cell receives the large axosomatic ending, formed by the calyx of Held. The morphological features of the principal cell and the calyx endings are so distinctive and have been so thoroughly described at the light microscopic level that it has been possible to identify features of their synaptic organization with electron micrographs and microelectrode recordings (Ramón y Cajal, 1909, Morest, 1968, in press, Li and Guinan, 1971, Guinan et al., 1972a, 1972b, Jean-Baptiste and Morest, unpublished observations). The chief morphological features are schematized in Fig. 3.

The calyx-principal cell synapses probably represent the highest degree of synaptic specificity possible, since they apparently establish a series of one-to-one connections between the cells of the IN region and MNTB. Consequently, the tuning curves, identified with the principal cells, are narrow, and a tonotopic sequence extends across the nucleus. The calyciferous axons, ranging up to 12 µm in diameter, are among the largest found in the cat's brain. Not surprisingly, the response latencies are among the shortest for units in the SOC. The preterminal axons and the calyx ending itself are probably the largest in the mammalian brain. Perhaps for this reason it has been possible in extracellular unit recordings to identify complex waveforms that probably correspond to pre- and postsynaptic events. These identifications have been confirmed with orthodromic and antidromic stimulation experiments. For these units, a presynaptic positivity is <u>always</u> followed by a postsynaptic negativity; thus it is likely that most, if not all, of the calyx synapses are excitatory - a conclusion in harmony with current speculations on the cytological features of excitatory synapses (Fig. 3: inset). These features and experimental findings indicate a high degree of synaptic security at the calyx-principal cell junction, in effect, a one-to-one input-output function. For this reason, the time-pattern of response of MNTB(P) units fits with the idea that the cells, forming the calyciferous axons, correspond to the units, recorded in the region of the IN, with response patterns similar to those of AN units.

Although the calyx appears to function as a perfectly secure synapse under the conditions so far explored, one cannot conclude that no opportunity for signal transformation exists. There are a number of other inputs to the principal cells by way of smaller, but more numerous, synaptic contacts on the body and dendrites. The activity of these inputs, the origins of which are largely unknown, could provide mechanisms for interactions with other neurons. Furthermore, the calyciferous axon forms a number of morphologically heterogeneous collaterals, just as the AN branches do in the CN. One kind of collateral arises from the calyx itself and forms many small boutons on the neighboring cell bodies of principal neurons (Fig. 3: CC-P). If these collateral endings should be inhibitory, they could provide for a surrounding field of inhibition. Another set of axonal branches, the precalycine collaterals, arises from the preterminal portions of the calyciferous axons and projects to DMPO, one of the main origins of the COCB. Since the principal cells of MNTB also project to DMPO, the neurons of the COCB would be in a position to sample portions of the input and output of the principal cells. How this would relate to the properties of the COCB and its proposed functions (Fex, 1962, Wiederhold and Kiang, 1970, Wiederhold, 1970) remains to be demonstrated.

Another type of unit in the MNTB is represented by the "off-response." This should correspond either to the stellate cell or the elongate cell. Both of these cell types have long dendrites that extend at

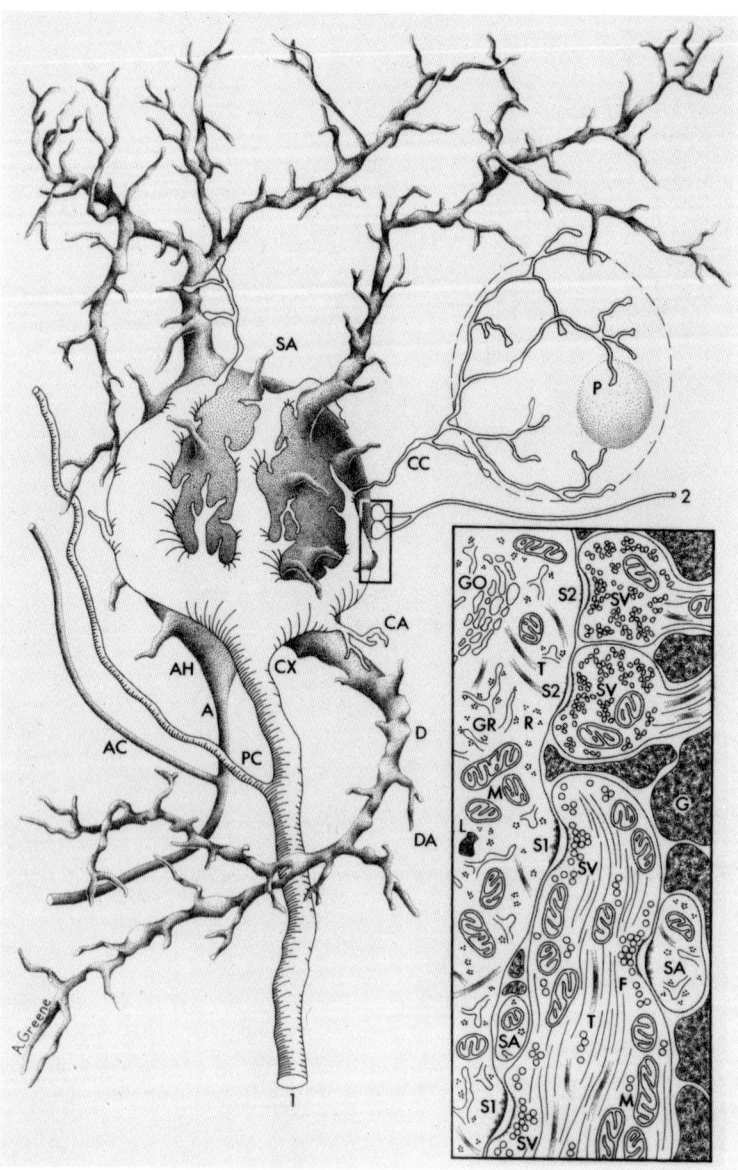

Fig. 3 A principal neuron of the medial nucleus of the trapezoid body: a drawing based on observations of Golgi impregnations and electron micrographs (Morest, 1968, in press, unpublished observations). Each principal cell

(Fig. 3 cont'd) body, about 35 μm in diameter, receives one, and only one, calyx (CX), the immense cup-shaped synaptic endings, formed by fibers, projecting from the contralateral ventral cochlear nucleus. Each calyciferous axon (1) forms one, and only one, calyx. Only principal cells receive the calyces. The calycine appendages (CA) are short extensions of the calyx that usually contact the body or proximal dendrites of the same cell as the primary ending. Thin collaterals of the calyx (CC) form a network of small terminal boutons, typically associated with the bodies of several nearby principal cells, one of which is shown at P. The body and dendrites (e.g., D) of the principal cell have a characteristic spiculated appearance, due to the somatic appendages (SA) and dendritic appendages (DA), which can also contact the calyx or its appendages. A number of thin axons (e.g., 2) form smaller synaptic endings on the cell body and dendrites. These fine axonal endings are especially numerous among the distal dendrites, where a conspicuous peridendritic plexus occurs (not shown here, but see Morest, 1968: Fig. 9). The origins of most of these small endings are undetermined, except for a small contingent, supplied by collaterals of the axons, projecting to the medial superior olive from the contralateral anteroventral cochlear nucleus. The axon (A) of the principal cell has a collateral (AC) that projects to the dorsomedial periolivary nucleus along with the precalycine collateral (PC) of the calyciferous axon. The other projection sites of the principal cell axon are uncertain but probably include the lateral superior olive. Abbreviations: 1, calyciferous axon; 2, thin afferent axon, forming small axosomatic endings on the principal cell body; A, initial segment of principal cell axon; AC, axonal collateral; AH, axon hillock; CA, calycine appendage; CC, calycine collateral; CX, calyx; D, dendrite of principal cell; DA, dendritic appendage; P, typical eccentric nucleus of principal cell body (outlined by dashes); PC, precalycine collateral; SA, somatic appendages.

(Fig. 3 cont'd) Inset: Cytological features of calycine synapses (S1) and one of several varieties of smaller axosomatic synapses (S2) (see also Lenn and Reese, 1966, in the rat, and Nakajima, 1971, in the bat). The calyx ending has relatively large, pale synaptic vesicles, about 0.050 μm in diameter, that gather at the synaptic complexes (S1), which are characterized by widened intercellular spaces, elevated postsynaptic surfaces, and greatly thickened postsynaptic membrane densities. Similar synaptic complexes involve the somatic appendages (SA). Contacts like those associated with electrical synapses have not been seen. The calycine processes are segregated from neighboring synapses by neuroglia (G). The smaller variety of synaptic ending, shown here, lacks filaments and contains smaller pleomorphic synaptic vesicles, which gather at synaptic complexes (S2), having a narrower synaptic cleft, flatter postsynaptic surface, and thinner postsynaptic density. Abbreviations for inset: F, neurofilaments; G, neuroglia; GO, Golgi apparatus; GR, granular endoplasmic reticulum; L, lysosome; M, mitochondria; R, ribosomes; SA, somatic appendages; SV, synaptic vesicles; S1, synapses of calyx; S2, synapses of small endings.

right angles to the "iso-frequency planes" of the MNTB and that contact a wide sector of the afferent fiber spectrum. Thus, not surprisingly, these units exhibit much wider tuning curves than observed for principal cells.

4. Discussion

In an understandable eagerness to explain experimental results in terms of neural connections, one sometimes forgets that a wiring diagram is, after all, a highly stylized convention that scarcely does justice to the actual structure of the brain. A schematic diagram of nuclei, connected by lines, may be a useful mnemonic device, but it does not imply that each nucleus performs a specific identifiable function. More likely, each part of the system plays significant roles in several different aspects of auditory behavior. A nucleus is not a self-contained unit but is only a convenient name for a topographic location. It does not even encompass a group of neurons except for cells with short axons (Golgi type II). Instead, it comprises a more or less distinct part of the neuropil (Herrick, 1948). Each part of the neuropil can be defined in terms of its synaptic organization, i.e., the particular arrangement of the synaptogenic portions of specific types of neurons. In other words, a nucleus in a wiring diagram consists of the axonal endings of certain neurons and the dendrites and cell bodies of certain others. Thus the spiral ganglion is probably not a functionally significant component of the wiring diagram of the auditory system. On the other hand, the spiral ganglion cells are, by virtue of their synaptic relations, as much a part of the PPVCN as the octopus-cell bodies. The locations of the cell bodies are essentially irrelevant to the wiring diagram, except when they happen to coincide with a particular population of synapses. Although this coincidence often occurs in the mammalian nervous system, it is by no means invariable, indeed is quite variable in lower vertebrates and not even reported in some invertebrates.

Even the basic concept of the wiring diagram, that one nucleus connects with another, is misleading. In fact, only individual neurons are connected. But as a general principle of vertebrate neuroanatomy, it seems useful to assume that certain types of neurons are connected to certain other types. Neverthless, it seldom happens that a sensory nucleus contains only one type of neuron, or that each type of neuron in one nucleus projects to each type of neuron in another nucleus and in exactly the same way. These considerations have important implications for the study of stimulus coding in the auditory system. The implications for a systematic analysis of unit response characteristics have been discussed in Paper I (Response Characteristics of Single Units).

For a systematic analysis, accurate information on the connections between auditory nuclei is necessary, but not sufficient. It is also necessary to define the precise relationships of the particular types of neurons in these connections. Some progress has been made in the case of the octopus-cell area of the PPVCN, the principal cells, receiving calyces, in the MNTB, and the neurons of the DMPO that contribute to the crossed olivocochlear bundle. Further progress must await more detailed morphological analyses at all levels of the auditory system.

In order for more detailed analyses to proceed, it will be necessary to work with a variety of anatomical methods, besides the traditional ones, including the Golgi methods, experimental degeneration and labelling methods, electron microscopy, and ultimately cytochemical techniques - in short, the entire technical arsenal of modern neuroanatomy. We have already referred to the inadequacy of the cytoarchitectonic approach in this field. Such an approach does not facilitate comparisons between the variety of morphological and physiological methods, demanded for a systematic analysis. It is a realistic consequence of this need that such schemes of parcellation, as those of Osen (1969) and of Harrison and Feldman (1970) in the CN, of Rose (1942) and Rioch (1929) in the medial geniculate body, and of Berman (1968) in the posterior colliculus require review in the light of other methods.

One of the most fascinating aspects of the present approach has been the opportunity to relate particular constellations of synaptic organization to specific response patterns. Initially it was not assumed that a particular type of unit would necessarily correspond to a morphological cell type. Nevertheless, the result obtained so far is that a correspondence between unit types and cell types has been documented in a number of cases.

Once such correspondences are established, one can investigate the neural mechanisms, involved in the generation of a particular pattern of responses. For example, one may now ask, what are the specific cellular mechanisms responsible for an "on" response from the octopus cells? This question has to be answered in terms of the synaptic organization of the cell and in terms of the physiological properties of its synapses. In doing so, the techniques of modern cell biology can be applied to the study of neural processes within a definable functional context, namely, that of stimulus coding in the auditory system.

In this approach one encounters problems that are basic to a functional analysis of any neural system.

Indeed the auditory system provides some exceptional opportunities to unravel some of these difficult problems. Ironically, this work is facilitated by the very complexity and high degree of specialization that distinguish the auditory system. However, the organizing principles of the auditory system may be no more complicated than those of other sensory systems. Although wiring diagrams seem to belie this prospect because of the sheer number of nuclear groups and pathways involved, the auditory nuclei of the brain stem, if more numerous, may have intrinsic organizations that are easier to analyze than those of other sensory systems. For example, the octopus cell area consists almost entirely of one type of neuron; the ventral nucleus of the medial geniculate body has only two types (Morest, 1971). In the visual and somesthetic nuclei there seems to be much more intermingling of morphologically heterogeneous types of neurons.

Consider, for example, the elaborate development of the axonal collaterals of auditory neurons. In the cochlear nucleus, individual auditory-nerve fibers send sizeable branches to each of the major subdivisions. Consequently, the same cochlear response patterns could be transmitted to morphologically distinct parts of the neuropil. This provides a uniquely controllable opportunity to define the role of different constellations of synaptic organization in the transformations of identical signal inputs. It may even be possible to dissect the relative functions of the axonal endings and the postsynaptic portions of the cochlear nucleus neurons, where different types of axonal endings contact the same cell type, as in the case of the octopus cell. A similar situation obtains in the case of the principal cell of the MNTB, due to the particular arrangement of the calyciform endings and their collaterals.

Other intriguing questions arise in relation to the finding that a single auditory-nerve axon can form two cytologically distinct types of synaptic contacts with the same octopus cell (Fig. 2). The features of these two types of endings, including the morphology of the synaptic vesicles, correspond to current notions of excitatory and inhibitory synapses (Gray, 1969). It has been suggested that such differences in vesicle and membrane morphology are cytological counterparts of different chemical transmitters (Uchizono, 1965, Walberg, 1965, Bodian, 1971). If one subscribes to this thinking, one may entertain the hypothesis that Dale's law does not apply to the auditory-nerve endings. It may also be that our current neurocytological concepts need serious revision. Insofar as the observed differences in synaptic morphology corresponded to different neurotransmitters, it would be necessary to explain how local conditions, at the level of the synaptic endings, favor the synthesis and/or release of one transmitter rather than another. On the other hand, even if the different types of endings released the same transmitters, the local responses of the postsynaptic cell might differ, as suggested by the striking morphological differences of the postsynaptic membranes (see Fig. 2: inset). These and other fascinating implications of the findings are now open for exploration with modern cytochemical, ultrastructural, and intracellular recording techniques.

Acknowledgments

Many people contributed to the preparation of these papers. A.B. Greene made the anatomical drawings. J.B. Brawer and M. Jean-Baptiste made available some of the results of their unpublished studies. W.B. Warr gave helpful advice. B.E. Norris, E.C. Moxon, J.H. DeBlois, T.R. Bourk, and P.R. Hochfeld helped in obtaining some of the data. G.S. Roberts and E.M. Marr gave editorial assistance.

This work was supported in part by the Public Health Service (Grants 5 R01 NS01344, 1 K04 NS42, 538, 2 R01 NS06115, 5 P01 GM-14940, 5 T01 GM-00406, and 5 S01 RR05485); in part by the Joint Services Electronics Program; in part by a National Science Foundation graduate fellowship; and in part by a Fannie and John Hertz Foundation predoctoral fellowship.

References

Berman, A.L. (1968). The Brain Stem of the Cat. A Cytoarchitectonic Atlas with Stereotaxic Coordinates. Univ. Wisconsin Press, Madison, Wisconsin.

Bodian, D. (1971). Presynaptic organelles and junctional integrity. J. Cell Biol. 48, 707-710.

Boudreau, J.C., and Tsuchitani, C. (1970). Cat superior olive S segment cell discharge to tonal stimulation. In: Contributions to Sensory Physiology. (W.D. Neff, ed.), pp. 143-213. Academic Press, New York.

Bruner, L. (1970). Electron microscopic studies of the cat cochlear nuclei. Thesis. Johns Hopkins Univ., Baltimore.

Caspary, D.M. (1971). Stimulus coding and the cytoarchitecture of the cochlear nuclei of the kangaroo rat, Dipodomys spectabilis. Thesis. New York Univ., New York.

Clark, G.M., and Dunlop, C.W. (1969). Poststimulus-time response patterns in the nuclei of the cat superior olivary complex. Exp. Neurol. 23, 266-290.

Cohen, E.S. (1972). Synaptic organization of the caudal cochlear nucleus of the cat: a light and electron microscopical study. Thesis. Harvard Univ., Cambridge, Mass.

Cohen, E.S., Brawer, J.R., and Morest, D.K. (1972). Projections of the cochlea to the dorsal cochlear nucleus in the cat. Exp. Neurol. 35, 470-479.

Conradi, S. (1969). Ultrastructure and distribution of neuronal and glial elements on the motoneuron surface in the lumbosacral spinal cord of the adult cat. Acta Physiol. Scand. Suppl. 332, 49-64.

DeRobertis, E. (1956). Submicroscopic changes of the synapse after nerve section in the acoustic ganglion of the guinea pig. An electron microscope study. J. Biophys. Biochem. Cytol. 2, 503-512.

Dowben, R.M., and Rose, J.E. (1953). A metal-filled microelectrode. Science 118, 22-24.

Fex, J. (1962). Auditory activity in centrifugal and centripetal cochlear fibres in cat. A study of a feedback system. Acta Physiol. Scand. 55, Suppl. 189, 1-68.

Fex, J. (1965). Auditory activity in uncrossed centrifugal cochlear fibres in cat. A study of a feedback system, II. Acta Physiol. Scand. 64, 43-57.

Gardner, D., and Kandel, E.R. (1972). Diphasic postsynaptic potential: A chemical synapse capable of mediating conjoint excitation and inhibition. Science 176, 675-678.

Godfrey, D.A. (1971). Localization of single units in the cochlear nucleus of the cat: an attempt to correlate neuronal structure and function. Thesis. Harvard Univ., Cambridge, Mass.

Goldberg, J.M., and Brown, P.B. (1969). Response of binaural neurons of dog superior olivary complex to dichotic tonal stimuli: some physiological mechanisms of sound localization. J. Neurophysiol. 32, 613-636.

Gray, E.G. (1969). Electron microscopy of excitatory and inhibitory synapses: a brief review. Progr. Brain Res. 31, 141-155.

Guinan, J.J., Jr., Guinan, S.S., and Norris, B.E. (1972a). Single auditory units in the superior olivary complex I: Responses to sounds and classifications based on physiological properties. Int. J. Neurosci. 4, 101-120.

Guinan, J.J., Jr., Norris, B.E., and Guinan, S.S. (1972b). Single auditory units in the superior olivary complex II: Locations of unit categories and tonotopic organization. Int. J. Neurosci. 4, 147-166.

Hall, J.L., II (1965). Binaural interaction in the accessory superior olivary nucleus of the cat. J. Acoust. Soc. Amer. 37, 814-823.

Harrison, J.M., and Feldman, M.L. (1970). Anatomical aspects of the cochlear nucleus and superior olivary complex. In: Contributions to Sensory Physiology. (W.D. Neff, ed.), pp. 95-142. Academic Press, New York.

Held, H. (1893). Die centrale Gehörleitung. Arch. Anat. Physiol., Anat. Abt., 201-248.

Herrick, C.J. (1948). The Brain of the Tiger Salamander. Univ. of Chicago Press, Chicago.

Kaiserman-Abramof, I.R., and Peters, A. (1972). Some aspects of the morphology of Betz cells in the cerebral cortex of the cat. Brain Res. 43, 527-546.

Katsuki, Y., Sumi, T., Uchiyama, H., and Watanabe, T. (1958). Electric responses of auditory neurons in cat to sound stimulation. J. Neurophysiol. 21, 569-588.

Katsuki, Y., Suga, N., and Kanno, Y. (1962). Neural mechanism of the peripheral and central auditory system in monkeys. J. Acoust. Soc. Amer. 34, 1396-1410.

Kiang, N.Y.S. (1965). Stimulus coding in the auditory nerve and cochlear nucleus. Acta Oto-Laryngol. 59, 186-200.

Kiang, N.Y.S., Pfeiffer, R.R., Warr, W.B., and Backus, A.S.N. (1965a). Stimulus coding in the cochlear nucleus. Ann. Otol. Rhinol. Laryngol. 74, 463-485.

Kiang, N.Y.S., Watanabe, T., Thomas, E.C., and Clark, L.F. (1965b). Discharge Patterns of Single Fibers in the Cat's Auditory Nerve. Res. Monogr. 35. M.I.T. Press, Cambridge, Mass.

Kiang, N.Y.S., Sachs, M.B., and Peake, W.T. (1967). Shapes of tuning curves for single auditory-nerve fibers. J. Acoust. Soc. Amer. 42, 1341-1342.

Kiang, N.Y.S. (1968). A survey of recent developments in the study of auditory physiology. Ann. Otol. Rhinol. Laryngol. 77, 656-675.

Lenn, N.J., and Reese, T.S. (1966). The fine structure of nerve endings in the nucleus of the trapezoid body and the ventral cochlear nucleus. Amer. J. Anat. 118, 375-390.

Li, R.Y.S., and Guinan, J.J., Jr. (1971). Antidromic and orthodromic stimulation of neurons receiving calyces of Held. Quart. Progr. Rep. 100, pp. 227-234. Research Laboratory of Electronics, M.I.T., Cambridge, Mass.

Lorente de Nó, R. (1933). Anatomy of the eighth nerve. III. General plan of structure of the primary cochlear nuclei. Laryngoscope 43, 327-350.

Lorente de Nó, R. (1937). The sensory endings in the cochlea. Laryngoscope 47, 373-377.

McDonald, D.M., and Rasmussen, G.L. (1971). Ultrastructural characteristics of synaptic endings in the cochlear nucleus having acetylcholinesterase activity. Brain Res. 28, 1-18.

Morest, D.K. (1964). The neuronal architecture of the medial geniculate body of the cat. J. Anat. (London) 98, 611-630.

Morest, D.K. (1965a). The laminar structure of the medial geniculate body of the cat. J. Anat. (London) 99, 143-160.

Morest, D.K. (1965b). The lateral tegmental system of the midbrain and the medial geniculate body: study with Golgi and Nauta methods in cat. J. Anat. (London) 99, 611-634.

Morest, D.K. (1968). The collateral system of the medial nucleus of the trapezoid body of the cat, its neuronal architecture and relation to the olivo-cochlear bundle. Brain Res. 9, 288-311.

Morest, D.K. (1971). Dendrodendritic synapses of cells that have axons: the fine structure of the Golgi type II cell in the medial geniculate body of the cat. Z. Anat. Entwicklungsgesch. 133, 216-246.

Morest, D.K. (1973). Auditory neurons of the brain stem. In: Advances in Oto-Rhino-Laryngology. (W.P. Work, M. Lawrence, and J.E. Hawkins, Jr., eds.), Vol. 19.

Morest, D.K., and Morest, R.R. (1966). Perfusion-fixation of the brain with chromeosmium solutions for the rapid Golgi method. Amer. J. Anat. 118, 811-832.

Moushegian, G., Rupert, A., and Whitcomb, M.A. (1964). Medial superior-olivary unit response patterns to monaural and binaural clicks. J. Acoust. Soc. Amer. 36, 196-202.

Nakajima, Y. (1971). Fine structure of the medial nucleus of the trapezoid body of the bat with special reference to two types of synaptic endings. J. Cell Biol. 50, 121-134.

van Noort, J. (1969). The Structure and Connections of the Inferior Colliculus. Van Gorcum & Co. N.V., Assen.

Osen, K.K. (1969). Cytoarchitecture of the cochlear nuclei in the cat. J. Comp. Neurol. 136, 453-484.

Osen, K.K. (1970). Course and termination of the primary afferents in the cochlear nuclei of the cat. An experimental anatomical study. Arch. Ital. Biol. 108, 21-51.

Osen, K.K. (1972). Projection of the cochlear nuclei on the inferior colliculus in the cat. J. Comp. Neurol. 144, 355-372.

Pfeiffer, R.R. (1966a). Anteroventral cochlear nucleus: Waveforms of extracellularly recorded spike potentials. Science 154, 667-668.

Pfeiffer, R.R. (1966b). Classification of response patterns of spike discharges for units in the cochlear nucleus: tone burst stimulation. Exp. Brain Res. 1, 220-235.

Polyak, S.L., McHugh, G., and Judd, D.K. (1946). The Human Ear in Anatomical Transparencies, p. 105. Sonotone Corporation, Elmsford, New York.

Price, G.R. (1972). Comment on intracochlear potentials recorded with micropipets. III. Relation of cochlear microphonic potential to stapes velocity. J. Acoust. Soc. Amer. 51, 2059-2061.

Ramón y Cajal, S. (1909). Histologie du système Nerveux de l'Homme et des Vertébrés, Vol. I, pp. 754-838. Instituto Ramón y Cajal, Madrid.

Rasmussen, G.L. (1960). Efferent fibers of the cochlear nerve and cochlear nucleus. In: Neural Mechanisms of the Auditory and Vestibular Systems. (G.L. Rasmussen and W. Windle, eds.), pp. 105-115. C. C. Thomas, Springfield, Ill.

Rasmussen, G.L. (1964). Anatomic relationships of the ascending and descending auditory systems. In: Neurological Aspects of Auditory and Vestibular Disorders. (W.S. Fields and B.R. Alford, eds.), pp. 5-19. C. C. Thomas, Springfield, Ill.

Rasmussen, G.L. (1967). Efferent connections of the cochlear nucleus. In: Sensorineural Hearing Processes and Disorders. (Graham, ed.), pp. 61-75. Little, Brown and Co., Boston, Mass.

Rioch, D. McK. (1929). Studies on the diencephalon of carnivora. Part I. The nuclear configuration of the thalamus, epithalamus, and hypothalamus of the dog and cat. J. Comp. Neurol. 49, 1-119.

Rose, J.E. (1942). The thalamus of the sheep: cellular and fibrous structure and comparison with pig, rabbit, and cat. J. Comp. Neurol. 77, 469-523.

Rose, J.E. (1960). Organization of frequency sensitive neurons in the cochlear nuclear complex of the cat. In: <u>Neural Mechanisms of the Auditory and Vestibular Systems</u>. (C.L. Racmussen and W. Windle, eds.), pp. 116-136. C. C. Thomas, Springfield, Ill.

Rupert, A.L., Moushegian, G., and Whitcomb, M.A. (1968). Olivo-cochlear neuronal responses in medulla of cat. <u>Exp. Neurol</u>. <u>20</u>, 575-584.

Spoendlin, H. (1972). Innervation densities of the cochlea. <u>Acta Oto-Laryngol</u>. <u>73</u>, 235-248.

Stotler, W.A. (1953). An experimental study of the cells and connections of the superior olivary complex of the cat. <u>J. Comp. Neurol</u>. <u>98</u>, 401-431.

Uchizono, K. (1965). Characteristics of excitatory and inhibitory synapses in the central nervous system of the cat. <u>Nature (London)</u> <u>207</u>, 642-643.

Vincenzi, L. (1900). Nuove ricerche sui calici di Held nel nucleo del corpo trapezoide. <u>Anat. Anz</u>. <u>18</u>, 344-348.

Walberg, F. (1965). A special type of synaptic vesicles in boutons of the inferior olive. <u>J. Ultrastruct. Res</u>. <u>12</u>, 237.

Warr, W.B. (1966). Fiber degeneration following lesions in the anterior ventral cochlear nucleus of the cat. <u>Exp. Neurol</u>. <u>14</u>, 453-474.

Warr, W.B. (1969). Fiber degeneration following lesions in the posteroventral cochlear nucleus of the cat. <u>Exp. Neurol</u>. <u>23</u>, 140-155.

Warr, W.B. (1972). Fiber degeneration following lesions in the multipolar and globular cell areas in the ventral cochlear nucleus of the cat. <u>Brain Res</u>. <u>40</u>, 247-270.

Weiss, T.F., and Peake, W.T. (1973). Cochlear potential response at the round-window membrane of the cat - a reply to the comment of G.R. Price. J. Acoust. Soc. Amer. (In press).

Wiederhold, M.L. (1970). Variations in the effects of electric stimulation of the crossed olivocochlear bundle on cat single auditory-nerve-fiber responses to tone bursts. J. Acoust. Soc. Amer. 48, 966-977.

Wiederhold, M.L., and Kiang, N.Y.S. (1970). Effects of electric stimulation of the crossed olivocochlear bundle on single auditory-nerve fibers in the cat. J. Acoust. Soc. Amer. 48, 950-965.

DISCUSSION

BRUGGE: You talked about firing patterns characterizing your units and said that the patterns can change with intensity and with frequency. To what extent do you see this variability within response areas? Are you characterizing your units only on the basis of patterns obtained at characteristic frequency or do you employ other criteria?

KIANG: We characterize units in terms of a profile of how they behave with respect to a great many different stimuli rather than a single histogram. That is the point of that one slide showing histograms as a function of intensity.

BRUGGE: In other words those cells in the octopus cell region are not strictly onset units but throughout the response area you might expect to see more complicated patterns. Is that correct?

KIANG: For low frequency stimuli, the "on" units will respond throughout the stimulus duration in a phase-locked manner.

BRUGGE: Is it correct that one of the patterns among many within a response area might be an onset response?

KIANG: Yes.

BRUGGE: Is this also true then for other units such as those which you call pausers or choppers? Do they keep one characteristic firing pattern at all intensities and frequencies in the response area?

KIANG: No, not if you mean by character the appearance of a single histogram. One needs to distinguish carefully between descriptions of response patterns and unit types. Some confusion is generated by using the same descriptive terms for both. For example in the deep DCN different patterns may be exhibited by one unit for stimuli in different frequency ranges.

BRUGGE: So there is not homogeneity within a region?

KIANG: No, I very carefully specified the regions in which there seems to be relative homogeneity of unit types. The DCN as a whole is not a homogeneous region, but units in the fusiform cell layer in the DCN are almost all either "pauser" or "buildup" units.

ZWISLOCKI: What is the onset time in the tone bursts that you use?

KIANG: 2 1/2 msec but if one uses say 5 msec or 10 msec onset times one would still get virtually the same results.

ZWISLOCKI: Do you have any work going on with intracellular recordings which would probably help a little bit in determining the input-output relationships?

KIANG: John Guinan in our lab had tried that for a while but he was discouraged by the fact that he never could get reasonable resting potentials. That is why you see so much reference in the literature to quasi-intracellular or semi-intracellular recordings because they are really not sure that they are intracellular in these recordings.

ZWISLOCKI: Well, you are going to do some intracellular recording.

KIANG: No, not necessarily. In fact, even if the

electrode is intracellular it is not so clear that
one would necessarily get an idea of what the input
to the whole cell is.

ZWISLOCKI: But it would provide you additional information.

KIANG: Yes, of course.

EVANS: Looking at your post-stimulus time histograms,
I would guess that the anesthesia you used was barbiturate.

KIANG: Throughout all of these studies we used dial
urethane anesthesia.

EVANS: That fits with our data. Without anesthesia,
or under chloralose, one obtains a quite different
picture of the dorsal cochlear nucleus from that obtained under barbiturate (Evans and Nelson, 1973).
In particular one obtains a greater preponderance of
inhibition in the frequency response areas and PST
histograms.

KIANG: We do even in these preparations. What I have
not tried to do here is to show you everything that
we find in the nucleus. I have greatly simplified the
story and have limited the points where the signal
tracing idea seems to be applicable.

EVANS: I am aware of that, but it is just the fact
that if, for example, you use the unanesthetized preparation, the majority of post-stimulus time histograms from cells in the region of the dorsal cochlear
nucleus would look completely different from the
overall picture that you have given us. For example,
there would be a preponderance of neurons showing inhibitory rather than excitatory PST histograms.

KIANG: If you say that to be true of the fusiform

cell layer, that would be interesting, but if you speak in terms of the whole dorsal cochlear nucleus, the localization is not fine enough to expect a clear description of unit types. I am not saying that anesthesia is not an important element. It obviously is, but assuming the level of anesthesia to be approximately the same for all these different regions, you still can trace activity through a normal chain. Who can say whether in the unanesthetized animal they would be the same. Very likely they would not.

EVANS: Dr. Kiang, what is the highest characteristic frequency you got in either the area of the Held endbulbs in AVCN or in the medial nucleus of the superior olivary complex?

KIANG: In the medial superior olive the highest characteristic frequencies are above 20 kHz.

BRUGGE: Would you regularly see the whole spectrum?

KIANG: This nucleus seems to have mainly units with low characteristic frequencies.

BRUGGE: But it would be unusual to find something about 10 or 12 kHz.

KIANG: Yes, but not impossible. We have not made a complete grid map of the MSO so that there might be regions that have not been matematically explored.

BRUGGE: Goldberg and Brown (1968) reported units with characteristic frequencies up to around 11 kHz in the medial nucleus of the superior olivary complex in the dog. Osen (1970) reported that the large spherical cells in anterior portion of AVCN anyway may not receive input from the whole cochlear nerve. Would you agree with that?

KIANG: I do not think that the evidence is that good

yet. We have some difficulties with Osen's classification of spherical cells. Whether the distinction between large and small spherical cells holds is certainly not yet settled. I think the AVCN is one region where the cytology has not yet been well described. Certainly one finds high frequency units in the AVCN including high frequency units with complex wave forms. Whether any of these units corresponds to what Osen calls large spherical cells is unknown.

References

Evans, E.F., and Nelson, P.G. (1973). The responses of single neurones in the cochlear nucleus of the cat as a function of their location and the anesthetic state. Exp. Brain Res. (In press).

Goldberg, J.M., and Brown, P.B. (1968). Functional organization of the dog superior olivary complex: an anatomical and electrophysiological study. J. Neurophysiol. 31, 639-656.

Osen, K.K. (1970). Course and termination of the primary afferents in the cochlear nuclei of the cat. An experimental anatomical study. Arch. Ital. Biol. 108, 21-51.

STUDIES OF PHASE-LOCKED COCHLEAR OUTPUT IN CELLS OF THE ANTEROVENTRAL NUCLEUS IN THE COCHLEAR COMPLEX OF THE CAT

J.E. Rose, M.M. Gibson,
L.M. Kitzes and J.E. Hind

Laboratory of Neurophysiology,
University of Wisconsin,
Madison, Wisconsin
USA

We shall summarize here some of our results concerning discharges of single neurons in the anteroventral nucleus of the cochlear complex. We shall consider only those low-frequency neurons which preserve (with great precision) the phase information provided by the temporal discharge pattern of auditory nerve fibers when the latter respond to low-frequency stimuli.

A majority but not all neurons encountered in the anteroventral nucleus exhibit phase-locked response. The response areas and other discharge characteristics of such neurons are very similar to those of auditory nerve fibers and we are uncertain at the present time whether any reliable signs of transformation can be proven to exist. Because of this similarity one may wonder whether our records from the anteroventral nucleus might actually have been obtained from terminals of acoustic nerve fibers. For several reasons, we think, this was not the case. First, there is often recorded preceding the spike a complex waveform which is reasonably interpreted as a presynaptic event. Secondly, it would be difficult to understand how our relatively large indium microelectrode with a tip of some 5 to 7 μ could routinely record potentials from a nerve terminal and remain in contact with it for many hours. Thirdly, we often record simultaneously two easily distinguishable spikes which militates against their being derived from auditory fiber terminals. Finally, we occasionally observe negative potentials with a strikingly short rise-time, so short that the discharges are hardly audible and require an upper cut off frequency well in excess of 10 kHz for undistorted recording. Such potentials are phase-locked but they usually disappear after a short time. It seems possible that these latter potentials may derive, in fact, from nerve terminals.

While we thus believe that most of our records stem from anteroventral cells, the uncertainty as to the exact source of the discharges does not raise any serious physiological problem for the purposes of the present study. For, if we record the phase-locked potentials from anteroventral cells we obviously observe cochlear output faithfully relayed at least as far as its time structure is concerned; on the other hand, if records should stem from nerve terminals we observe this output directly before transformation.

The essential reason for selecting the anteroventral cells as a source of information about the cochlear output was the ease with which we can maintain an anteroventral neuron under observation for many hours. Since we felt that a large number of measurements on the same neuron is essential to gain better insight into the previously observed nonlinear behavior of auditory nerve fibres, an extensive examination of the phase-locked responses of anteroventral neurons seemed potentially rewarding.

The main objective of this study was thus to determine - with a degree of detail not attained in auditory nerve fibers - how the amplitudes of the two primaries of a two-tone complex interact when the sound pressure level of one or both of them is varied.

For each neuron we first determined its response area in the form of iso-sound-pressure contours. Guided by this knowledge, appropriate frequencies were selected and delivered at different sound pressure levels, both as single pure tones and in combination as a complex periodic sound. The latter consisted always of two primaries locked precisely in some ratio of small integers. Stimuli were usually 5 or 10 seconds in duration, often repeated to generate a fairly large sample. All measurements were done on the resultant period histograms. By matching the shape of the histograms an effective stimulating waveform was constructed since it is our belief that the time structure of the response reflects to a reasonable approximation unidirectional elevations of such a waveform. The latter was always a combination of two sinusoids of the given frequencies; we have expressed the amplitudes of the primaries in terms of the heights of the two sinusoids.

The center line for the constructed waveform was made either to coincide with the abscissa of the histogram or it was moved above or below it as suggested by a given set of data. However, the position of the center line of the waveform, once chosen, was usually kept constant for all data from the same neuron even though some error is probably introduced by such a procedure.

The main results are as follows:

(1) When a complex periodic sound is presented and the sound pressure levels of the two component primaries are adjusted so that one of them dominates the response, it is then always possible to make the other primary dominant by increasing its sound pressure level. The only restrictions are that each primary, when presented alone, must produce an undistorted response and the fixed sound pressure level should not be so high that the necessary sound pressure levels for the other primary cannot be delivered.

Significantly, the level of the discharge rate provides no restrictions. The statement holds true both for those (fairly rare) neurons whose discharge rate is hardly changed from spontaneous level by variations of stimulus strength as well as for all other neurons whose discharge rate is a function of the sound pressure level until the saturation discharge rate is reached. Specifically, it matters not at all if both primaries are at a sound pressure level that greatly exceeds the level sufficient to cause saturation rate. It is still true that the effective stimulating amplitude of either component can be reduced to a small value merely by increasing the sound pressure level of the other component.

(2) In synthesizing the waveform for a complex

periodic sound it is advantageous to enter as one
component a waveform which has the same amplitude
and essentially the same phase angle as the sinusoid
which matches the response to one primary when it is
presented alone. We have found that the waveform of
the second primary must then be given an amplitude
which is either equal to or smaller than the amplitude of the waveform which matches this primary when
it is delivered alone.

(3) Since such matchings can be done consistently
when the sound pressure level of one primary is
gradually raised in small steps, one is lead to
assume that one component frequency, if sufficiently
intense, either may attenuate the other component in
the stimulating waveform or may act as if it did.
The decrease in amplitude of one primary caused by
the presence of the other in the complex periodic
sound can be expressed in decibels and we propose to
use it as a measure of the <u>attenuating or damping
power</u> of the primary whose amplitude is undiminished.
If there is no amplitude diminution the attenuating
powers of both primaries are equal, either because
both are at zero level (which is often the case at
low sound pressure levels) or because the attenuating
power of one primary reached the level of that of the
other. In either case the amplitudes of both primaries as established for the tones alone simply add
to produce a matching waveform for the complex periodic sound.

(4) Some limited generalizations seem justified by
the data at hand. Thus: A. At any moderate sound
pressure level the attenuating power is probably
greatest at or near the best frequency of the neuron.
B. One factor which may determine the value of attenuating power of a given frequency is the distance
of its point of maximal amplitude on the cochlear
partition from the locus of the best frequency.
C. When a complex periodic sound is presented and
the sound pressure level of both primaries is successively augmented but with the intensity ratio maintained constant, the attenuating power of the originally less efficient frequency rises faster that that
of the other primary when absolute sound pressure
levels become high. D. For some neurons within limited frequency and intensity ranges the attenuating
power of a component frequency in a complex periodic

sound can be predicted fairly closely by examining responses to this tone alone as its sound pressure level is raised in small steps from threshold to saturation level. For any given step the attenuating power is about equal to the deficit, expressed in decibels, between the growth of amplitude and the increase in sound pressure level. E. A frequency can have an attenuating power at a sound pressure level at which it is quite ineffective in producing spikes when it is presented alone.

(5) There is a need to differentiate between threshold for spike discharges for a given frequency and the threshold for interaction of this frequency in the complex periodic sound. The latter can be defined as the lowest sound pressure level at which a given frequency measureably affects the time structure and spike counts in a response to a complex periodic sound. Threshold for interaction can be at least some 20 to 30 decibels lower than the discharge threshold.

(6) The number of spikes produced by a complex periodic sound seems to depend essentially on the magnitude of the component waveforms and how they combine in phase. The magnitude of each component in turn depends on the effectiveness of the respective component in the response area and the relation of its attenuating power to the attenuating power of the other component. Thus a frequency at the margin of the response area which is only slightly effective in producing spikes may drastically reduce the spike count to a complex periodic sound in comparison with the count produced by a more efficient primary acting alone if the attenuation power of the marginal frequency is higher than that of the more efficient primary.

DISCUSSION

ZWISLOCKI: If this suppression is not neural, what is it?

ROSE: Mechanical, as a first guess.

ZWISLOCKI: Well, I do not see how it could be mechanical but I see how it could be neural.

ROSE: There are great difficulties in considering it neural.

ZWISLOCKI: Could not all this have to do with the so-called relative refractiveness and the probability of firing? Sometimes it is very difficult to distinguish the sinusoidal shapes from some kind of probability curve, maybe a little skewed, and especially when you are in the range of saturation. Then, if you wanted to explain this strictly on the basis of linearity or nonlinearity of the system, you would expect some peak clipping. You do not get any peak clipping. On the other hand, if you think in terms of probability and in terms of relative refractoriness, I think, it is possible to make a reasonable model to explain your results.

GREEN: Did I not see in the last graphs that the second tone actually turned the fiber off?

ROSE: It was not zero but 3 spikes, which is close enough to zero.

GREEN: Who is making all of those fibers refractory, those three spikes?

ROSE: Certainly, at 19 spikes per 10 seconds, there are still 2 spikes per second which is quite a devilish refractory period.

THE FREQUENCY SELECTIVITY OF THE COCHLEA

E.F. Evans[1] and J.P. Wilson

University of Keele
Staffordshire
England

1. Introduction

The problem of the frequency selectivity of the cochlea has in recent years generated considerable experimental and theoretical activity. Hitherto, the correspondence between the broad frequency selectivity of the cochlear partition observed by von Békésy (1944) and the broadly tuned frequency threshold curves obtained in the first successful measurements in the cochlear nerve (of the guinea pig) by Tasaki (1954), had led to the conclusion that the poor mechanical frequency selectivity of the cochlea represented the input to the central nervous system (e.g., von Békésy, 1969, 1970; Whitfield, 1967). Measurements on cochlear nerve fibers of the cat, however, by Katsuki et al. (1958), Kiang et al.(1965, 1967) de Boer (1969) and Evans et al. (1970) indicated that frequency threshold curves ("tuning curves") could be obtained which were very substantially sharper than the frequency response functions of von Békésy. With the advent of Mössbauer techniques, allowing measurements to be made of the frequency response of the basal end of the guinea pig cochlea (Johnstone and Boyle, 1967, Johnstone et al., 1970), and new measurements on single cochlear nerve fibers in the guinea pig (Evans 1970a, 1972a, b), it has been possible to make quantitative comparisons of the mechanical and neural cochlear frequency selectivities in the same species (e.g., Evans, 1971, 1972a, b). These indicated that the guinea pig cochlear nerve fibers could be as sharply tuned as those of the cat, and that a discrepancy of up to an order of magnitude existed between the relatively broadly tuned basilar membrane response and the much more sharply tuned

---

[1] Medical Research Council Research Group.

cochlear fibers. More recent Mössbauer measurements of basilar membrane motion in the squirrel monkey by Rhode (1971) have led some to conclude that there is no real discrepancy between the mechanical and neural data (e.g., Johnstone and Sellick, 1972). The present paper therefore attempts to review the present situation. In addition, it will compare measures of the frequency selectivity of the cochlear nerve with certain psychophysical data relating to the frequency selectivity of the auditory system.

The neurophysiological data discussed here were obtained from two series of studies on single fibers of the cochlear nerve, in the guinea pig (Evans, 1970a, b, 1972a, b), and in the cat in collaboration with J. Rosenberg (Evans et al., 1970, 1971, Evans and Wilson 1971, Wilson and Evans, 1971). Full details of recording technique are to be found in Evans (1972b). Briefly, using ultrafine micropipettes, recordings were made from several hundred single cochlear fibers in the pentobarbitone anesthetized preparation. Special attention was paid to maintaining the physiological condition of the animals, of particular importance in the guinea pig. Fibers were positively identified on grounds of latency, spike polarity and histology. Stimuli were delivered by condenser microphone driver in a closed system, and stimulus levels monitored by a probe tube microphone at the tympanic membrane. Frequency threshold curves (FTCs) were determined in two ways. In the guinea pig, the classical method was adopted, using visual and aural criteria of threshold of response to gated tonal stimuli. In the cat, the FTCs were determined in great detail by a semi-automatic plotting method. The stimuli in each case were pure tones of 100 msec duration and 5 msec rise and fall times, with repetition rate 4/sec. All FTCs were corrected for the frequency response of the sound system to threshold dB SPL at the tympanic membrane and, with the exception of those in Fig. 1, in the closed bulla condition.

2. Neural versus mechanical frequency selectivity of the cochlea: cochlear sharpening

Fig. 1 illustrates the problem facing attempts to reconcile the mechanical and neural frequency selectivities of the cochlea. The lower curves, arbitrarily arranged in the sound level dimension to meet the abscissa, are from measurements of the basilar mem-

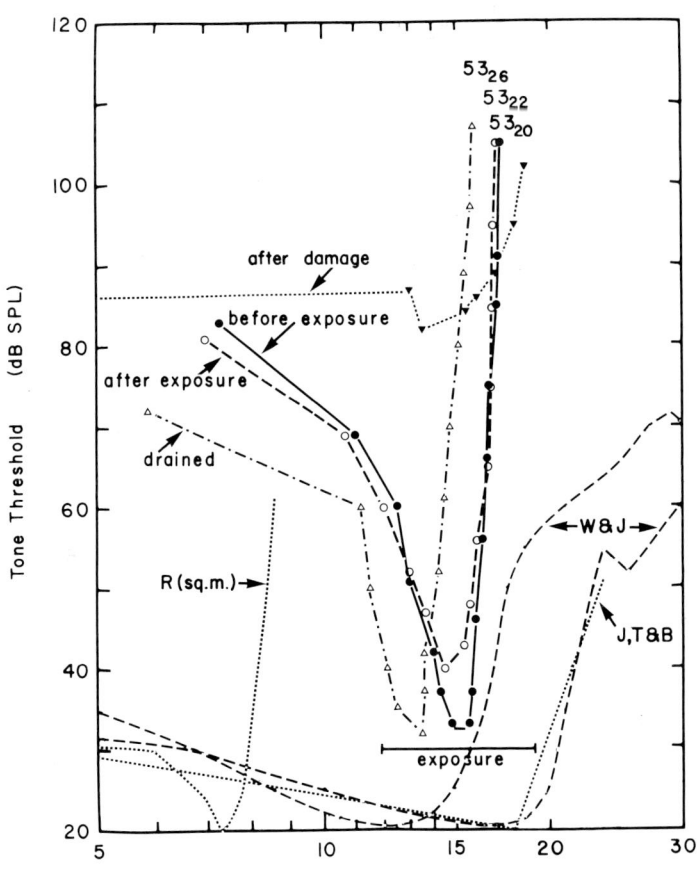

Fig. 1 Comparison of neural FTCs and mechanical frequency response functions

Lower curves: frequency response of basilar membrane at four positions, in squirrel monkey and guinea pig, expressed in terms of stimulus level required to maintain a constant arbitrary amplitude of vibration.
R: from Rhode (1971) Fig. 7, 0.003 μm criterion (see text) squirrel monkey, 7.4 kHz optimal frequency.
W & J: from Wilson and Johnstone (1972), guinea pig, 12 and 17 kHz.
J, T & B: from Johnstone et al. (1970), guinea pig, 18 kHz.   (cont'd)

(Fig. 1, cont'd)
Upper curves: frequency threshold curves of 4 cochlear fibers in the guinea pig, corrected to SPL at the tympanic membrane in the open bulla condition, (Evans, 1970b).
Solid curve: fiber 53_{20}, obtained with cochlea intact.
Dashed curve: fiber 53_{22}, obtained after opening scala tympani of first turn and removing round window ("exposure" indicates approximate range of optimal frequencies subserved by exposed basilar membrane).
Dotted and dashed line: fiber 53_{26}, obtained after draining perilymph from exposed region of scala tympani.
Dotted line: fiber obtained after slight damage to spiral lamina.

brane mechanical frequency response, by Rhode (1971) in the squirrel monkey, and in the guinea pig by Johnstone et al. (1970), and Wilson and Johnstone (1972; and to be published). Above these curves are plotted the FTCs of cochlear nerve fibers, one (solid line) obtained in the intact cochlea and three (interrupted lines) under the same conditions of opening of the basal turn of the cochlea necessary for the mechanical measurements of Johnstone et al. (1970), Wilson and Johnstone (1972), and (Evans, 1970b). The similarity between the curves of fibres 53_{20}, 53_{22}, and 53_{26} indicates that opening the scala vestibuli of the first cochlear turn and draining the perilymph do not significantly alter the frequency response characteristics of the cochlea. (The anomalous fourth curve will be referred to later).

These FTCs are characteristic of cochlear fibers in cat, guinea pig and monkey, with characteristic frequencies (CFs) above about 3 kHz. On a logarithmic frequency scale they are asymmetrical, with cut-offs rising steeply on either side of the minimum threshold at least for the first 40 dB or so, but thereafter the slope of the low frequency cut-off abruptly decreases to less than 10 dB/octave. The high frequency cut-off is considerably steeper than the low frequency cut-off but, unlike the latter, it continues to steepen with stimulus intensity, in some cases approaching slope values of 1000 dB/octave.

The slope values of the mechanical frequency response functions, on the other hand, are substantially lower, particularly on the low frequency side.

The mechanical frequency response taken from Rhode's data is substantially different from the other basilar membrane curves shown in Fig. 1. Unlike Johnstone et al. (1970) and Wilson and Johnstone (1972), Rhode found significant non-linearities in the basilar membrane response with signal levels of 70 dB SPL and above. This means that the slopes of the low and high frequency cut-offs of his curves depend on signal level and whether a constant SPL or amplitude of vibration is specified. Thus, for constant SPL, Rhode gives values of about 10 dB/octave and 50 - 150 dB/octave respectively, which are consistent with the data of Johnstone et al. and Wilson and Johnstone. However, if a constant amplitude criterion (e.g., 0.003 μm, Fig. 7 of Rhode, 1971) is used for deriving the filter function, the sharper curve illustrated in Fig. 1 is obtained, with slopes of about 30 and 250 dB/oct. respectively.

More broadly tuned cochlear nerve functions can be obtained if the cochlear partition is interfered with, as in the uppermost plot of Fig. 1. In addition, similarly broadly shaped FTCs have been obtained in the guinea pig cochlear nerve under conditions where the cochlear blood supply was inadequate through low systemic blood pressure or partial constriction of the internal auditory artery, and where the round window whole nerve (AP) responses had a pathologically high threshold. The frequency response of these pathological FTCs resembles those of the basilar membrane.

Fig. 2 allows a quantitative comparison to be made between the slopes of the low frequency cut-offs of several hundred cochlear nerve FTCs obtained from cat, guinea pig, and squirrel monkey (derived from the neural firing rate versus tone frequency curves of Rose et al. (1971) using near threshold isorate criteria), and of the frequency response functions obtained for the cochlear partition by von Békésy (1944), Rhode, Johnstone et al, and Wilson and Johnstone (as in Fig. 1). The slopes in each case were computed for the region of the cut-off between 5 and 25 dB of the tip. The slope values for the cochlear

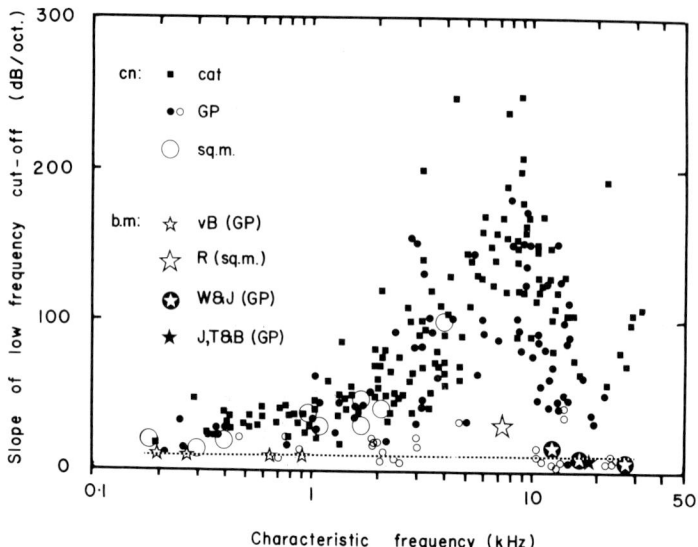

Fig. 2 Comparison of slope of low-frequency cut-off between neural FTCs and mechanical frequency response functions.

Slope values (in dB/octave) measured over the region 5-25 dB above minimum threshold for several hundred cochlear nerve fibers (cn) of cat (Evans and Wilson, 1971), guinea pig (GP: Evans, 1972b), and squirrel monkey (sq.m.: from Rose et al., 1971), and plotted against their characteristic frequencies. Small open circles: values from pathological G.P. cochleas (see text). Analogous values from basilar membrane data of von Békésy (1944: vB), Johnstone et al. (1970: J, T & B), and Wilson and Johnstone (1972: W & J) in the guinea pig, and Rhode (1971: R) in the squirrel monkey.

fiber populations increase with characteristic frequency, reaching maximum values of between 100 - 300 dB/octave at CFs of 5 - 15 kHz. The slope values for the mechanical data, on the other hand, remain below 10 dB/octave, with the exception of the point derived from Rhode's data (30 dB/octave, restricted to 10 dB of the tip, see Fig. 1). Thus, with the exception of the low values for the cochlear fibers obtained in pathological guinea pig cochleas (small open circles; vd. above) the neural low frequency slopes are up to 50 times steeper than the mechanical values.

Analogous measurements of the high frequency slopes of cat (Evans and Wilson, 1971) and guinea pig (Evans, 1972a, b) cochlear nerve fiber FTCs gave slope values ranging from about 100 to 600 dB/octave at the optimal CF (8 - 10 kHz) compared with 100 - 200 dB/octave for the analogous values of the mechanical functions. These comparisons, made within 25 dB of the tip of the frequency response functions, do not take into account the severe discrepancy which exists between the slopes of the high frequency cut-offs at higher threshold stimulus levels. In the case of the cochlear nerve fibers, the slopes become progressively steeper; in the studies of Rhode (1971) and Wilson and Johnstone (1972) the basilar membrane cut-offs reach a plateau at 40 dB or so above the tip (see Fig. 1).

A common and convenient way of expressing the relative sharpness of the FTCs is to use the "$Q_{10}dB$" value, that is, the CF divided by the bandwidth at 10 dB above minimum threshold (Fig. 3). Again, these values reach a maximum for fibers of intermediate CF (about 8 kHz) where a range of values of between 4 to 10 is obtained. With the exception of fibers from pathological guinea pig cochleas (small open circles), these values are up to an order of magnitude greater than those of the basilar membrane.

In all these comparisons, the basilar membrane data of Rhode from the squirrel monkey are inconsistent with the other mechanical data. As has been mentioned above, this discrepancy derives from the non-linearity encountered by Rhode at sound levels of 70 dB SPL and above. Such a non-linearity was specifically not found by von Békésy or by Johnstone and colleagues, or by Wilson and Johnstone (1972). The latter authors, in particular, using a very sensitive capacitive probe device, were able to measure basilar membrane motion amplitudes in healthy guinea pig cochleas with sound levels as low as 40 dB SPL. They were able to demonstrate non-linearities only at sound levels in excess of 110 dB SPL and then only at frequencies above the peak sensitivity. Clearly there is a need for further measurements of the basi-

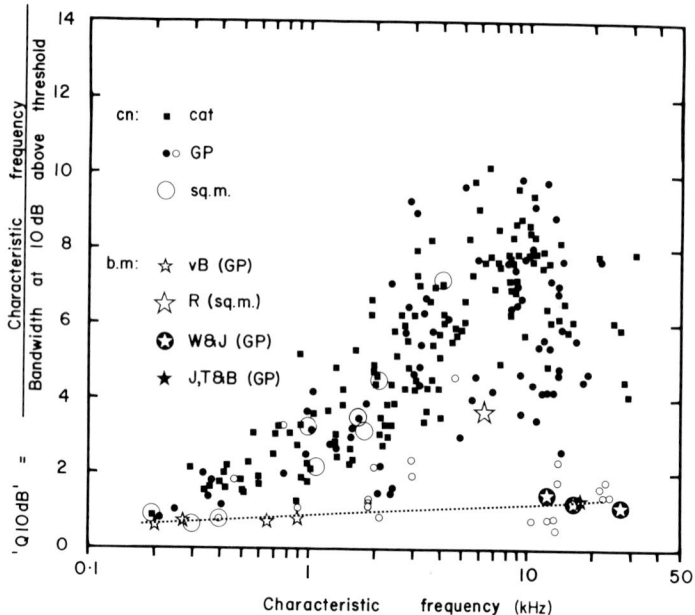

Fig. 3 Comparison of relative sharpness (Q_{10} dB) of neural and mechanical frequency response functions.

Values for several hundred cochlear nerve fibers of cat, guinea pig and squirrel monkey compared with those from basilar membrane data. Symbols and sources as in Fig. 2.

lar membrane motion, particularly in the intermediate frequency region of the cochlea, to settle this issue. This discrepancy notwithstanding, the data of Figs. 1 to 3 indicate that a considerable degree of extra filtering is required in the guinea pig, squirrel monkey and cat cochlea to account for the observed neural frequency selectivity. Other, less likely, possibilities of course remain, namely (a) that all the existing measurements of the basilar membrane response are grossly in error; (b) that the motion of the basilar membrane does not represent the effective mechanical input to the hair cell transducer mechanism, but that other mechanical (more highly frequency selective) structures are involved.

3. Mechanism of frequency sharpening: evidence for a "second filter".

Many mechanisms for cochlear sharpening have been proposed, ranging from mechanical processes (e.g., Huggins and Licklider, 1951) through innervation pattern models (e.g., Nieder, 1971) to lateral inhibition (e.g., von Békésy, 1960, 1970, Furman and Frishkopf, 1964). No model yet proposed appears to account entirely satisfactorily for the physiological and anatomical data available. Whatever the exact mechanism may turn out to be, evidence is accumulating which would implicate a second sharply tuned filter existing beyond the relatively broadly tuned filter of the basilar membrane (Evans, 1972a, b; Wilson and Johnstone, 1972).

Such a two-filter system was first proposed to account for certain properties of the cochlear combination tone, $2f_1-f_2$, and the two-tone suppression observed in the cochlear nerve (Goldstein, 1967, 1970, Pfeiffer 1970, Smoorenburg, 1972). In these cases an "essential" (i.e., level independent) non-linear process was envisaged to be "sandwiched" between a broadly tuned input (basilar membrane) filter and a sharply tuned "second" filter.

Circumstantial evidence for a sharply tuned second filter has been obtained from the above-mentioned studies of the cochlear nerve, particularly in the guinea pig. Firstly, both cat and guinea pig cochlear nerve show a wide variation in frequency selectivity from fiber to fiber. Thus, in the same animal and between fibers of common CF, differences in cutoff slope and bandwidth up to a ratio of 5:1 may be found (vd. Figs. 2 and 3) which cannot be accounted for by experimental error. Secondly, in the guinea pig, there has been the finding of a population of high threshold, broadly tuned fibers, in cochleas with evidence of circulatory insufficiency (Evans, 1972a, b). The broad tuning of these fibers resembles that of the basilar membrane (Figs 1, 2 and 3). Occasional fibers with similar properties have been found in the basal turn of apparently normal guinea pig cochleas, interspersed with low threshold sharply tuned fibers (Evans, 1972b; see section 5). If the narrow frequency selectivity of the cochlear nerve merely reflected sharp mechanical tuning of the basilar membrane we should expect the tuning properties of the cochlear nerve (a) to be uniformly distributed, i.e., to be similar for all fibers originating from the same portion of the cochlea, and (b) not to be so severely degraded by influences such as anoxia. On the contrary, the data suggest that each cochlear fiber is preceded by a second, sharply tuned but physiologically vulnerable filter "private" to that fiber.

It is an interesting question whether the differences in frequency selectivity can be related to the minimum threshold of the fibers concerned, after excluding the pathologically high threshold broadly-tuned fibers. Unfortunately, there are insufficient data to conclusively answer the question in fibers of common CF in the same animal, although the trend in one guinea pig yielding some of the narrowest bandwidths found in the present experiments is in the direction that the sharper the FTC, the lower the threshold. Pooling the data from all animals, an approximate

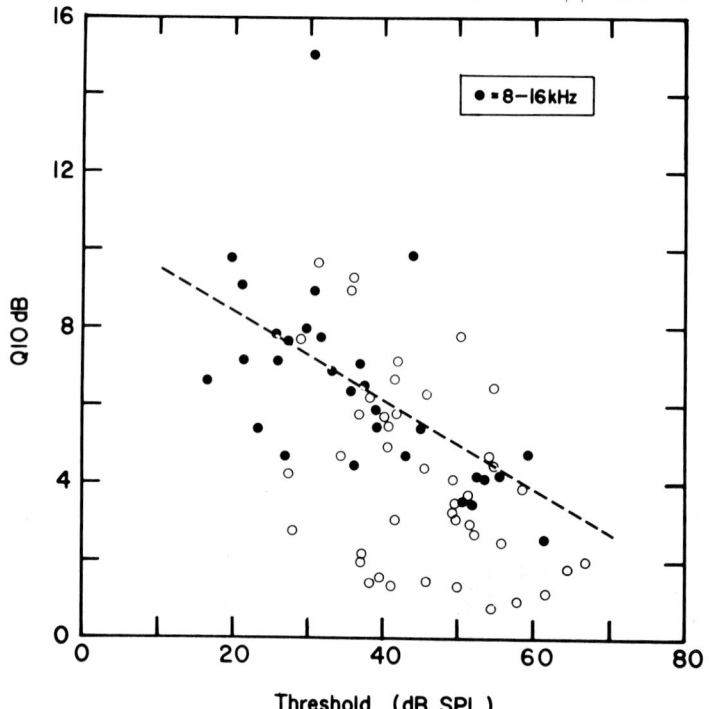

Fig. 4 Relative sharpness (Q_{10} dB) versus minimum threshold of cochlear fiber FTCs in guinea pig. (cont'd)

(Fig. 4, cont'd)
Cochlear fiber population of Evans (1972b) excluding fibers with pathologically high thresholds (see text). Filled circles: fibers with characteristic frequencies limited to the octave 8-16 kHz. Dashed line: regression of Q_{10} dB on threshold for solid points.

inverse relationship appears, as shown in Fig. 4. However, such a relationship would be expected on account of the roughly similar dependence of the two variables on characteristic frequency (Evans, 1972b). Limiting the data, therefore, to fibers with CFs in the octave 8-16 kHz, where there exists the greatest range of Q_{10} dB and threshold values, one obtains the solid points of Fig. 4. The regression of Q_{10} dB on threshold had a negative slope of 0.12 which was significantly different from zero ($p<0.005$; Evans, 1972b). Reducing the sample further to match the high and low halves of the Q_{10} dB population for characteristic frequency did not significantly alter the regression. These observations are consistent with an active filtering process such as one employing positive feedback.

Fig. 5 summarizes a hypothetical scheme incorporating such a second filter in an attempt to account for the existing mechanical, cochlear microphonic and cochlear nerve data. There is evidence that the intermediate non-linearity responsible for the $2f_1-f_2$ combination tone (the essential non-linearity of Goldstein, 1967, 1970) may not be closely coupled to the basilar membrane. Using the capacitive probe technique, Wilson and Johnstone (1972) found that the level of the $2f_1-f_2$ distortion component in the basilar membrane vibration was more than 40 dB below the level predicted from psychophysical and **physiological** results (Goldstein 1967, 1970, Goldstein and Kiang, 1968), although admittedly in a different frequency region. Similarly, Dallos (1969) could not find a component in the differentially recorded cochlear microphonic (CM) which could account for the level and properties of the $2f_1-f_2$ distortion product hitherto assumed to be generated by interaction of the primaries and distributed along the basilar membrane to the site of the transduction. The correspondence between the amplitude and phase aspects of Dallos' differentially recorded CM data (Dallos, this volume) and the basilar membrane data of Wilson and

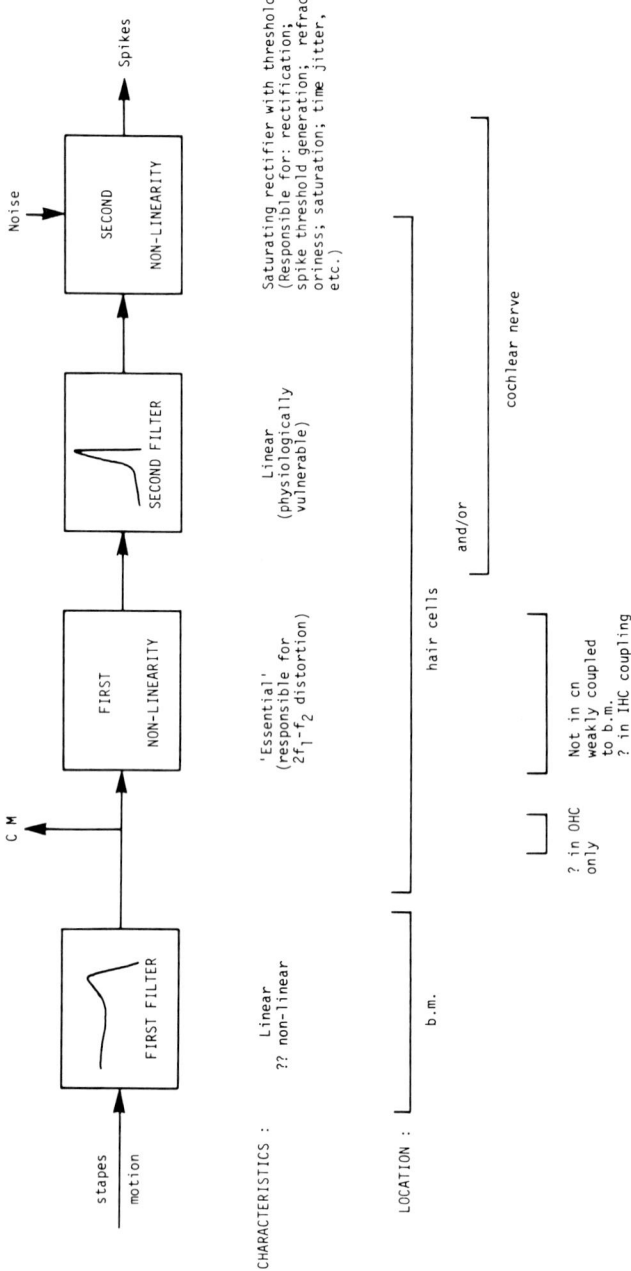

Fig. 5 Summary scheme for arrangement, characteristics and location of functional mechanisms between stapes motion and cochlear nerve response.

Johnstone (1972) further suggests that the CM reflects the basilar membrane vibration amplitude and is generated prior to the essential non-linearity. Contrary to the mechanical data, however, the CM amplitude saturates at modest sound levels. The recent data from Dallos et al. (1972) open up the exciting possibility that the CM may reflect the activity of the outer hair cells only and that the inner hair cells may be coupled less directly to the basilar membrane and reflect the velocity of basilar membrane displacement. Because Spoendlin (1969, 1971) has shown that the great majority of afferent cochlear nerve fibers innervate inner hair cells only, it becomes thereby possible to envisage how such grossly different behavior can be exhibited by CM and cochlear nerve fibers without relegating the CM to the category of an epiphenomenon, particularly in view of the correspondence between the properties of the two in other respects (Pfeiffer and Molnar, 1970). Goldstein (1972) has summarized the evidence for the stimulus-like combination tone $2f_1-f_2$, and therefore the essential non-linearity, being generated prior to the cochlear nerve impulse generating mechanism.

The location of the second filter has few constraints at present, however. The considerations of the preceding paragraph allow the possible intervention of an hydromechanical "second filter" between the basilar membrane outer hair cell complex and inner hair cell transducer as suggested by Tonndorf (e.g., 1970) and Steele (pers. comm.). On the other hand, it is not easy to see how such a mechanism could be physiologically vulnerable. Hence a more likely (or less unlikely) site would be in the hair cell/hair cell innervation, perhaps involving inner → outer hair cell interactions.

Clearly more experimental information is required on the nature of the second filter. The next section summarizes a series of experiments made in collaboration with J. Rosenberg (Evans et al., 1970, 1971, Evans and Wilson, 1971, Wilson and Evans, 1971) to examine the possibilities that the second filter might be non-linear in nature and might involve lateral inhibition.

4. Nature of second filter

4.1 The filter does not appear to be non-linear

Furman and Frishkopf (1964) have advanced non-linear inhibition as a possible sharpening mechanism for the cochlea. A simple test for linearity in a filtering process is to compare the response of the filter to pure tone and broadband noise signals. The response of a linear filter to a broadband signal is equal to the sum of the responses to the individual frequency components. The ratio between the power transmitted by the filter from a pure tone at the optimal pass frequency and from a broad band noise spectrum of equal overall power is simply:

$$10 \log_{10} \frac{\text{Bandwidth of noise signal}}{\text{Effective bandwidth of the filter}} \text{ in dB.} \quad (1)$$

The effective bandwidth of a linear filter is approximately the half-power ("3 dB down") bandwidth, but can be derived exactly by integrating the area under the attenuation curve expressed in linear power versus linear frequency co-ordinates (e.g., Fig. 6). This paradigm can be applied to cochlear nerve fibers in spite of their manifestly non-linear response (i.e., the existence of a threshold and saturation, etc., expressed by the "second non-linearity" of Fig. 5) by utilizing a constant response criterion for comparing the relative effectiveness of tone and noise stimulation. In practice, the FTC was determined in great detail, especially around the tip, and immediately afterwards the threshold to a broadband noise stimulus was measured, using the same criterion for threshold. Both of these were done semi-automatically. The decibel difference between the noise threshold and the threshold for a tone at the CF is plotted for 118 fibers of the cat cochlear nerve with CFs ranging from 0.27 - 31 kHz in the upper section of Fig. 7 (M values). Treating the FTC as a linear filter attenuation curve (Fig. 6), its effective bandwidth was computed. From this the threshold difference between noise and tone signals was calculated according to the expression above. This value was computed for each cochlear fiber and the results are shown in the middle section of Fig. 7 (C values). In

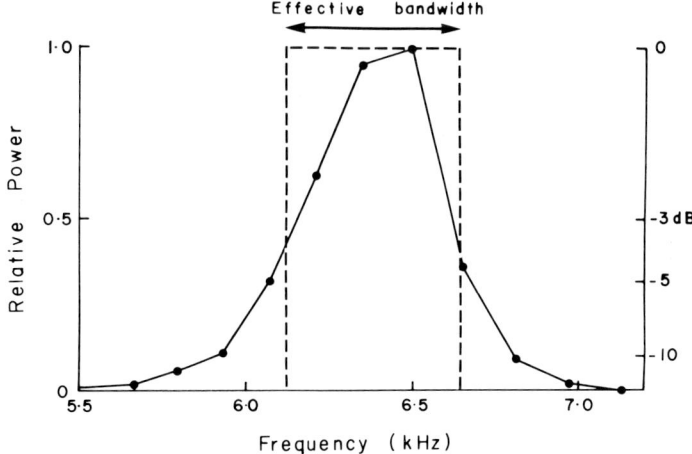

Fig. 6   Cochlear nerve FTC considered as linear filter function

Plot of FTC from cat as attenuation function in linear relative power and linear frequency co-ordinates. "Effective bandwidth" represents the width of a rectangular filter function of equal area, from which the response to a broad-band noise signal can be calculated.

the lower section of Fig. 7 the differences between the corresponding measured and computed values are plotted. There is reasonably close clustering of the data points about zero. This suggests that, within the limits of experimental error (compounded in many cases by transient shifts in threshold during the measurements) and within the rather limited dynamic range of the method (10-20 dB), the overall frequency filtering characteristics of the cochlea (and by implication the second filter) act as a linear filter of bandwidth consistent with the characteristics of the pure tone FTC.

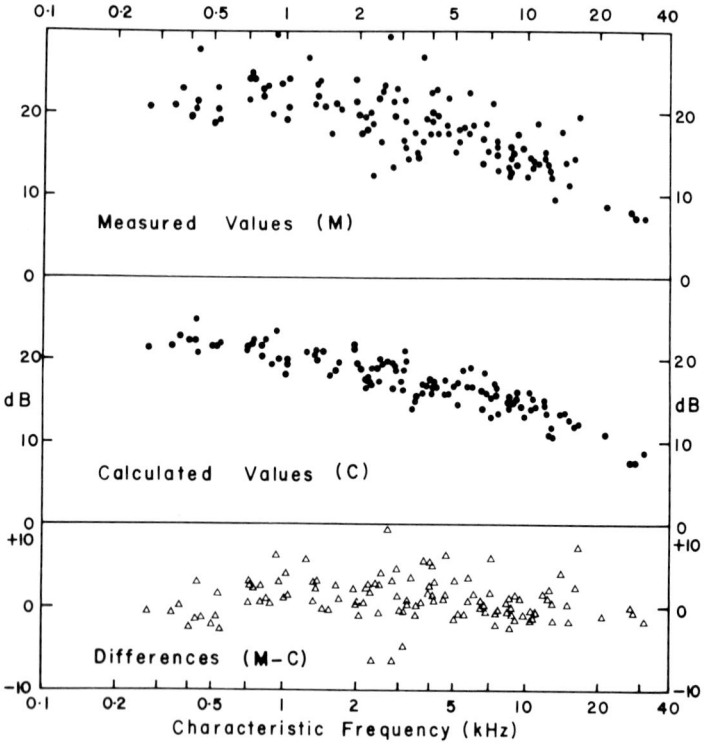

Fig. 7 Difference between noise and tone thresholds for 118 cochlear fibers from 5 cats. (Evans and Wilson, 1971).

(M): Measured values in dB of level of noise threshold above tone threshold at CF.
(C): Corresponding values computed from FTC of each fiber (bandwidth of noise: 21.5 kHz).
(M-C): Differences between corresponding measured and calculated values.

This derivation is based on r.m.s. power measurement, whereas it is possible that the neural threshold may depend on peak amplitude. Simulation of a linear filter followed by a peak amplitude detector indicated that an error of about 4 dB could be introduced. However, the error became negligible if broadband or low-pass filtered noise was added at the detector stage to simulate physiological levels of "spontaneous discharge" (i.e., from 0-100 spikes/sec).

An additional test of linearity is afforded by the second series of experiments, designed to examine the cochlear filtering process for evidence of lateral inhibition.

4.2 Lateral inhibition is not involved

Campbell, Robson and colleagues (e.g., Campbell and Robson, 1968, Campbell et al., 1969) have measured the response of the visual system to luminosity gratings. They obtained maximal responses when the spacing of the grating corresponded to the geometry of the inhibitory surround. We have utilized an acoustic grating stimulus in psychophysical experiments (Wilson 1967, 1970) and, by analogy with Campbell's experiments, used it to look for evidence of lateral inhibition in the cochlear filtering process (Wilson and Evans, 1971). This acoustic "grating" is generated by mixing a uniform broadband noise signal with a delayed version of itself. A spectrum is thereby produced with a sinusoidal distribution of energy, i.e., with peaks and valleys of energy spaced on a linear frequency scale according to the delay (see thin solid outlines in Fig. 8, and note linear power and frequency co-ordinates). Inversion of the phase of the delayed noise produces an inverted spectral envelope (interrupted outlines, Fig. 8).

The principle of the experiment is to measure how well a cochlear fiber can differentiate between the peaks and valleys of differently spaced spectra. The FTC was first plotted in great detail and the threshold for broadband noise determined, as above. The mean level of the grating stimulus was set about 10dB

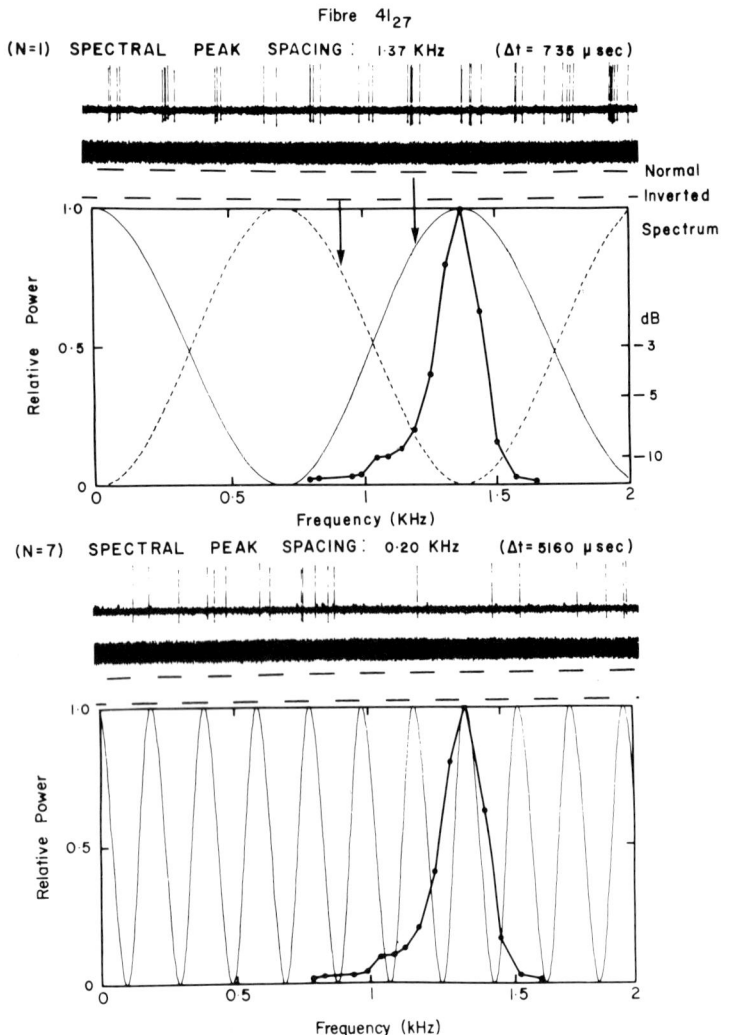

Fig. 8 Determination of the response of a cat cochlear nerve fiber to two acoustic gratings (comb-filtered noise).

(a) Upper half. Widely spaced acoustic grating. Thin continuous sinusoid: evelope of "normal" noise spectrum, with first peak coincident with CF of FTC (plotted as filter function as in Fig. 6: thick   (cont'd)

(Fig. 8,cont'd) continuous line). Dashed sinusoid: envelope of "inverted" spectrum. Continuous film records: spike discharge pattern, waveform of signal, and alternation pattern of normal and inverted spectra at 5/sec., respectively. Note burst of spike discharge evoked during periods when peak of (normal) spectrum was coincident with the cochlear fiber CF.

(b) Lower half. Finely spaced acoustic grating. Peak spacing 0.2 kHz. Envelope of normal spectrum only shown (thin sinusoid); otherwise as in (a). Note moderate rate of discharge unrelated to alternation of normal and inverted spectra.

above the noise threshold level. The delay of the noise addition was set at $1/CF$ so that the first energy peak of the spectrum lay at the CF of the unit (Fig. 8a). This produced, as expected, a brisk spike discharge response (continuous film record of Fig. 8a). After 100 msec the spectrum was inverted for an identical period so that a spectral "valley" lay over the CF of the FTC, producing only a small response. The spectrum was alternated in this manner 5 times a second, thus producing alternating bursts of response. The ratio of spike discharge for normal versus the inverted spectra was determined over a 10 sec period of alternation. The time delay was then increased successively to $2/CF$, $3/CF$ etc., to enable firing ratios to be obtained at progressively finer spacings of the acoustic gratings. Eventually a point was reached (Fig. 8b) where the fiber could not distinguish between the peaks and valleys of the spectrum, and the firing ratio corresponding to the spectral alternations became unity. The FTC filter had reached the limit of its resolving power. Next, the fiber was subjected to alternating levels of noise (the steps ranging from 3 to 20 dB) at the same mean signal level and repetition rate as in the grating situation, and the firing ratios determined as a function of the magnitude of the noise steps. This allowed the firing ratios obtained under conditions of the grating stimulus to be converted into equivalent "contrasts" in dB.

On the basis that the cochlear fiber FTC represents

the filter function of a linear filter it is possible to compute the ratio of powers passed by such a filter from the normal and inverted spectra. This was done by computing the sum of the cross-multiplications between the attenuation function of the filter (solid outline at 1.37 kHz in Fig. 8a and b) and the respective normal and inverted spectral envelopes for each grating stimulus. Hence we derive a theoretical value of "contrast" for each spacing of the grating.

In Fig. 9 the results of such computations (filled

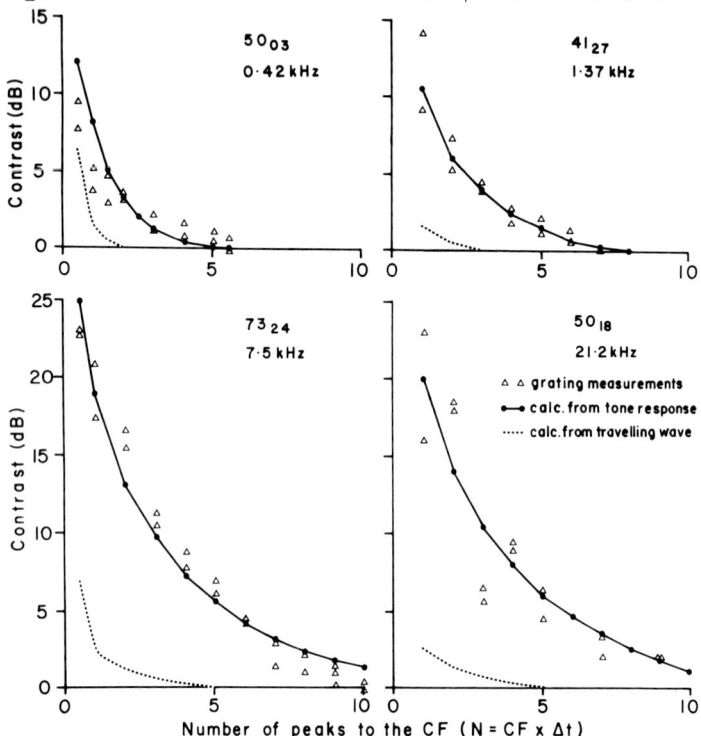

Fig. 9 Resolving power functions for 4 cat cochlear fibers.

Measured "contrasts" between normal and inverted acoustic grating spectra (open triangles), as a function of the spacing of the grating spectra, compared with values computed from the cochlear nerve FTC (continuous line and solid points) and compared with values derived from the (cont'd)

(Fig. 9, cont'd) appropriate basilar membrane frequency response (dotted lines). Abscissa denotes fineness of spacing of grating in terms of the number of peaks between zero frequency and the CF of the fiber. CF indicated in kHz to right of each plot.

circles and lines) are compared with the contrast ratios determined in the experiment (triangles) for 4 cochlear fibers of widely differing CF. These data are representative of comparisons which have been made on 38 cat cochlear fibers. The abscissa in each case represents the fineness of the grating pattern in terms of the number of peaks of the spectrum between zero frequency and the CF of the fiber (equivalent to the noise delay multiplied by the CF).

The close agreement between calculated and measured values at all spacings of the comb-filtered noise stimuli indicates again that the cochlear filter is acting as if it were a linear filter. Furthermore, such a comparison over all spacings is a sensitive test for lateral inhibition, which would be expected to reduce the response to widely spaced gratings and to enhance that to intermediate gratings (vd. Fig. 4.14 of Ratliff, 1965). Thus, we can exclude sharpening mechanisms involving linear lateral interaction.

For comparison, the interrupted curves in each case represent the response computed for the basilar membrane filter, and serve to emphasize the discrepancy between neural and mechanical selectivity.

4.3 The second filter is not likely to be level dependent

Both the above measures were taken within 10-20 dB of threshold. The question arises whether the conclusions can be justified for higher stimulus levels. Indeed, it could be concluded that the apparent broadening of the frequency response of cochlear fibers at high stimulus levels (shown in plots of the discharge rate as a function of frequency, Rose et al., 1971) indicates otherwise. However, this apparent broadening derives from the saturation of response and the limited dynamic range of the firing rate of cochlear fibers (second non-linearity of Fig. 5). In fact, if isorate contours (i.e., analogous plots to the FTCs but with higher rate criteria) are derived from the frequency versus discharge rate plots, these do not show any signs of systematic changes in bandwidth, at least within the range before saturation precludes accurate measurement (e.g., Sachs and Kiang, 1968, Evans, Rosenberg and Wilson, unpublished data; measurements on data of Rose et al., 1971). Furthermore, a few of our experiments with the acoustic gratings (b above) have been repeated at higher stimulus levels with similar results.

De Boer (e.g., 1969), using a technique of "reverse correlation" between the waveform of a wide band noise stimulus and the spike discharge pattern of cat cochlear fibers, has also shown that for frequencies up to the limit of phase-locking in the cochlear nerve (ca. 4 kHz) the cochlea behaved as if it were a linear filter with a comparable frequency response to that of the neural FTC. Our results with broad-band and acoustic grating stimuli extend this conclusion to frequencies and fibers with CFs above 4 kHz. De Boer (1969) claimed that the filter functions were largely independent of stimulus level, in one case over a range of 60 dB.

We may conclude, therefore, that at least over the dynamic range of cochlear fibers (30-50 dB), there is no evidence of changes in the characteristics of the cochlear filter with stimulus level.

4.4 Linear filtering in the face of non-linear processes in the cochlea

The question arises how the above findings can be reconciled with the many evidences for non-linearities in the cochlea (e.g., threshold and saturation of cochlear nerve response: Kiang et al, 1965, 1969; the combination tone $2f_1-f_2$: Goldstein 1967, 1970; two-tone suppression in the cochlear nerve: Sachs and Kiang 1968; combination click effects: Goblick and Pfeiffer 1969; etc.).

The methods of sections 4.1 and 4.2 above were designed to eliminate the effects of the non-linearities related to the spike generation process (i.e., the "second non-linearity" of Fig. 5). In section 4.1 this was effected by utilizing a constant response criterion for comparing the relative effectiveness of tone and noise stimulation. In section 4.2 the comparisons between measured and computed "contrasts" were made after appropriately correcting the nerve response for its level-dependent non-linearity.

The correlation method of de Boer (which gave rise to similar conclusions to those above) is also able to yield information on the nature of the cochlear filter independent of ensuing transducer/spike generator non-linearities (de Boer, 1968).

A problem is, however, raised by the non-linearities assumed for the present purposes to precede the second filter (i.e., the "first non-linearity" of Fig. 5), and to account for the combination tone $2f_1-f_2$, and possibly the two-tone suppression phenomenon (vd. section 3 above). In order to look specifically for evidence of two-tone suppression effects, a further experiment was carried out, combining the acoustic grating stimulus with a steady noise background in such a way that "two-tone" effects should have been emphasized (Wilson and Evans, to be published). No evidence of such effects was revealed, and the results again corresponded with the predictions from a linear filter model.

For the effects of the combination tone $2f_1-f_2$, it would appear that a portion of the energy of the primaries is transferred downwards on the frequency scale to the frequency $2f_1-f_2$. In the case of the broadband noise signal, it would seem reasonable to assume that an equal proportion of energy is shifted downwards throughout the spectrum. In the case of the acoustic grating signal, the effect would be to shift energy downwards from peak to peak throughout the spectrum. Thus, in both cases, the filter would "see" approximately the same energy distribution as if the combination components had not been generated.

It is not clear, however, why the effects of the two-tone suppression phenomenon do not appear in our results, unless the phenomenon is restricted to pure-tone stimuli.

We can therefore only conjecture at this stage that these phenomena are either (a) such that their effects are obscured by the nature of the stimuli we are using; (b) too weak to be observed under the conditions of our experiments; or (c) that the noise-like nature of our signals linearize the cochlear system. That the second interpretation may be the case is supported by the finding of Goldstein et al. (1971) that cat cochlear nerve FTC, phase, and latency data are interrelated in a manner similar to that which would be predicted for a linear filter system followed by a memory-less transducer.

5. Comparison of neural and psychophysical frequency selectivity

Wilson (Wilson and Evans, 1971) has made psychophysical measurements of the human frequency resolving power for acoustic gratings. Briefly, the subject's task was to decrease the spacing of an acoustic grating stimulus until he could no longer resolve the individual peaks, i.e., distinguish the signal from uniform noise. The limits of frequency resolving power were determined at a number of frequencies (by appropriate filtering of the grating signal) and are plotted as the interrupted line in Fig. 10. For com-

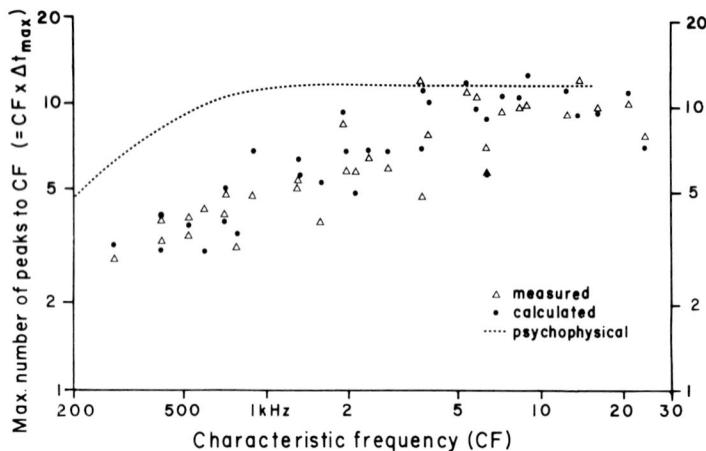

Fig. 10 Comparison of psychophysical and cat cochlear nerve fiber resolving powers for acoustic gratings.

Resolving power expressed as maximum number of peaks of acoustic grating stimulus (between zero frequency and frequency of measurement) which can be resolved, as a function of the frequency of measurement. Data for human subjects: interrupted line; for 33 cochlear fibers: measured (triangles) and computed (filled circles) values. (Wilson and Evans, 1971).

parison, the limit of resolving power for each of the
cat cochlear fiber population (i.e., in the grating
spacing corresponding to a contrast of 0.7 dB, the
minimum contrast psychophysically discernible, vd.
Wilson and Evans, 1971) is shown. Both measured and
computed values are given. The agreement between the
two sets of data is good for frequencies above 4 kHz,
but at lower frequencies the neural values fall significantly below the psychophysical results. This may
indicate a species difference, or that in spite of
attempts to exclude them, non-spectral (e.g., temporal) factors entered into the psychophysical judgement in the low frequency region. Preliminary results
of psychophysical experiments using a masking paradigm favor the latter interpretation.

In Fig. 11 the effective bandwidths (computed as in

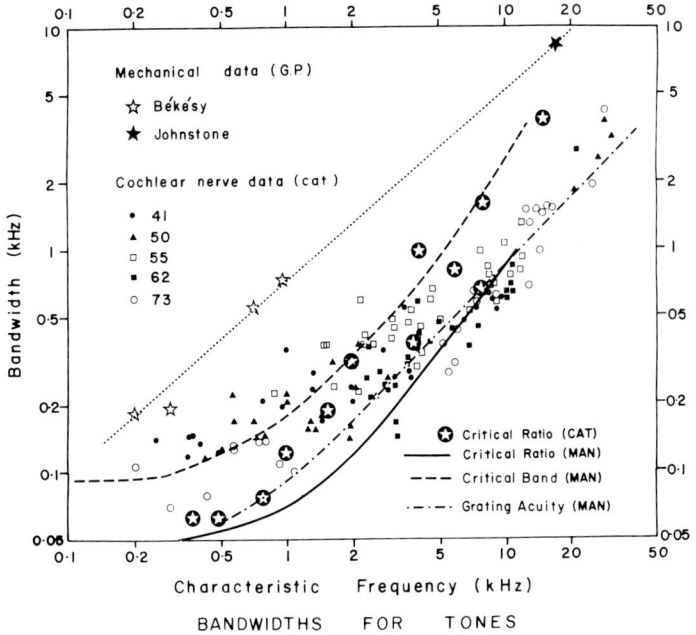

BANDWIDTHS FOR TONES

Fig. 11 Comparison of effective bandwidths of cat
cochlear fibers with psychophysical and
behavioral measures of frequency selectivity

Effective bandwidths computed for 140 cat
cochlear fibers from 5 cats, plotted against
their characteristic frequencies. (cont'd)

(Fig. 11, cont'd) Dotted line: effective bandwidths computed for basilar membrane response curves of von Békésy (1944) and Johnstone et al. (1970). Enclosed stars: behavioral measurements of critical ratio in cat (Watson, 1963). Solid line: critical ratio values for man (Hawkins and Stevens, 1950). Dashed line: critical band values for man (Zwicker et al., 1957). Dotted and dashed line: resolving power expressed as effective bandwidth from acoustic grating measurements (Wilson and Evans, 1971).

section 4.1 above) of 140 cochlear fibers from 5 cats have been plotted against the CFs of the fibers. For comparison, three psychoacoustic measurements of frequency selectivity have been plotted (solid and interrupted lines) and data points (enclosed stars) from behavioral determinations of critical ratio in cat (Watson, 1963). The dashed line represents the value of the critical band for man, from Zwicker et al. (1957), and the solid line shows the critical ratio values from Hawkins and Stevens (1950). The latter is approximately 2.5 times less than the former (Scharf, 1970). The dashed-dotted line represents effective bandwidths corresponding to the grating acuity psychoacoustic measurements above.

Also for comparison, the effective bandwidths of the basilar membrane frequency response functions of von Békésy (1944) and Johnstone et al. (1970) have been computed (open and closed stars respectively).

The similarity between these various measures of behavioral and human psychophysical frequency selectivity and the range of effective bandwidths of cochlear nerve fibers, together with the agreement noted in Fig. 10 suggests the conclusion that the frequency selectivity of the auditory system is already determined within the cochlea.

It has been pointed out in section 3 that, in pathological conditions of the guinea pig cochlea, the FTCs have been found to be abnormally wide. The fact that this can also occur in apparently normal cochleas in a few fibers of high characteristic frequency (Evans, 1972b) may correlate with the finding of sporadic loss of outer hair cells in the basal turn of healthy guinea pigs (J. Wersäll, pers. comm.). There is, furthermore, some evidence that abnormally broadly tuned FTCs may be obtained in cochleas with hair cell damage induced by kanamycin administration (Fig. 10 of Kiang et al., 1970).

Inasmuch as these situations may serve as animal models of sensorineural deafness in man, they may well correlate with the finding of abnormally wide critical bands in patients with end-organ deafness (e.g., de Boer, 1959, Scharf and Hellman, 1966). Thus the degradation of speech intelligibility found in these cases even after correction for elevated thresholds may reflect a broadening of the cochlear and hence psychophysical bandwidths. This would result in the inability of the auditory system to resolve the important formant frequencies of the speech signal.

6. Summary

(a) The frequency selectivities of single cochlear fibers of cat, guinea pig and squirrel monkey are substantially narrower than analogous measurements of basilar membrane motion by optical, Mössbauer and capacitive probe techniques. This inference is based on measurements of the slopes of the cut-offs of the frequency threshold curves, and the 10 dB and effective bandwidths.

(b) Evidence is advanced that this discrepancy in frequency selectivity may be brought about by the operation of a second filter located between the basilar membrane and the cochlear nerve spike generation process, but not tightly coupled to the basilar membrane. This second filter appears to be physiologically vulnerable and may be "private" to each cochlear fiber.

(c) Investigations of the nature of the second filter (via the overall cochlear filtering properties) indicate that it acts as if it were a linear filtering mechanism and in a manner not determined by lateral interaction (o.g., inhibitory) mechanisms. The filter properties appear to be relatively independent of stimulus level.

(d) Comparisons are made of cochlear nerve, behavioral and psychophysical frequency selectivity. The agreement is sufficiently close for the tentative conclusions to be drawn that the frequency selectivity of the auditory system is already determined at the level of the cochlear nerve, and that it may become degraded in cases of end-organ deafness.

Acknowledgements

We are grateful to Dr. J. Rosenberg for collaboration in the cat cochlear nerve experiments, and to Mr. J.S. Corbett for technical assistance. Grants from the M.R.C. and the S.R.C. made possible the data analyses and computations thereon.

References

Békésy, G. von (1944). Über die mechanische Frequenzanalyze in der Schnecke vershiedener Tiere. Akust. Z. 9, 3-11.

Békésy, G. von (1960). Experiments in Hearing. McGraw-Hill, New York.

Békésy, G. von (1969). Resonance in the cochlea? Sound 3, 86-91.

Békésy, G. von (1970). Travelling waves as frequency analysers in the cochlea. Nature (London) 225, 1207-1209.

Campbell, F.W., and Robson, J.G. (1968). Applications of fourier analysis to the visibility of gratings. J. Physiol. 197, 551-566.

Campbell, F.W., Cooper, G.F., and Enroth-Cugell, C. (1969). The spatial selectivity of the visual cells of the cat. J. Physiol. 203, 223-235.

Dallos, P. (1969). Combination tone $2f_1-f_h$ in microphonic potentials. J. Acoust. Soc. Amer. 46, 1437-1444.

Dallos, P., Billone, M.C., Durrant, J.D., Wang, C-y., and Raynor, S. (1972). Cochlear inner and outer hair cells: functional differences. Science 177, 356-358.

De Boer, E. (1959). Measurement of critical bandwidth in cases of perception deafness. In:Proc. Int. Congr. Acoust., 3rd, Vol. 1, pp. 100-102.

Elsevier, Amsterdam.

De Boer, E. (1968). Reverse correlation I. A heuristic introduction to the technique of triggered correlation with applications to the analysis of compound systems. Proc. Kon. Ned. Akad. Wetensch. 71, 472-486.

De Boer, E. (1969). Reverse correlation II. Initiation of nerve impulses in the inner ear. Proc. Kon. Ned. Akad. Wetensch. 72, 129-151.

Evans, E.F. (1970a). Narrow "tuning" of cochlear nerve fibre responses in the guinea pig. J. Physiol. 206, 14-15P.

Evans, E.F. (1970b). Narrow "tuning" of the responses of cochlear nerve fibres emanating from the exposed basilar membrane. J. Physiol. 208, 75-76P.

Evans, E.F. (1971). Does frequency sharpening occur in the cochlea? Proc. Int. Union Physiol. Sci. 9, 167.

Evans, E.F. (1972a). Does frequency sharpening occur in the cochlea? Symposium on Hearing Theory, 1972, pp. 27-34. IPO Eindhoven, Holland.

Evans, E.F. (1972b). The frequency response and other properties of single fibres in the guinea pig cochlea. J. Physiol. 226, 263-287.

Evans, E.F., and Wilson, J.P. (1971). Frequency sharpening of the cochlea: the effective bandwidth of cochlear nerve fibres. Proc. Int. Congr. Acoust., 7th, Vol. 3, pp. 453-456. Akademiai Kiado, Budapest.

Evans, E.F., Rosenberg, J., and Wilson, J.P. (1970). The effective bandwidth of cochlear nerve fibres. J. Physiol. 207, 62-63P.

Evans, E.F., Rosenberg, J., and Wilson, J.P. (1971). The frequency resolving power of the cochlea. J. Physiol. 216, 58-59P.

Furman, G.G., and Frishkopf, L.S. (1964). Model of neural inhibition in the mammalian cochlea. J.

Acoust. Soc. Amer. 36, 2194-2207.

Goblick, T.J. Jr., and Pfeiffer, R.R. (1969). Time-domain measurements of cochlear non-linearities using combination click stimuli. J. Acoust. Soc. Amer. 46, 924-938.

Goldstein, J.L. (1967). Auditory non-linearity. J. Acoust. Soc. Amer. 41, 676-689.

Goldstein, J.L. (1970). Aural combination tones. In: Frequency Analysis and Periodicity Detection in Hearing (R. Plomp and F.G. Smoorenburg, eds.), pp. 230-245. Sijthoff, Leiden, The Netherlands.

Goldstein, J.L. (1972). Evidence from aural combination tones and musical notes against classical temporal periodicity theory. Symposium on Hearing Theory 1972, pp. 186-208. IPO Eindhoven, Holland.

Goldstein, J.L., and Kiang, N.Y.S. (1968). Neural correlates of the aural combination tone $2f_1-f_2$. Proc. IEEE 56, 981-992.

Goldstein, J.L., Baer, T., and Kiang, N.Y.S. (1971). A theoretical treatment of latency, group delay and tuning characteristics for auditory-nerve responses to clicks and tones. In: Physiology of the Auditory System (M.B. Sachs, ed.). National Educational Consultants, Baltimore.

Hawkins, J.E. Jr, and Stevens, S.S. (1950). The masking of pure tones and of speech by white noise. J. Acoust. Soc. Amer. 22, 6-13.

Huggins, W.H., and Licklider, J.C.R. (1951). Place mechanisms of auditory frequency analysis. J. Acoust. Soc. Amer. 23, 290-299.

Johnstone, B.M., and Boyle, A.J.F. (1967). Basilar membrane vibration examined with the Mössbauer technique. Science 158, 389-390.

Johnstone, B.M., and Sellick, P.M. (1972). The peripheral auditory apparatus. Quart. Rev. Biophys. 5, 1-58.

Johnstone, B.M., Taylor, K.J. and Boyle, A.J. (1970).
Mechanics of the guinea pig cochlea. J. Acoust.
Soc. Amer. 47, 504-509.

Katsuki, Y., Sumi, T., Uchiyama, H., and Watanabe, T.
(1958). Electric response of auditory neurons in
cat to sound stimulation. J. Neurophysiol. 25,
569-588.

Kiang, N.Y.S., Watanabe, T., Thomas, E.C., and Clarke,
L.F. (1965). Discharge Patterns of Single Fibers
in the Cat's Auditory Nerve, Res. Mongr. 35.
M.I.T. Press, Cambridge, Mass.

Kiang, N.Y.S., Sachs, M.B., and Peake, W.T. (1967).
Shapes of tuning curves for single auditory
nerve fibers. J. Acoust. Soc. Amer. 42,
1341-1342.

Kiang, N.Y.S., Baer, T., Marr, E.M., and Demont, T.D.
(1969). Discharge rates of single auditory nerve fibers as functions of tone level. J. Acoust.
Soc. Amer. 46, 106.

Kiang, N.Y.S., Moxon, E.C., and Levine, R.A. (1970).
Auditory nerve activity in cats with normal and
abnormal cochleas. In: Sensorineural Hearing
Loss (G.E.W. Wolstenholme and J. Knight, eds.),
pp. 241-268. Churchill, London.

Nieder, P. (1971). Addressed exponential delay line
theory of cochlear organisation. Nature (London)
230, 255-257.

Pfeiffer, R.R. (1970). A model for two-tone inhibition of single cochlear nerve fibers. J. Acoust.
Soc. Amer. 48, 1373-1378.

Pfeiffer, R.R., and Molnar, C.E. (1970). Cochlear
nerve fiber discharge patterns: relationship
to the cochlear microphonic. Science 167,
1614-1616.

Ratliff, F. (1965). Mach Bands. Holden-Day, San Francisco.

Rhode, W.S. (1971). Observations of the vibration of
the basilar membrane in squirrel monkeys using

the Mössbauer technique. J. Acoust. Soc. Amer. 49, 1218-1231.

Rose, J.E., Hind, J.E., Anderson, D.J., and Brugge, J.F. (1971). Some effects of stimulus intensity on response of auditory nerve fibers in the squirrel monkey. J. Neurophysiol. 34, 685-699.

Sachs, M.B., and Kiang, N.Y.S. (1968). Two-tone inhibition in auditory nerve fibers. J. Acoust. Soc. Amer. 43, 1120-1128.

Scharf, B. (1970). Critical bands. In: Foundations of Modern Auditory Theory Vol. 1., (J.V. Tobias, ed.), pp. 159-202. Academic Press, New York.

Scharf, B., and Hellman, R.P. (1966). Model of loudness summation applied to impaired ears. J. Acoust. Soc. Amer. 40, 71-78.

Smoorenburg, G.F. (1972). Combination tones and their origin. J. Acoust. Soc. Amer. 52, 615-632.

Spoendlin, H. (1969). Structural basis of peripheral frequency analysis. In: Frequency Analysis and Periodicity Detection in Hearing (R. Plomp and F.G. Smoorenburg, eds.), pp. 2-36. Sijthoff, Leiden, The Netherlands.

Spoendlin, H. (1971). Degeneration behaviour of cochlear nerve. Arch. Klin. Exp. Ohr-Nas Kehlk-Heilk 200, 275-291.

Tasaki, I. (1954). Nerve impulses in individual auditory nerve fibres of guinea pig. J. Neurophysiol. 17, 97-122.

Tonndorf, J. (1970). Cochlear mechanics and hydrodynamics. In: Foundations of Modern Auditory Theory Vol. 1., (J.V. Tobias, ed.) pp. 205-254. Academic Press, New York.

Watson, C.S. (1963). Masking of tones by noise for the cat. J. Acoust. Soc. Amer. 35, 167-172.

Whitfield, I.C. (1967). The Auditory Pathway. Arnold, London.

Wilson, J.P. (1967). Psychoacoustics of obstacle detection using ambient or self-generated noise. In: Les Systèmes Sonars Animaux (R.G. Busnel, ed.), pp. 89-114. Jouy-en-Josas.

Wilson, J.P. (1970). An auditory after-image. In: Frequency Analysis and Periodicity Detection in Hearing (R. Plomp and F.G. Smoorenburg, eds.), pp. 303-315. Sijthoff, Leiden, The Netherlands.

Wilson, J.P. and Evans, E.F. (1971). Grating acuity of the ear: psychophysical and neurophysiological measures of frequency resolving power. Proc. Int. Congr. Acoust., 7th, Vol. 3, pp. 397-400. Akademiai Kiado, Budapest.

Wilson, J.P., and Johnstone, J.R. (1972). Capacitive probe measure of basilar membrane vibration. Symposium on Hearing Theory 1972, pp. 172-181. IPO Eindhoven, Holland.

Zwicker, E., Flottorp, G., and Stevens, S.S. (1957). Critical bandwidth in loudness summation. J. Acoust. Soc. Amer. 29, 548-557.

DISCUSSION

TONNDORF: Dr. Evans, I would like to make a suggestion here about what this second filter may physically represent. Something which many of us keep forgetting is that the input to the hair cells is not given by the traveling wave directly, but rather by the shear wave. In model experiments and also of course in von Békésy's original observations, the envelopes over the two events were not identical. My associate, Dr. Khanna has subjected this problem to a computer simulation (Khanna et al., 1968). In the conversion from traveling waves to shear waves it turns out that these simulated envelopes were exactly like yours; that is, the lefthand slope became considerably steeper. I would therefore suggest that there is a good chance that what you showed us so beautifully today is physically related to the shear wave envelope rather than to the traveling wave envelope.

EVANS: I agree in principle to the suggestion, but I am not aware of any such simulations generating envelopes with slopes above 100 dB/octave.

DAVIS: I shall ask Dr. Evans if he thinks that the shear wave mechanism which Dr. Tonndorf has suggested as a physical basis of that second filter will qualify for your second characteristic, namely the vulnerability. I do want to know what you think that second filter is.

EVANS: We have tried many models and ideas and frankly we have not come up with any one model which accounts satisfactorily for the physiological and the anatomical data. In answer to your first part, I agree that it is difficult to envisage a shearing wave system that would be physiologically vulnerable, but then we know so little about what is actually possible in the cochlea.

KOHLLÖFFEL: If I understand you rightly you conclude from your experiment that the cochlear output is basically linear as far as tuning is concerned. Taking your stimulus situation I find it a little puzzling that you could not observe any "two-tone interaction" type effects since you probably cover inhibitory bands, at least partially. Could it not be that the absence of nonlinearity in your case simply means a lack of sensitivity of your technique. You go through a rather complicated series of steps, e.g. using the noise-intensity function for calibration, which may just lead to a loss of sensitivity and resolution.

EVANS: I do not think we lose resolution. The only conclusion that we have come to is that while we are not denying the existence of two-tone inhibition, the effect of this phenomenon is slight compared with the effect of stimulation over the characteristic frequency of the fiber in the experimental paradigm that I have described. In fact we did a second series of analogous experiments where we deliberately tried to exploit the two-tone suppression phenomenon by stimulating the fiber all the time with a low level of noise and then arranging the peaks of the grating spectrum so that they would preferentially stimulate the two-tone suppression side bands. To our surprise plots of the overall response to this stimulus, as a function of the spacing of the grating spectrum, showed no systematic deviations from those computed from the pure tone frequency threshold curves, as in Fig. 9 of my paper. On the other hand, similar experiments we have carried out on units in the dorsal cochlear nucleus did demonstrate the lateral inhibition there.

GREEN: I take it that all these measurements of the grating spectra were made under continuous stimulation. I wonder if you would like to comment on the results obtained by Houtgast, (Houtgast, 1972), who finds lack of inhibition under continuous stimulation but considerable evidence for inhibition using a pulsation technique, in which he alternates the signal and the noise.

EVANS: We have discussed this with him but I think we

are as much at a loss as he is to explain the significance of the difference between his two sets of stimulus conditions. It is possible that his measurements of "pulsation threshold" involve both forward and backward masking phenomen. The latter almost certainly are a function of processes at a higher level than the cochlear nerve.

References

Houtgast, T. (1972). Psychophysical experiments on grating acuity. Symposium on Hearing Theory 1972, pp. 50-57. IPO Eindhoven, Holland.

Khanna, S.M., Sears, R.E., and Tonndorf, S. (1968). Some properties of longitudinal shear waves: A study by computer simulation. J. Acoust. Soc. Amer. 43, 1077-1084.

CONSIDERATIONS OF NONLINEAR RESPONSE PROPERTIES
OF SINGLE COCHLEAR NERVE FIBERS

Russell R. Pfeiffer and Duck On Kim

The Washington University
St. Louis, Missouri
USA

1. Introduction

Nonlinearities of the peripheral auditory system have been receiving increased amounts of attention in recent years. Prior to approximately 1960, very little data were available from single cochlear nerve fibers, but nonlinear characteristics such as the limiting of spike discharge rate for high signal level (Tasaki, 1954) and refractoriness were known. Subsequently, the improvement of recording techniques led to the acquisition of considerable data while the introduction of statistical methods made it possible to characterize the stochastic response activity of the cochlear nerve fibers in convenient ways (Gerstein and Kiang, 1960, Rodieck et al., 1962, Kiang et al., 1962, Rupert et al., 1963, and Nomoto et al., 1964). Statistical measures became to be considered as response patterns of the single fibers. Nonlinear phenomena such as "rectification" of excitation inferred from certain response patterns (Kiang et al., 1965, Brugge et al., 1969), and more subtle characteristics, such as the "depletion effect" described by Gray (1966), developed during the mid-60's. As late as 1964, however, there existed controversy as to whether or not two-tone inhibition or suppression could be demonstrated for single cochlear nerve fibers (Kiang et al., 1962, Rupert et al., 1963). Key work by Sachs (1966) dispelled any doubt about the existence of two-tone suppression, but the responsible mechanisms remained unknown.

During these periods, it was generally assumed by most investigators that elements peripheral to the hair cells were linear (e.g., Békésy, 1960, Flanagan, 1965, Weiss, 1966). The limited available data on basilar-membrane mechanics (Békésy, 1960) as well as more extensive data on the external and middle ear mechanics (Wiener et al., 1966, Guinan and Peake, 1967) influenced most investigators to assume linearity for all of these mechanical elements. Consequently, there was a severe constraint such that any and all nonlinear phenomena were to be accounted for by either complex innervation or complex properties of the hair cells or characteristics of spiral ganglion neurons (e.g., Furman and Frishkopf, 1964, Furman, 1965, Klatt, 1964, Lynn and Sayers, 1970). On the other hand, there have been early attempts (Tonndorf, 1958 and 1970) to explain nonlinear phenomena observed in electrophysiological experiments on the basis of nonlinear cochlear hydrodynamics. These latter studies suggested that nonlinearities in the cochlear hydrodynamics may be significant, but were not able to offer a unified account of the nonlinear phenomena observed in the response patterns of single cochlear nerve fibers outlined here. Rhode's (1971) discovery that the motion of the basilar membrane was nonlinear eliminated the severe constraint outlined above.

Throughout the decade perhaps the most confusing situation was the discrepancy between the available data about basilar-membrane motion and the response properties of single cochlear nerve fibers. When considering the characteristics in the frequency-domain, there was concern about how the poor frequency selectivity or low Q (Békésy, 1960) of basilar-membrane motion developed or produced sharp or high Q response areas (e.g. Kiang et al., 1965) of single cochlear nerve fibers. Correspondingly, in the time-domain, there was a discrepancy between the number of cycles in the calculated impulse response of the basilar membrane (Flanagan, 1965) and the larger number of peaks in the post-stimulus time (PST) histogram of responses of single cochlear nerve fibers to click stimuli. These inconsistencies provided motivation to seek further details of the properties of the basilar-membrane motion or to explore possible schemes of cochlear innervation or electrophysiological interaction to achieve the so-called "neural sharpening." Techniques to measure directly basilar-membrane motion at stimulus levels in the normal physiological range were under development (Johnstone and Boyle, 1967). Anatomical studies of the cochlear receptors were receiving more attention (e.g., Engström et al., 1966, Spoendlin, 1966, and Iurato, 1967). And finally, electrophysiological studies closely related to the topic were underway (e.g. Sachs, 1966).

It was believed that a detailed description of the impulse response of the basilar-membrane would help to resolve the reported differences in Q of membrane motion and neural response. Still under the assumption that the basilar-membrane motion was linear, Goblick and Pfeiffer (1968) attempted to measure indirectly its impulse response. They only managed, however, to uncover two new nonlinear phenomena that were not only seemingly disjointed from each other, but were not easily related to other known facts about the peripheral auditory system. These latter measurements added to the list of describable nonlinear phenomena observed in the response patterns of single cochlear nerve fibers, and increased the difficulty of providing a unified description or model of this peripheral system. These and other data such as those of Sachs, 1966, Gray, 1966, Goldstein and Kiang, 1968, Pfeiffer and Molnar, 1970, and Anderson et al., 1971, placed severe restrictions on models. The result was that models were developed to address particular nonlinear phenomena because unification of the known facts and details of the nonlinear phenomena was difficult. On the other hand, these restrictions coupled with Rhode's evidence of basilar-membrane nonlinearity provided a new basis for modelling the basilar-membrane motion (Kim, 1972) which led to an improved situation for understanding possible relationships between seemingly disjointed nonlinear phenomena of the peripheral auditory system.

We attempt in this paper to outline the nonlinear phenomena observed in response patterns of single cochlear nerve fibers that we consider must be addressed when attempting to develop a unified analysis of the operation of the auditory system peripheral to the brain stem. We will propose plausible sources of these phenomena in terms of the components of the system as outlined in Fig. 1.

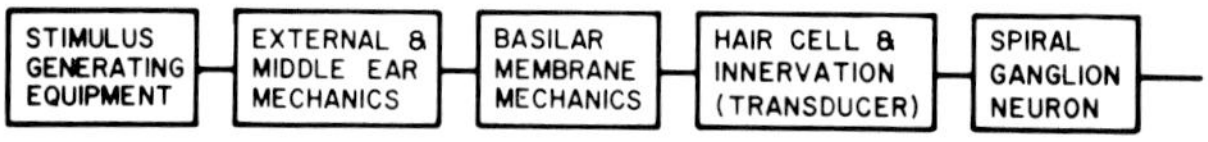

Fig. 1 A simple block diagram of the peripheral auditory system. This configuration appears to be adequate to evaluate the origin and probable cause of nonlinearities observed in response patterns of single cochlear nerve fibers. The stimulus generating equipment is included to emphasize that it can have significant effects in the analysis and interpretation of response patterns especially when considering subtle nonlinear properties.

We will briefly describe some models that were only partially effective and propose a relatively comprehensive model for activities of single cochlear nerve fibers. We believe that a detailed and sound understanding of the nonlinear phenomena and their sources is necessary in order to determine if they are functionally significant or if they are merely seductive epiphenomena.

2. Review of nonlinear phenomena

Single Tone Stimulation

Among the earliest reported nonlinearities was the relationship between signal level and spike-discharge rate of single fibers. The spike discharge rates generally increase with signal level, then reach a maximum rate and then occasionally decrease slightly with further increases in signal level (Fig. 2) (Tasaki, 1954, Nomoto et al., 1964, Kiang et al., 1965, Rose et al., 1971). This phenomenon is probably not due to limitations of the neuron (Moxon, 1968) but may be attributable to either limiting of the motion of the basilar membrane or to a saturation of the transducer. Identification of which of these is the dominant factor is, at present, difficult. We note, however, that some similarities do exist between limiting curves obtained for different frequencies from a given fiber (Fig. 2) (Nomoto et al., 1964, Rose et al., 1971) and corresponding data obtained from measures of basilar-membrane motion (Fig. 3) (Rhode, 1971).

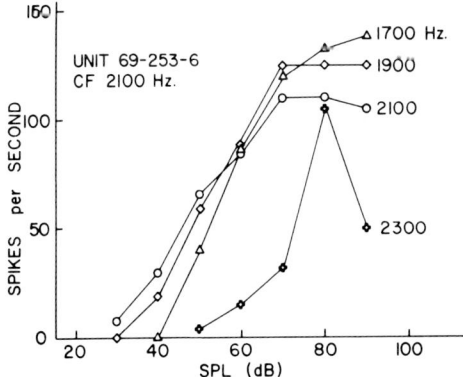

Fig. 2 Spike discharge rate of single cochlear nerve fiber versus sound pressure level of a single sinusoidal stimulus for four different frequencies. These curves are derived from Fig. 2 of Rose et al., 1971. Note that each of the curves saturates, and that they cross over each other such that the most effective frequency decreases with increases in signal level. Analogous trends were observed for amplitude of motion of points on the basilar-membrane (Rhode, 1971). See Fig. 3.

The limiting curves of Fig. 2 can be derived from plots of spike discharge rate versus frequency for fixed levels of stimulation (Fig. 4). These latter spike rate plots show a decrease in "Q" with increases in signal level. It will be shown later that this decrease in "Q" with signal level is consistent with properties of response patterns of single fibers to transient stimuli. Note in Figs. 2 and 4 that the frequency of the stimulus to which the neuron is maximally responsive decreases with signal level. In other words, the "limiting" nonlinearity is frequency dependent. This along with the decrease in Q with

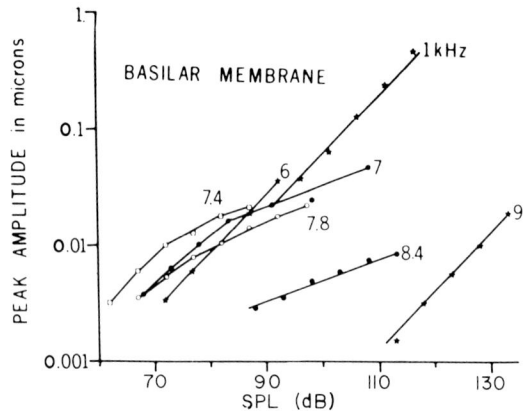

Fig. 3 Peak amplitude of motion of a point on the basilar-membrane versus sound pressure level for seven different frequencies of sinusoidal stimulus. From Fig. 7, Rhode, 1971. Compare with Fig. 2.

signal level is consistent with corresponding observations of the amplitude of motion of a point on the basilar-membrane (Rhode, 1971).

The above measures of spike rates are relatively crude in that they pay no attention to the temporal structure of the spike train. More detailed considerations of response to sinusoidal stimuli can be obtained by examining period histograms. It has been shown under certain conditions that there is a close correspondence between the shape of the period histogram and the time waveform of the sinusoidal stimulus (Brugge et al., 1969). From the period histograms one can measure input-output amplitude and phase relationships of the fundamental and generated harmonic components (Pfeiffer and Molnar, 1970). Fig. 5 shows a series of period and compound period histograms for one fiber as a function of signal level. For low levels, these histograms resemble a sinusoid, but as stimulus level is increased deviations from a sinusoidal shape occur.

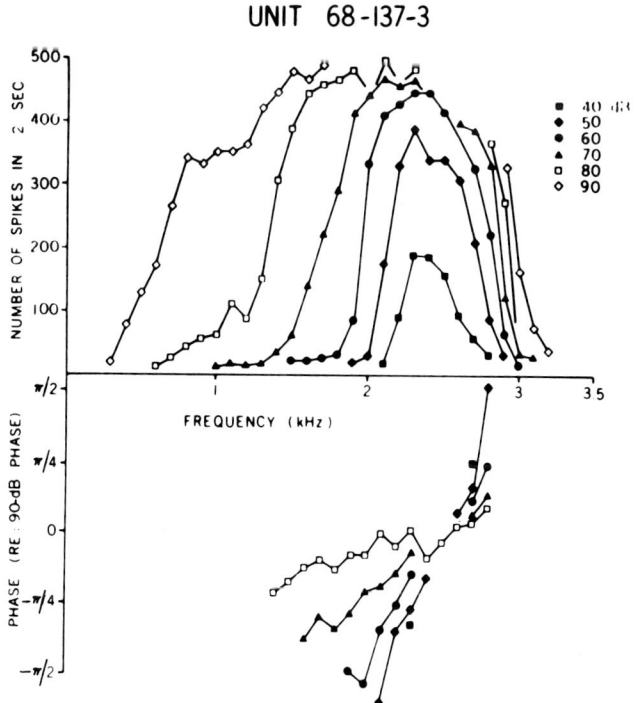

Fig. 4 Spike-discharge rate (upper part) and phase angle of the period histogram (lower part) of a single cochlear nerve fiber versus frequency of sinusoidal stimulus for six sound pressure levels. The numbers in the inset indicate sound pressure levels re SPL. The phase angle is relative to that at 90 dB SPL, and the phase lag is considered positive. Note the apparent decrease in "Q" and reduction in most effective frequency with increases in signal level. From Anderson et al., 1971.

We have found that well known properties of a neuron (i.e., spike generation and refractoriness) are adequate to simulate the distortions observed in the period histograms of responses to single sinusoids. Fig. 5 shows the similarity between period histograms obtained from a model neuron and those obtained from a single cochlear nerve fiber. The model neuron was a variable threshold device with properties as

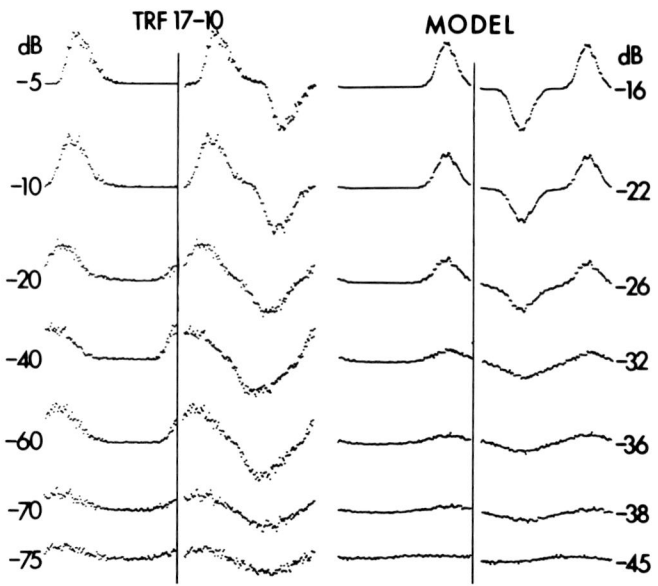

Fig. 5 Column 1: Period histograms of responses to continuous sinusoidal stimulation for a cochlear nerve fiber. Note that at low levels the response pattern resembles a sinusoid, but as level is increased, only one-half cycle of the stimulus is effective (rectification). The shape of the response pattern for the excitatory half cycle is further distorted as is emphasized in the <u>compound</u> period histograms of these same data (column 2). The compound histograms were constructed by shifting the period histogram one-half period and algebraically subtracting it from the original (compare to Fig. 9).

Column 3 and 4: Comparable data obtained from the output of the analog model shown in Fig. 7. The properties of the model are such that the input to the model neuron is essentially sinusoidal. The distortions shown are therefore generated by the model neuron.

described in Fig. 6. The close correspondence suggests to us that these distortions may be properties of the neuron.

Care must be taken when studying period histograms

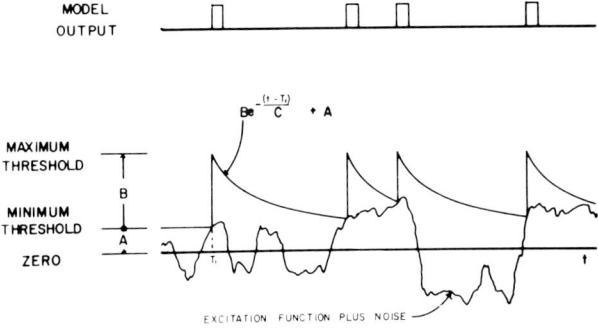

Fig. 6 Principle of operation of a variable threshold device used to simulate a neuron. The input is a continuous waveform consisting of signal plus noise. The noise is used to simulate spontaneous activity. The exponential decay of the variable threshold simulates refractoriness. Shown from bottom to top are: the summed input to the device, the instantaneous threshold, and the pulse output of the model. These operations are similar to those modelled on a digital computer by Weiss, 1966. The data in Fig. 5, columns 3 and 4, were obtained from an analog device (designed by C.E. Molnar) with the properties shown here. From Matthews, 1972.

of the responses to high level sinusoidal stimulation administered at frequencies far below the characteristic frequency (CF)[1] because harmonic distortions generated by the earphone can cause considerable response even though they may be 40-70 dB down from the fundamental! A similar caveat is also appropriate for studies using multiple tones.

Period histograms are an extremely useful and accurate means of obtaining details of phase relation-

---

[1] The characteristic frequency (CF) is defined as that frequency to which a nerve fiber is most sensitive. For a point on the basilar-membrane the CF is defined, by us, to be the limiting value of the most effective frequency as stimulus amplitude approaches zero. This latter definition is necessary because the frequency to which the membrane is most responsive is a function of signal level.

ships between response patterns and the stimulus. It has been shown that the phase angle measured from the period histogram systematically changes as a function of both the signal level and the ratio of stimulus frequency to the CF (Fig. 4) (Anderson et al., 1971), an observation that is inconsistent with a linear system. We believe that this nonlinear phase property is related to the basilar-membrane motion and is not attributable to the hair cell or to the neuron, first because if it were, the phase changes observed would not likely be related to the CF of the neuron, especially in light of Spoendlin's results (1970, 1972) indicating that 95 percent of the spiral ganglion neurons innervate single hair cells, and second because this nonlinear phase characteristic has been observed from a nonlinear model of basilar-membrane motion based in part on Rhode's data (Kim, 1972).

Two-Tone Stimulation

A simple extension from single to double sinusoidal stimulation leads to several additional nonlinear interactions. Perhaps the one that has received most attention to date is two-tone "inhibition" or "suppression." Sachs (1966) has studied in detail and described in functional form the effects on the response of one tone by the presence of a second. Although it has been suggested that such interaction may be due to complex interconnections (lateral inhibition) of sensory cells and primary neurons (Furman and Frishkopf, 1964) the recent anatomical results of Spoendlin (1970, 1972) do not show such

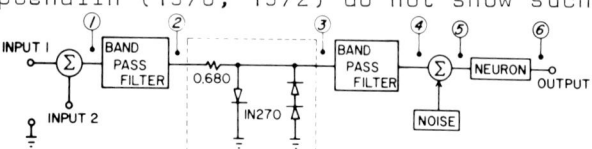

Fig. 7   An analog model for single cochlear-nerve fiber activity. The model consists of a "bandpass" nonlinearity (BPNL)(Blachman, 1964) with neuron (see Fig. 6) and a noise input to simulate spontaneous activity. The model cannot account for all experimentally observed nonlinear properties of single cochlear nerve fibers but can simulate qualitatively or quantitatively a surprising number of reported properties. From Pfeiffer, 1971.

interconnections. On the basis of a study of bandpass nonlinear (BPNL) model (Fig. 7) it has been suggested that the two-tone interaction is a result of signal suppression rather than neurological inhibition, and also that the phenomenon occurs peripheral to the neuron (Pfeiffer, 1970). Although it remains to be seen whether or not two-tone suppression can be directly observed in basilar-membrane motion, at least one model based on data to date demonstrates the phenomenon when one tone is at the CF and the other tone is above the CF (Kim, 1972).

Under certain conditions, it has been demonstrated that two-tone stimulation can also lead to the generation of a large number of combination tones, e.g., (f_2-f_1), $(2f_1-f_2)$, $2f_1$, (f_1+f_2), and $2f_2$ (Goldstein and Kiang, 1968, Littlefield, pers. comm.). One $(2f_1-f_2)$, has received particular attention because of its psychophysical interest (Goldstein, 1967). Among those combination tones noted above, the $(2f_1-f_2)$ is the only one that is prominent in the output of the BPNL model without neuron (point 4 of Fig. 7) as well as in the output of a nonlinear model of basilar-membrane motion (Kim et al., 1972). In contrast, the model neuron (Fig. 6) generates all of the above combination tones except $(2f_1-f_2)$ (Fig. 8). This suggests that the $(2f_1-f_2)$ combination tone is generated at the level of the basilar-membrane while the others are generated medial to it.

Single Click Stimulation

Histograms of responses to clicks of opposite polarity (rarefaction and condensation) are consistent with rectification of the resultant oscillatory vibration of the basilar membrane, as is shown in Fig. 9. The uniform interleaving of the preferred times of discharge as illustrated in Fig. 9 occurs for fibers with CF between a few hundred Hz up to several kHz. At lower frequencies there are still preferred times of discharge, but the precise interleaving is lost (Fig. 10) (Pfeiffer and Kim, 1972). This latter anomalous response property may be due to the presence of the helicotrema lying along the apical turn of the cochlea. It has also been suggested that the anomaly may be due to differences in velocity of propagation for opposite polarity clicks (Schroeder, pers. comm.); the two possibilities may be related.

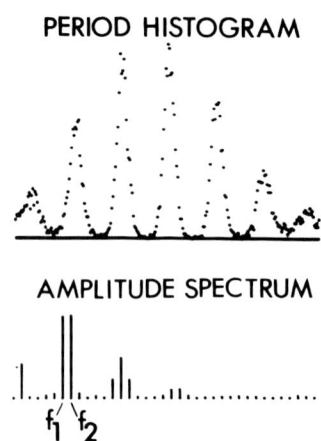

Fig. 8 Top: period histogram of the responses of the variable threshold device (model neuron) due to two-tone stimulation. The stimulus consists of two equal-amplitude sinusoids, f_1 at 600 Hz and f_2 at 700 Hz (phase difference π radians). The period of the histogram is $1/(f_2-f_1)$. Spontaneous activity of the model neuron was set at 43 pulses per second. The mean pulse rate during stimulation was 73 pulses per second.
Bottom: Amplitude spectrum of the Fourier transform of the period histogram. The mean value (dc component) of the spectrum has been set to zero for convenience (left-most dot). Each component is an integer multiple of the fundamental, (f_2-f_1). The first major compo-
(cont'd)

(Fig. 8, cont'd) nent of the spectrum is (f_2-f_1) followed by f_1, f_2, $2f_1$, f_1+f_2, and $2f_2$ respectively. Note that the $(2f_1-f_2)$ component is negligible.

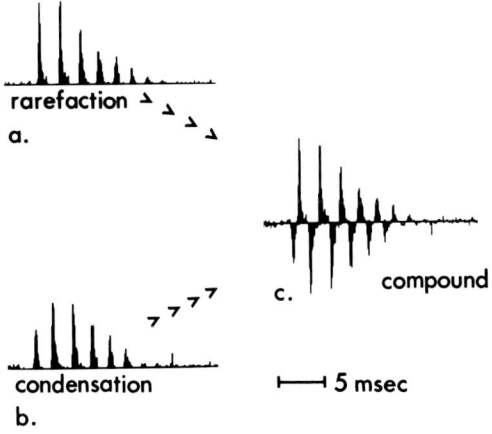

Fig. 9 Poststimulus time (PST) histograms of responses to click stimuli.

a.) PST histogram of responses to rarefaction clicks.

b.) PST histogram of responses to condensation clicks for the same nerve fiber and for the same stimulus amplitude as for Part a.

c.) A combination of Parts a and b (compound PST histogram) except the histogram for condensation clicks b has been inverted and put in time registration with the histogram for rarefaction clicks a. From Goblick and Pfeiffer, 1969.

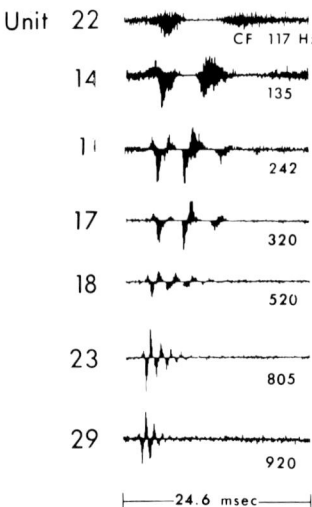

Fig. 10 Compound PST histograms from several different fibers from one cat providing examples of the loss of interlacing of the preferred times of discharge of rarefaction clicks and condensation clicks with decreases in the characteristic frequency of the fibers. From Pfeiffer and Kim, 1973.

The response patterns to continuous single tone stimulation (steady state) for these fibers with low CF do not exhibit any comparable anomalies.

For most of cochlear nerve fibers having CF below a

few kHz, increases in the signal level of the click i) have little effect on the number of peaks in the response pattern (at least for levels above 65 dB SPL) (Fig. 11), but ii) cause a distinct change in

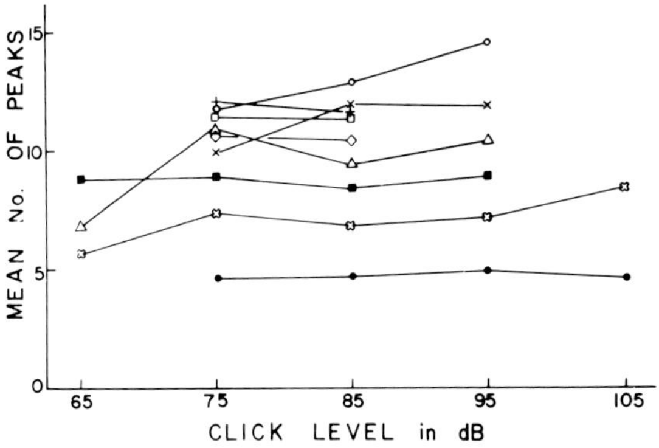

Fig. 11 Mean number of peaks in the compound PST histogram versus click level. Each of the curves corresponds to a different characteristic frequency band: ●, 0-0.3 kHz; ☒, 0.3-0.5 kHz; ■, 0.5-0.7 kHz; Δ, 0.7-0.9 kHz; ◇, 0.9-1.1 kHz; x, 1.1-1.3 kHz; □, 1.3-1.5 kHz; +, 1.5-1.7 kHz; o, 1.7-2.0 kHz. These data were obtained from more than 800 different cochlear nerve fibers. From Pfeiffer and Kim, 1973.

the shape of the envelope of the response pattern such that the crest of the envelope occurs earlier at higher levels (Kiang et al., 1965; Pfeiffer and Kim, 1973). These two characteristics are also demonstrated in the recovered-probability response patterns by Gray (1967) and therefore suggest that these effects occur peripherally to the neuron. This contention is consistent with the measurements of basilar-membrane motion by Rhode (1971) that illustrates a decrease in "Q" with signal level.

Combination Click Stimulation

The nulling experiments of Coblick and Pfeiffer (1969), using click pairs, demonstrated that the effects on the response to the first click by the presence of a second click were nonlinear both as a function of the amplitude of the first click and as a function of the time separation between the clicks of the click pair. These effects were denoted as "amplitude" and "temporal" nonlinearities respectively. The nonlinearities were measured by precisely controlling the time and amplitude of the second click to selectively null a particular peak in the compound PST histogram of the responses to the click pairs. The experiments were designed on the premise that the mechanical excitation was linear and that zero input to the transducer would yield zero output of the neuron (excluding spontaneous activity). The results indicated that either or both of these two assumptions were invalid. Nonlinear models were explored in attempts to arrive at a configuration that would simultaneously mimic the "amplitude" and "temporal" nonlinearities as manifested in these experiments. For some time there was only one model (Fig. 15) which, to the best of our knowledge, had characteristics consistent with the nulling data of

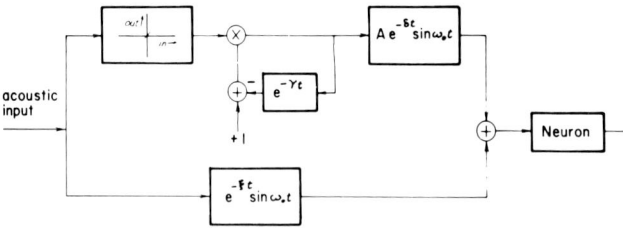

Fig. 15 A two-channel model devised to mimic the nonlinearities observed in the click-pair nulling experiments. This model was the result of extensive search to find any scheme that would simultaneously duplicate the seemingly complex "amplitude" and "temporal" nonlinearities. It was viewed with interest, for some time mainly because it was the only model that seemed to work. But it is phenomenological, relatively complex and unappealing because it is quite limited.

Goblick and Pfeiffer. Subsequently, Rhode (1971) observed that the mechanical excitation was not linear, but it remained to show (Kim, 1972) a possible relationship between the nonlinearities described by Rhode and those observed in the click-pair experiments.

The nulling technique used in the click pair experiments provided very precise descriptions of these

nonlinear characteristics. Fig. 12a shows plots of
the click ratios in dB that nulled particular peaks
in the compound PST histogram for several different
fibers when the level of the first click was held
constant. It can be observed that these curves are
essentially the same in shape. From Fig. 12b one can
derive that a curve for a given fiber translates up
or down with changes in signal level of the first
click. The curves of Fig. 12a must be translated
downward with increases in level of the first click,
at least above about 70-75 dB SPL. The data are consistent with the observation of the change in enve-

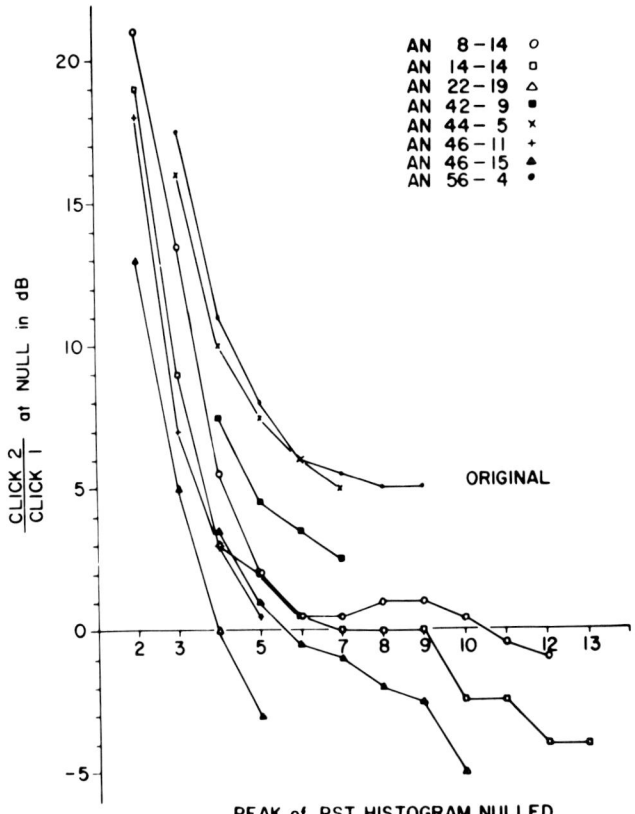

Fig. 12 a.) Plots of stimulus conditions necessary
to obtain a null in the compound PST histogram versus peak being nulled. Each curve
corresponds to data obtained from a given
fiber.

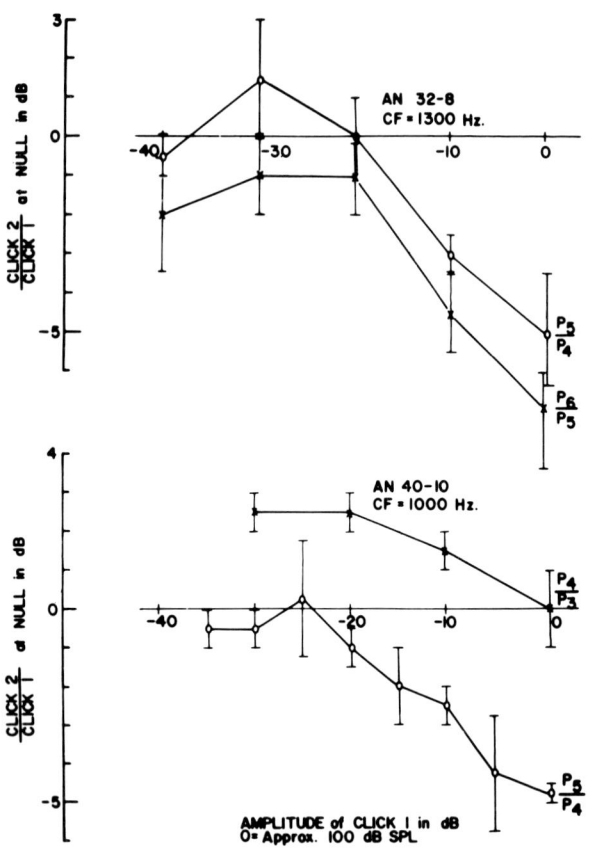

b.) Plots of click pair stimulus settings necessary to maintain a null of a particular peak of the compound PST histogram versus the level of the first click. Data for two different peaks are shown for each of two fibers. The curves for a given fiber are similar and are separated by equal amounts over the entire range (within measurement brackets).

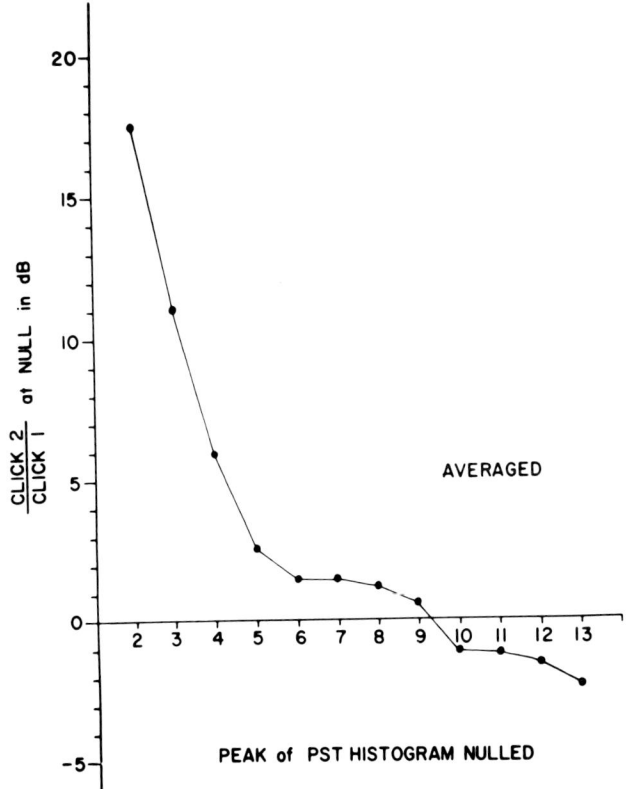

c.) The average of stimulus conditions necessary to obtain a null in the compound PST histogram versus peak being nulled. All from Goblick and Pfeiffer, 1969.

lope shape with signal level as observed in response patterns to single clicks in that the crest of the envelope (which occurs at the peak number where the curves of Fig. 12a intersect the abscissa) shifts towards earlier and earlier peaks with increases in signal level.

From data such as shown in Fig. 12d, we obtained an average curve for the click ratio necessary to null a peak vs. peak number (Fig. 12c). From data such as in Fig. 12b, we estimated that the average curve would shift downward at a rate of about 5 dB for each 20 dB increase in signal level above about 75 dB

SPL. These data were compared to results from measurements of mechanical motion of the basilar membrane by Békésy (1960) and Rhode (1971). Estimates of the envelope of the click response of the basilar-membrane at different signal levels were obtained by assuming that the shifted curves of Fig. 12c provided ratios of <u>amplitudes</u> of adjacent peaks. Fig. 13

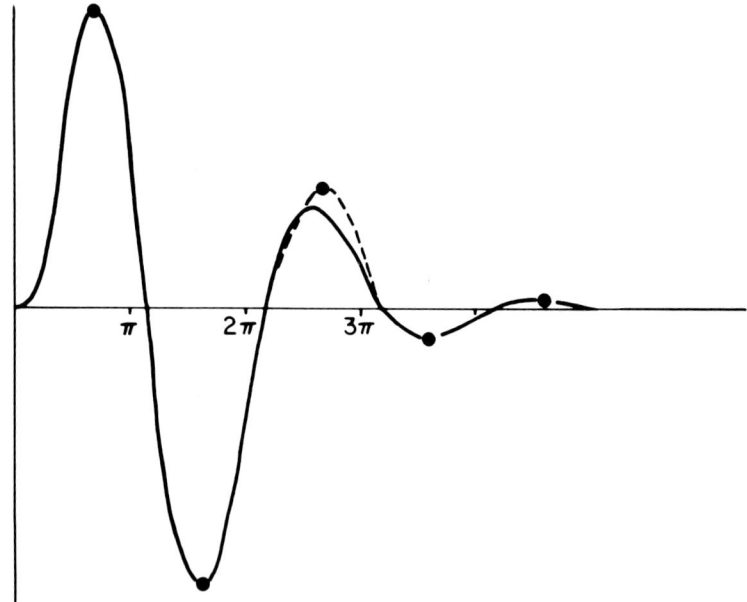

Fig. 13   Impulse response of basilar-membrane motion as calculated by Flanagan (1965) (solid line). Flanagan's calculations were based on data by Békésy (1960) obtained at high levels of sinusoidal stimulation (130-140 dB SPL). Estimated impulse response of the basilar membrane as derived from extrapolated data obtained from click-pair nulling experiments of Goblick and Pfeiffer (1969)(dashed line). The extrapolation was based on data as in Fig. 12 and was estimated for 135 dB SPL. The curve of Fig. 12c was shifted downward 18.2 dB from which the relative amplitudes of adjacent peaks of the impulse response were derived (●'s). The locations of the zero crossings were arbitrarily set equal to those of the solid line.

shows estimated relative amplitudes of the first five peaks of the click response at level estimated to be 130-140 dB SPL. They are plotted on top of the impulse response of the basilar-membrane calculated by Flanagan (1965) from his ad hoc model of Békésy's basilar-membrane measurements (1960) obtained under sinusoidal stimulation at high levels, perhaps 130--140 dB SPL. In addition, we obtained plots of the Fourier transforms of click responses estimated from three different translations of the curve in Fig. 12c corresponding to 135, 95 and 75 dB SPL and compared them to the corresponding data from Flanagan's ad hoc model and from Rhode's basilar-membrane measurements from the monkey respectively (Fig. 14).

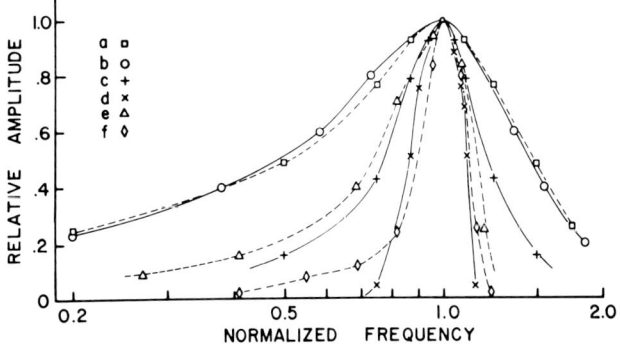

Fig. 14 Amplitude response of basilar-membrane motion. Both amplitude and frequency are normalized. a.) basilar-membrane model by Flanagan (1965), based on high level sinusoidal stimulation (approximately 130-140 dB SPL, Békésy, 1960). b.) estimated amplitude response based on Fourier transform of extrapolation of data obtained from click-pair nulling experiments by Goblick and Pfeiffer (1969)(see Fig. 13). Estimated stimulus level 135 dB SPL. c.) same as in (b) but estimated stimulus level is 95 dB SPL. d.) same as in (b) but estimated stimulus level is 75 dB SPL. e.) from direct measurements of basilar-membrane motion using Mössbauer technique by Rhode (1971). Signal level 90 dB SPL. f.) same as in (e) but signal level 70 dB SPL. Compare a to b, c to e, and d to f. Note that the Q of the amplitude response is a function   (cont'd)

(Fig. 14,cont'd) of signal level, and that the "amplitude" nonlinearity observed in the response patterns of single cochlear nerve fibers in the click-pair nulling experiments is consistent with mechanical nonlinearities.

The close correspondence between changes in the amplitude response calculated for three different signal levels, from the "amplitude" nonlinearity data of the single cochlear nerve fiber discharge pattern, suggests that the "amplitude" nonlinearity may be attributable to the basilar-membrane mechanics.

3. Discussion

For some time it has been difficult to determine if the various nonlinearities as observed in response patterns of single cochlear nerve fibers were related to each other or if they were results of independent nonlinear mechanisms. Several "nonlinearities" have been observed, most have been described in detail, some have been modelled successfully; but none have been fully understood. Recent results from direct observations of mechanical motion (Rhode, 1971); studies of anatomical material (Spoendlin, 1970, 1972); electrophysiological measurements (Gray, 1966, Goblick and Pfeiffer, 1969, Anderson et al., 1971); and inferences from modelling efforts (Pfeiffer, 1971, Kim, 1972) provide motivation to investigate the origins of and the possible interrelationships between the seemingly unrelated nonlinear phenomena. We attempt here, to examine the majority of these nonlinear phenomena and to suggest where each may originate when considering the peripheral system to be represented as in Fig. 1. Great simplifications in understanding the nonlinear properties of this system could be realized if one were to know the essential contribution of each of the subsystems.

Table 1 lists 15 nonlinearities or nonlinear phenomena as seen in spike discharge patterns of single cochlear nerve fibers along with suggestions of their origins. We do not claim that the list is exhaustive, or that the suggested origins are necessarily conclusive.

We attribute items 1, 3, and 10 of Table 1 to basilar-membrane mechanics because each has been observed directly by Rhode (1971). The remaining items that

TABLE 1. Summary of nonlinear phenomena seen in responses of single cochlear nerve fibers, and an estimate of the component of the peripheral auditory system responsible for the generation of each phenomenon. References are not necessarily exhaustive.

NONLINEAR PHENOMENA	REFERENCE FOR SINGLE FIBER DATA	SUGGESTED ORIGIN
1. Decrease in Q with increase in stimulus level.	e.g., Rose et al., 1971	Basilar membrane mechanics
2. Changes in phase angle of response with stimulus level of single tone.	Anderson et al., 1971	Basilar membrane mechanics.
3. Changes in the most effective frequency with stimulus level.	e.g., Anderson et al., 1971	Basilar membrane mechanics
4. Two-tone suppression.	e.g., Sachs and Kiang, 1968	Basilar membrane mechanics
5. Generation of the combination tone, $(2f_1-f_2)$.	Goldstein and Kiang, 1968	Basilar membrane mechanics
6. Changes in shape of the envelope of click response with stimulus level.	e.g., Gray, 1966	Basilar membrane mechanics
7. Amplitude nonlinearity in response to combination clicks.	Goblick and Pfeiffer, 1969	Basilar membrane mechanics
8. Temporal nonlinearity in response to combination clicks.	Goblick and Pfeiffer, 1969	Basilar membrane mechanics
9. Anomalous response to clicks of opposite polarity when CF<350-500 Hz.	Pfeiffer and Kim, 1973	Basilar membrane mechanics

TABLE 1 (cont'd)

NONLINEAR PHENOMENA	REFERENCE FOR SINGLE FIBER DATA	SUGGESTED ORIGIN
10. Saturation or limiting.	e.g., Tasaki, 1954; Pfeiffer and Molnar, 1970	Basilar membrane mechanics or transducer
11. Rectification.	e.g., Brugge et al., 1969	Transducer or Neuron
12. Generation of the combination tones (f_2-f_1), (f_1+f_2), $2f_1$ and $2f_2$.	Littlefield (unpublished)	Transducer or Neuron
13. Harmonic distortion in response to single tones.	Pfeiffer and Molnar, 1970	Neuron
14. Effects of Refractoriness.	Gray, 1966	Neuron
15. Generation of spike trains.	(Obvious)	Neuron

we also attribute to basilar-membrane mechanics are each supported by the anatomical data of Spoendlin (1970, 1972) showing simplicity of innervation as well as failure of the model neuron (variable threshold device Fig. 6) to produce such phenomena. Some items receive further support in that they are properties of the BPNL model without neuron (nos. 1, 4, 5, and 10); some items are supported by results of comparing calculation and extrapolations of the electrophysiological data of Goblick and Pfeiffer (1969) with the mechanical data of Rhode (1971) and with Flanagan's (1965) model based on Békésy's (1960) data (nos. 1, 6, and 7); but most items (nos. 1, 2, 3, 4, 5, 6, 7, 8, and 10) receive considerable support because they all have been demonstrated to be properties of a nonlinear model of basilar-membrane motion that incorporates a single nonlinearity (Kim, 1972) (Fig. 16). Finally, item 9 is suggested to be mechanical in origin first because the frequency range corresponds to the location of the

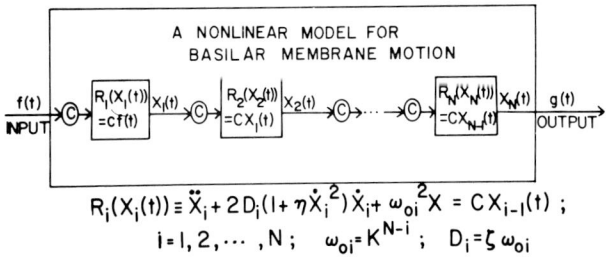

$$R_i(X_i(t)) \equiv \ddot{X}_i + 2D_i(1+\eta \dot{X}_i^2)\dot{X}_i + \omega_{oi}^2 X = CX_{i-1}(t) ;$$
$$i=1,2,\cdots,N ; \quad \omega_{oi} = K^{N-i} ; \quad D_i = \zeta \omega_{oi}$$

Fig. 16 A block diagram of a nonlinear model for basilar-membrane motion. The input f(t), corresponds to the displacement of the stapes and the output, g(t), corresponds to the displacement of a point on the basilar-membrane. Approximate representation for displacements of different points (one point at a time) on the basilar-membrane whose characteristic frequencies are above 500 Hz can be achieved by normalizing the time scale with respect to the period of the characteristic frequency associated with the point on the basilar-membrane under study. Parameter values of the model are: N=10, K=33/32, C=1.25, η=256, ζ=0.25. Note that the model consists of ten cascaded elements, each of which is defined by the second-order nonlinear differential equation shown in the figure. From Kim, 1972.

helicotrema, and second, because the hair cells and neurons along the cochlear duct have an apparent uniformity.

The remaining nonlinearities (items 11-15) we attribute to the transducer or neuron. At low signal levels and for fibers with moderate or high spontaneous rates, say 20/sec or more, period histograms, for clicks and sinewaves, do not indicate rectification but merely a modulation of the spike rate (Littlefield et al., 1972). For these conditions the effects of the nonlinearities listed in items 11, 12, 13, and 14, are not very great. On the other hand, for moderate to high levels of two-tone stimulation, the (f_1+f_2), (f_2-f_1), $2f_1, 2f_2$, and $(2f_1-f_2)$ distortion components appear as significant components in period histograms. Of these, (f_1+f_2), (f_2-f_1), $2f_1$, and $2f_2$, may be a direct result of the rectification.

The distortions of the period histograms for single tone stimulation (item 13) were attributed to the neuron simply because a sinewave input to our variable threshold device yielded similar histograms to those obtained from single cochlear nerve fibers (Fig. 5). This correspondence was detected in our studies of the BPNL with neuron. We found that in case of the stimulus frequency near the CF, the nonlinearity between the linear band-pass filters was inconsequential with respect to the harmonic content of the signal entering the neuron because the input to the neuron is essentially sinusoidal due to the second narrow band-pass filter; the nonlinearity, on the other hand, is the key to two-tone suppression. We have not been able to relate this important second filter to any anatomical structures, but we have developed a nonlinear model of basilar-membrane motion that has overall properties that include those of the BPNL. Hence, under conditions of high level single-tone stimulation, the basilar membrane motion may be nearly sinusoidal even though its amplitude is being limited (Kim, 1972).

Perhaps one of the major causes of difficulties in interpretation has been the assumption that the basilar-membrane mechanics were linear. If the assessments outlined in Table 1 are correct, it is easy to see that much may occur prior to and independent of excitation of the sensory cells. The nonlinearities that remain for the transducer and neuron are essentially rectification, refractoriness and, of course, spike generation.

Given the waveform of motion of the basilar membrane at the site of the hair cell associated with the nerve fiber being observed and also given that there is point innervation between the spiral ganglion neuron and inner hair cell receptor, as reported by Spoendlin (1970, 1972), it appears that one can qualitatively predict the effects that the last two subsections (denoted in Fig. 1) have on the response patterns as represented by PST histograms. Rectification of the waveform (Brugge et al., 1969, Goblick and Pfeiffer, 1969), possible saturation effects of the transducer, and effects on period histograms due to the neuron (Gray, 1966; Pfeiffer and Molnar, 1970; Matthews, 1972) are nonlinearities that are not too difficult to evaluate. On the other hand, the nonlinearities manifested in the first ten properties listed in Table 1, are more complex and their effects on a general form of stimulus are more difficult to predict. The key appears to be in the further understanding of basilar-membrane mechanics.

Throughout this paper we have noted that the nonlinear model of basilar-membrane motion developed by Kim (Fig. 16) simulates a considerable number of nonlinear phenomena. Further, this model is compatible with the model neuron as described in Fig. 6 to the extent that we have been able to propose the origins of the nonlinear phenomena as in Table 1. Thus, we suggest that at the present time, the most comprehensive model for nonlinear response characteristics of single cochlear nerve fibers is a cascade of the basilar-membrane model of Fig. 16 and the variable threshold device of Fig. 6 along with, if one desires, the appropriate adjustments for external and middle ear mechanics.

Spiral ganglion cells that innervate the outer hair cells may receive inputs from several receptors (Spoendlin 1970, 1972). In those cases, the relationships between the associated response pattern and the motions of the basilar membrane could be more complex. On the other hand, the relation may be as simple as a superposition or summation of several waveforms each from one of the outer hair cells being innervated by the spiral ganglion cell (Pfeiffer and Kim, 1973). At any rate, if 95 percent of the spiral ganglion cells innervate inner hair cells as reported by Spoendlin, it is most likely that data used in this paper were derived from that majority group.

The study of the nonlinear characteristics of the peripheral system has led to the examination of some subtle properties of the response patterns. As more detailed questions are asked, more demands are placed on the quality of the stimulus. For example, the combination click studies of Goblick and Pfeiffer (1969) necessitated a distortion compensating driver-amplifier to ensure independence between click level and click polarity (Molnar et al., 1968). Stimulus generating devices with much lower harmonic distortions are necessary, however, when studying effects of two-tone stimulation or of high level single-tone stimulation lest we study the combination tone generating qualities of the stimulus apparatus or the response properties to stimulus harmonics respectively. In particular, responses of fibers to high level stimulation at frequencies far below the CF must be questioned, because the second, third, and other harmonics, although many tens-of-dB down from the fundamental, may be well within the response area of the fiber. Under similar conditions, studies of two-tone interaction may be distorted by unexpected interactions between harmonics of the second tone falling within the response area, and the often used first tone at the CF.

Finally, one might raise the question as to whether or not these nonlinear phenomena are functionally significant in the process of hearing. Prior to any conclusions, more precise descriptions and sound understanding of the phenomena are necessary.

Acknowledgment
We wish to acknowledge the kind assistance and collaboration with our colleagues in our laboratory and in particular with Dr. Charles E. Molnar.

This work was supported in part by several grants from the National Institutes of Health.

References

Anderson, D.J., Rose, J.E., Hind, J.E., and Brugge, J.F. (1971). Temporal position of discharges in single auditory nerve fibers within the cycle of a sine-wave stimulus: frequency and intensity effects. J. Acoust. Soc. Amer. 49, 1131-1139.

Békésy, G.v. (1960). Experiments in Hearing. McGraw-Hill, New York.

Blachman, N.M. (1964). Band-Pass Nonlinearities. IRE Transactions on Information Theory IT-10, pp. 162-164.

Brugge, J.F., Anderson, D.J., Hind, J.E., and Rose, J.E. (1969). Time structure of discharges on single auditory nerve fibers of the squirrel monkey in response to complex periodic sounds. J. Neurophysiol. 32, 386-401.

Engström, M., Ades, M.W., and Anderson, A., (1966). Structural Pattern of the Organ of Corti. Almquist and Wiksell, Stockholm.

Flanagan, J.L., (1965). Speech Analysis, Synthesis, and Perception. Academic Press, New York.

Furman, G.G. (1965). Cochlear sensory-field effects based on inter-unit coupling. Electronic Res. Lab. Rep. No. 65-19. Univ. of California, Berkeley.

Furman, G.G., and Frishkopf, L.S., (1964). Model for neural inhibition in the mammalian cochlea. J. Acoust. Soc. Amer. 36, 2194-2201.

Gerstein, G.L., and Kiang, N.Y.S., (1960). An approach to the quantitative analysis of electrophysiological data from single neurons. Biophys. J. 1, 15-28.

Goblick, T.J., Jr., and Pfeiffer, R.R., (1968). A test for cochlear linearity from cochlear nerve spike discharges in response to combination click stimuli. J. Acoust. Soc. Amer. 44, 363.

Goblick, T.J., Jr., and Pfeiffer, R.R., (1969). Time domain measurements of cochlear nonlinearities using combination of click stimuli. J. Acoust. Soc. Amer. 46, 924-938.

Goldstein, J.L., (1967). Auditory nonlinearity. J. Acoust. Soc. Amer. 41, 676-689.

Goldstein, J.L., and Kiang, N.Y.S., (1968). Neural correlates of the aural combination tone $2f_1-f_2$. Proc. IEEE. 56, 981-992.

Gray, P.R. (1966). A statistical analysis of electrophysiological data from auditory nerve fibers in cat. Tech. Rep. No. 541. Research Laboratory of Electronics, M.I.T. Cambridge, Mass.

Gray, P.R., (1967). Conditional probability analysis of the spike activity of single neurons. Biophys. J. 7, 759-777.

Guinan, J.J., Jr., and Peake, W.T., (1967). Middle ear characteristics of anesthetized cats. J. Acoust. Soc. Amer. 41, 1237-1262.

Iurato, S., (1967). Submicroscopic Structure of the Inner Ear. Pergamon Press, New York.

Johnstone, B.M., and Boyle, A.J.F., (1967). Basilar membrane vibration examined with the Mössbauer technique. Science 158, 389-390.

Kiang, N.Y.S., Watanabe, T., Thomas, E.C., and Clark, L.F., (1962). Stimulus coding in the cat's auditory nerve: a preliminary report. Ann. Otol. Rhinol. Laryngol. 71, 1009-1026.

Kiang, N.Y.S., Watanabe, T., Thomas, E.C., and Clark, L.F., (1965). Discharge Patterns of Single Fibers in the Cat's Auditory Nerve. Res. Monogr. 35. M.I.T. Press, Cambridge, Mass.

Kim, D.O., (1972). A nonlinear model for basilar membrane motion and related phenomena of single cochlear nerve fibers. Thesis. The Washington Univ., St. Louis, Mo.

Kim, D.O., Molnar, C.E., and Pfeiffer, R.R. (1972). A Nonlinear Model for Basilar Membrane Motion. Meet. Acoust. Soc. Amer., 84th.

Klatt, D.M., (1964). Theories of aural physiology. Communication Sci. Lab. Rep. No. 13. Univ. of Michigan, Ann Arbor.

Littlefield, W.M., Pfeiffer, R.R., and Molnar, C.E., (1972). Modulation index as a response criterion for discharge activity. J. Acoust. Soc. Amer. 51, 93.

Lynn, P.A., and Sayers, B.McA., (1970). Cochlear innervation, signal processing, and their relation to auditory time-intensity effects. J. Acoust. Soc. Amer. 47, 525-533.

Matthews, J.W., (1972). A nonlinear analog model of the peripheral auditory system. Thesis. The Washington Univ., St. Louis, Mo.

Molnar, C.E., Loeffel, R.G., and Pfeiffer, R.R., (1968). Distortion compensating, condenser-earphone driver for physiological studies. J. Acoust. Soc. Amer. 43, 1177-1178.

Moxon, E.C., (1968). Auditory nerve responses to electric stimuli. Quart. Progr. Rep. No. 90. Research Laboratory of Electronics, M.I.T. Cambridge, Mass.

Nomoto, M., Suga, N., and Katsuki, Y., (1964). Discharge pattern and inhibition of primary auditory nerve fibers in the monkey. J. Neurophysiol. 27, 768-787.

Pfeiffer, R.R., (1970). A model for two-tone inhibition of single cochlear nerve fibers. J. Acoust. Soc. Amer. 48, 1373-1378.

Pfeiffer, R.R., (1971). A nonlinear model for single cochlear-nerve fiber activity. In: Physiology of the Auditory System (M.B. Sachs, ed.), pp. 125-131. National Educational Consultants, Inc., Baltimore.

Pfeiffer, R.R., and Goblick, T.J. Jr., (1969). A model for responses of single cochlear nerve fibers to click pair stimuli. International Biophysics Congress of the International Union for Pure and Applied Biophysics, 3rd, p. 180. Cambridge, Mass.

Pfeiffer, R.R., and Kim, D.O., (1973). Response patterns of single cochlear nerve fibers to click stimuli: descriptions for cat. J. Acoust. Soc. Amer. (In press).

Pfeiffer, R.R., and Molnar, C.R., (1970). Cochlear nerve fiber discharge patterns: relationship to the cochlear microphonic. Science 167, 1614-1616.

Rhode, W.S., (1971). Observations of the vibration of the basilar membrane in squirrel monkeys using the Mössbauer technique. J. Acoust. Soc. Amer. 49, 1218-1231.

Rodieck, R.W., Kiang, N.Y.S., and Gerstein, G.L., (1962). Some quantitative methods of studying spontaneous activity of single neurons. Biophys. J. 2, 351-368.

Rose, J.E., Hind, J.E., Anderson, D.J., and Brugge, J.F., (1971). Some effects of stimulus intensity on response of auditory nerve fibers in the squirrel monkey. J. Neurophysiol. 34, 685-699.

Rupert, A., Moushegian, G., and Galambos, R., (1963). Unit responses to sound from auditory nerve of the cat. J. Neurophysiol. 26, 449-465.

Sachs, M.B., (1966). Auditory nerve fiber responses to two-tone stimuli. Thesis. M.I.T. Cambridge, Mass.

Sachs, M.B., (1969). Stimulus-response relation for auditory-nerve fibers: two-tone stimuli. J. Acoust. Soc. Amer. 45, 1025-1036.

Sachs, M.B., and Kiang, N.Y.S., (1968). Two-tone inhibition in auditory nerve fibers. J. Acoust. Soc. Amer. 43, 1120-1128.

Spoendlin, H., (1966). The organization of the cochlear receptor. S. Karger, Basel-New York.

Spoendlin, H., (1970). Structural basis of peripheral frequency analysis. In: Frequency Analysis and Periodicity Detection in Hearing (R. Plomp and G.F. Smoorenburg, eds.), pp. 2-40. A.W. Sijthoff Leiden, The Netherlands.

Spoendlin, H., (1972). Innervation densities of the cochlea. Acta oto-laryngol.73, 235-248.

Tasaki, I., (1954). Nerve impulses in individual auditory nerve fibers of guinea pig. J. Neurophysiol. 17, 97-122.

Tonndorf, J., (1958). Harmonic distortion in cochlear models. J. Acoust. Soc. Amer. 30, 929-937.

Tonndorf, J., (1970). Nonlinearities in cochlear hydrodynamics. J. Acoust. Soc. Amer. 47, 579-591.

Weiss, T.F., (1966). A model of the peripheral auditory system. <u>Kybernetik</u> <u>3</u>, 153-175.

Wiener, F.M., Pfeiffer, E.E., and Backus, S.N., (1966). On the sound pressure transformation by the head and auditory meatus of the cat. <u>Acta oto-laryng.</u> <u>61</u>, 255-269.

Figures 3, 4, 9, 10, 11, and 12 reproduced by permission of Journal of the Acoustical Society of America.

Figure 7 reproduced from PHYSIOLOGY OF THE AUDITORY SYSTEM edited by M.B. Sachs, 1971, by permission of National Educational Consultants, Inc., Baltimore.

DISCUSSION

DALLOS: I would like to comment on the basilar membrane model which I understand is supposed to describe correctly a variety of nonlinear phenomena. You made the statement that it accounts for the $2f_1-f_2$ phenomenon, for example. It appears to me that there is extremely good evidence today that indicates that $2f_1-f_2$ is not contained in the basilar membrane motion. This partially comes from my numerous microphonic experiments, partially from the measurements of Wilson and Johnstone (1972) with the capacitive probe.

PFEIFFER: I have no answer to that.

ZWISLOCKI: You said that the model was based on Rhode's data and then you show a curve that agrees with Békésy's data. These data are very different in the way of selectivity.

PFEIFFER: If one accepts that the Q value decreases with signal level, you end up with a low Q-curve at high levels that is not inconsistent with Békésy's results. I might add, there is one item that we have not considered, and that is the change in Q value with changes in frequency. Rhode's data are at a higher frequency than Békésy's. I do not know how this may influence the results.

DALLOS: Do you have any responses to clicks at low levels?

PFEIFFER: No, normally the click responses that we looked at were obtained at higher levels because we needed a large number of spike discharge responses. Generally our clicks were delivered about 30 or 40 dB above the click threshold for a given fiber.

EVANS: I would like to follow on from Peter Dallos's question and ask, what are the frequency filtering capabilities of your model?

PFEIFFER: It depends on how many boxes you put in cascade. The upper end slope of the model is about 120 dB per octave and the lower end is much less. The results can be rather easily manipulated by either having more or fewer boxes in cascade. The end result was in fact designed to match Rhode's data.

EVANS: The reason I asked is that I wondered if your $2f_1-f_2$ component had the right dependence on the frequency ratio of the primaries. That was the crucial finding which I think led Goldstein to propose a 2-filter model in the first place.

PFEIFFER: Well, we are presently looking at the combination tone problems, but we are not quite ready to say anything. Details like that are, of course, being looked at. I might point out that the model is not much different from Ted Evans's model; it is just that the boundary between the hair cell and the mechanics is shifted. It is conceivable that the basilar membrane model as we call it, may be a model of something more than the basilar membrane. The reason that we stopped at the basilar membrane, and included no more, was that the model duplicated the characteristics of published data of basilar membrane mechanics very well.

EVANS: Of interest is your point about the change in Q value with level. Now, one does not see this if one looks at the tuning of fibers above threshold in the form of isorate contours.

PFEIFFER: What about those curves such as Anderson's (Anderson et al., 1971) which show spike rate as a function of tone frequency at various levels?

EVANS: Right. These do get broader at high levels, but in fact if you replot them as isorate contour curves, they get a little sharper with stimulus level, if anything.

Is it possible also that we are referring to different stimulus levels? In other words, are you talking about levels above 70 dB SPL? I am considering here levels of up to 20-30 dB above a fiber's threshold.

PFEIFFER: I think most of these data are obtained at levels above 70 dB although the details pertaining to combination tones are for levels below that.

ZWISLOCKI: I have been pleading for quite some time that the so-called tuning curves and the iso-intensity curves are nonlinearly related to each other and therefore it is not possible to draw the same conclusion from both. It seems to me that the tuning curves are not tuning curves whatsoever. They are constructed in a way that does not reflect the distribution of neural response to a given stimulus. This would be true if they were linearly related but they are not. Thus if you want to see the distribution of neural response for a given stimulus you have to look at the frequency of firing as a function of frequency for constant intensity and not the trading between frequency and intensity for constant firing rate.

EVANS: I would agree that it is not possible to draw the same conclusions from iso-rate (tuning) curves and iso-intensity curves. The point is that if you have a black box model of a cochlear filter followed by a nonlinearity (namely that responsible for the saturative function of the fiber) then to get at the tuning characteristics of that filter, it is the tuning curve which is the appropriate curve to use and not the rate versus frequency function.

References

Anderson, D.J., Rose, J.E., Hind, J.E., and Brugge, J.F. (1971). Temporal position of discharges in single auditory nerve fibers within the cycle of a sine-wave stimulus: frequency and intensity effects. J. Acoust. Soc. Amer. 49, 1131-1139.

Goldstein, J.L., (1967). Auditory nonlinearity. J. Acoust. Soc. Amer. 41, 676-689.

Wilson, J.P., and Johnstone, J.R. (1972). Capacitive probe measures of basilar membrane vibration. Symposium on Hearing Theory 1972, pp. 172-181. IPO Eindhoven, Holland.

CODING OF AMPLITUDE MODULATED SOUNDS
IN THE COCHLEAR NUCLEUS OF THE RAT

Aage R. Møller

Karolinska Institute
Stockholm
Sweden

1. Introduction

Most previous neurophysiological studies on the function of the ascending auditory pathway have been conducted with simple and often static sounds such as pure tones and clicks as stimuli. Because of the great complexity of the auditory system and the lack of understanding of the details in the structure of the auditory nervous system, it is not possible to deduce how the responses are to such complex and time varying stimuli as natural sounds on the basis of the responses to simple static sounds. It is therefore of basic interest to study how changes in amplitude and spectrum of a sound are coded in the nervous system.

It has been shown earlier that rapid changes in stimulus intensity are enhanced in several other sensory neural systems. Sinusoidally intensity modulated stimuli have been used to study the dynamic properties of the sensory neural transmission in vision quantitatively (see e.g. Cleland and Enroth-Cugell, 1966) in proprioception (see e.g. Matthews and Stein, 1969) and the transmission between neurons (see e.g. Watanabe, 1962, Terzuolo and Bayley, 1968). The dynamic properties of these systems have been described quantitatively by gain functions or by transfer functions showing the ratio between the modulation of the stimulus (or the stimulus itself if the system responds to low frequency stimuli) and the frequency modulation of the recorded neural discharges. Such gain functions often show a peak at a certain modulation frequency. This means that these neural systems are "tuned" to a certain modulation frequency at which small changes in stimulus intensity are enhanced in the neural discharge pattern of individual neurons compared with slower or more rapid changes (see e.g. Ratliff et al., 1967, Ratliff et al., 1969).

In the present paper the dynamic characteristic of single units in the cochlear nucleus is described on the basis of responses to amplitude modulated tones and noise. The justification of the use of linear systems theory in analysis of the responses is discussed with regard to the linearity and stationarity of the system.

The dynamic characteristics are described by transfer functions showing the ratio between the degree of frequency modulation of the neural discharge rate and the degree of amplitude modulation of the sound. This ratio is plotted as a function of modulation frequency. The recording technique and surgical procedure have been described earlier (Møller, 1969, 1971) as has the processing of the recorded responses (Møller, 1972, 1973). The material presented in this paper is based on recordings from 97 units in 32 animals.

2. Experimental Results

2.1 Responses to sinusoidal modulated tones

Fig. 1 shows a cycle histogram of the responses to sinusoidally amplitude modulated tone. Two periods of the modulation are included. It is seen that the modulation of the sound is clearly reproduced in the cycle histogram and that a sinusoidally amplitude modulated tone gives rise to a discharge frequency which in a first approximation is sinusoidally modulated. Similar histograms showing one period of the modulation and covering a larger range of modulation frequencies are seen in Fig. 2 together with a graph showing the ratio (in dB), between the relative amplitude of a sine wave, which fits the cycle histogram, and the modulation of the sound. The phase angle between the modulation of the sound and the modulation of histograms is also shown. It is seen that there is a pronounced peak in the transfer function around a modulation frequency of about 300 Hz. This means that amplitude changes with frequencies around this peak are enhanced in the discharge pattern. In this unit a 10 % change in amplitude (1 dB) gave rise to as much as 30 % change in the discharge frequency when the modulation frequency was 300 Hz.

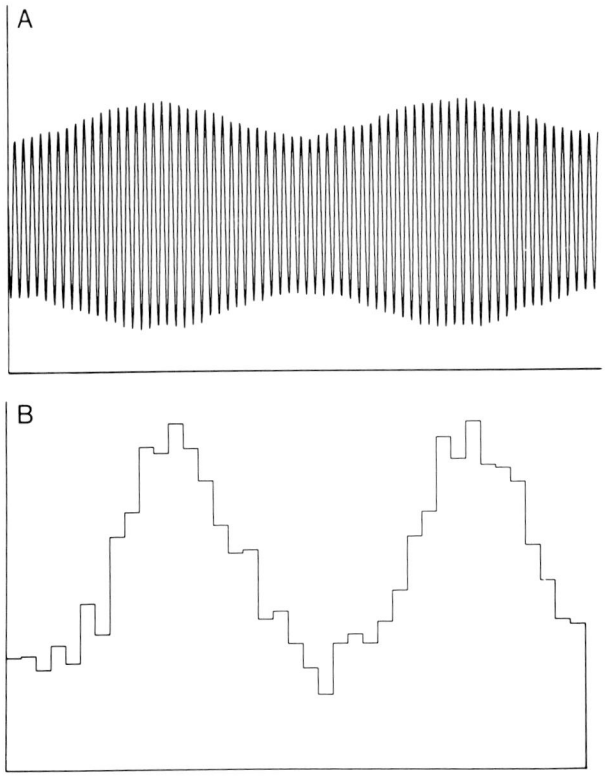

Fig. 1 Sample of a sinusoidal amplitude modulated tone (A) used as stimulus together with a histogram of the response from a unit in the cochlear nucleus (B). Two periods are shown. Modulation frequency was 200 Hz and modulation depth was 10 %.

At a low modulation frequency (10 Hz) it was about 3 %. The transfer function to amplitude modulated tones thus gives the impression of a "tuning" of the units to a particular modulation frequency. In the response shown in Fig. 2, this "tuning" is fairly pronounced. This is typical for many units but some units show a less pronounced peak and the transfer functions of such units resemble low pass functions with a cut-off frequency which varies from unit to unit in the range of 400 to above 1000 Hz.

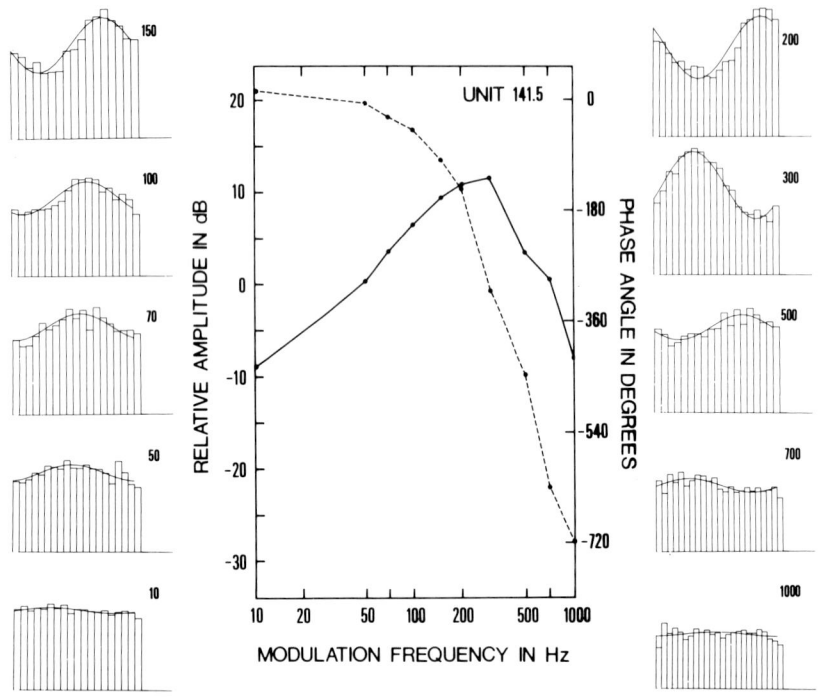

Fig. 2 Cycle histograms of the discharges in response to amplitude modulated tones at different modulation frequency (indicated by legend numbers). The smooth curves are sine waves that fit the histograms according to the least mean square criterion.

The middle graph shows the relative amplitude of the sine wave that fits the histogram divided by the relative amplitude of the modulation of the tone stimuli i.e. the gain function. The phase angle between the modulation and these sine waves is also shown as a function of modulation frequency. The modulation of the stimulus tone was 10 % and its frequency was equal to the CF of the unit (30.0 kHz). The stimulus intensity was 60 dB SPL and the threshold of the unit was 45 dB SPL (From Møller 1972).

In many units the transfer function with regard to
amplitude modulation is of a rather unchanged shape
within a large range of sound intensities. In other
units there is a systematic change in shape. Usually
the peak in the transfer function becomes sharper as
intensity is increased. In this latter type of units
an increase in sound intensity results in a marked
decrease in the modulation of the neural discharge
frequency for low modulation frequencies.

Fig. 3 shows the transfer functions of a typical unit
of the first mentioned type obtained at three different sound intensities and Fig. 4 shows in a similar
way the transfer functions of a typical unit of the
latter type.

The results shown in Figs. 1-4 were all obtained in
experiments where the frequency of the tone which was
modulated (carrier) was equal to the characteristic
frequency of the unit (CF). The transfer functions in
response to amplitude modulated tones are, however,
rather independent of the carrier frequency provided
that it is within the response area of the unit. This
is illustrated in Fig. 5 which shows transfer functions of a unit at three different carrier frequencies, above, at and below the CF of the unit.

2.2 Nonlinearity

It is of interest to investigate whether the transfer
functions obtained with sinusoidal modulation constitute a general description of the dynamic properties of the system. That would be the case if the
system were linear. In such a case the response to
stimulation with any waveshape could be precisely
predicted from knowledge about the stimulation and
the transfer function of the system. It is therefore
important to study to what extent the system under
study behaves in the same way as a linear system.

When the input to a nonlinear system is a sine wave,
the waveshape of the output is likely to be a distorted
sine wave. One way to study the linearity of a system
would therefore be to measure the harmonic content of
the output when the input is a pure sine wave.

Fig. 6 shows the relative amplitude of the modulation
of the histograms of a unit in response to an amplitude modulated tone at CF. In addition to the funda-

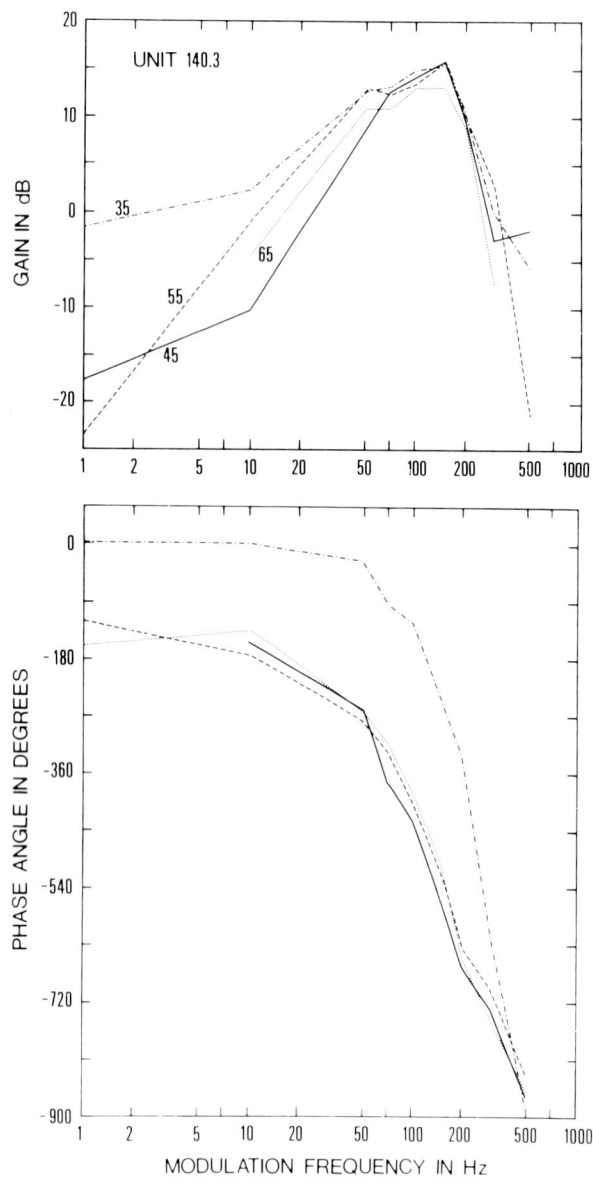

Fig. 3 Gain functions obtained at different sound
intensities (given in dB SPL on the individual curves). The CF of the unit was 15.2 kHz
and its threshold was about 20 dB SPL. The
modulation was 10 %. The firing rate   (cont'd)

(Fig. 3, cont'd) of this unit had its maximum value at 40 dB SPL. Above that level the firing rate decreased again. (From Møller, 1972.)

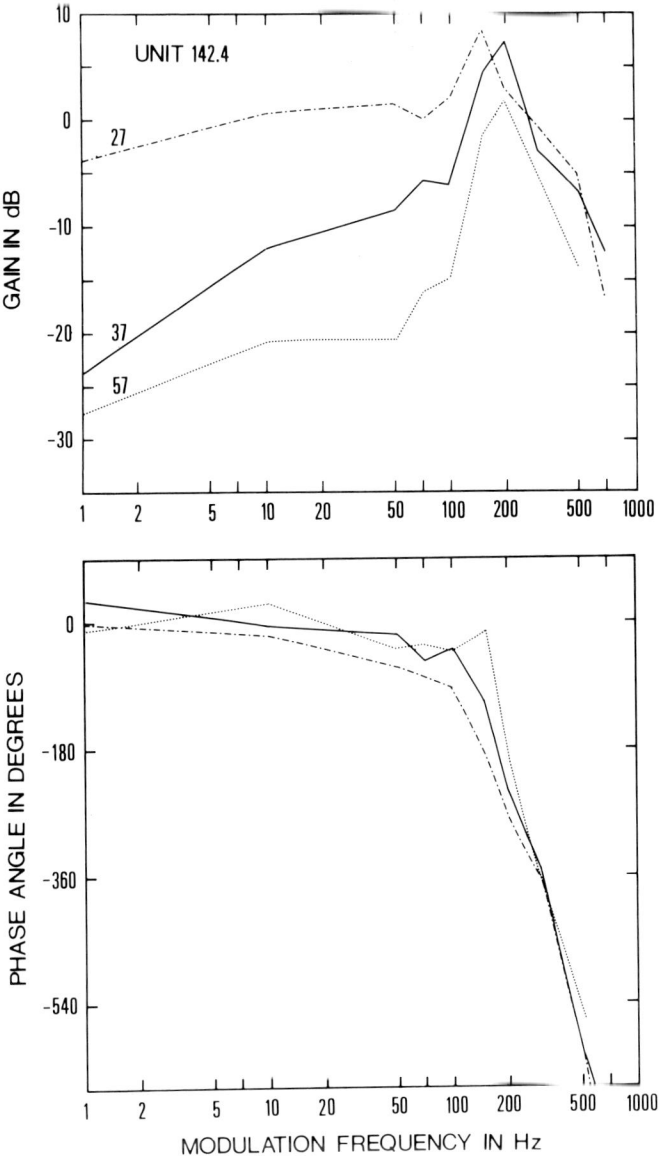

Fig. 4 Gain functions similar to those in Fig. 3. The CF of this unit was 21.9 kHz and (cont'd)

(Fig. 4, cont'd) its threshold was about 17 dB SPL. The modulation was 30 %. (From Møller 1972).

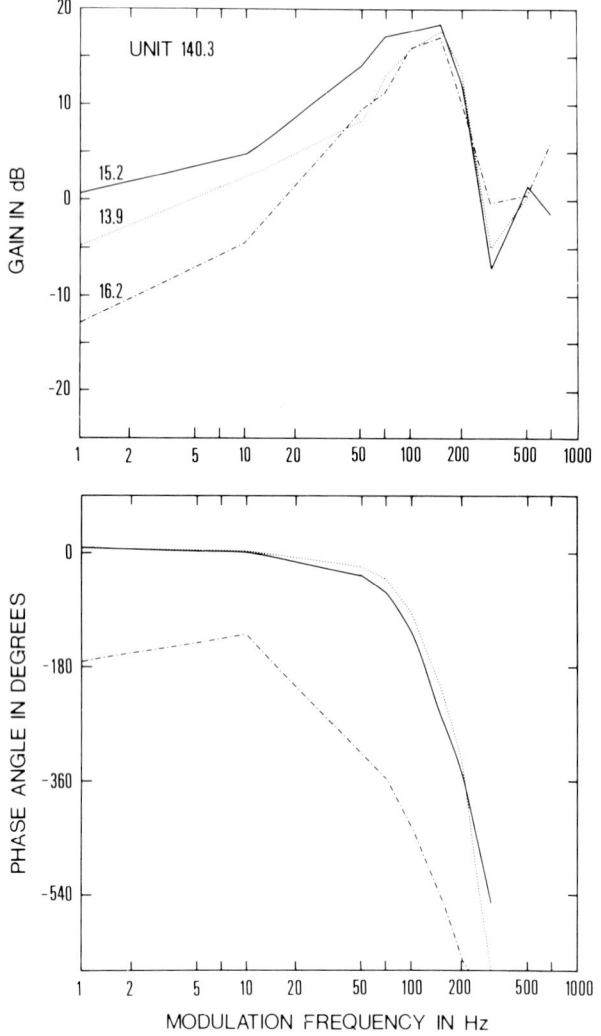

Fig. 5 Gain functions based on the responses to amplitude modulated tones of three different frequencies indicated by legend numbers (in kHz). The modulation was 10 % and the CF of the unit was 15.2 kHz. The sound intensity at 13.9 kHz was 55 dB, at 15.2 kHz   (cont'd)

(Fig. 5, cont'd) 35 dB and at 16.2 kHz 45 dB SPL. (From Møller, 1972).

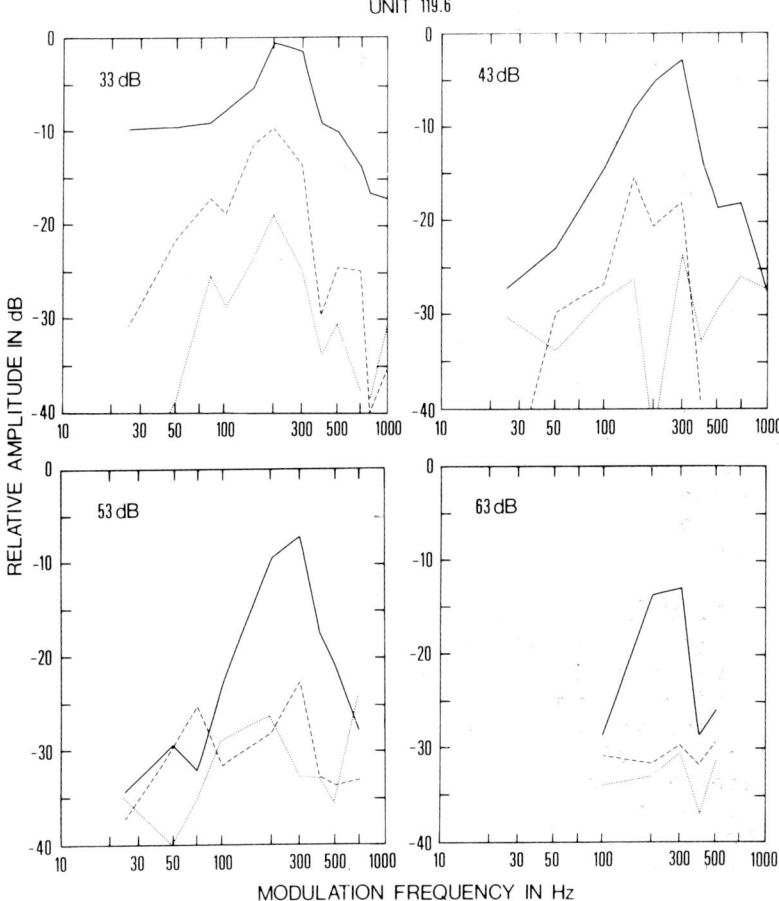

Fig. 6   Relative amplitude of the fundamental frequency (solid line) of the second (dashed line) and third harmonic (dotted line) wave of the modulation of the discharges in response to amplitude modulated tones at four different intensities (given in each graph in dB SPL). The modulation of the stimulus tone was 15 % and the threshold of the unit at CF (23.2 kHz) was 20 dB SPL. (From Møller, 1972).

mental frequency of the modulation the content of second and third harmonics are shown. These data were obtained by fitting three sine waves at the same time to the cycle histograms of the responses. The frequency of the fundamental sine wave was equal to the modulation; the frequency of the two other was twice and three times respectively of that of the fundamental frequency.

It is seen from Fig. 6 that the second harmonic is more than 10 dB below the amplitude of the fundamental frequency in most of the frequency ranges studied. The third harmonic is about 20 dB below the amplitude of the fundamental. These data thus indicate that this neuron under these circumstances exhibits only a low and fairly insignificant nonlinearity.

On the other hand, the fact that different sound levels result in transfer functions of different shapes shows that the system does not work as a linear system over a large intensity range. For small variations in amplitude around a certain operating point, however, the system seems to work in very much the same way as a linear system.

2.3 Response to noise modulated sounds

The complexity of the system studied, however, makes it of value to investigate the dynamic properties with different methods. After all, sine waves are rather special waveshapes which do not occur as natural stimulation. Testing the dynamic properties of a system with sine waves means that the system is studied with only one frequency at a time. The result is the obscuring of any possible interactions between different spectral components.

It has been shown earlier that the transfer function of a linear system can be evaluated statistically on the basis of the responses to any stochastic input, when this input contains reasonably much energy in the frequency range of interests. Using stochastic signals as input the transfer function of a linear system is the cross-spectrum between the input and the output of the system divided by the autospectrum of the input. Since the transfer function is based on the cross-spectrum between input and output the possible inherent noise in the system under test is reduced because it is uncorrelated with the input.

Furthermore, this method makes it possible to compute coherence functions. These show to what extent the output is caused by the actual input to the system. This is of importance in systems with inherent noise where the output may be a result of the inherent noise rather than the input.

There are, however, some difficulties in applying this technique in studies of the dynamic properties of sensory neural systems. Due to the large variability in the discharge frequency large samples of data have to be processed and because of the large bandwidth required (about 1500 Hz) the sampling rate must be high. Consequently analyses become very expensive with regard to computer time. These difficulties can however be overcome by the use of pseudorandom noise instead of normal noise. This makes it possible to reduce the statistical variability of the recorded discharge pattern by the averaging process of cycle histograms which are locked to the periodicity of the noise. Instead of computing the cross-correlation over the entire recording period this procedure reduces the computation to one such noise period (Møller, 1973). Fig. 7 shows a period of the pseudorandom noise used together with the amplitude of the tone modulated with that noise. A histogram of the responses to a tone modulated with noise and the computed cross-correlation between one period of the pseudorandom noise and the histogram is also shown in Fig. 7.

Typical transfer functions computed from cross-correlograms of the noise and the histograms of the responses to amplitude modulated tones in single units in the cochlear nucleus are seen in Fig. 8 together with transfer functions obtained using sinusoidal amplitude modulation. As seen, there is a good agreement between the results obtained with those two different methods. This in itself indicates that the system studied behaves reasonably similarly to a linear system under the actual experimental circumstances. The high values of the coherence spectrum, at least in the middle part of the frequency range investigated, constitute a further support for that statement.

A further advantage of determining the transfer function on the basis of stochastic signals is that it

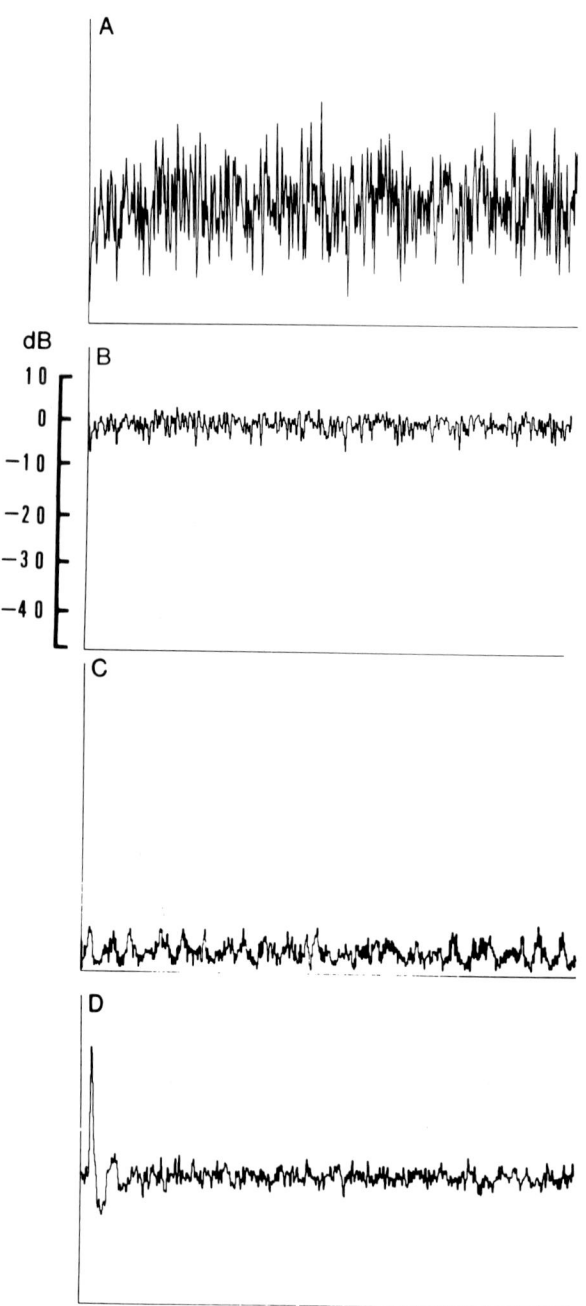

Fig. 7

One period of pseudorandom noise (A) together with the amplitude (in dB) of a sound modulated with the noise (B). The modulation depth was 30% RMS. C. shows a histogram of the responses to a tone amplitude modulated with that noise and D. shows the cross-correlation between the noise and the histogram.

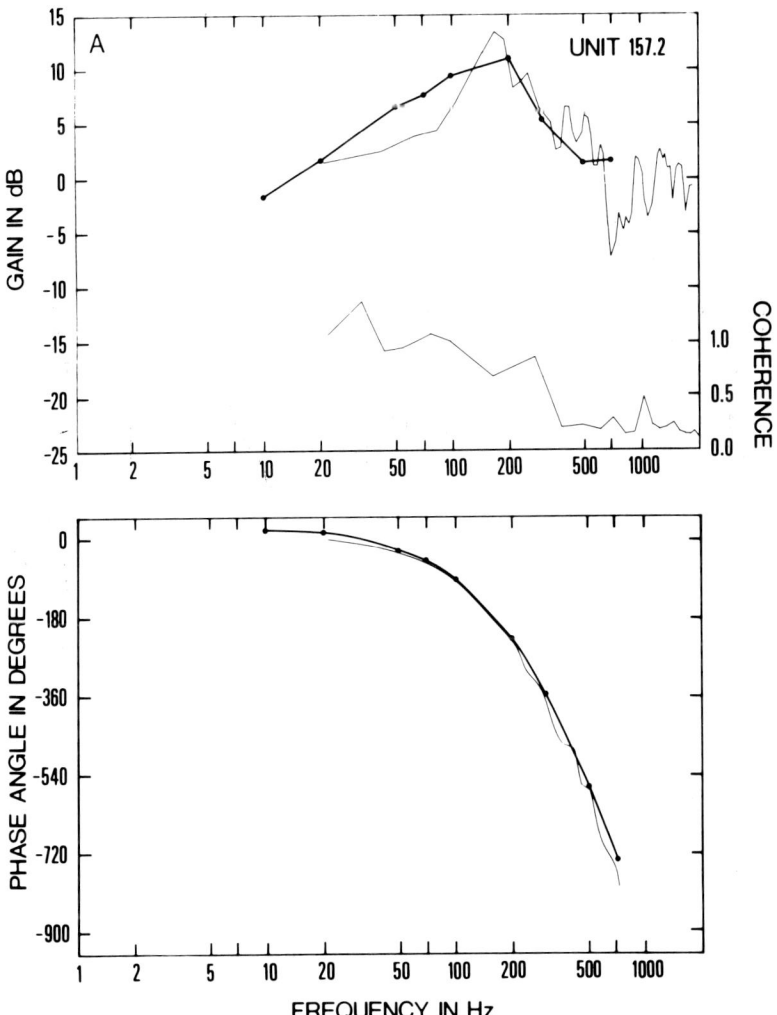

Fig. 8 Gain functions obtained on the basis of the responses of sinusoidally modulated tones (thick lines) and to tones modulated with pseudorandom noise (thin lines). Upper part of each graph shows gain (in dB) and coherence spectrum (lower thin lines). Lower part of the graphs shows the phase angle (in degrees).

A. Sound intensity 50 dB SPL, threshold at CF 30 dB SPL CF 24.4 kHz. 5 minutes of data were

(Fig. 8A cont'd) processed. Mean discharge rate: 147 discharges per second.

B, C, D: CF 12.8 kHz, threshold at CF 28 dB SPL. Each graph is based on 10 minutes of recording.

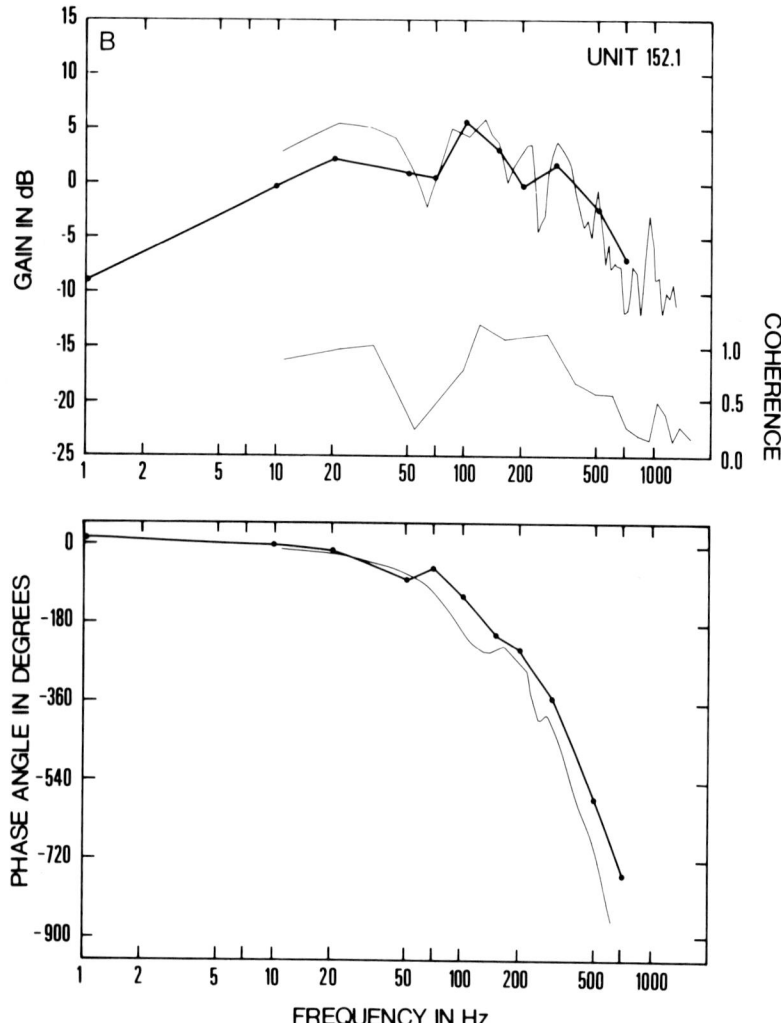

B. Sound intensity 38 dB SPL. Mean discharge rate: 43.2 discharges per second.

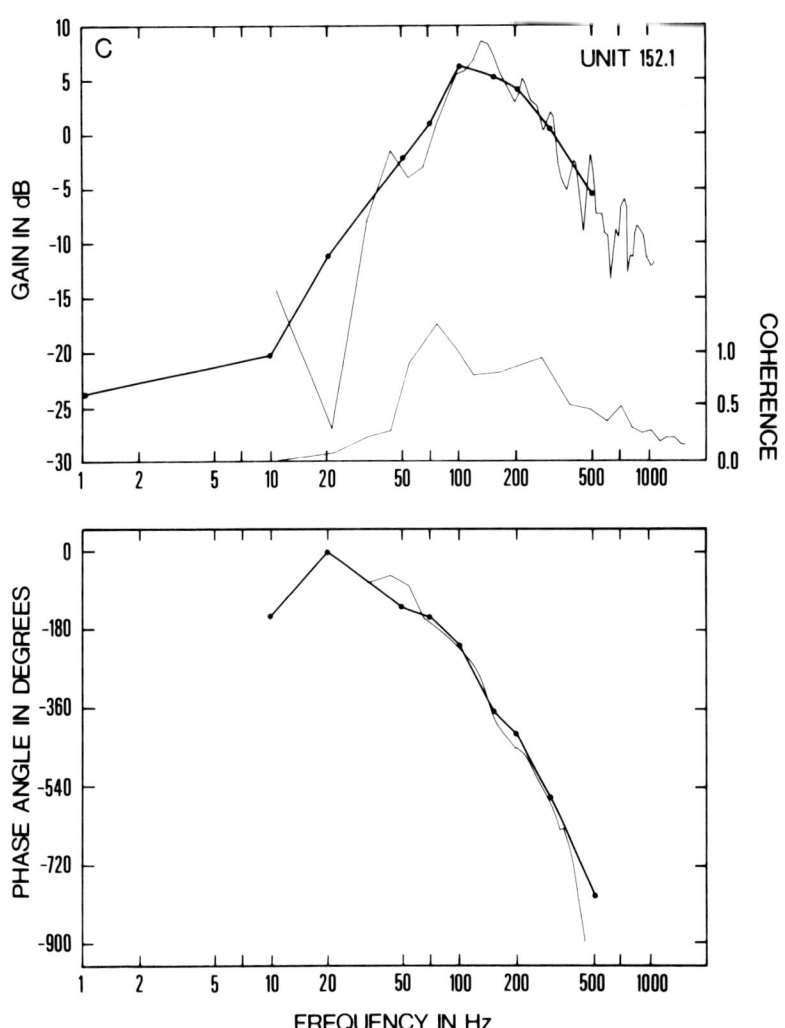

C. 58 dB SPL. 47.7 discharges per second.

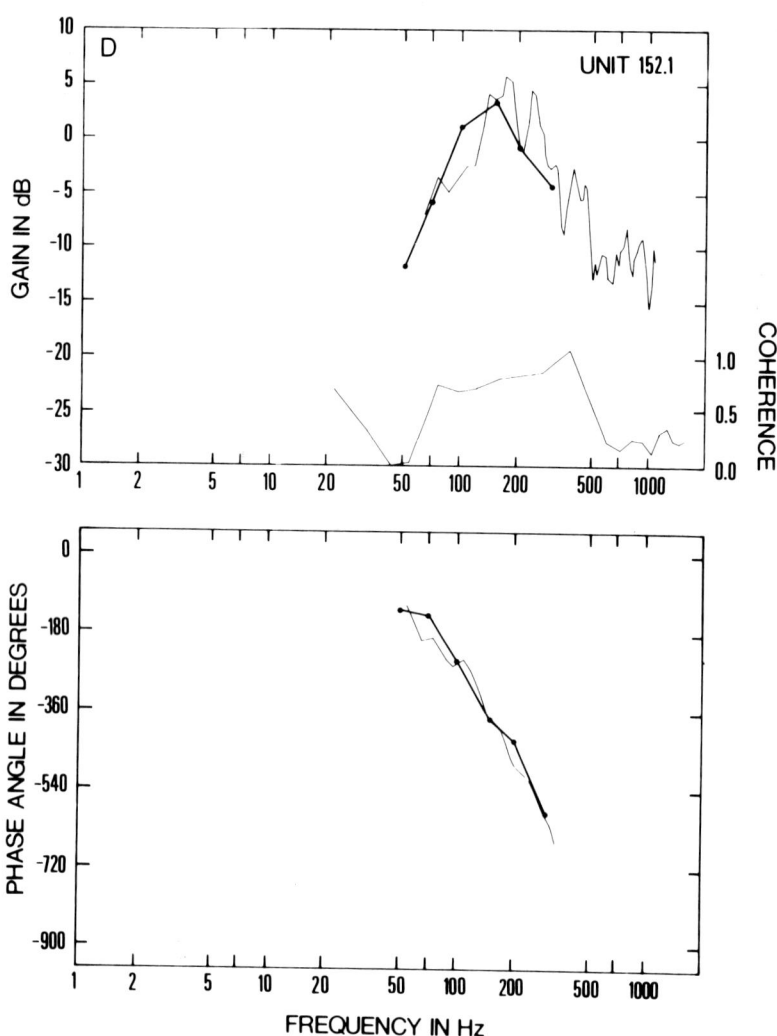

D. 78 dB SPL, 50.0 discharges per second. (From Møller, 1973).

enables the determination of the transfer function of
the system in one single experimental run. The frequency resolution achieved by this method is also
higher than what is practically obtainable using sinusoidal input at discrete frequencies. This is of
particular advantage when the long time stationarity
of the response pattern is questionable.

2.4 Stationarity

The longer the samples for obtaining the transfer
functions, the less becomes the variance of each estimate of the transfer ratio. However, in case the
properties of these neurons are not stationary over
a long time, this averaging will introduce an unanticipated effect of also averaging the properties of
the neurons. If there are narrow peaks in the transfer
function of the units and if the frequency of these
peaks varies during the recording session these peaks
will appear broadened if data are averaged over long
times. The peaks will hence be lower than they would
have been if their frequency location had been constant during the recording period.

The dynamic properties of some of the units in the
cochlear nucleus obtained on basis of the responses
to noise modulated tones show several such peaks in
their transfer functions in addition to the main peak
which is seen in nearly all units. These other peaks
appear in the frequency range above the main peak and
they do not seem to be particularly stationary. When
e.g. a 10 min. recording session is split up into
shorter periods these peaks are often seen to vary in
both amplitude and in frequency. This is illustrated
in Fig. 9 which shows the transfer function obtained
during a 10 min. recording together with those obtained during the first and last 5 min. respectively
of this recording. It is seen that these higher order
peaks in the transfer functions vary in location and
height in these two recording periods. Consequently,
the transfer functions computed on the basis of 10
min. of recording do not contain as many peaks as do
each of the 5 min. functions.

2.5 Dynamic properties of inhibitory tones compared with excitatory tones

Most units in the cochlear nucleus show pronounced
inhibitory areas on both sides of their excitatory

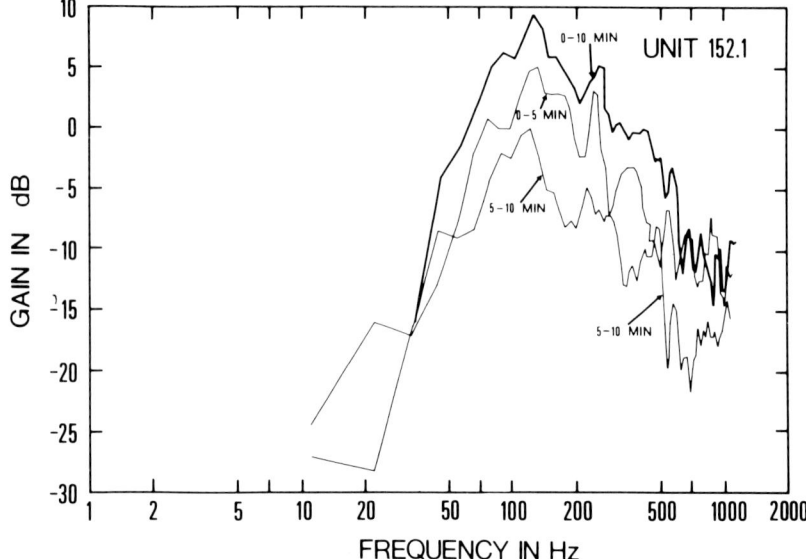

Fig. 9 Gain functions based on different lengths of recordings. The stimulus was a 12.8 kHz tone amplitude modulated with pseudorandom noise (CF of the unit was 12.8 kHz). The intensity of the tone was 48 dB SPL (20 dB above threshold). The curves for 0-5 min were shifted downwards 5 dB and the 5-10 min curve downwards 10 dB in order to facilitate comparison. Mean discharge rates were 52.4 and 48.0 discharges per second respectively. (From Møller, 1973).

response areas. The presence of those inhibitory areas is most easily demonstrated when a tone the frequency of which is slightly higher or lower than the CF of the units is added to a tone at CF. The addition of such a tone usually reduces the rate of firing evoked by the tone at CF.

It is of interest to study the dynamic properties of these inhibitory areas and compare them with those of the excitatory areas. This has been done by presenting two tones simultaneously, one at CF and one with a frequency above or below CF at a frequency where maximal inhibition occurs. Either the excitatory or the inhibitory tone was then amplitude modulated with pseudorandom noise and the evoked unit responses were analyzed in the same way as was done for single tones.

The results of two typical experiments are seen in Fig. 10-14. The transfer functions are shown in Figs. 11 and 13 and Figs. 10 and 12 show the cross-correlograms on which the transfer functions were based. The

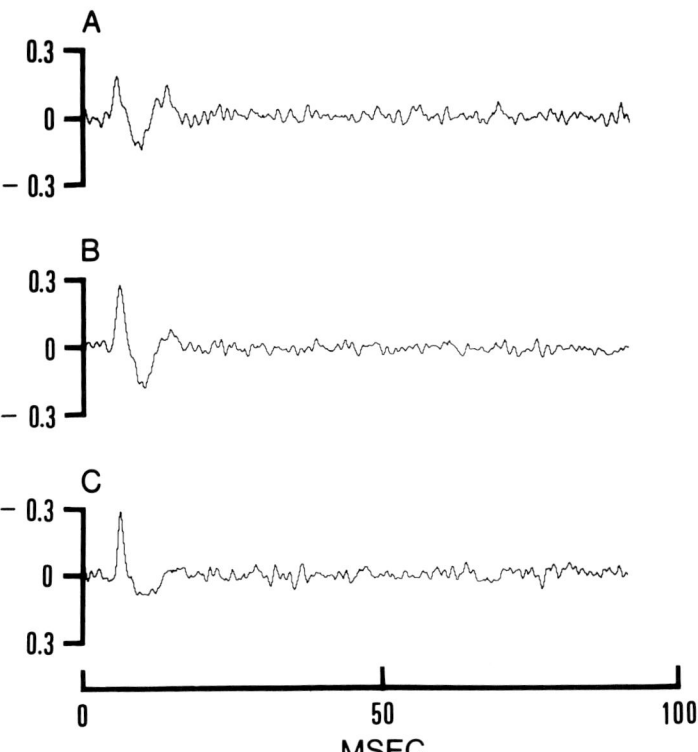

Fig. 10 Cross-correlograms obtained on the basis of responses to pseudorandom noise modulated tones. A: Correlogram representing the responses to a single tone at CF. B: shows similar results when an inhibitory tone was added. C: correlogram obtained when the inhibitory tone was modulated. (In order to facilitate comparison the lower curve was inverted to show negative correlation upwards).

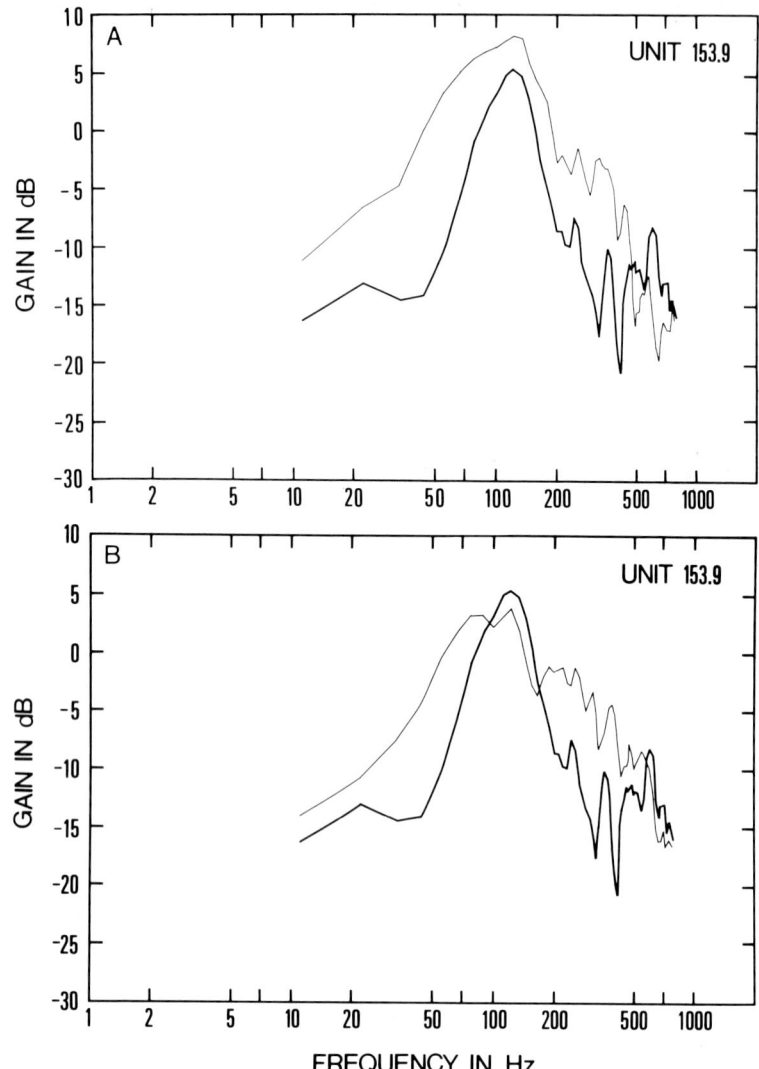

Fig. 11 Transfer function computed on the basis of the correlograms shown in Fig. 10. The thick line represents the case in which a single tone at CF was modulated. In A the thin line represents modulation of an excitatory tone in the presence of an inhibitory tone and in B the thin line represents modulation of the inhibitory tone.

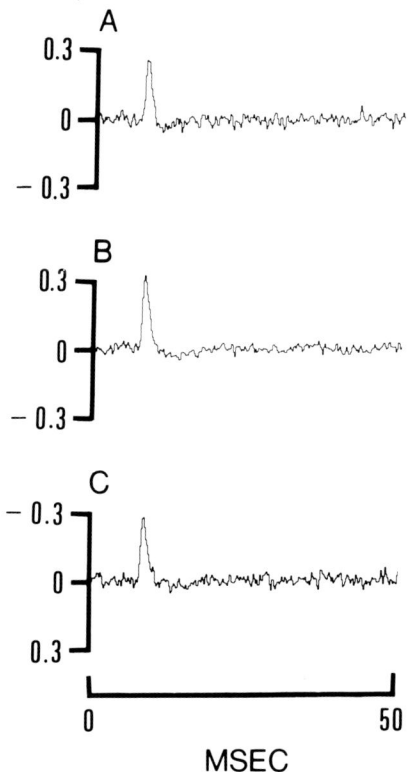

Fig. 12 Same as Fig. 10 for another unit.

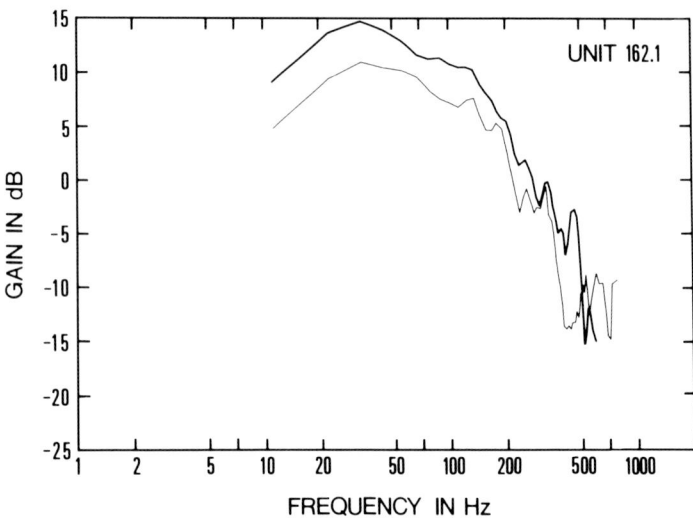

Fig. 13 Transfer functions computed on the basis of the correlograms in Fig. 12. The thick line represents the transfer function when the excitatory tone was modulated (corresponding to B in Fig. 12) and the thin line represents modulation of an inhibitory tone in presence of an excitatory tone.

upper graphs (A in Fig. 10 and 12) show the results when only one tone with frequency equal to the CF of the unit was presented and the middle curves (B) show the results obtained when an inhibitory tone was added. The lower traces (C) show the cross-correlograms obtained when the inhibitory tone was modulated. These three correlograms are similar in shape in both units. Also the transfer functions based on the cross-correlograms of the three stimulus situations show great similarity in shape but the absolute value of the gain is less when the inhibitory tone is modulated compared to modulation of the excitatory tone in presence of an inhibitory tone or of a single excitatory tone.

The results are usually only little dependent on the relationship between the intensity of the inhibitory and excitatory tones as long as both influence the firing pattern of the neuron. The inhibitory tone can be increased more than 20 dB relative to the excitatory tone without affecting the shape of the transfer function very much. The absolute value of the gain may change as a result of varying the intensity relation between the two tones.

3. Discussion

It is interesting to note that the modulation of the discharge frequency of the neurons as a result of a modulation of the intensity of a sound is greatly dependent on the frequency of the modulation. Furthermore, at the modulation frequency at which maximal change in discharge frequency occurs a 1 dB modulation e.g. can give rise to as much as a 50 % change in discharge frequency. This is the case over a large intensity range even in the range where the unit's mean discharge frequency depends very little on the mean sound pressure level. There is thus a considerable enhancement of changes in the intensity of a sound at the level of the cochlear nucleus. Although we do not know how these changes in discharge frequency can be transmitted further up in the ascending auditory pathway it is of interest to see that small changes in the intensity of a tone are so well represented over such large intensity ranges.

It is also worth noting that the waveshape of a change in intensity is reproduced with little non-linear distortion only in the discharge frequency. A modulation with a complex waveform will, however, not be reproduced with an unchanged waveshape in the discharge frequency because of the frequency dependent characteristic of the transfer from amplitude change to change in neural discharge frequency. Certain frequency components are enhanced and others are suppressed.

The fact that the transfer functions obtained on the basis of modulation of an inhibitory tone are almost identical in shape to those obtained from modulation of an excitatory tone indicates that the inhibitory inflow to the neurons studied is transmitted through an equal number of neurons from the cochlea as are the excitatory input. It is not clear whether this inhibition is established in the cochlear nucleus neurons or whether it is identical to the inhibition (or suppression) in single primary fibers where the excitatory response areas have been found to be "sandwiched" between inhibitory areas. (Nomoto et al., 1964, Sachs and Kiang, 1969).

Acknowledgement

This work was supported by the Swedish Medical Research Council (Project no 14 - X - 90).

References

Cleland, B., and Enroth-Cugell, C. (1966). Cat ganglion cell responses to changing light intensities: Sinusoidal modulation in the time domain. Acta Physiol. Scand. 68, 365-381.

Matthews, P.C.B., and Stein, P.B. (1969). The sensitivity of muscle spindle afferents to small sinusoidal changes of length. J. Physiol. 200, 223-243.

Møller, A.R. (1969). Unit responses in cochlear nucleus of the rat to pure tones. Acta Physiol. Scand. 75, 530-541.

Møller, A.R. (1971). Unit responses in the rat cochlear nucleus to tones of rapidly varying frequency and amplitude. Acta Physiol. Scand. 81, 540-556.

Møller, A.R. (1972). Coding of amplitude and frequency modulated sounds in the cochlear nucleus of the rat. Acta Physiol. Scand. 86, 223-238.

Møller, A.R. (1973). Statistical evaluation of the dynamic properties of the cochlear nucleus units using stimuli modulated with pseudorandom noise. Brain Res. (in press).

Nomoto, M., Suga, N., and Katsuki, Y. (1964). Discharge pattern and inhibition of primary nerve fibers in the monkey. J. Neurophysiol. 27, 768-787.

Ratliff, F., Knight, B.W. Toyoda, J., and Hartline, H.K. (1967). Enhancement of flicker by lateral inhibition. Science, 158, 392-393.

Ratliff, F., Knight, B.W. and Graham, N. (1969). On tuning and amplification by lateral inhibition.

Proc. N.A.S. <u>62</u>, 733-740.

Sachs, M.B., and Kiang, N.Y.S. (1968). Two-tone inhibition in auditory-nerve fibers. <u>J. Acoust. Soc. Amer.</u> <u>43</u>, 1120-1128.

Terzuolo, C.A., and Bayley, E.J. (1968). Data transmission between neurons. <u>Kybernetik</u> <u>5</u>, 83-85.

Watanabe, I. (1962). Response of an abdominal ganglion of the crayfish to electrical stimulation with sinusoidal frequency change. <u>J. Fac. Sci. Hokkaido Univ. Ser VI Zool.</u> <u>15</u>, 93-102.

DISCUSSION

SCHWARTZKOPFF: I wonder if you can tell me whether this function you were studying is something bound to the area of the cochlear nucleus or whether you think it is more general. I am asking this because we have found modulation responses up to 500 Hz in the forebrain of the bird.

MØLLER: I know of only a few studies of the responses to modulated tones. One is by Ted Evans (Evans and Nelson, 1966). I think you may find a similar type of responses in many places of the nervous system. I do however, not think that you get the same type of clear responses if you go one of more stages higher in the auditory nervous system.

ZWISLOCKI: Can you define what you mean by "linear system" here? It seems to me that a simple intensity response function of a neuron shows that it is extremely nonlinear.

MØLLER: I would not call the system linear system but rather say that it *behaved* like a linear system under certain circumstances. The reason we are so interested in this question is of course that we in a simple way can get a general description of the properties of a system that behaves like a linear system. Under those circumstances in which it works like a linear system, the transfer function describes the dynamic properties of the system entirely.

GREEN: Do you find any correlation between the characteristic frequency of the cells and the apparent time window that you determine from the impulse response of the cells?

MØLLER: No, I have not seen any correlation at all. Those units I showed you had a characteristic frequency ranging from something like 5 kHz to 30 kHz.

TONNDORF: This may be a naive question, but does not the introduction of what you called a pseudorandom noise, with its regular repetition, result in a line spectrum?

MØLLER: The pseudorandom noise precisely as you noted, generates a line spectrum, where the difference between the lines equals the periodicity of the noise. One can then select the periodicity in accordance with the spectral resolution one wants. As you know you can trade spectral resolution for statistical stability of each spectral estimates. The higher the resolution is the more variable become the estimates for the same amount of data.

EVANS: I do not agree with Aage Møller that we will find the kind of linearity that he has been talking about in many places in the auditory system. For example, in the cochlear nucleus complex itself, it is very much harder to find linearities of the sort that he has been describing in the dorsal nucleus compared with the neutral. I would like to ask where were your records from, have you made such a subdivision of your results?

MØLLER: No, I have not. I have tried to sample the cochlear nucleus as evenly as possible with all the drawbacks that this would entail, but I have not found much difference I must say. If one looks at the distortion in the histograms of the response to sinusoidally modulated sounds one is astonished that almost 100 % modulation can take place with very little contents of harmonics.

Reference

Evans, E.F., and Nelson, P.G. (1966). Responses of neurons in cat cochlear nucleus to modulated tonal stimuli. J. Acoust. Soc. Amer. 40, 1275-1276.

V
NEURAL CODING AT HIGHER LEVELS

TIME DEPENDENT FEATURES OF ADEQUATE SOUND STIMULI AND THE FUNCTIONAL ORGANIZATION OF CENTRAL AUDITORY NEURONS

G.V. Gersuni and I.A. Vartanian

Pavlov Institute of Physiology
of the Academy of Sciences of the USSR
Leningrad, USSR

In his work "Die Lehre von den Tonenempfindungen" (1863) Helmholtz considered a pure tone to be the most simple and adequate stimulus for investigation of human audition. Such a view was based on Helmholtz's renowned assumption about the properties of the cochlea as a frequency analyzer and the specificity of nervous structures connected with differently localized parts of the cochlea for pitch sensations.

In idealization, such a pure tone stimulus could be considered as infinite (stationary in amplitude and spectrum). Argumentation that such an idealized stationary signal does not fit to mechanisms operating in the auditory system at the present time would be a mere truism. A search for mechanisms which operate with signals restricted in time and characterized by different time dependent phenomena is typical for contemporary hearing studies. But in spite of numerous investigations along this line performed by different methods (psychophysical, neurophysical, biophysical), general features of such a mechanism, especially in the central divisions of the auditory system, are far from clear (discussions and literature in reviews and symposia: Erulkar et al., 1968, Plomp and Smoorenburg, 1970, Møller, 1972).

One question among others which seem to be important in the search for auditory mechanisms is that of sound features, which are to be considered as specially adapted (adequate) for the functioning of the auditory system. The data necessary for consideration of this problem can be derived from evaluation of features of natural sounds and their sources. Sounds emitted by animals can be considered as natural sounds used as signals in different forms of behavior.[1] As a result of numerous studies of acoustical emission in different animal groups (Sebeok, 1968), a general assumption of interdependence between features of bioacoustical signals and properties of hearing in biologically and ecologically related groups and in special forms of behavior is widely accepted (Marler and Hamilton, 1967).

Especially advanced are studies along this line on such special forms of behavior as echolocation (Griffin, 1958, Marler and Hamilton, 1967, Airapetianz and Konstantinov, 1970, Erulkar, 1972) and ecologically related more simple species and forms of behavior (escape behavior) (Roeder and Treat, 1961).

Some forms of echolocating signals, such as frequency modulation, high rate of pulses, were stressed and the perception of such sounds was specially analyzed by neurophysiological methods (Suga, 1968, Grinnell, 1969). But there are many other animal groups with well developed hearing and sound emission abilities, which do not possess such specialized forms of acoustical behavior as found in bats or dolphins; first are to be mentioned such common subjects for neurophysiological and behavioral studies, as cats, white rats, monkeys, and dogs. The sounds emitted by these and many other animals are widely used in their communication behavior. If one tries to determine the general task which the auditory system performs in different forms of behavior (including as a special case echolocation), one comes to the conclusion that recognition of the sound source properties is to be considered as such a general task (for discussion, see Bergeijk, 1967, Gersuni, 1972). A question arises: is it possible to evaluate some general features of sounds emitted by biological sources which are to be considered as specially adapted (adequate) for such a functioning of the auditory system?

---

[1] Natural sounds caused by non-biological events on the earth are not evaluated. The probable assumption is accepted that such sounds can be considered as background noises.

MECHANISMS IN HEARING

In this report consideration of this question, which serves as an introduction to a neurophysiological study, will be restricted to data on sound emission obtained in our laboratory on such experimental animals as white rats, cats and monkeys (Cebus capucinus). Only a few, but as we think, typical, examples are presented (Figs. 1 and 2). Segmentation in time is a feature common to all signals. There are different forms, orders and values of time segmentation. The signals presented in Figs. 1 and 2 show a first order segmentation which can be characterized by: 1) single pulse durations, 2) intervals between pulses, 3) pulse-repetition rates (see Table 1). The time structure within the pulses is characterized by different forms of segmentation: a) intrapulse amplitude modulation (AM) (see Fig. 1a, b, c; Fig. 2b); b) an intrapulse click amplitude and frequency modulation, if the pulses are formed by clicks (Fig. 2d). Some signals (for instance, cat purr Fig. 2c) consist of periodically amplitude modulated click series. In such a signal two time orders are most clearly seen: the low rate amplitude modulation of the click series, and the intracycle (intragroup) click rate (Fig. 2c, d). Separate pulses can form a well-defined pulse train (group). The capuchin orienting call presents an example of such a pulse train organization. Intertrain intervals appear (Fig. 2a) (for more detail, see Malt'sev, 1970, Gersuni and Malt'sev, 1973). In Table 1, some characteristics of time structure of different signals presented in Fig. 1 and 2 are given. The spectral characteristics of the signals can be seen from dynamic spectrograms (Fig. 1, 2) and spectrographic sections (Fig. 3). The data show that pulses of different signals are filled with a mixture of harmonics and bands of noise and have different spectral maxima. The shift to high frequencies is most evident in the pain cry of an infant rat (Fig. 1a, Fig. 3c), and the shift to low frequencies in the orienting calls of the capuchin and in the pain cry of the cat (Fig. 3a and Fig. 3e, respectively).

Frequency modulation (FM) is not significant in the samples of single pulses, but is characteristic for the pulse train of the orienting call (Fig. 2a). A schematic representation of features of bioacoustical signals derived from the data of Figs. 1, 2 and 3 is given in Fig. 4b-g. In Fig. 4a a non-interrupted pure tone signal ("classical") is presented for comparison. In Fig. 4b the general features of a bioacoustical signal: segmentation in time (interruption) and filling of individual pulses with tone mixtures are presented. In Fig. 4c-g schemes of differently time-structured signals are given.

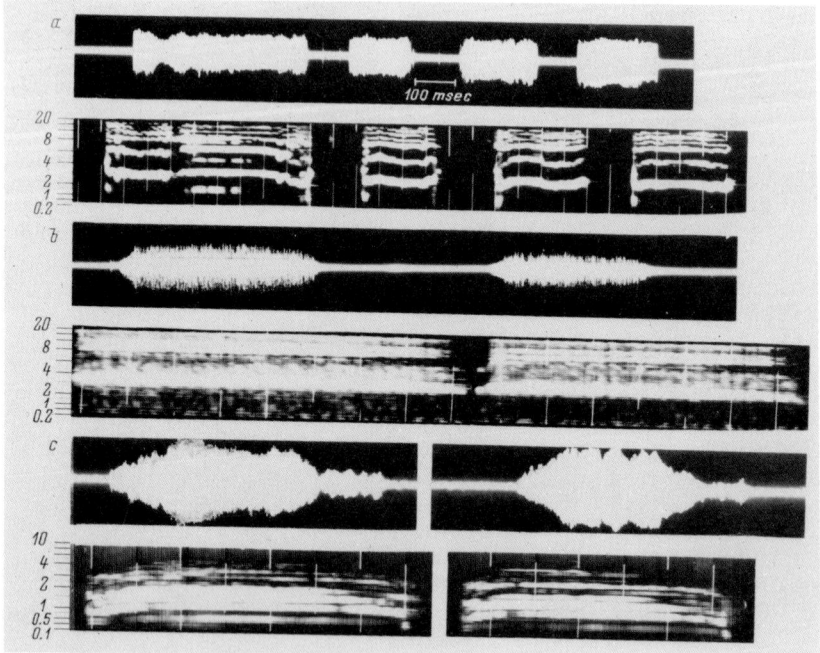

Fig. 1 Oscillogram and dynamic spectrograms of pain cries. The pain cries are elicited by electric stimulation of the skin. a. infant white rat (17 days). Above - oscillogram; below - spectrogram. Number on the left of the spectrogram: frequency in kHz; vertical white lines indicate time intervals (50 msec). b. adult white rat. Time calibration - oscillogram - the same as in a; spectrogram - vertical white lines, time intervals (100 msec). c. cat. Time calibration the same as in b. Two separate pulses are shown. Interval between pulses, 900 msec. Note the difference in the calibration time of oscillograms and spectrograms (After Gersuni and Malt'sev, 1973).

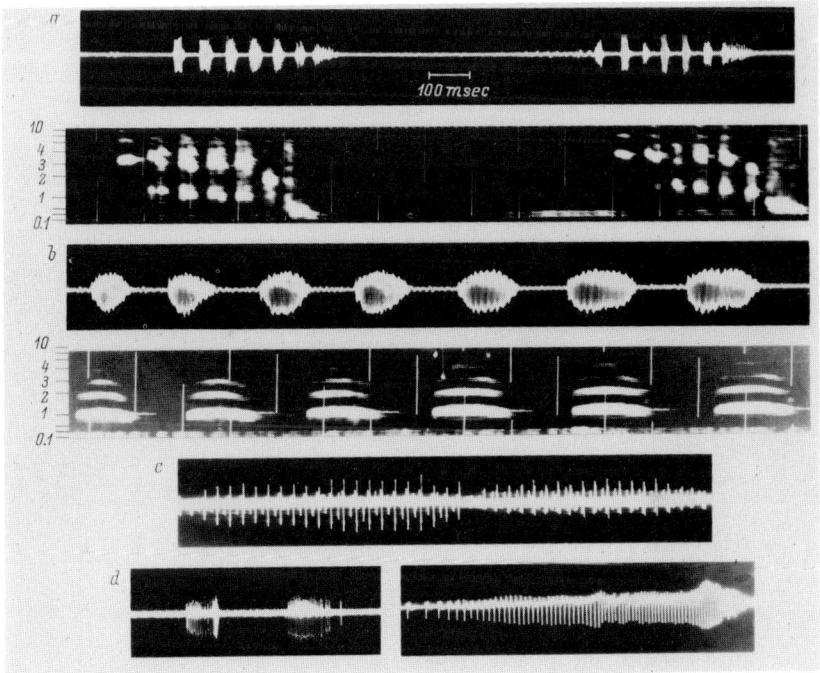

Fig. 2 Oscillograms and dynamic spectrograms.
a. Orienting call of Cebus capucinus, b.
isolation call of a male Cebus capucinus.
White vertical lines on dynamic spectrograms
mark 100 msec, c. Oscillogram of cat purring
formed by AM clicks, d. Oscillograms of pain
click pulses of an infant white rat (4
days); left - two click pulses, right - one
click pulse (different time calibration).

Time calibration bar - 100 msec - on the
top oscillogram for a, b, c, d (left);
for d (right) the same length of the calibration bar indicates 10 msec (After
Malt'sev, 1970).

Table 1 Characteristics of time structure of different signals presented in Figs. 1 and 2.

NN	Animal	Signal	Duration of single pulse (msec.)	Intervals between pulses (msec.)	Pulse repetition rate (Hz)	Intrapulse time segmentation
1.	infant white rat (17 days)	pain cries	40-420	150-300	1.3-5.0	Low frequency non periodical amplitude changes.
2.	adult white rat	pain cries	210-600	120-500	0.9-3.0	Deep AM; bursts of 1.5-5 msec. duration
3.	adult cat	pain cries	540-850	880-3100	0.25-0.6	Low frequency non periodical amplitude changes; at the end high frequency AM (about 300/sec.)
4.	monkey (cebus capucinus)	orientation call	19-64	37-67	15-20	AM in the last pulse
5.	-"-	isolation call	60-216	110-123	3.5-4.5	—
6.	cat	purring[1]	690-720	—	1.4	AM click series; repetition rates 27-33 per sec.
7.	infant white rat (4 days)	pain click pulses	25-225	150-300	1.4-3.0	AM and FM click series; repetition rates 200-800 per sec.

[1] one purr-cycle is considered as a pulse.

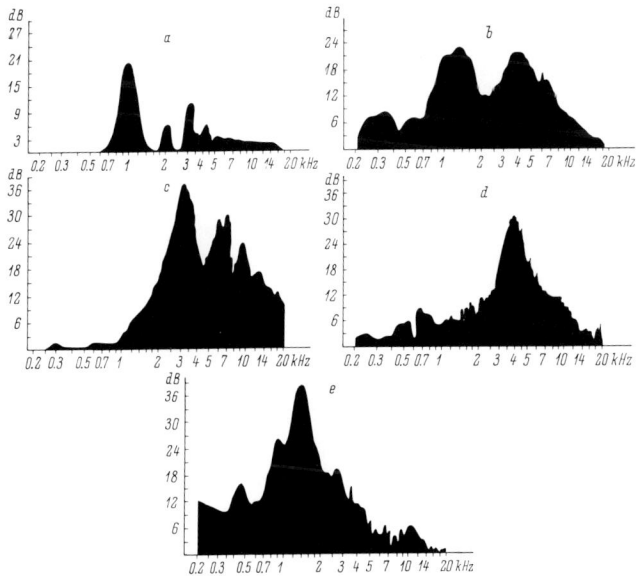

Fig. 3 Spectrographic sections of sound pulses emitted by monkey (Cebus capucinus), white rat and cat. Ordinate: amplitude in dB; abscissa: frequency in kHz (measurements by Bruel and Kjaer analyzer, type 2107). The spectrographic sections were taken in the middle of a pulse. a. Cebus capucinus orienting call (middle of the third pulse), b. Cebus capucinus isolation call, c. Infant rat pain cry, d. adult rat pain cry, e. cat pain cry (After Gersuni and Malt'sev, 1973).

One phenomenon which is important for biologically emitted sounds was not considered above. This phenomenon is the movement of biological sound-emitters and receivers. The movement of the sound source or the receiver determines acoustical cues which are important for localization of the sound source. There are many acoustical cues used in different cases of sound source localization by binaural and monaural perception (Altman, 1972, Erulkar, 1972). One, the most simple and evident cue of sound source localization, valid not only for binaural, but also for monaural perception, is a cue for distance (Coleman, 1963), as it is reflected by amplitude changes caused by movement of the sound source, relatively to the receiver (or vice versa). In Fig. 4h amplitude changes of a signal emitted by a moving source are presented. The signal is formed by short pulses (for instance, click-filled pulses as presented in Fig. 4e). It is assumed for simplification that the source (animal) moves at a constant speed (v) along a straight line trajectory. The changes of the sound pressure at a point r_o (minimal distance between the source and the receiver) are shown by the envelope of the amplitudes of the pulses.[1]

The conclusion about the prime importance of segmentation in time (interruption, amplitude modulation) is really only a statement of facts well known in bioacoustical and connected behavioral studies, especially in lower vertebrates (Anura -Littlejohn and Loftus-Hills, 1968) and insects (Orthoptera - Popov, 1972). But in neurophysiological studies on the neuronal level, especially in such commonly used animals as cats, white rats, and monkeys, reactions of central auditory neurons to interrupted or amplitude modulated signals are rarely dealt with in existing data, in contradistinction to reactions to frequency modulated signals (reviews by Møller, 1972, Erulkar, 1972).

The task of this report is to present data on reactions of central auditory neurons to signals with different time structures: 1) AM pure tones and white noise; 2) AM clicks and short noise pulses. The latter are signals with two different time orders of segmentation. Schemes which show, in approximated form, click modulated bioacoustical signals (Fig. 4e, g, h) can serve at the same time as models of the signals used in experiments (Fig. 5).

---

[1] For the calculation, the following assumptions are accepted. The sound source is pointlike, the medium homogenous and unlimited. If values of $v = 2$ m/sec and $r_o = 1$ m are accepted, the horizontal calibration bar on the time axis corresponds to 0.5 sec. The duration of the whole signal in this case is about 4 sec. If we change the speed in the range from 0.5 to 10 m/sec (the values suitable for many groups of animals including rats, cats, monkeys), the form of the envelope remains valid; the values of the time calibration, correspondingly, are to be changed. We are greatly indebted to Prof. W.K. Labutin for the calculation.

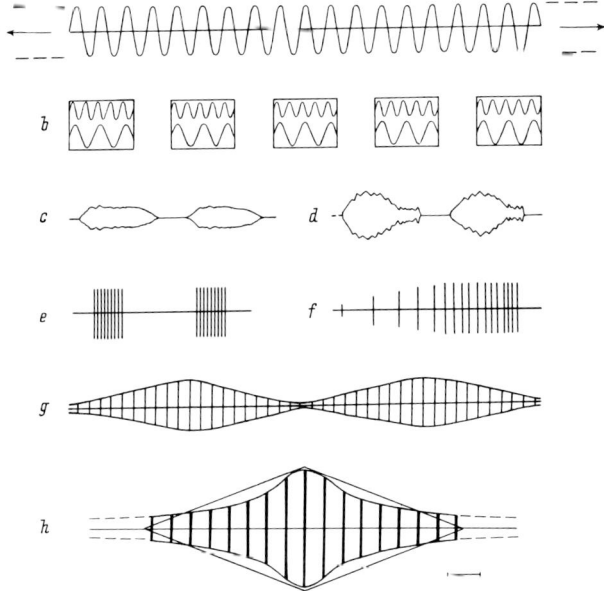

Fig. 4 Scheme of sounds emitted by white rats and cats presented in Figs. 1 and 2. For comparison, a stationary ("classical") tone is shown (a).

b. Interrupted sounds: pulse train; each pulse contains harmonics with different amplitude maxima. c., d. Pulses of different forms, intervals and spectral maxima. e. Two orders of time segmentation; intervals between click train pulses and intrapulse intervals between clicks. f. Frequency and amplitude modulated click train pulse. g. Sinusoidally amplitude modulated click series. Two time orders: 1) rate of AM, 2) intracycle rate. h. Sound pressure (amplitude) changes dependent on the sound source motion with a constant speed. Ordinate: Sound pressure, abscissa: time. The central black vertical bar (maximum sound pressure) corresponds to the point of the distance minimum (r_o) between the moving source and the ear. Horizontal bar = time calibration. See text.

2. Methods

Experiments were performed on white rats. Single unit activity from colliculus inferior was recorded extracellularly.

2.1 Sound stimuli

The following sound stimuli were used. 1) sinusoidally amplitude modulated (AM) tones and white noise bursts (the depth of modulation about 90-95%, burst duration - 600-1000 msec). The rates of modulation varied from 1 to 100 Hz. The carrier tone frequencies were established according to the unit tuning curve; the characteristic frequency (CF) of higher and lower frequencies was used. The form of the AM tone burst is shown in Fig. 5A(1,2). 2) clicks and short white noise pulses (duration 5 msec) triangularly or sinusoidally modulated. The repetition rates (r.r.) of clicks and noise pulses varied from 5 to 30/sec, according to the optimal r.r., established in preliminary determinations. In most units the limits of the optimal r.r. were from 20 to 30/sec. The following were the durations of triangularly modulated short pulse trains: 3.74, 2.91, 2.22, 1.24 sec. Two forms of triangularly modulated signals were used, one with a rise from a minimum to a maximum of amplitude values and a subsequent fall, another with a fall from maximum to minimum of amplitude values and a subsequent rise. These two symmetrically reversed forms of AM pulse trains are shown in Fig. 5A(3,4). 3) a. non-modulated tones and noise bursts of the same durations as the AM bursts; b. non-modulated clicks and short pulse trains as shown in Fig. 5A(5); c. short tone and noise bursts (80-100 msec and 2-5 msec duration) used for the classification of units.

Pure tones, white noise (bandwidth 0.02-20 kHz), and short rectangular pulses (2.0 msec) were amplitude modulated by a special device. An electronic switch determined the selected number of modulation cycles. For triangular AM (depth 100%) the device could perform a selection of any part of the modulation cycle. In the triangular AM series only 1 or 0.5 cycles were used as stimuli. Intensity of the stimuli was controlled by an attenuator with 1 dB steps.

The signal was switched on and off in zero phase of the modulation cycle (Fig. 5A(1,2)). A special electrostatic earphone for rats constructed by the engineer A.M. Lichnitsky was used. The tube of the earphone was inserted in the external auditory meatus of the rat. The length of the tube was 10 mm; the outer diameter was 3.5 mm. The closed volume formed by the tube and the auditory meatus of the rat was estimated (mean value) as 100 mm^3.

The frequency characteristics of the whole sound generating system were measured by a Brüel and Kjaer probe condenser microphone (4135) connected by a special chamber to the tube of the earphone (closed volume including the tube was about 100 mm^3). The frequency characteristic of the sound generating system is shown in Fig. 5B. The sound pressure level

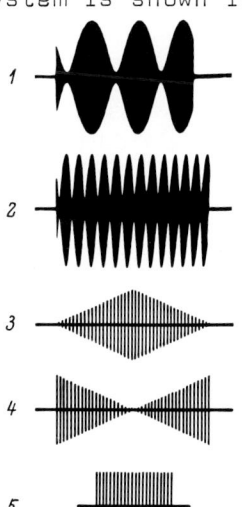

Fig. 5 Amplitude modulated (AM) sounds (electrical form).

5A. 1, 2. Sinusoidal AM bursts of different repetition rates. Stimuli 1 and 2 are formed by 3 and 13 cycles. Stimuli are switched on and off in zero-phase of the modulation cycle.

3,4,5. Short noise pulse trains (5 msec) 3,4. Triangular AM pulse trains; 5. Non-modulated (rectangular) pulse train.

All stimuli are symmetrical to the time axis.

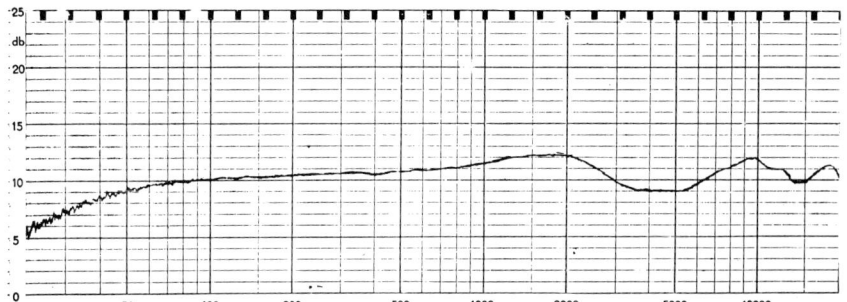

Fig. 5B. Frequency characteristic of the sound generating system.

in the range of frequency from 0.1 to 20 kHz shows fluctuations which do not exceed ± 2 dB. The maximal sound pressure level (zero dB of attenuation) corresponded to 78 dB re 0.0002 µbar for the frequency of 4 kHz. SPL's from 40 to 75 dB were used in the majority of experiments with AM sounds.

2.2 Surgical preparation

The experiments were carried out on white rats weighing 180-220 g, anesthetized with chloralose (30 mg per kg) and urethan (500 mg/kg), given intraperitoneally. After the onset of narcotic sleep, tracheotomy was performed. The cochlea, contralateral to the side of the stimulation, was destroyed. After removal of the soft tissues, the bone over the parietal region was removed and the dura was incised. When the hemisphere was displaced forward the inferior colliculus was clearly seen. The inferior colliculus was covered with a layer of warm vaseline oil. The animal's head was fixed in a headholder. In order to minimize the respiratory and pulsation movements of the brain tissue, cisternal drainage was carried out through the cisterna magna and the inferior colliculus was covered with a 4-5% agar solution in physiological saline. During the experiments the body temperature of the animal was maintained at a constant level $(37-38^{\circ}$ C).

2.3 Recording of the impulse activity

The preparation was placed in an acoustically isolated chamber. Tungsten microelectrodes with tip diameters less than 1μ and an equivalent resistance of 10 to 20 megohms measured at 1000 Hz were used. The electrodes were mounted on a hydraulic microdriver. Insertion of the electrode was accomplished in steps of $1-2\mu$ by the experimentator situated outside the chamber. The location of the electrode tip was estimated from the depth of the electrode insertion; in most cases histological control was exercised by the method of Fox and Eichman (1959). Electrode placement covered most areas of the inferior colliculus with the majority of the units being recorded from the central nucleus of the inferior colliculus. Extracellular potentials of the units were amplified by UBP-1-02. The impulse activity was recorded with a MEZ-28A magnetic tape recorder. A reliable separation of the impulse activity from the background activity was achieved with the aid of a threshold device. Subsequently an automatic analysis of the impulse activity was performed. 256 channels were used for recording PST histograms (post stimulus time). Simultaneously a dots display was used (Wall, 1959).

2.4 Experimental procedure

2.4.1 Preliminary series

1) The search for a responding unit was carried out by a probe white noise burst. 2) Determinations of tuning curves of the unit were performed. The tuning curves were measured by tone bursts of 100-200 msec duration. 3) Classification of the unit type. For classification different criteria were used (Rose et al., 1963, Radionova, 1971a, 1971b, Gersuni et al. 1971, Vartanian and Snetkov, 1970). The criterion generally accepted is the discharge pattern obtained on stimulation with a tone or noise burst of suprathreshold intensity. At the level of the inferior colliculus units with discharge patterns designated as onset pattern neurons (Rose et al., 1963, Gersuni et al., 1971) are common. The same pattern designated as transient (Møller, 1969, 1971) exists in the units at the level of cochlear nuclei (Radionova, 1971a, 1971b). The other quite different discharge pattern is designated as a sustained discharge (Rose et al., 1963). In this work we accepted as most suitable for rapid determination a differentiation of discharge patterns among the three groups: sustained discharge, burst discharge and onset discharge (Fig. 6 I, II, III). Other criteria specially used in our laboratory were time-dependent threshold criteria: 1) duration threshold shift (Fig. 6 a_1, b_1, c_1); 2) time rise threshold shift (Fig. 6 a_3, b_3, c_3) (for different frequencies see Fig. 6 a_4, b_4, c_4; a_5, b_5, c_5); 3) intensity-latency shift (Fig. 6 a_2, b_2, c_2) (see in more detail Vartanian and Snetkov, 1970, Gersuni, 1971, Radionova, 1971a, Maruseva, 1971).

As was shown, a high correlation exists between different time dependent criteria and intensity-latency shift (Gersuni et al., 1971). In this work for classification of the unit, two criteria were systematically determined: 1) the pattern of the discharge to the characteristic frequency (CF) or white

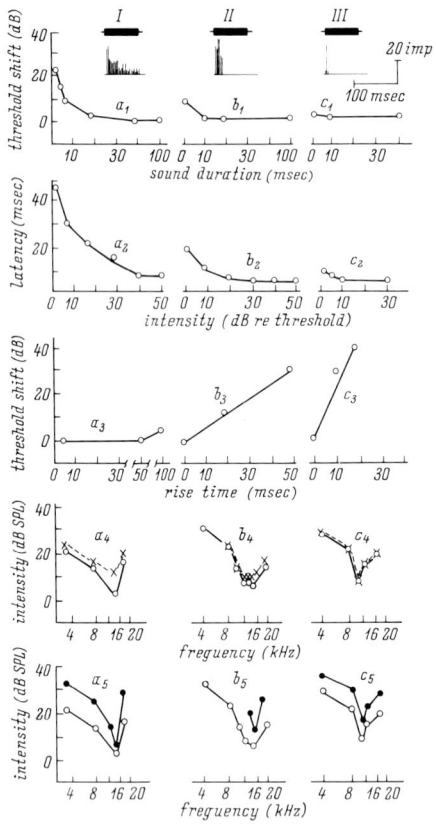

Fig. 6 Response characteristics used for classification of collicular units.

I, II, III - types of discharge patterns: sustained (I), burst (II), onset (III). Stimuli: sound bursts of 80 msec duration. Time dependent threshold characteristics and latency-intensity characteristics for different types of units. a_1, b_1, c_1 - threshold duration curve for three types of units. On the ordinate the zero indicates the threshold for a 100 msec duration sound burst. a_2, b_2, c_2 - latency as a function of intensity levels re threshold for a sound burst of 100 msec duration. a_3, b_3, c_3, - threshold shift dependent on the time-rise constant (τ) of the exponentially rising signal. On the ordinate zero indicates the threshold for a stimulus with a (cont'd) rectangular envelope (rise time less 0.2 msec). a_4, b_4, c_4 - tuning curves obtained with tone bursts of two durations (100 msec - open circles; 2 msec crosses and dashed line; ordinate - zero - SPL 0.0002 μbar. a_5, b_5, c_5 - tuning curves obtained with 100 msec tone bursts with two different time-rise constants (τ), open circles - rectangular envelope (time-rise less 0.2 msec), filled circles for a_5 - rise time 70 msec, for b_5 - 10 msec, for c_5 - 8 msec. The coordinate scales are the same as for a_4, b_4, c_4. For a_1-c_1, a_2-c_2, a_3-c_3 characteristic frequency (CF) or white noise bursts were used.

For the classification procedure used in this work the discharge patterns (I, II, III) and threshold differences between sound bursts of different durations (100 and 2 msec) i.e. temporal summation index (TSI) or threshold duration shift (TDS) were established for all units.

noise burst (Fig. 6 I, II, III); 2) the differences between threshold values of sound bursts (CF or white noise) of two durations (threshold duration shift - TDS): 200 msec and 2 msec. These differences are largest for a unit with a sustained discharge (about 20 dB, Fig. $6a_1$) and minimal for units with onset discharge (1-2 dB, Fig. $6c_1$). For the burst discharge unit the intermediate values of time duration threshold shift were obtained (about 10 dB, Fig. $6b_1$). For threshold determinations a probability of response of 0.5 was accepted.

In experiments with trains of clicks and short noise pulses a rapid determination of an optimal repetition rate was performed. The criteria for an optimal rate were a) full synchronization 1 to 1 to the rate of stimulation and rate of discharge bursts, b) the stability of the discharge during 0.5-1.0 sec of stimulation, c) the largest number of impulses per stimulus as can be rapidly estimated on the oscillographic screen. These rates were used in the succeeding main series.

2.4.2 Main series

Two main series of experiments were performed accordingly with two types of AM signals (see section 2.1).

1) In the first series the reactions of units to sinusoidal AM signals of different rates and carrier frequencies were investigated.

2) In the second series the reactions of units to trains of short noise pulses, with the repetition rate established from preliminary experiments were investigated.

As a quantitative criterion of the discharges of units, with different types of PST histograms, number of spikes per stimulus was used. The time used for a unit investigation was not less than one hour. In this report data are presented which were obtained on 336 units of the inferior colliculus of white rats.

3. Results

3.1 Unit impulse activity on stimulation with AM white noise bursts and click trains

In Fig. 7 PST histograms of impulse activity of two typical units: one (A) with sustained discharge and a threshold duration shift of about 10 dB; the other (B) with an onset discharge and minimal threshold duration shift (TDS) (2 dB) are presented for different rates of AM. The unit A-117 responds with discharges well synchronized with the rate of modulation beginning from low frequencies (see also Fig. 9). A one to one synchronization is observed until the rate of 50/sec. But a diminution of the spike number per cycle in the sequence of the cycles begins and is evident at the rates of 30 and 50/sec. At low rates (5-10/sec) the responses as judged by spike number per cycle are relatively stable. The spike count per the whole time of stimulation is maximal for the rates 30-50/sec. The unit B-133 with an onset discharge begins to respond only at frequencies higher than 30/sec in contrast to the unit A-117 which responds to much lower rates of AM. To respond only to higher rates of sinusoidal AM signals is a characteristic of onset units. The maximal number of spikes per stimulation time is reached at 90/sec. The diminution of spikes during the stimulation time which at the lower levels of the auditory system is called adaptation is most prominent for the units B-133 and A-117.

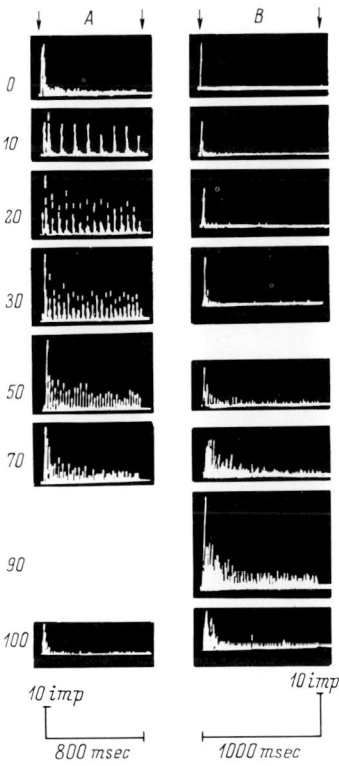

Fig. 7 PST histograms of firing patterns of two units to different rates of sinusoidal AM noise bursts.

A - unit N 117 with a sustained discharge. Temporal summation index (TSI) - 11 dB. B - unit N 133 with an onset discharge, TSI - 2 dB. Numbers on the left indicate modulation rates in Hz. 0 - non-modulated noise burst. Intensity - 55 dB. The zero reference level for a noise burst is accepted as equivalent to the voltage established for the 0.0002 µbar reference level of a tone of 4 kHz. Threshold for the non-modulated noise burst for unit A - 13 dB, for unit B - 23 dB. On the bottom the vertical calibration bar indicates number of impulses. Arrows on the top - duration of stimulation. Number of stimulation (N) = 25.

As can be seen from Fig. 6 for the onset units an increase of threshold with the increase of the time-rise of stimuli is characteristic. As long as the amplitude of the sound burst sine-modulated by low frequency grows slowly the unit does not respond to such a stimulus; the unit begins to respond to higher frequency of modulation, i.e. to a stimulus with a higher rise time.

In Fig. 8 responses (dot display) of three units with different discharge patterns (onset, burst and sustained, and threshold duration shifts (TDS) 1.5 and 12 dB, respectively) to AM noise bursts (left column) and click trains (right column) are presented. The AM frequency is 5 Hz, the click repetition rate, 30/sec. The onset unit (N 119) does not respond to the noise burst with a low rate of AM. The burst discharge unit (N 115) responds to each cycle of modulation, but there is a diminution of spike number per cycle to the third and fourth cycles (Table 4). The sustained discharge unit N 117 responds to each cycle; the number of spikes per cycle and the response phase timing fluctuate (see also Table 4 and PST histogram for the same unit - Fig. 7A). Quite different discharge patterns are seen by stimulation with AM click trains (right column, Fig. 8). The onset discharge unit (N 119) responds to each modulation cycle, but the click rate (30/sec) is evidently too high for a full 1:1 reproduction. For units 115 and 117 there is a perfect reproduction of each click in the cycle sequences. The discharges are stable during the whole time of stimulation (especially for unit 117, Table 4). Note that for unit 117 the click rate 30/sec coincides with the frequency of sinusoidal AM which shows a well synchronized and relatively stable response pattern (Fig. 7A). For this unit the rate of repetition of 30/sec can be evaluated as optimal according to two criteria: 1) spike number per stimulus duration, 2) stability of spike number in the train (no adaptation)(Table 4).

In Fig. 9 the values for optimal rates of AM noise bursts established according to the maximal spike number per burst are given for 44 units. The optimal rate for most units lies in the range 20-30/sec. There exists a difference in the distribution of optimal rates among the three different groups of units. The shift to high rates (80-100/sec) is observed only in onset units with minimal threshold duration shift. The optimal rate for burst discharge units is lower than for sustained discharge units.

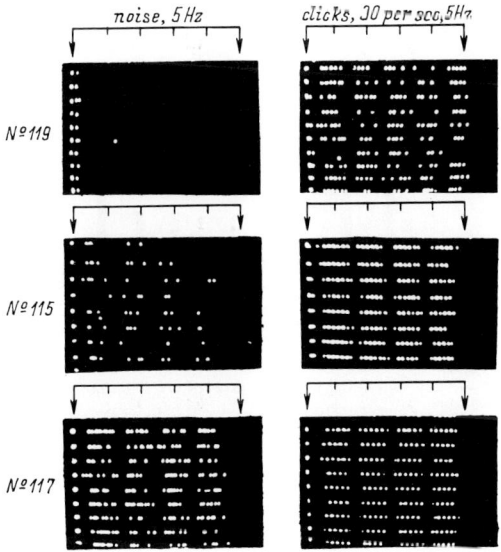

Fig. 8 Firing patterns for three different units, to AM noise burst and AM click trains. Each dot represents the occurrence of a spike, excluding the first dot on the left which indicates the onset of the stimulus. On the left - unit number, on the top of each oscillogram time calibration - 200 msec. The arrows indicate 1 sec stimuli for the oscillograms on the left - sinusoidal AM noise burst; rate of modulation 5 Hz; on the right, click train; repetition rate 30 sec; sinusoidal AM repetition rate - 5 Hz. Responses to four cycles of AM are presented; for the unit 119 only, responses to five cycles are presented (on the right, top). N 119 - unit with an onset discharge pattern; TSI less than 1 dB, intensity 58 dB; threshold 13 dB. N 115 - unit with a burst discharge; TSI - 8 dB; intensity 55 dB; threshold 13 dB. N 117 - unit with a sustained discharge, TSI 11 dB; intensity 55 dB; Threshold 13 dB.

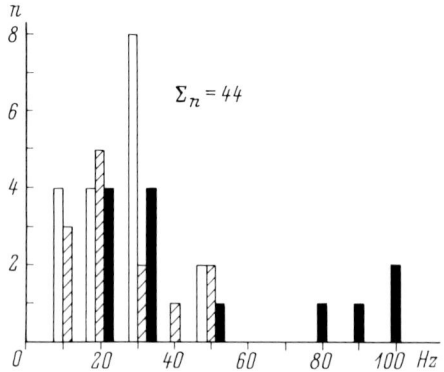

Fig. 9 Optimal repetition rates for a sample of 44 collicular units; white bars - units with a sustained discharge pattern; black bars - onset discharge units; shaded bars - burst discharge units. Abscissa: repetition rates of sinusoidal AM tones of CF and noise bursts which give an optimal discharge (see text). Ordinate: number of cases.

The data presented in Fig. 8 also show how much the unit discharge pattern is dependent on the time structure of the stimulus. It is evident that the designation used for different discharge patterns is meaningful only under restricted conditions, i.e. stimulation with non-modulated relatively short bursts of noise or tones of frequency characteristic (CF) for the unit (see the following section 3.2).

3.2 Stimulation with AM tone bursts

In Fig. 10 PST histograms and graphs showing spike number for two carrier frequencies are presented. One carrier frequency coincides with the CF of the unit (14 kHz); the other is higher (19 kHz). The unit gives a sustained discharge to a non-modulated tone of the CF (a pause after the initial discharge burst is seen). A maximal number of spikes and full synchronization of responses are observed at the rate of AM 30/sec (for the CF). A quite different discharge pattern is seen for the higher carrier frequency (19 kHz). For this the response is seen as modulation of background (spontaneous) activity most evident for the rate of 5/sec. For higher rates and non-modulated tone a depression of spontaneous activity is seen (the level of spontaneous activity is 136 impulses on the ordinate scale). In Fig. 11 another unit (burst discharge pattern) is presented; the carrier frequencies are 12 kHz (CF) and 16 kHz. A response during the whole time of stimulation is observed only for the tone of CF amplitude modulated at the rate of 50/sec. The drastic influence on the unit response of the combination of two parameters: 1) carrier frequency, 2) modulation rate, is clearly seen. It is important to note that this characteristic feature of the unit activity becomes evident only when stimulated with a train of pulses (modulation cycles). In Figs. 12-14 data for another unit with a burst discharge are shown. The carrier frequencies in this experiment are shifted in relatively small steps from the CF of the unit (6.0 kHz) to higher and lower frequencies. In Fig. 12 PST histograms for 6 carrier frequencies and 3 rates of AM are presented. Responses to non-modulated tone bursts for the same frequencies are given for comparison. An optimal response to the modulation rate 20/sec is seen for the CF (6.0 kHz) of the unit (tuning curve, Fig. 13a). For all modulation rates (5, 10, 20/sec) at the CF, the unit discharges are observed at each cycle in the cycle train during the whole time of stimulation (1 sec). The shift from the CF in the carrier determines a fall of the optimal modulation rate of the discharge (Figs. 12, 14). One can see the more powerful influence of the shift to the high frequency side (Fig. 12). The number of spikes per stimulus duration (Fig. 13b) shows that the frequency selectivity of the responses rises to a maximum for the modulation rate 20/sec. One can see that the phenomenon is observed only when the number of impulses reaches a value not less than 50-70; this spike number is obtained by low suprathreshold intensity levels. The values of the frequency bands (Fig. 13b) for the level of 100 spikes per stimulus duration are - 2600 Hz (for 5/sec modulation rate), 2000 Hz (for 10/sec) and 500 Hz (for 20/sec).

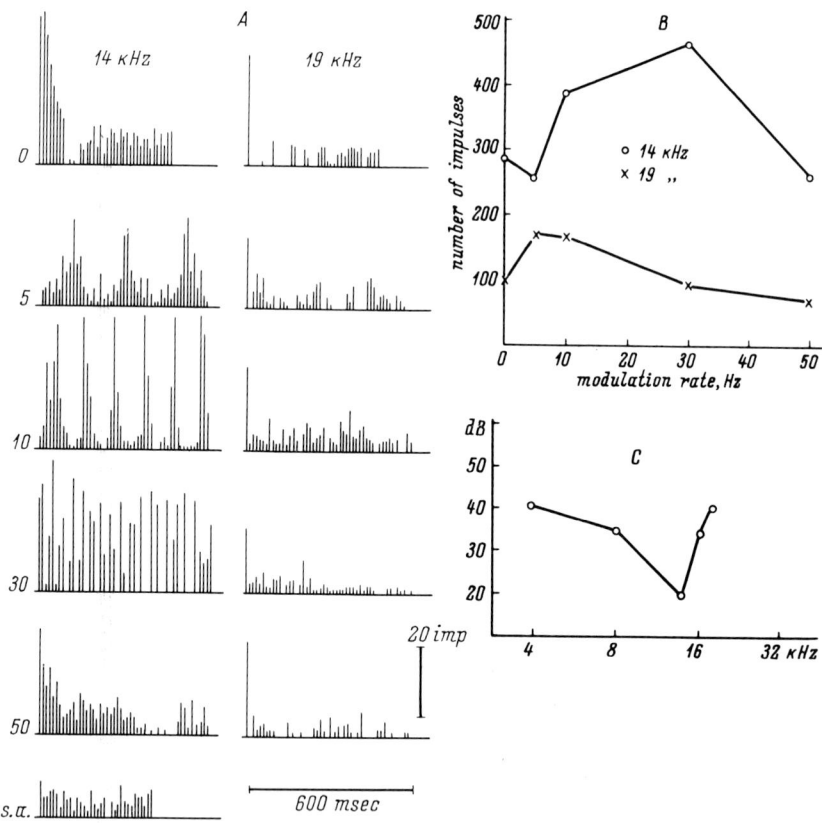

Fig. 10A. PST histograms of responses of unit N 87 with a sustained discharge to AM tones of characteristic frequency (14 kHz) and a higher one (19 kHz). TSI for CF - 16 dB, for 19 kHz - 4 dB; intensity 55 dB; threshold for CF - 18 dB. Numbers on the left of the histograms - modulation rates (Hz). 0 - non-modulated tone burst. S.a. - spontaneous activity. Vertical calibration bar - number of impulses.

Fig. 10B. Total number of impulses (20 presentations of the stimulus) for the CF (14 kHz) and 19 kHz at different modulation rates.

Fig. 10C. Threshold tuning curve. Abscissa: frequency; ordinate: 0.0002 dB SPL

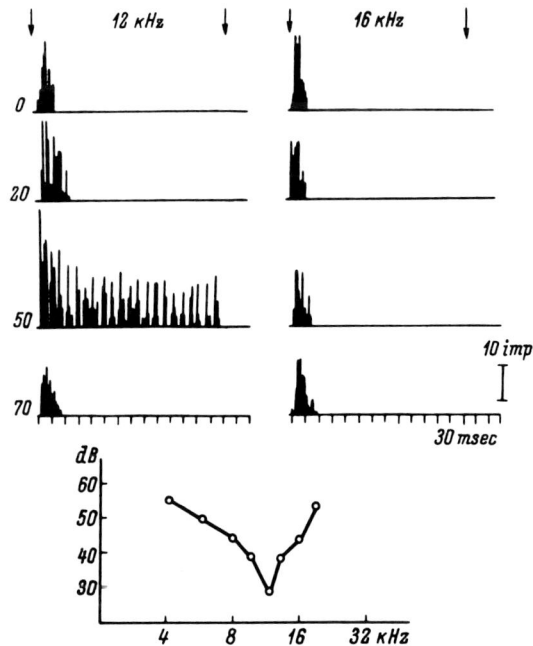

Fig. 11 PST histograms of responses of unit N 75 with a burst discharge to AM tones of CF (12 kHz) and a higher one (16 kHz) of different modulation rates (numbers on the left). 0 - non-modulated tone burst. Arrows mark the beginning and the end of stimulation. Intensity level - 65 dB; TSI for CF - 16 dB, for 16 kHz - 7 dB. C. Threshold tuning curve. Coordinates - same as in Fig. 10C.

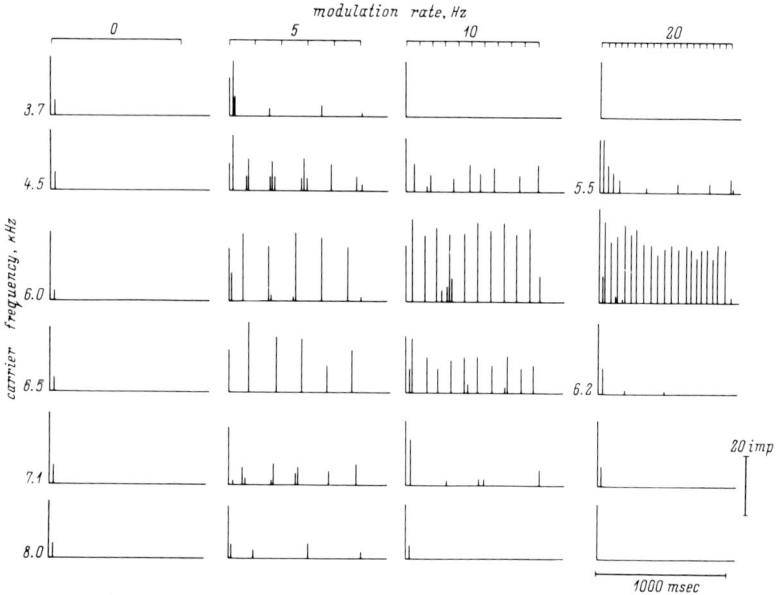

Fig. 12 PST histograms of unit N 124 to AM tones of different carrier frequencies (numbers on the left) and modulation rates (numbers on the top). 0 - non-modulated tone bursts. Horizontal lines on the top indicate the time of stimulation, the short vertical bars mark modulation cycles (zero phase). N = 20. Intensity: 60 dB. CF = 6.0 kHz. TSI for CF = 10 dB. Thresholds - see tuning curves (Fig. 13A).

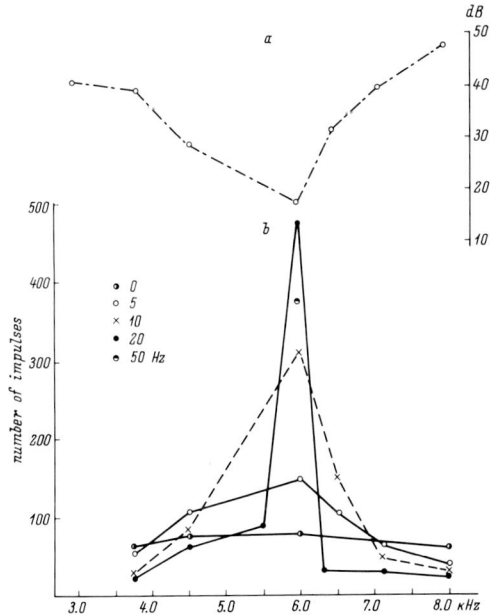

Fig 13 A. Threshold tuning curve of unit N 124 (PST histograms in Fig. 12). B. Number of impulses as function of carrier frequencies at different modulation rates. Abscissa: carrier frequencies; ordinate: total number of impulses per 20 presentations. Parameters - modulation rates. 0 - non-modulated tone bursts. Maximum of impulse number is seen for the CF (6.0 kHz) at the rate of modulation 20/sec.

In Fig. 14 the number of impulses as a function of modulation rates for different carrier frequencies is presented. The shift of the optimal rates of the unit from 20/sec to 10/sec determined by the shift of the carrier frequency from 6.0 kHz (CF) to 6.5 kHz is well seen.

In Fig. 15 data for a unit with an on and off discharge pattern for two frequencies - 10 kHz (CF) and 20 kHz are presented. The optimal modulation rate, as judged by the maximal spike number, is for the CF (10kHz) - 100/sec, for 20 kHz, 30/sec. For this unit with extremely low threshold at CF, the intensity

levels for the carrier frequencies are established at
equal suprathreshold values (40 dB above threshold);
as can be seen from the tuning curve this value corresponded to the SPL - 20 dB for the CF (10 kHz) and
57 dB for 20 kHz. In spite of such large differences
of SPL, the differences between responses at different carrier frequencies are similar to that observed
in other units, stimulated with sounds of equal SPL,
but different suprathreshold intensities (Fig. 10-14). These data suggest that above a certain suprathreshold level the intensity is not critical for the
features of the unit response determined by the modulation rates and the frequencies of the carrier. In
Fig. 16 spike counts as a function of modulation rate
for two intensity levels (in two units A and B) are
presented. One can see on this figure that the curves
for different intensities have a similar shape, but
lie on different spike count levels.

The data presented in Figs. 10-16 characterize the
features of the unit responses as stimulated with
trains of cycles. The question about the unit response characteristics related to a single modulation
cycle was not considered here. This question was
specially studied by Nelson et al. (1966); see also
Gersuni and Vartanian (1969).

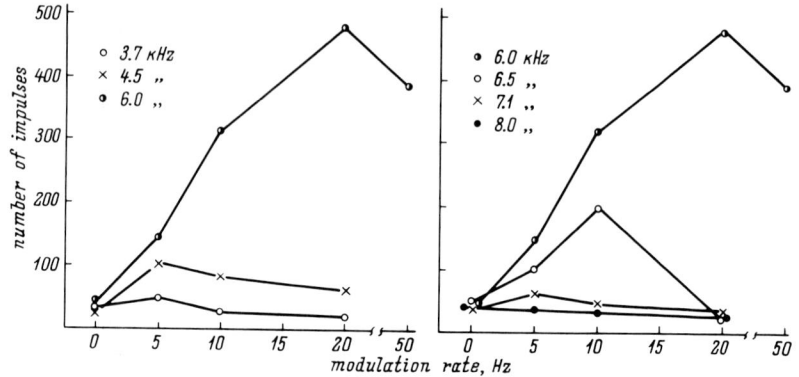

Fig. 14 Number of impulses as function of modulation
rate for different carrier frequencies (unit
N 124, see Figs. 12, 13). On the left - data
for CF (6.0 kHz) and two lower frequencies;
on the right - for CF and three higher frequencies. Note the shift of the optimal modulation rate. N = 20.

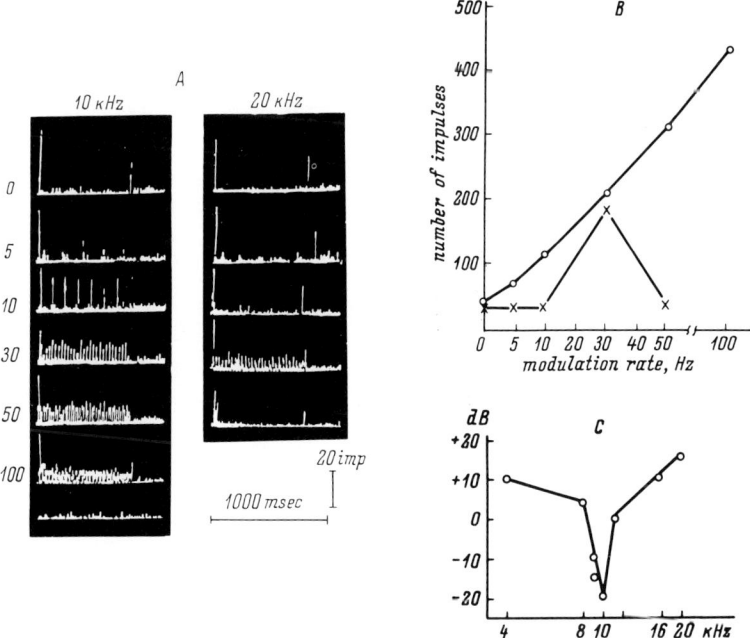

Fig. 15 A. PST histograms of unit responses with on-off discharge to AM tones of different carrier frequencies; CF (10 kHz) and a higher one (20 kHz). Intensity - for both frequencies 40 dB above threshold. TSI for CF = 7 dB; for 20 kHz - 4 dB. The bottom histogram (left) - spontaneous activity (N = 50). Designations as in other figs.

Fig. 15 B. Number of impulses as a function of modulation rate. CF = 10 kHz (circles), 20 kHz (crosses). N = 20.

Fig. 15 C. Threshold tuning curve. The thresholds are extremely low.

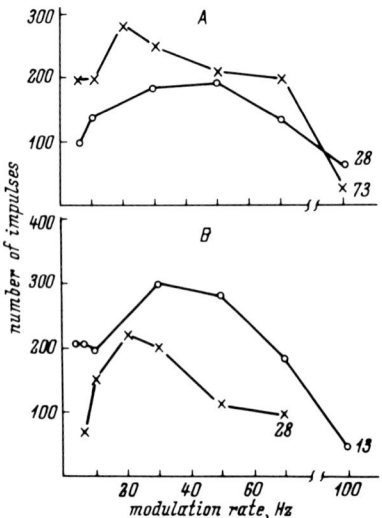

Fig. 16 Number of impulses as function of modulation rate for different intensity levels for two units: monotonic (A) and non-monotonic (B) spike-intensity relation. Ordinate: number of impulses per 10 presentations of the stimulus (noise bursts - duration 660 msec). Numbers 28, 73 for A and 28, 13 for B indicate the SPL in dB. Threshold for a non-modulated noise burst for unit A = 13 dB, for unit B = 4 dB.

In this paper we will only consider some characteristics of the responses related to a single modulation cycle. In Figs. 17 and 18 responses of two units (with high and low levels of spontaneous activity) to AM tones are presented. The unit with a high level of spontaneous activity (SA) (Fig. 17) is stimulated by AM tones with three carrier frequencies - 12 kHz (CF) 6.0 kHz and 20 kHz. The modulation rate is 3/sec. The shape of the response corresponds to the form of the modulation cycle. The maximum of the spike number is related to the point of the maximal amplitude of the modulation cycle (270°). There is a diminution of SA at the point of the minimum (90°) and at the end of the stimulation (the stimulus is formed by two cycles). At the carrier frequency 6.0 kHz, the response begins later than for the CF; a diminution of the SA between cycles and after the end of the stimulation is observed. At the higher carrier frequency (20 kHz) the maximum of the depression of the SA coincides with the point of the amplitude maximum of the modulation cycle (270°). Two peaks in the histogram coincide - one with the point of amplitude minimum and the other with the end of stimulation; a long aftereffect (facilitation of SA) is observed. Such a powerful inhibitory influence and aftereffect facilitation are characteristic for high frequency carriers.

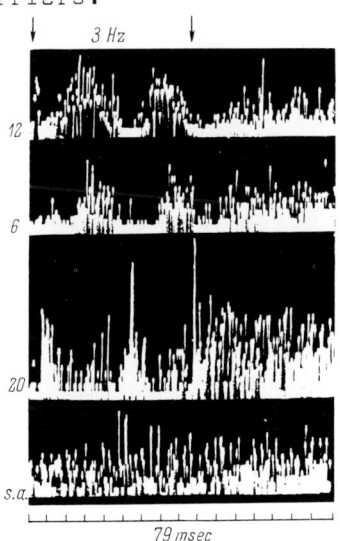
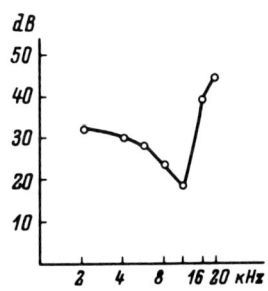

Fig. 17 PST histograms of the responses of a unit with a high level of spontaneous activity (S.a.). Responses to sinusoidal AM tones of different carrier frequencies. Numbers on the left - carrier frequencies (kHz). Modulation rate 3 Hz. Arrows indicate stimulus duration. Intensity 65 dB re 0.0002 μbar. Right - threshold tuning curve. CF = 12 kHz.

Histograms of a unit without spontaneous activity are presented in Fig. 18. On the left data about stimulation with non-modulated tone bursts of different frequencies are shown (CF - 13 kHz). On the right data for the AM tones are presented. The same powerful influence on discharge pattern at the carrier frequency higher than the CF of the unit is seen. An increase of the delay time due to a shift of the response to the later parts of the cycle, a diminution of spike number and a fall of responses from the first to the fourth cycles evidently express the inhibitory influence of the high frequency carrier. It is important to note that such inhibitory influences of the higher carrier frequency are more clearly manifested in stimulation by AM bursts.

3.3 Stimulation with AM pulse trains

In these series short noise pulse trains triangularly AM were used. (Duration of the trains 3.74, 2.22, 1.24 sec). The optimal pulse rate was established for each unit, in preliminary measurements. Two shapes of triangularly AM modulated stimulus were used: rise-fall and fall-rise. As the maximal amplitude in the train for a given sound pressure level was the same, the difference in duration determined an equivalent change of the speed of the rise and fall of the amplitude. The stimulus is symmetrical in respect to the time axis (see section 2).

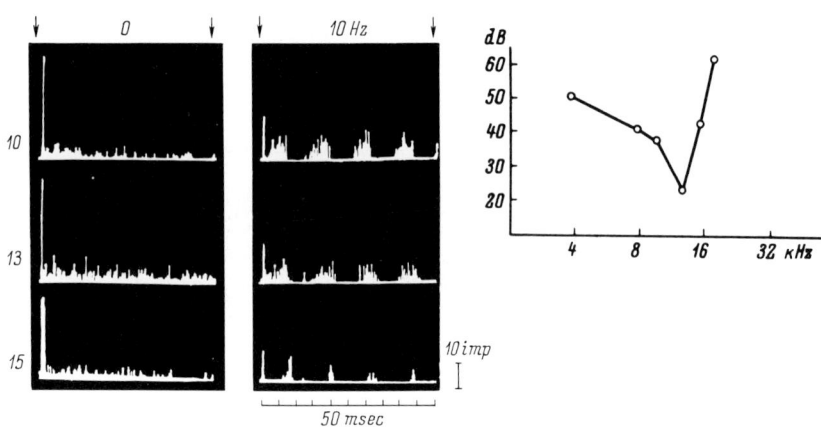

Fig. 18   PST histograms of unit responses without a background (spontaneous) activity. Responses to AM tones (modulation rate 10 Hz) of different carrier frequencies (numbers on the left - kHz) and non-modulated tone bursts (0). Arrows indicate stimulus duration. Intensity - 65 dB. N = 30. Right: threshold tuning curve. CF = 13 kHz.

In Fig. 19 PST histograms for a unit stimulated by AM pulse trains are presented. The responses of the unit in all conditions of stimulation (different durations, intensities, directions) reflect the symmetrical form of the stimuli. However, some asymmetry is observed in the responses to a long duration (3.74 sec), low intensity (38 dB) stimulus with a fall-rise form. Evidently the observed diminution of the response to the rise-fall branch is due to adaptation. The response to an equivalent shorter stimulus (1.24 sec) does not show such an asymmetry. At the bottom of Fig. 19 the responses to a train of pulses (on the left) and to a continuous noise burst (on the right) with a rectangular envelope (duration 0.62 sec) are shown. At the lower intensity (38 dB) for the pulse train a facilitation and for the continuous burst an adaptation are seen. At higher intensity (63 dB) a slight diminution of the response in time for the pulse train, and a more pronounced adaptation for the continuous stimulus are observed.

In Fig. 20 responses of a non-monotonic unit are presented. The symmetrical responses are observed at the low intensity level (33 dB, 10 dB above threshold) for both durations. At higher intensity levels (most pronounced at 73 dB, i.e. at 50 above threshold) there is a diminution in the whole number of impulses included in the response. At these high levels, a prevalence of the response to the first half of the stimulus over the second half is noted (the left PST histograms). For the fall-rise shape a reverse picture is observed especially evident for the long duration stimulus at the intensity level 73 dB.

The PST histograms for the long and short duration stimuli for both units (Figs. 19 and 20) do not show any substantial differences. As changes of duration determine equivalent changes of the speed of rise and fall of the amplitude, the conclusion can be drawn that the speed of the amplitude changes is not a determinative parameter for the activity of these units. A quite different picture is observed for responses of units presented in Figs. 21 and 22.

In Fig. 21 responses of a unit for pulse train stimuli of different durations (3.74 and 1.24 sec) at the same SPL (73 dB-45 dB above threshold for rectangular pulse train) are presented. For stimulus

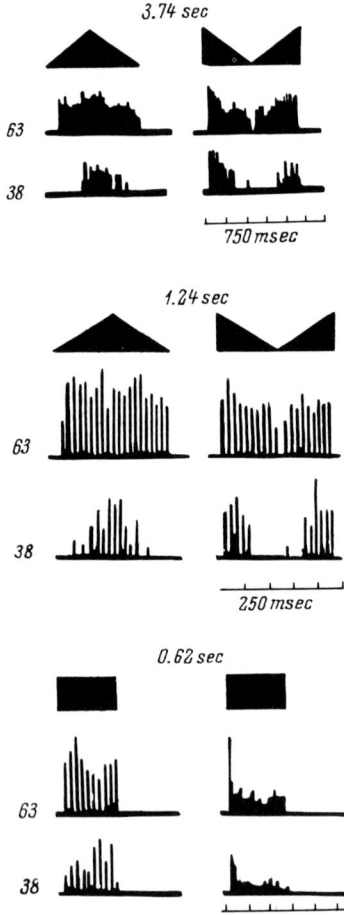

Fig. 19 PST histograms of unit (N 17/2) responses to AM noise pulse trains (pulse duration 5 msec; repetition rate 16/sec). The form of the triangular AM pulse trains is shown by black triangles; separate pulses in the train are not shown. (See Fig. 5A 3, 4, 5 and Fig. 22). Pulse train duration 3.74 and 1.24 sec. The quadrangles (duration 0.62 msec) show on the left a non-modulated (rectangular) pulse train; on the right - a continuous noise burst. Numbers on the left - SPL in dB. Threshold for rectangular puls train - 28 dB. N = 25. Symmetrical form of responses of the units.

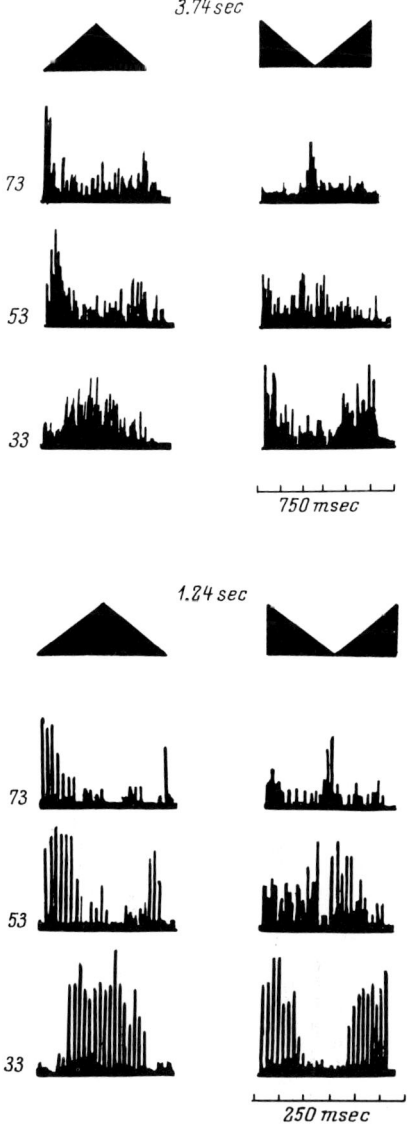

Fig. 20 PST histograms of unit N 10/2 responses to triangular AM noise pulse trains; repetition rate 20/sec. Numbers on the left - SPL in dB. Pulse train durations 3.74 and 1.24 sec. Threshold for the rectangular pulse train - 28 dB. Symmetrical form of responses for low intensity stimuli.

duration of 3.74 sec the PST histograms are of the usual symmetrical shape. An off-response is also observed. For the 1.24 sec stimulus the response becomes nonsymmetrical, arising mostly at the half of the stimulus with a fall of the amplitude. For this duration (1.24 sec) the speed of amplitude changes is three times faster than for the longer stimulus (3.74 sec). At such a speed the response of the unit becomes unidirectional; the unit responds only to the diminution of the amplitude. It is important that this unidirectional response to the diminution of the amplitude is preserved for stimuli with different sequences of the rise-fall and the fall-rise halves. The response for rectangular pulse train (1.1 sec duration) shows a tendency toward facilitation. So, the unidirection phenomenon cannot be determined by adaptation.

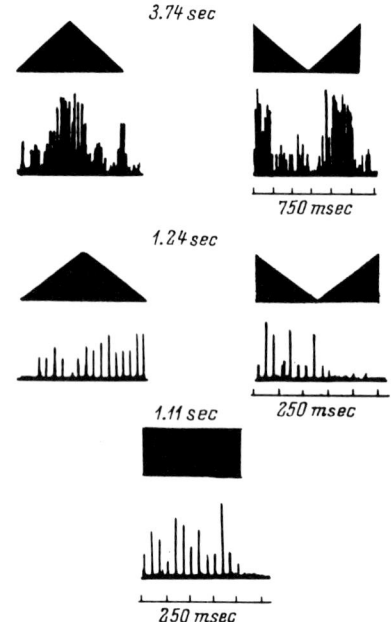

Fig. 21   PST histograms of unit N 12/2 responses to triangular AM noise pulse trains (durations 3.74 and 1.24 sec) and non-modulated (rectangular) pulse train (1.1 sec). Repetition rate 10/sec. SPL - 73 dB. Threshold for rectangular pulse train - 28 dB. An asymmetrical response; maximum to the rise-fall direction of amplitude changes (duration of the pulse train 1.24 msec).

In Fig. 22 responses of another unit are presented. The stimuli for this unit were constant in duration and shape and only varied in intensity (73, 63, 53 dB). The unit is non-monotonic and responds to non-modulated (rectangular) pulse train with a maximal discharge to the low intensity stimulus (53 dB). At the intensity of 73 dB the unit responds only with an initial burst during the first 100 msec of stimulation.

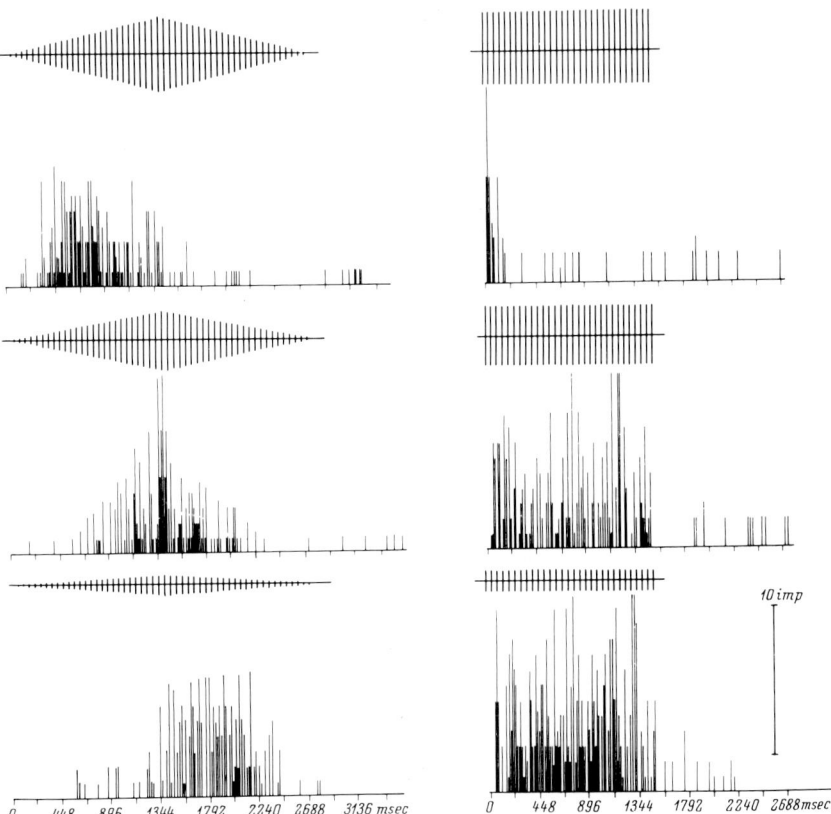

Fig. 22   PST histograms of unit N 29/1 responses to triangular and rectangular noise pulse trains. Repetition rate 10/sec. SPL top histograms - 73 dB, middle - 63 dB, bottom - 53 dB, threshold for rectangular pulse train 43 dB. N = 12. In this experiment, random phase switching for subsequent stimuli was used. Timing of the response to different segments of the signal is seen.

The responses for the triangularly modulated pulse trains at three different intensity levels show drastic differences in timing of the discharge. For 73 dB the response is nonsymmetrical and is timed to the rising half of the stimulus. At 63 dB the response is symmetrical. At 53 dB the response is asymmetrical, and is timed to the falling half of the stimulus. In that case, contrary to the data of Fig. 21, the duration of the stimulus was constant and the speeds of the amplitude changes were determined by the intensity levels. In Table 2, data are presented which permit evaluation of the dependence of the spike count and timing of the unit discharge on two parameters of the stimulus: 1) amplitude (sound pressure) level, and 2) speed of amplitude changes. For the non-modulated (rectangular) pulse train the maximal number of spikes is about six times greater at the lowest intensity (53 dB) than at the highest (73 dB). The spike count is largely dependent on the intensity; the dependence is inverse, as is typical for this non-monotonic unit. For the triangularly AM pulse trains the dependence of the spike number on the intensity is not a characteristic feature of the unit responses. For such stimuli the timing of the responses to different phases of the AM pulse trains is typical. For these triangularly AM stimuli the speed of amplitude changes (dA/dt) and not the amplitude differences (ΔA) must be accepted as a parameter which determines such a response feature as the timing of the discharge. The data for these two units show that changes of speed can lead to the nonsymmetrical responses and timing of the response to the fall-rise half (Fig. 21, Fig. 22, bottom) or to the rise-fall half (Fig. 22, top) of the pulse trains. Unidirectional responses to amplitude changes (to a diminution and to a rise of amplitude) are interesting from the biological point of view. Such units may be involved in detection of the direction of the movement of the sound source relative to the ear.

If one accepts the relation between sound pressure and the distance of the sound source which moves with a constant speed (see Fig. 4, h), it becomes possible to estimate the speeds of the sound motion, according to the data of Table 2. The obtained values of speeds of the sound source motion lie in the range of speeds of animal motions.

Table 2   Spike count. Unit N 29/1. Fig. 22

	Form of the noise pulse-train			
	Triangular-duration 2.9 sec		Rectangular-duration 1.6 sec	
SPL.[1] dB	Speed of amplitude changes μbar/sec.	Number of impulses per 12 presentations	SPL.dB	Number of impulses per 12 presentations
73	0.614	220	73	63
63	0.194	179	63	234
53	0.061	264	53	393

The triangular stimuli of the given duration (2.9 sec.) are equivalent (if the approximation presented on Fig. 4h is accepted) to a definite speed value (3.4 m/sec) of a sound source motion

[1] Sound pressure levels are given for the central pulse in the train (amplitude maximum). The 0 reference level is accepted as equivalent to the voltage established for a 0.0002 μbar reference level of a tone of 4 kHz.

The question of units' responses to the direction and the speed of the amplitude changes needs further investigation. In the sample of 52 units investigated with triangularly AM pulse trains we found such unidirectional responses to amplitude changes in only 5 units. It is important to differentiate such responses which depend on the direction of amplitude changes from the phenomena of diminution of the discharge in time (adaptation). The latter phenomenon is the most common determinant for the nonsymmetrical type of responses. In the sample of 52 units, nonsymmetrical responses were observed in 25. In 16 units the nonsymmetrical form of the responses could be ascribed to the diminution of the discharge as a function of the stimulation time (adaptation).

In Fig. 23 a unit with a nonsymmetrical response due to adaptation is presented. The responses are observed only during the first half of the stimulus for durations 3.74 and 2.22 sec irrespective of the direction of amplitude changes. For the shortest stim-

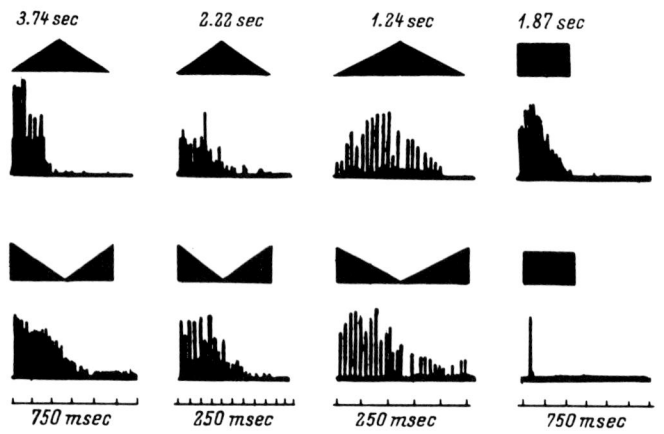

Fig. 23 PST histograms of responses to units N 6/2 to triangular and rectangular noise pulse trains. Repetition rate 20/sec. Numbers on the top - durations of stimuli. SPL - 73 dB; threshold for the rectangular pulse train - 35 dB. The quadrangles (duration of the stimulus 1.87 sec) indicate: on the top - noise pulse train; on the bottom - continuous noise burst. Asymmetrical responses of the unit, irrespective of the direction of amplitude changes.

ulus (1.24 sec) facilitation is observed in the responses for the first rise and fall halves of the stimuli and subsequent diminution of the responses for the second half, irrespective of the direction of amplitude changes. For the rectangular pulse trains (duration 1.87 sec, Fig. 23, top) the diminution of the response begins after 0.6 sec of stimulation. For the continuous rectangular noise burst (Fig. 23, bottom) there is only an initial discharge which lasts not more that 100 msec. For pulse trains of different duration and direction of AM the responses last from 1.2 to 2.5 sec. The data presented in Fig. 23 show how much the diminution of the discharge, as a function of stimulation time, is dependent on the time characteristics of the stimuli.

3.4 The dependence of adaptation on some time characteristics of the stimuli

In Table 3 data are presented concerning the adaptation phenomena as observed with different sound stimuli: continuous bursts, AM bursts and pulse trains. The adaptation phenomena are evaluated by the spike number counts (N_1 and N_2) for two time segments of the stimulus: one from the moment of initiation to the middle point of the time axis, the other from the middle point to the end. Data for four units are presented. The relation (K) between spike numbers N_2/N_1 can serve as a simple indicator of changes of the unit responses dependent on the duration of the stimuli. The data presented in Table 3 show clearly that AM clicks or pulse trains give the more stable responses, with a minimum of adaptation (maximum K values).

In Table 4 spike numbers are evaluated for the sequence of modulation cycles which form the stimulus (from the first to the fourth cycles). Data are presented for three units stimulated by low rate AM sound bursts and click trains. The responses to AM click trains show for all units a more stable response for the four-cycle sequence.

4. Discussion

4.1 Repetition rates and intervals in the pulse train optimal for auditory units' responses

In the investigation of central auditory neurons, trains of pulses formed by deep AM tone or noise

Table 3 Adaptation phenomena observed with different sound stimuli.

Unit Number	Type of discharge to a noise or CF burst.	AM Stimuli carrier	modulation rate (Hz)	Sound pressure Level	N_1	N_2	$K=\frac{N_2}{N_1}$	T time of spike count (msec.)
55	sustained	contin.noise contin.noise click train 30/sec.	0 3 3	68 dB	660 190 190	240 100 185	0.36 0.53 0.98	666 - " - - " -
87	sustained	contin. tone 14 kHz (CF) click train 80/sec.	80 0	55 dB	209 550	85 480	0.4 0.9	480 - " -
119	onset	contin.noise contin.noise click train 30/sec.	0 5 5	58 dB	20 20 100	0 0 80	0 0 0.8	400 - " - - " -
133	onset	contin.noise contin.noise click train 90/sec.	0 90 5	55 dB	20 420 189	0 200 161	0 0.47 0.84	500 - " - 400

[1]) N_1 is the number of impulses counted in the first, and N_2 in the second halves of the time segment (T).

Table 4   Impulses per modulation cycle

Unit number	Type of discharge to noise burst	AM stimuli carrier	AM stimuli modulation rates Hz	Number of impulses per modulation cycle [1] N_1	N_2	N_3	N_4	$K = \dfrac{N_4}{N_1}$ [2]
119	onset	continious noise	5	1.1	0	0	0	0
		click train 30/sec.	5	4.6	3.4	3.7	3.0	0.65
115	burst	continious noise	5	2.35	2.25	1.75	0.87	0.32
		click train 30/sec.	5	6.75	6.0	5.7	5.1	0.75
117	sustained	continious noise	5	6.1	5.1	5.7	4.9	0.83
		click train 30/sec.	5	4.9	5.0	5.1	5.0	1.02

1) mean values; 8-10 stimulations. See Fig. 8.
2) see Table 3.

bursts or by AM trains of short noise pulses and clicks were used. The experimental data showed that pulse rates which give a discharge at every pulse in the train and a maximum of spike number per the whole train, could be established for every unit. Such optimal rates were unexpectedly low (from 10 to 30/sec for most units, range of variations from 10 to 100 per sec). Such a parameter as pulse rate is not sufficient per se to characterize the time structure of a signal. Intervals between pulses and pulse durations must be known. For rectangular short noise pulses used in the experiments (pulse duration 5 msec) with optimal rates of 20-30/sec, the values of intervals were 45 and 28 msec. If one compares these interval values characteristic for most units with the data obtained by measurements of the recovery time by a pair of clicks or short pulses, a good correspondence appears. So, two-click intervals necessary for a 100% recovery of the response for the second click for rat collicular units with different discharge patterns were as follows: a) for onset discharge units, about 10 msec, b) for burst discharge units, 30 msec, c) for sustained discharge units, 52 msec (mean 27 msec) (Maruseva, 1971).

Two-click intervals for a 100% recovery obtained in evoked potential recording (the first positive wave) at the collicular level in cats and white rats give values about 40-60 msec (Altman and Maruseva, 1965, Vartanian et al., 1966). There are data that show that not only a 100% recovery but also facilitation phenomena are characteristic for such optimal rates and corresponding intervals between pulses; so a fall of thresholds to short noise pulse trains (rates 20-30/sec, pulse duration 2 msec) was obtained (Altman, 1969). Such facilitation on threshold and low suprathreshold levels for repetition rates 20-30/sec was also observed in experimental series (Figs 21, 22) with AM trains of short pulses. From these data it is evident that intervals between pulses which give a full recovery and facilitation of unit activity are characteristic for an optimal rate of a pulse train. Inhibitory influences which are typical for a shift of the carrier frequency of AM tones from the CF of the unit must decrease the optimal modulation rate of the pulse train.

Measurements of the recovery time by a pair of short tone pulses showed that the intervals necessary for a 100% recovery increase to a large degree when the frequency of the first tone pulse is shifted from CF to a higher one. In such cases an increase of the recovery time from a mean value of 30 msec to 70 msec is typical (Vartanian and Gersuni, 1972). In cases of repetitive stimulation when both parameters: i.e., repetition rate and intervals between pulses, can be adequately measured (in our experimental series AM trains of short rectangular pulses) optimal intervals of a pulse train which give a maximum number of spikes per train and a constant number of spikes per each pulse in the train, as mentioned above, lie in the range from 28 msec to 45 msec. The time structure of sounds segmented by intervals lying in this range is well reproduced in the discharge patterns in the great majority of units with different types of discharge (Fig. 8). A discharge pattern for such sound stimuli is most stable and shows a minimum of adaptation for the whole train duration.

It is important to compare our data obtained at the collicular level with responses of other parts of the auditory system to trains of pulses of AM sounds. Unfortunately data for AM sounds are scanty. Responses of cochlear units of rats to a train of tone pulses at a constant frequency (CF of the unit) with different repetition rates (from 0.1 to 100/sec) and durations were investigated by Møller (1971). The spike number for the whole pulse train and relative height of peaks in the histograms as a function of repetition rates were presented (for two units). A response maximum at definite repetition rates was clearly seen. For one unit the optimal response was observed at r.r. of 3-7/sec; for another at 50/sec.

Optimal rates for frequency modulation established for the same unit were found in the same range of values as for AM. Taking the differences between the stimuli used in both studies into consideration, it can be concluded that ranges of optimal rates and intervals between pulses are quite comparable for collicular and cochlear units.

It is not the intention here to review data on responses of units at higher levels of the auditory system to AM sounds. It should only be noted that at the level of the medial geniculate body, repetition rates of 10-15/sec are reproduced by several types of units (Altman et al., 1970); for some units such rates as 100-120/sec are reproduced (Aitkin and Dunlop, 1968). Reproduction of such repetition rates as 5-10/sec is usual for auditory cortex. Much higher repetition rates are reproduced as studied by evoked potentials.

In short, the reproduction of the time structure of sounds segmented by intervals which lie in the range optimal for collicular and cochlear units is evidently possible for some units at the higher levels of the auditory system.

4.2 Timing of unit responses to different segments of AM pulse trains

For triangularly AM pulse trains discharge patterns of symmetrical and asymmetrical forms were observed. The asymmetrical responses could be divided into two different types. One type could be characterized by a decrease in spike number especially pronounced in the second half of the triangular train, irrespective of the direction of the amplitude changes. For the other type, a timing of the response dependent on the direction of amplitude changes (rise-fall or fall-rise) irrespective of the sequence of the two halves was characteristic. Arguments were presented that in the latter case, the parameter which determines the timing of the response to the fall or to the rise segments of the pulse train is the speed of amplitude changes (dA/dt). Owing to the time structure of the stimuli (AM pulse trains) long lasting responses to slow amplitude changes (about 0.6 to 0.067 μ bar per sec) were observed. Such low speeds of amplitude changes as were discussed earlier (see Fig. 4h) are characteristic for a decrease or an increase of distance between a sound source, which moves at a speed of 2-8 meters/sec and the ear. Such speeds are characteristic for animal movements. It can be assumed that unidirectional responses for such speeds of amplitude changes (Fig. 21, 22) can be used as indicators for the direction of changes in the distance between the animal and a moving sound source. In such cases the shift of the response to different segments of a triangularly AM pulse train reaches values as great as 1500 msec

(Fig. 22, bottom). Such time shifts of the responses of collicular units to different segments of AM pulse trains are larger than that obtained by stimulation with sinusoidally AM tones, especially studied by Nelson et al. (1966).

Considerations of the possible mechanisms of such a time shift run along the same line as argued by Nelson et al. (1966) and Erulkar et al. (1968). Such phenomena are to be considered as a result of excitatory and inhibitory influences with different time courses and thresholds. From the data presented in Figs. 21 and 22 one can suppose that thresholds for inhibitory influences are higher and that the maximum of these influences is reached with a significant delay relative to the excitatory ones. Data which show a delay of the rise of inhibitory influences relative to the excitatory ones were obtained in different series of experiments on the collicular units of rats. A decrease of inhibitory influences is observed by shortening the stimulus duration in such series as spike count-intensity determinations (Maruseva, 1971) and two-tone inhibition measurements (Vartanian, 1972). That a discharge pattern of a unit depends on the interrelation between inhibitory and excitatory inputs stimulated by AM trains of pulses is evidently difficult to cast any doubt upon (Erulkar et al., 1968, Gersuni and Vartanian, 1969). Our data at the present time are not sufficient to lead into further discussion of this question.

4.3 Bioacoustical pulse trains and afferent impulse flow

Bioacoustical signals are complex sounds, formed by a train of pulses. In mammals the bioacoustical pulse trains arise as a result of complex coordinated patterns of muscle activities of a sound generating system which includes different organs. The speech generating mechanism in man can be considered as a special and most advanced organization of complex patterns of muscle activities of different organs which lead to sound production (Lieberman, 1968, Christovich and Kozhevnikov, 1972). Different patterns of muscle activities of the sound generating system are characteristic for different forms of behavior in animals. Evaluating even such simple features of the time structure of the bioacoustical pulse trains as presented in Table 1 (interval between pulses, pulse duration, pulse rates) and the data obtained in the investigation of single central auditory neurons with AM sounds, the question arises as to how the properties of the bioacoustical emitters and receivers are matched.

In our sample of bioacoustical pulse trains (Table 1) the first order intervals between pulses and pulse rates are limited by a minimum interval of about 35-40 msec and pulse rates of about 15-20/sec.

Data obtained in such extensively studied animals as echolocating bats during different stages of hunting behavior show that the pulse rates in the train lie in the range from 4-5 to 100-150 per sec (intervals from 6 to 125 msec) for two families of bats (review Airapetianz and Konstantinov, 1970).

In the investigation of the responses of central auditory neurons to repetitive sounds such mean values of optimal intervals and repetition rates were obtained: intervals: 28-45 msec, rates: 20-30/sec. (The criteria accepted for an optimal discharge to a pulse train were given earlier). The data obtained in two click measurements of intervals necessary for a 100% recovery of the unit discharge (mean values 27 msec; the range of variation for different types of units from 10 to 50 msec) lie in the same range. The values presented for intervals and rates characterize the repetitive stimuli which give rise to such repetitive discharges of central auditory units which reproduce the time structure of the pulse train during long lasting stimulation; (the discharge can be characterized by a maximum number of impulses per stimulation time). The values of intervals and rates of such optimal repetitive stimuli lie in the same ranges which are characteristic for the bioacoustical pulse trains (especially for the upper limits of the rate values). These values of intervals and rates of the bioacoustical pulse trains evidently reflect the time pattern of muscle activities of the sound generating organs.

We think that the data presented support the optimal intervals and low frequency repetition rates as indices of properties of central auditory neurons which are adapted to perception of such signals.

It is important to note that the optimal low frequency rates are most clearly demonstrated in the investigations of Møller (1971) of the responses of units in the rat cochlear nucleus. The low frequency optimal rates are similar for the cochlear and collicular units.

In conclusion it is necessary to note that in the investigations of the problem of the recognition of complex sounds, especially of such sounds as the bioacoustical signals, the data on single units are to be considered only as a part of a coordinated neurophysiological and behavioral study.

References

Airapetiantz, E. Sh., Konstantinov, A.I. (1970). Echolocation in Nature. Nauka, Leningrad.

Aitkin, L.M., and Dunlop, C.W. (1968). Interplay of excitation and inhibition in cat medial geniculate body. J. Neurophysiol. 31, 44-61.

Altman, J.A. (1969). Responses of the posterior colliculi units of the cat to lateralization of rhythmic acoustic stimuli. J. Higher Nervous Activity (Moscow) 19, 59-70.

Altman, J.A. (1972). Sound localization (neurophysiological mechanisms). Nauka, Leningrad.

Altman, J.A., and Maruseva, A.M. (1965). Evoked potentials of the auditory system. J. Higher Nervous Activity (Moscow) 15, 539-549.

Altman, J.A., Syka, I., and Shmigidina, G.H. (1970). Neuronal activity in the medial geniculate body of the cat during monaural and binaural stimulation. Exp. Brain Res. 10, 81-93.

van Bergeijk, W.A. (1967). The evolution of vertebrate hearing. In: Contributions to Sensory Physiology. (W.D. Neff, ed.), Vol. 2, pp. 1-49. Academic Press, New York.

Chistovich, L.A., and Koshevnikov, V.A. (1972). Speech perception. In: Physiology of Sensory Systems. (G.V. Gersuni, ed.), Part 2, pp. 427-514, Nauka, Leningrad.

Coleman, P.D. (1963). An analysis of cues to auditory depth perception in free space. Psychol. Bull. 60, 302-315.

Erulkar, S.D. (1972). Comparative physiology of spatial localization of sound. Physiol. Rev. 52, 257-360.

Erulkar S.D., Nelson, P.G., and Bryan, J.S. (1968). Experimental and theoretical approaches to neural processing in the central auditory pathway. In: Contributions to Sensory Physiology (W.D. Neff, ed.), Vol. 3, pp. 149-189. Academic Press, New York.

Fox, C.A., and Eichman, I. (1959). A rapid method for locating intracerebral electrodes. Stain Technol. 34, 39-42.

Gersuni, G.V. (1971). Temporal organization of the auditory function. In: Sensory Processes at the Neuronal and Behavioral levels. (G.V. Gersuni, ed.), pp. 85-114. Academic Press, New York.

Gersuni, G.V. (1972). General characteristics of hearing in vertebrates. In: Physiology of Sensory Systems. (G.V. Gersuni, ed.), Part 2, pp. 150-157. Nauka, Leningrad.

Gersuni, G.V., and Malt'sev, V.P. (1973). Some general characteristics of impulse sequences in bioacoustical signals. J. Evol. Biochem. Physiol. 9, 2. (In press).

Gersuni, G.V., and Vartanian, I.A. (1969). Responses of specialized neurons of the colliculus inferior of rats to amplitude modulated sounds. J. Evol. Biochem. Physiol. 5, 207-217.

Gersuni, G.V., Altman, J.A., Maruseva, A.M., Radionova, E.A., Ratnikova, G.T., and Vartanian, I.A. (1971). Functional classification of neurons in the inferior colliculus of the cat according to their temporal characteristics. In: Sensory Processes at the Neuronal and Behavioral levels. (G.V. Gersuni, ed.), pp. 157-179. Academic Press, New York.

Griffin, D.R. (1958). Listening in the Dark. Yale Univ. Press. New Haven, Conn.

Grinnell, A.D. (1969). Comparative physiology of hearing. Ann. Rev. Physiol. 31, 545-575.

Helmholtz, H. (1863). Die Lehre von den Tonempfindungen als physiologische Grundlage für die Theorie der Musik. Citation 5th ed. Vieweg and Son, Braunschweig, 1896.

Lieberman, P. (1968). Primate Vocalization and human linguistic ability. J. Acoust. Soc. Amer. 44, 1574-1584.

Littlejohn, M.I., and Loftus-Hills, J.J. (1968). An experimental evaluation of premating isolation call in the Anura. Evolution, 22, 659-663.

Malt'sev, V.P. (1970). On sound signalization in Cebus capucinus. J. Evol. Biochem. Physiol. 6, 64-73.

Marler, P.R., and Hamilton. W.J. (1967). Mechanisms of Animal Behavior. John Wiley and Sons, New York.

Maruseva, A.M. (1971). Temporal characteristics of the auditory neurons in the inferior colliculus. In: Sensory Processes at the Neuronal and Behavioral Levels. (G.V. Gersuni, ed.), pp. 181-200. Academic Press, New York.

Møller, A.R. (1969). Unit responses in the rat cochlear nucleus to repetitive, transient sounds. Acta Physiol. Scand. 75, 542-551.

Møller, A.R. (1971). Unit responses in the rat cochlear nucleus to tones of rapidly varying frequency and amplitude. Acta Physiol. Scand. 81, 540-556.

Møller, A.R. (1972). Coding of sounds in lower levels of the auditory system. Quart. Rev. Biophys. 5, 59-155.

Nelson, P.G., Erulkar, S.D., and Bryan, I.S. (1966). Responses of units of the inferior colliculus to time-varying acoustic stimuli. J. Neurophysiol. 29, 834-860.

Plomp, R., and Smoorenburg, G.F. (eds.)(1970). Frequency Analysis and Periodicity Detection in Hearing. A.W. Sijthoff, Leiden, The Netherlands.

Popov, A.V. (1972). Sound signals in Orthoptera, Gryllidae, from South districts of Europe and part of USSR. Entomol. Rev. 51, 17-36.

Radionova, E.A. (1971a). Two types of neurons in the cat's cochlear nuclei and their role in audition. In: Sensory Processes at the Neuronal and Behavioral Levels. (G.V. Gersuni, ed.), pp. 135-155. Academic Press, New York.

Radionova, E.A. (1971b). Functional Characteristics of the Cochlear Nuclei Neurons and Audition. Nauka, Leningrad.

Roeder, K.D., and Treat, A.E. (1961). The reception of bat cries by the tympanic organ of noctuid moths. In: Sensory Communication. (W.A. Rosenblith, ed.), pp. 545-560. M.I.T. Press, Cambridge, Mass.

Rose, J.E., Greenwood, D.D., Goldberg, J.M., and Hind, J.E. (1963). Some discharge characteristics of single neurones in the inferior colliculus of the cat. I. Tonotopical organization, relation of spike counts to tone intensity and firing patterns of single elements. J. Neurophysiol. 26, 294-320.

Sebeok, T.A. (ed.)(1968). Animal Communication. Indiana Univ. Press, Bloomington, Indiana.

Suga, N. (1968). Analysis of frequency-modulated and complex sounds by single auditory neurons of bats. J. Physiol. 198, 51-80.

Vartanian, I.A. (1971). Impulse activity of neurons of the rat's inferior colliculus in response to amplitude-modulated sound signals. In: Sensory Processes at the Neuronal and Behavioral Levels.

(G.V. Gersuni, ed.), pp. 201-220. Academic Press, New York.

Vartanian, I.A. (1972). Dependence of inhibitory areas in the inferior colliculus neurons on time characteristics of sound signals. Neurophysiol. (Kiev) 4, 236-244.

Vartanian, I.A., and Gersuni, G.V. (1972). Responses of auditory neurons in the inferior colliculus to amplitude-modulated sounds with changing carrier frequency and modulation rate. Neurophysiol. (Kiev) 4, 12-22.

Vartanian, I.A., and Snetkov, V.I. (1970). Effect of the time rise of acoustic stimulus on unit activity of inferior colliculus. Neurosci. Translations, 16, 63-73.

Vartanian, I.A., Lebedeva, Z.P., and Maruseva, A.M. (1966). Electrical reaction of the inferior colliculus in the rat under the action of brief sound signals (clicks). Bull. Exp. Biol. Med. (Moscow), 2, 3-6.

Wall, P.D. (1959). Repetitive discharge of neurons. J. Neurophysiol. 22, 305-320.

FEATURE EXTRACTION IN THE AUDITORY
SYSTEM OF BATS

Nobuo Suga

Washington University
St. Louis, Missouri
USA

1. Introduction

1.1 Information-Bearing Elements in Animal Sounds

In orthopterans, the species-specific song is generally recognized by the rhythm of pulsatory sounds. The detail of the frequency spectrum of each pulsatory sound is not essential for the recognition of the species-specific song (Autrum, 1955, Busnel et al., 1956, Walker, 1958). In other words, acoustic information is given by the envelope of amplitude-modulated carrier waves. The carrier wave is important only for the effective stimulation of a receptor. For instance, certain species of grasshoppers produce pulsatory sounds, the energy of which is concentrated at frequencies higher than 10 kHz. Their auditory neurons are not sharply tuned to many different frequencies and show no phase-locked response to the carrier wave, but show a response synchronized with each pulsatory sound, i.e., amplitude-modulation of the carrier wave (e.g. Katsuki and Suga, 1960, Suga and Katsuki, 1961, Suga, 1966). Furthermore, some central auditory neurons are specialized for responding to pulsatory sounds at a particular temporal pattern (Adams, 1969). Thus, the amplitude-modulation of the carrier wave, i.e., the species-specific rhythmic movement of the elytra, conveys the most essential information for the recognition of a species. This is the commonly accepted theory (Dumortier, 1963), although physiological studies on peripheral (Katsuki and Suga, 1960, Popov, 1965, Michelsen, 1966, 1971) and central auditory neurons of certain insects (Horridge, 1961, Suga and Katsuki, 1961, Yanagisawa et al., 1967, Adams, 1969, Kalmring et al., 1972) suggest the possibility of some analysis of carrier frequency. Some fishes produce sounds which are probably used for communication. These sounds usually consist of frequencies lower than a few kHz (Fish and Mowbray, 1970, Tavolga, 1960). Saccular neurons, which do not show a sharp tuning curve, discharge impulses well synchronized with each wave of low frequency pure tones (Enger, 1963, Furukawa and Ishii, 1967, Grozinger, 1967). Behavioral experiments indicate that the goldfish can discriminate a 3.5 % change of about 500 Hz (Jacobs and Tavolga, 1968). If fishes do actually communicate with low frequency acoustic signals, both the carrier and its envelope may be important for the recognition of a species-specific sound. In the bullfrog (Rana catesbeiana), not only the envelope of the amplitude modulated carrier sound, but also the spectrum of the carrier is important for the recognition of the species-specific croak (Capranica, 1966). The peripheral auditory system of the bullfrog is specialized for the reception of his croak. Inhibition occurring at the receptor plays an essential role in the recognition of the communication sounds (Frishkopf and Goldstein, 1963). In many birds (Konishi, 1963, 1965, Nottebohm, 1968) and mammals (Winter et al., 1966, Jürgens and Ploog, 1970), acoustic signals for communication are highly elaborated, and the analysis of sound spectrum changing with time is undoubtedly essential for acoustic communication.

Human speech sounds consist of various phonemes combined in different sequences and are consequently very complicated. The sonograms of these speech sounds, however, exhibit the following three basic features or components: (1) constant frequency (CF) component, (2) noise component, and (3) frequency-modulated (FM) component (Fig. 1A). These are called three types of "information-bearing elements". The sonogram of a consonant consists of a vertical bar indicating the scatter of sound energy over many frequencies. This is called a "fill", i.e., noise burst. The sonogram of a vowel consists of several horizontal bars, which are called "formants". The formant is a spectral peak characterizing a vowel. The lowest is called the first formant (F_1), the second-lowest is the second formant (F_2), and so on. These may simply be considered CF (or pure-tone) components. Not all of the components of human speech sounds which appear in the sonogram

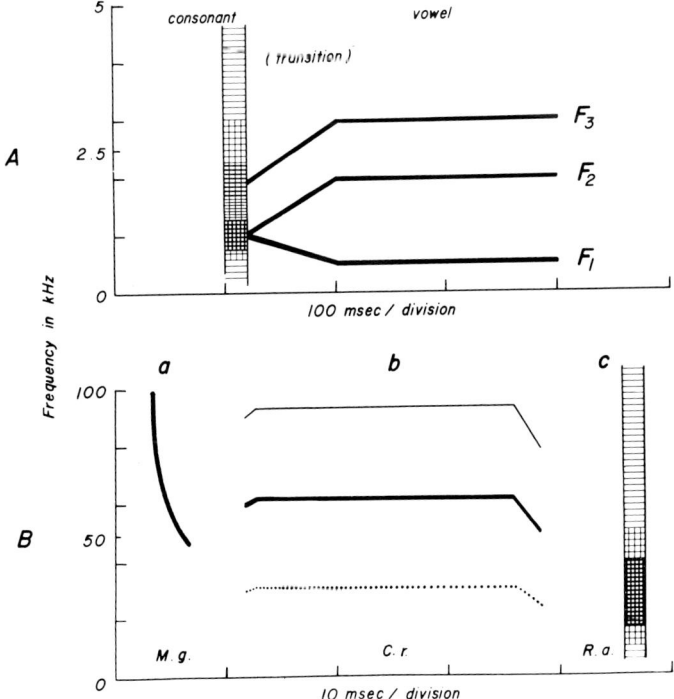

Fig. 1 Schematic presentation of three types of information-bearing elements in human speech sounds (A) and three types of orientation sounds used by different species of bats (B). The ordinates and abscissas respectively represent frequency in kHz and time in msec. In A, a sonogram of a monosyllabic word is presented. F_1, F_2 and F_3, respectively, represent the first, second and third formants of the vowel. In B, a, b, and c represent sonograms of orientation sounds of the gray bat (Myotis grisescens), mustache bat (Chilonycteris rubiginosa) and fruit bat (Rousettus amplexicaudatus stresemanii), respectively.

are information-bearing elements. Vowels are identified mainly by F_1 and F_2, although F_3 has some influence on word identification. When these two phonemes are combined to form a monosyllabic word, a new component called a "transition" will appear. The transition is an FM component since its frequency changes with time (Fig. 1A; Potter et al., 1966). This FM component is very important for identification of some monosyllabic words. Plosive consonants (k, t, p, g, d, and b) are identified not only by their fills, but also by the transition before F_2 of a following vowel. The transition of F_1 provides a distinction between voiced (g, d, and b) and voiceless plosive consonants (k, t, and p). Some fricative consonants, such as "f" and "th", are also identified mainly by the transition of F_2. Fricative consonants "s" and "sh" are, however, distinguishable from other consonants because of their high energy noise bursts, concentrated around 2-3 kHz and above 4.4 kHz, respectively (Denes and Pinson, 1963). Nasal sounds (m and n) and glides (w, j, r, and l) are somewhat similar to vowels. The glides, however, always contain FM components (Potter et al., 1966). Human speech sounds, thus, consist of the three types of information-bearing elements. It should be noted, however, that speech recognition is accomplished not only by acoustic cues, but also linguistic, semantic and circumstantial cues (Denes and Pinson, 1963).

These three types of information-bearing elements are also found in sounds produced by acoustically specialized animals. For example, toothed whales and porpoises emit very short noise bursts for echolocation and sounds consisting of FM and/or CF components for communication (Bastian, 1967, Norris et al., 1967). For echolocation, the little brown bat (Myotis lucifugus) and the gray bat (Myotis grisescens) emit short FM sounds, in which the frequency always sweeps from high to low (Fig. 1, B a; Griffin, 1958). In the orientation sound of the greater horseshoe bat (Rhinolophus ferrumequinum), frequency rises 1-12 kHz in the initial part and reaches a long plateau of 83 kHz. Then, it drops by 13-16 kHz. Thus, the orientation sound consists of CF and FM components (Schnitzler, 1968). In this sound, overtones are nearly absent. The orientation sound of the mustache bat (Chilonycteris rubiginosa) also consists of CF and FM components, but it has prominent overtones (Fig. 1, B b; Schnitzler, 1970). African fruit bats (Rousettus aegiptus and R. emplexicandatus stresemanii) emit short noise bursts (Fig. 1, B c; Kulzer, 1956, Grinnell and Hagiwara, 1972). The frequencies of predominant components in orientation sounds greatly vary from species to species, ranging between about 5 and

150 kHz. Such differences in acoustic signals emitted are related to their acoustic behavior and habitat (Griffin, 1971).

Echoes returning from objects at different places overlap each other and show complex envelopes and structures which differ from those of an outgoing sound. The bats analyze these complex echoes from different aspects for echolocation. Each of the three types of signals (CF tones, FM sounds, and noise bursts) has both advantages and disadvantages as orientation sounds. A CF sound is an ideal signal for the measurement of change in the distance between a bat and a target, i.e., for the measurement of the relative velocities of a moving target, but not for target-ranging, echo-localization, and analysis of targets. When the size of a target is larger than the wavelength of a signal, the CF sound is also a very good signal for echo-detection, because the reflected sound energy is highly concentrated at a particular frequency, and it effectively stimulates auditory neurons tuned to that frequency. A short noise burst (or click) is good for echo-ranging and echo-localization, but not for the measurement of velocity, because of a wide scattering of sound energy for many frequencies. An FM sound is suited for echo-detection, -ranging, and localization, and analysis of targets, because of the systematic change in wavelength. Information about the change in distance to a target is also obtained with the FM signal, although it is very inferior compared with that obtained with a CF signal (Cahlander, 1964, Schnitzler, 1968, 1970, Altes and Titlebaum, 1970, Simmons, 1971a, b, 1973a, b). Since all bats using FM signals emit brief sounds at a high repetition rate during the approach and terminal phases in insect hunting and landing, the information about the change in distance to a target is always available for them on the basis of change in the interval between the emitted signal and echoes. For echolocation, FM sounds are probably a better signal than CF sounds and noise bursts. As a matter of fact, all microchiropterans use FM sounds or sounds with FM components for echolocation, and the bats which emit CF plus FM sounds apparently are more specialized for echolocation than the others. Since bats use relatively simple acoustic signals for echolocation, which is absolutely indispensable for their survival, their auditory systems may be suited to neurophysiological studies on the recognition of the three types of information-bearing elements in animal sounds.

As described above, the three types of information-bearing elements are present in the sounds emitted by humans and acoustically specialized animals, and these are also found in the sounds produced by many other animals. All animal sounds are modulated in amplitude. Therefore, the following three common questions may be asked concerning the feature extraction from complex acoustic pattern: (1) how do single auditory neurons respond to each element isolated from complex sounds? (2) how do single auditory neurons respond to these elements when they are within complex sounds? and (3) how do single neurons respond to amplitude-modulated sounds?

1.2 Assumptions for Feature Extraction from Acoustic Signals

Since the mammalian auditory system has many band-pass filters in the cochlea, the power spectrum of acoustic signals is analyzed in the cochlea. The outputs of the filters are coded by primary auditory neurons. Spatial and temporal patterns of discharges of primary auditory neurons change with the sound spectrum. Psychological phenomena in hearing can be thus correlated with these patterns of discharges of primary auditory neurons to a significant extent. Intervening processes between excitation of primary auditory neurons and psychological phenomena are decoding of or feature extraction from coded signals. Concerning the neural basis of pattern recognition, two opposing assumptions are conceivable. In one extreme assumption, recognition of a particular acoustic signal is directly related to the spatial and temporal patterns of discharges of auditory neurons at higher levels, but not to the activities of neurons specialized to respond exclusively to that acoustic signal. In other words, "feature detectors" are not necessary for the recognition (e.g. Nottebohm, 1972). If one makes this assumption, one may extensively study temporal patterns of nerve discharges, tuning curves (or excitatory response areas) of single neurons, and tonotopic organization. In the other extreme assumption, the presence of higher order neurons specialized to respond to particular acoustic signals is essential for the recognition of the signals. If one takes this assumption, one may extensively look for single neurons which exclusively respond to one of various types of acoustic patterns. In the frog retina, there are neurons highly specialized for responding to particular types of visual signals which are meaningful for the frog (Lettvin et al., 1961). In the visual systems of cats and monkeys, such specialized neurons are not found in the retina, but in the cerebral cortex. Simple, complex and hyper-complex neurons have been found in visual cortices (Hubel and Wiesel, 1962, 1965, 1968). In the auditory system, there are several nuclei between the auditory nerve and cortex. It is highly probable that higher-order auditory neurons show specialization for particular acoustic signals as shown by higher-order visual neurons. In the present paper, the author presents evidence that the auditory system of a bat has "feature detectors", i.e., neurons specialized for responding to one of the three types of information-bearing elements.

Since the specialized visual neurons are not found with a diffuse light illumination, but with various other types of photo-stimuli, specialization of auditory neurons for feature extraction cannot be studied by using only either pure tones or click sounds. One has to deliver meaningful sounds produced by an experimental animal and sounds emitted by its predators and preys. When a neuron responding exclusively to a particular animal sound is found, one has to examine whether any single component in it is insufficient to excite the neuron and which combination of two or more components is actually necessary for the excitation of the neuron. In an alternative way, the three types of the information-bearing elements are delivered either separately or in a particular combination, and one can examine whether there are neurons showing specialization in responding to a particular acoustic pattern. In my experiments, the latter method was employed.

My experiments had been performed with the following three assumptions: (1) For the recognition of high frequency CF tones, to which single neurons cannot show phase-locked responses, single neurons should have very narrow tuning curves and should be specialized to respond only to CF tones. For the recognition of low frequency CF tones, phase-locked discharges may take an important role. In bats, orientation sounds are higher than 10 kHz, and their ears are sensitive to ultrasonic signals, so that phase-locked responses to the signals may be absent. (2) When the frequency of sound sweeps from high to low, primary auditory neurons with a high best frequency are the first to be stimulated; subsequently those with a lower best frequency are excited. When the direction of frequency sweep is reversed, these neurons are stimulated in the opposite order. For the recognition of FM sounds, the brain should contain neurons which exclusively respond to FM signals and which can detect the order, speed, and functional form in which peripheral auditory neurons with different best frequencies are excited. (3) For the recognition of a noise burst, the brain must contain neurons which can detect the number of peripheral auditory neurons with different best frequencies which are being stimultaneously excited. (4) For the recognition of AM sounds, the brain should contain neurons, of which not only spectrum of a carrier, but also its envelope is an important factor for excitation. The bats have auditory neurons specialized to exclusively respond to certain types of sounds, i.e., feature detectors. The population of such specialized neurons in the brain may, however, be different from species to species, depending on what types of sound an animal uses for echolocation and/or communication and also on the postnatal experience of the animal.

In the present paper, the problems in feature extraction are discussed on the basis of the data obtained from anesthetized bats of the genus Myotis during the last several years (Suga, 1964a, b, 1965a, b, c, 1968, 1969a, 1970, 1971 and unpublished data, Suga and Schlegel, 1973).

1.3 Classification of Single Neurons in Terms of Responses to Three Types of Information-Bearing Elements

In general, mammalian cochleas show such broad threshold curves that any sounds, which can excite the cochleas, are coded by primary auditory neurons, regardless of their acoustic features. Thus, extensive information processing should be performed in the brain. At higher levels of the auditory system, neurons with different properties have been found. For the description about properties of single neurons, it is convenient to classify them and to give names to them, although there are no discrete groups, but continuous spectrums of properties. Here, single neurons are classified in terms of their responses to three types of information-bearing elements.

At first, single neurons may be divided into two major groups: (A) neurons responding to a single component in complex sounds and (B) neurons responding only to particular combinations of two or more components in complex sounds. Group A may be divided into three subgroups: (i) units responding to three types of elements (CF tones, FM sounds, and noise bursts) of complex sounds, (ii) units responding to two of these elements, and (iii) units responding to only one of the three. Since neurons which were definitely in group B were not found, a classification of neurons belonging to group A only are shown in Table 1, in which (i)-(iii) are divided into seven classes.

Each class may be further divided on the basis of responses to sounds different in either frequency, intensity, time, or spatial domains. Characteristics of neurons in the frequency domain are often expressed by whether their excitatory response areas are narrow or wide or by whether their best frequencies are high or low. This expression is, however, unsatisfactory because it disregards inhibitory response areas which play an essential role for recognition of complex sound. In most neurons in the inferior colliculus, responses to FM sounds sweeping upward or downward by one octave across an excitatory area of a given unit with its best frequency at the center of the frequency sweep are highly correlated with the presence of excitatory and inhibitory areas. Therefore, the responses to the FM sounds are useful in classifying neurons in the frequency domain. Neurons are called "asymmetrical (or directional) units" if their responses to FM tone pulses differ by more than 10 dB in threshold depending on the direction of frequency sweep; otherwise, neurons are called "symmetrical (or non-directional) units". In Table 1, generalized, CF-deaf, noise-deaf, and FM-specialized neurons may be further divided into two groups: directional and non-directional for FM.

The relation between the number of impulses and the intensity of sound (called an impulse-count function) shows a continuous spectrum from monotonic to non-monotonic function. In the extreme case of non-monotonic impulse-count function, an "upper-threshold" appears, above which a neuron fails to respond. Thus,

Table 1[1]

Classification of neurons in terms of responses to three types of information-bearing elements: CF (or pure) tone, FM sound, and noise bursts.

Type	% in I.C.	% in A.C.
(i) Units responding to three elements Pure, FM and noise		
Generalized		
Symmetrical	66	47
Asymmetrical	16(21)	12(30)
Upper-threshold	4(8)	12
(ii) Units responding to two elements		
(a) FM and noise	2	
(b) Noise and Pure	0	
(c) Pure and FM	1	
(iii) Units responding to one element		
(a) Pure	8(9)	15
(Upper-threshold)		
(b) FM	2	14
(c) Noise	1	

1) Approximate percentages of 9 types of neurons sampled in the dorsal and central regions of the inferior colliculus are given in this table (Suga, 1969a). When the auditory cortex was studied, pure tones and FM sounds were used, but noise bursts were not used. Thus, some of the CF- and FM-specialized neurons might be FM-deaf and CF-deaf units, respectively, as indicated by the oblique dotted lines on the right (Suga, 1965c). Some neurons showed properties belonging to more than one category. When these neurons were counted twice, percentages of certain types of neurons increased as shown in parentheses.

for showing qualitatively the characteristics of neurons in the intensity domain, neurons may be classified depending on whether these show upper-threshold or not. Since animal sounds are always modulated in amplitude, it is also important to study responses of single neurons to sounds amplitude-modulated in various ways.

Characteristics of neurons in the time domain such as response pattern and recovery cycle may also be included in this classification. In terms of response patterns, neurons are often called either tonic or phasic units. This simple, rather arbitrary classification is often convenient, because tonic neurons are considered to be specialized for detection of stimulus magnitude and phasic ones, to be specialized to detect the rate of amplitude modulation. At higher levels, however, there are various types of response patterns, and a response pattern of a single neuron changes with the frequency and intensity of sound, so that classification becomes complicated (Katsuki et al., 1962, Evans and Whitfield, 1964, Greenwood and Maruyama, 1965, Pfeiffer, 1966, Suga, 1969a). A classification in terms of recovery cycles appears to be also possible because single neurons at higher levels show a wide spectrum of recovery curves (Friend et al., 1966, Suga and Schlegel, 1973). Animal sounds often consist of a series of complex sounds or noise bursts, so that it is important to study recovery cycles of auditory neurons.

Furthermore, auditory neurons may be classified in terms of directional sensitivity or binaural interaction. An ideal classification of responses of auditory neurons to signals with four domains (frequency, intensity, time, and space) is thus very complicated and difficult because there are almost no available data which contain a complete description of properties of single neurons in these four domains. Available data usually tell us about properties of neurons in terms of a certain aspect. In my experiments described below, for instance, recovery cycles and binaural interaction are not studied. Some generalized neurons, which appear to be unimportant in terms of analysis of the information-bearing elements, may be specialized for detecting a particular acoustic rhythm or for sound localization, but such information has not yet been obtained.

2. Materials and Methods

<u>Myotis grisescens</u>, <u>M</u>. <u>lucifugus</u>, <u>M</u>. <u>sodalis</u>, and <u>M</u>. <u>yumanensis</u> were caught in caverns and old houses. All these animals belonging to the family Vespertilionidae emit short downward-sweeping FM sounds for echolocation. The bats (about 6-7 g) were anesthetized by intraperitoneal injection of sodium pentobarbital (45 mg/kg). Ether was used at the initial phase of the operation to limit movement of the animal, if necessary. The operation and the recording of single unit activity were carried out for about 8 hours in a sound-proofed room at 35-37°C, often without any additional anesthetic because the animal did not move unless the skin was touched. After pushing aside the temporal muscles, a small hole was made in the skull over either the inferior colliculus (I.C.) or the auditory cortex (A.C.) for the insertion of a micropipette electrode filled with 3M-KCl solution. In order to expose the cochlear nucleus (C.N.), the skull over the lateral portion of the cerebellum was chipped away, and the cerebellum was partly aspirated with a small grass pipette connected with a vacuum pump. The auditory nerve (A.N.) is located immediately ventral to the C.N., so that action potentials of single neurons in both the C.N. and A.N. could be recorded during a nearly perpendicular insertion of the microelectrode into the C.N. from its dorso-lateral surface. The bat was mounted on a small metal plate after the operation. The skull was held fast by four sewing needles fixed on four micromanipulators. The microelectrode mounted on a micromanipulator was advanced hydraulically from outside the sound-proofed room. An indifferent silver wire electrode was placed on the neck muscles through wet cotton. Single unit activity was amplified and was displayed on an oscilloscope screen.

In order to deliver the three types of information-bearing elements, sound stimuli were generated as described in the previous papers (Suga, 1965a, 1968, 1969a). Since the methods have been changed during the last several years, the most often used methods are concisely described below. The voltage-controlled wave generator produced a continuous sine wave, the frequency of which was constant or modulated linearly or exponentially with time according to the voltage signal from a home-made sweep-function generator. In order to have only the frequency modulated or unmodulated portion as a short tone burst, the continuous sine wave was formed into a short electric signal corresponding to a tone pulse by a home-made electronic switch driven by pulses synchronizing with the voltage signal from the sweep-function generator. The duration and rise-decay time of the tone pulse were kept at 4.0 and 0.5 msec, respectively, unless otherwise stated (Fig. 2, A a). Since the rise-decay time

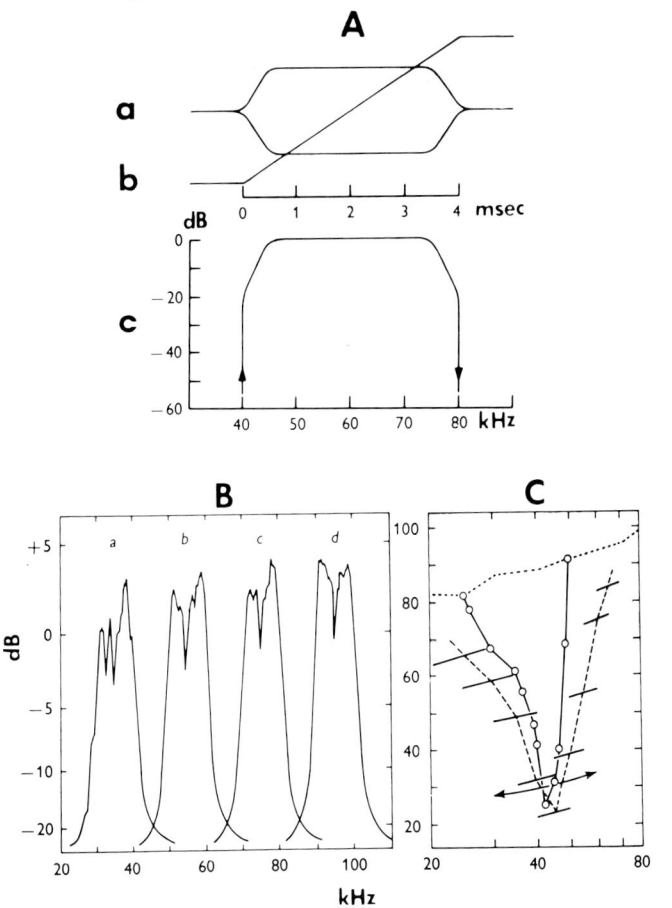

Fig. 2 A: The relationship between frequency and amplitude modulations in an FM sound. a: Envelope of a tone burst. b: Voltage signal to modulate the frequency of the tone burst. c: Relationship between frequency sweep and amplitude modulation of the FM sound. The ordinate and abscissa represent amplitude (cont'd)

in dB and frequency in kHz, respectively (Suga, 1968).

B: Spectra of four noise bursts delivered with a loudspeaker. The bandwidth of the noise bursts is set at 10 kHz. The abscissa represents the frequency of sound in kHz and the ordinate represents the amplitude of sound in dB; the reference level of dB is arbitrary (Suga, 1969a).

C: Thresholds of a symmetrical neuron for noise bursts in comparison with those for pure and FM tone bursts. The uppermost dotted line shows the frequency-response curve of the condenser loudspeaker. The area above a tuning curve (open circles) is the excitatory area of the neuron. The arrow shows the direction and range of frequency sweep of a 4 msec FM sound. The threshold of the neuron for it is represented by the vertical position of the solid arrow. Thus, the double-headed arrow in C means that the neuron showed the same threshold (about 30 dB SPL) to FM sounds sweeping either upward or downward between 30 and 60 kHz. If a neuron did not respond to an FM sound at any amplitude, it is shown by a dashed arrow on the frequency-response curve of the loudspeaker. If a neuron showed an upper-threshold for an FM sound, the upper-threshold is shown by a dotted arrow. The bars represent the frequency bands of 4 msec noise bursts. The threshold of the neuron for the noise burst is represented by the vertical position of the solid bar. If the neuron did not respond to a noise burst at any amplitude, it is shown by a dashed bar on the frequency-response curve of the loudspeaker. If a neuron showed an "upper-threshold", it is represented by a dotted bar. The abscissa and ordinate respectively represent the frequency of sound in kHz and stimulus amplitude at threshold in dB referred to 0.0002 dyne/cm^2 r.m.s. (Suga, 1969a).

was 0.5 msec in order to minimize transients at the onset and cessation of the tone pulse, the amplitude of the FM signal to the loudspeaker was not uniform. The relation between frequency modulation and intensity is schematically shown in Fig. 2 A. In this figure, the frequency of an electric signal with an envelope shown in "a" is modulated by a linearly rising voltage indicated by "b". The modulation starts and ends when the amplitude of the signal is between 20 and 30 dB below the plateau. Therefore, the intensity of this signal changes with frequency sweep as shown by a curve in Fig. 2, A c. The tone pulse produced by this electric signal is called an FM sound sweeping from 40 to 80 kHz. The frequency in pure tones and FM sounds was always measured with electronic counters.

In order to deliver a noise burst with a sharply defined band in addition to pure or FM tone pulses, noise from a random noise generator was passed through a low pass filter at 5 kHz (18 dB/octave) and was applied to one input of a ring modulator. The second input of the modulator was supplied from a sine wave oscillator. The output of the modulator contained only sum and difference frequencies of the input signals. Therefore, the bandwidth of the noise was 10 kHz. The intensity of noise was always -18 dB at 5 kHz from the edge of the band. The center frequency of this noise was the same as that of the sine waves from the oscillator (Fig. 2, B). Harmonics from the modulator were eliminated with a low pass filter. The noise was then put into an electronic switch in order to shape a burst. The duration of the noise burst was 4 msec unless otherwise stated. The rise-decay time control of the electronic switch was set at 0.5 msec.

One of the above electric signals from the electronic switch was amplified by a 40 dB amplifier and a power amplifier after passing through a decade attenuator. Finally, the signal drove a solid-dielectric condenser loudspeaker with a 300 V bias potential, through a 40 dB power attenuator which was used in order to improve the signal-to-noise ratio when the sound was attenuated more than 40 dB. Thus the stimulus intensity was controlled by both the decade attenuator and the power attenuator.

The stimulating system consisted of two identical sets of such instruments as described above, so that two tone pulses which were independently controlled in frequency, intensity, duration, and rise-decay time could be delivered simultaneously or successively. The time separating two tone pulses was controlled by a Grass Co. stimulator. The repetition rate of a stimulus (or paired stimuli) was 1.5 per second which was low enough to minimize any aftereffect, i.e., an influence of a preceding stimulus. Two loudspeakers, one above the other, were placed 92.5 ± 0.2 cm from the bat's ears. The sound intensity at the bat's ears was determined with a Brüel and Kjaer calibrated condenser microphone 4135. All sound intensities in this article are expressed in dB SPL (sound pressure level referred to 0.0002 dyne/cm^2 r.m.s.). Some of the sounds delivered at available maximum intensity were analyzed by either a Kay Electric Co. sonograph or a Tektronix spectrum analyzer. In order to analyze sounds with the sonograph, they were recorded with a tape-recorder at a tape speed of 60 inches per second and were played back at 3 3/4 or 1 7/8 inches per second. In pure tones and FM sounds, acoustic transients at their onset and cessation were not noticeable in their waveforms displayed on a CRO screen and their sonograms. When pure tones and FM sounds were mixed in air, combination tones appeared in the sonogram, although these were very faint. The intensity within the FM sound was not uniform but varied with frequency even at a constant input voltage to the loudspeaker because of the frequency-response curve of the loudspeaker. Therefore, the intensity of the FM tone pulse had to be expressed as attenuation below the maximum intensity available from the loudspeaker, i.e., by a line parallel to the frequency-response curve (see Fig. 2, C). The amplitude spectra of 4 noise bursts with a 10 kHz bandwidth are shown in Fig. 2, B. The dip at the center of each amplitude spectrum was due to the frequency characteristics of a transformer in the ring modulator.

Responses of a single neuron to acoustic stimuli can be either excitation or inhibition, so that a response area can be either an excitatory or an inhibitory response area. In this paper, the excitatory response area is called "the excitatory area", and inhibitory response area, "the inhibitory area". When the response consists of a combination of excitation and inhibition, e.g., excitation followed by inhibition as in phasic on-response, the area for this type of response is also called the excitatory area. On the other hand, the area for off-response following inhibition is called the inhibitory area. When a neuron shows no spontaneous discharges, the inhibitory area is not measurable unless two sounds are delivered successively or simultaneously.

A threshold for excitation was defined as the lowest intensity of a sound which evoked 0.1-0.2 impulses per stimulus on the average, while a threshold for inhibition, as that reducing an average rate of impulse discharges higher than 0.5 per stimulus to less than 0.1 impulse per stimulus.

3. Results and Discussion

3.1 Differences in basic properties between peripheral and central auditory neurons

3.1.1 Peripheral auditory neurons

When a microelectrode was inserted into the cochlear nucleus from the dorsal side after aspiration of the cerebellum, single unit activity was recorded from the cochlear nucleus and then from the auditory nerve in the internal auditory meatus. It was, however, not decisive whether the activity was recorded from the nerve or the nucleus without histological studies after depositing some ions or dyes at the tip of the microelectrode.

Auditory nerve fibers and cochlear nuclear neurons usually showed tonic on-responses to tonal stimuli (Suga, 1964a, b, 1965a). Post-stimulus-time (PST) histograms always showed a peak at the beginning of the response and a gradual decay toward a plateau. Post-excitatory inhibition, following the tonic on-response was always observed when the neurons were spontaneously active (Fig. 3, A a). These tonic neurons responded to tonal stimuli regardless of any amplitude modulation, because of slow accommodation and adaptation. Unlike auditory nerve fibers, cochlear nuclear neurons appear to show some variety in response pattern. Eight percent of neurons studied showed not only excitatory responses, but also inhibitory responses to tonal stimuli. The inhibitory response was often followed by post-inhibitory rebound (Fig. 3, A b). The boundary between the excitatory and inhibitory areas was so sharp that the response pattern drastically changed from excitation to inhibition with a minor shift in frequency (Fig. 4, B). In thirteen percent of neurons studied, prominent after-discharges were observed when the sound pressure level was high (Suga, 1964a). When two pure tones

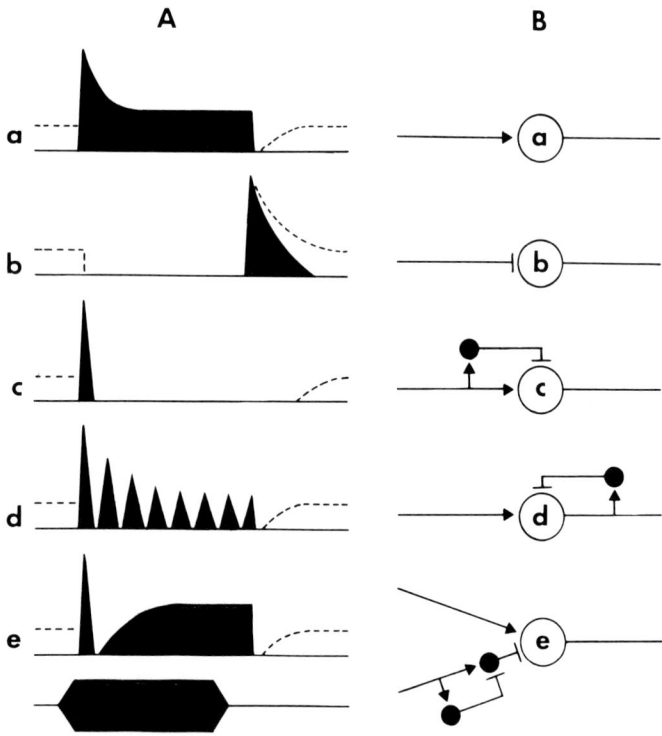

Fig. 3 Various types of response patterns of higher-order auditory neurons expressed by schematized PST histograms (filled areas in A) and the simplest neural networks producing these response patterns (B). When neurons show background activity, the PST histograms of their responses are the shaded areas plus the areas below the dashed lines. The envelope of a sound stimulus is shown on the bottom of A.

Aa: Tonic on-responses similar to the response pattern of a primary auditory neuron. Excitatory transmission as shown in Ba causes this response pattern. Ab: Off-response which is caused by inhibitory transmission as shown in Bb. Ac: Phasic on-response followed by an inhibitory period. This response pattern is produced by forward self-inhibition as shown by Bc or forward lateral inhibition. Ad: "Serrate on-response" which may be ex- (cont'd)

(Fig. 3, cont'd) plained by backward self-inhibition as shown by Bd or backward lateral inhibition. Ae: "Paused on-response". This response pattern is produced by two lower order neurons converging upon this neuron. One of them sends tonic excitatory bombardments the other sends phasic inhibitory bombardments through an inhibitory interneuron. In B, nerve fibers coming from the left side are assumed to be the axons of primary or primary-like auditory neurons. The arrow-head means an excitatory synapse and the "T" end, an inhibitory synapse. The postsynaptic neurons indicated by a, b, --- e show the response patterns shown in a, b, --- e in A, respectively.

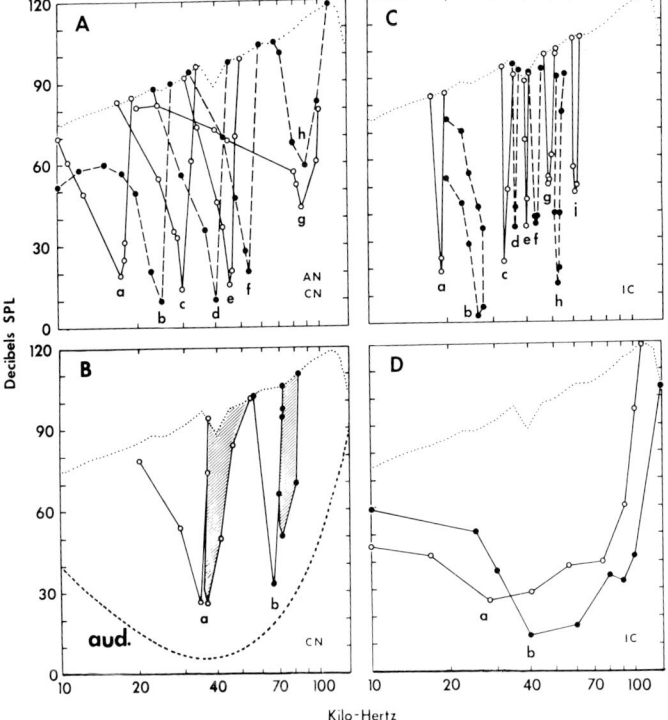

Fig. 4 A: Excitatory areas of eight neurons recorded from the auditory nerve and cochlear nucleus. Curve "aud" in B is the audiogram which is determined by the excitatory areas of (cont'd)

(Fig. 4, cont'd) the most sensitive of the 229 single neurons recorded at both the cochlear nucleus and inferior colliculus.

B: Excitatory (unshaded) and inhibitory (shaded) areas of two cochlear nuclear neurons, a and b. Sounds in the shaded areas inhibited background activity of these neurons.

C: Narrow excitatory areas of nine neurons in the inferior colliculus.

D: Broad excitatory areas of two neurons in the inferior colliculus. The uppermost dotted line shows the maximum available sound amplitude, i.e., the frequency-response curve of the loudspeaker. The ordinates and abscissas represent stimulus amplitude at threshold in dB SPL and frequency in kHz, respectively (Suga, 1964a, b, 1965a, and unpublished data).

were simultaneously delivered, most neurons studied showed "two-tone inhibition" (Frishkopf, 1964, Suga, 1965a, unpublished data).

The sharpness of a tuning curve of a single neuron has been expressed by a Q-value which is a best frequency divided by its bandwidth at 10 dB above a minimum threshold (Kiang, 1965). Q-values for excitatory areas of 256 single neurons in the cochlear nerve and nucleus ranged between 1.41 (BF = 30.4 kHz) and 21.6 (BF = 54.0 kHz). Seventy percent of them were between 4 and 12, and 16 percent were less than 4 (Fig. 5, A). The slope of a tuning curve of a primary auditory neuron was 300 dB/octave at frequencies higher than a best frequency and 100 dB/octave at frequencies lower than that (Fig. 4, A, Frishkopf, 1964). Auditory nerve fibers and cochlear nuclear neurons responded not only to pure tones, but also to FM sounds and noise bursts whenever a part of the sound energy fell into their excitatory area. The response pattern to FM sounds might slightly differ depending on directions of frequency sweep, but it was very rare to find a neuron which showed a difference of more than 10 dB in threshold due to direction of frequency sweep (Suga, 1965a). These neurons were thus not specialized for the analysis of one of the three types of information-bearing elements, and they were

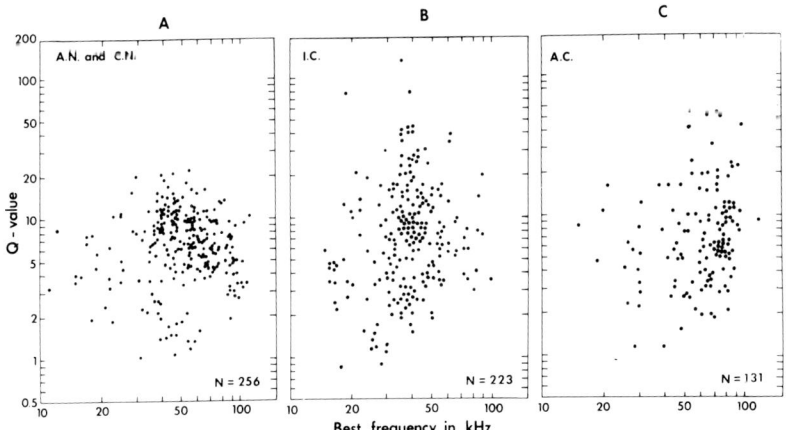

Fig. 5 Distributions of Q-values of single neurons in the auditory nerve plus cochlear nucleus (A), inferior colliculus (B), and auditory cortex (C). The ordinates and abscissas represent Q-values and best frequencies in kHz, respectively. The total number of neurons studied is 256 for graph A, 223 for graph B, and 131 for graph C.

naturally not specialized for responding only to a particular complex sound. In the animals which have to analyze acoustic signals from various aspects, such as target-ranging, echo-localization, target analysis, and communication, it is essential not to have specialized neurons in the cochlear nucleus. If the cochlear nucleus consisted of specialized neurons, information which is not extracted by the specialized neurons would be lost.

In cats, all auditory nerve fibers studied have shown tonic on-responses to acoustic stimuli. The PST histogram is characterized by a sharp peak at the beginning followed by a gradual decay until a plateau is reached. Q-values of these excitatory areas increase with best frequencies, from 0.9-5 at 0.5 kHz to 5-24 at 10 kHz. The scatter in Q-values is large at high best frequencies (Kiang, 1965). One might expect that Q-values of bats' auditory neurons were very large because of their high best frequencies. This is, however, not true in the bats of the genus Myotis (Fig. 5, A). Primary auditory neurons of cats and monkeys show inhibitory responses to simultaneous two-tone stimuli (Nomoto et al., 1964, Sachs and Kiang, 1968, Arthur et al., 1971). Neurons in the cochlear nucleus show various types of response patterns, but the predominant response pattern is a tonic on-response (Pfeiffer, 1966). Q-values of cochlear nuclear neurons show a tendency to be smaller than those of auditory nerve fibers (e.g., Møller, 1972). The cochlear nucleus appears to contain no neurons specialized for exclusively responding to one of the three types of information-bearing elements (Møller, 1969, in rats; Watanabe and Ohgushi, 1968, in cats).

3.1.2 Central auditory neurons

In echolocating bats, the auditory nuclei in the medulla and midbrain are enormously hypertrophied, but this is not true of either the medial geniculate body or the auditory cortex (Poljak, 1926). The severe bilateral ablation of the inferior colliculus (I.C.) causes the failure in echolocation, while the severe unilateral ablation of the I.C. and/or the bilateral ablation of the auditory cortex (A.C.) do not decrease the ability to echolocate fine wires. That is, the comparison of the activities in both lateral lemnisci (L.L.s) and/or I.C.s at the auditory nuclei or centers higher than the L.L. is dispensable for processing the information essential for the avoidance of fine wires. The analysis of echoes in the I.C. on one side seems sufficient (Suga, 1969b, c). These facts indicate that most information processing for echolocation is performed in (or before) the I.C. Thus, extensive effort has been devoted for the exploration of properties of I.C. neurons, and neurons specialized for responding to one of the three types of information-bearing elements have been found (Grinnell and McCue, 1963, Suga, 1964b, 1965a, 1968, 1969a). The properties of A.C. neurons have also been studied, and it has been found that the A.C. contains specialized neurons at a percentage higher than that of such neurons in the I.C. (Suga, 1965b, c).

In the I.C. and A.C., single neurons showed various types of response patterns to tonal stimuli as shown in Fig. 3, A: primary-like tonic on-response (a), off-response (b), phasic on-response (c), serrate on-response (d), and paused on-response (e). The predominant type was phasic on-response. The off-response and serrate on-response were rare. Not every neuron was necessarily characterized by one of the above response patterns. Some neurons varied in response pattern with frequency and intensity of a tonal stimulus, because the response pattern resulted from the interaction between excitatory and inhibitory neurons, each of which had a particular tuning curve (Suga, 1965c, 1969a). Furthermore, it has been found that response patterns of some neurons changed with the rate of intensity increase (Suga, 1971). The various types of response patterns were mainly due to the excitatory and inhibitory interaction. Thus, detailed studies of response patterns greatly help to explore a neural network in which a given neuron is involved. In Fig. 3 B, the basic neural network models are shown which could produce various types of response patterns different from those of primary (or primary-like) auditory neurons.

Unlike neurons in the cochlear nucleus, higher order neurons showed various shapes of excitatory areas (Figs. 4, 6, 7, and 8). In the I.C., Q-values for excitatory areas of 223 neurons ranged between 0.90 (BF = 28.2 kHz) and 122 (BF = 36.6 kHz). Twenty-six percent of them were less than 4, and 29 percent were larger than 12 (Fig. 5 B). Apparently, some I.C. neurons had a very broad excitatory area, while some others had a very narrow one (Fig. 4 C and D). The sharpest slope of a tuning curve measured was more than 2,000 dB/octave (Figs. 4 C and 6). The shapes of the tuning curves in Fig. 4 C and D are clearly different from those in Fig. 4 A. The distribution of Q-values in Fig. 5, however, does not necessarily give us such an impression. The bandwidth at 30 dB above minimum threshold appears better than the Q-value for showing a change in tuning curve. In the auditory cortex, neurons with either a very narrow or broad excitatory area have been found (Suga, 1965c).

The narrow excitatory area did not indicate that only the narrow frequency band of sound influenced the activities of neurons with such an area, because they usually had inhibitory areas also. If Q-values of these neurons were measured by including both the areas, the values would become smaller. Their responses to excitatory tones were modified by the stimulation of their inhibitory areas, so that these neurons were not a simple band-pass filter. As described below, the measurement of both the excitatory

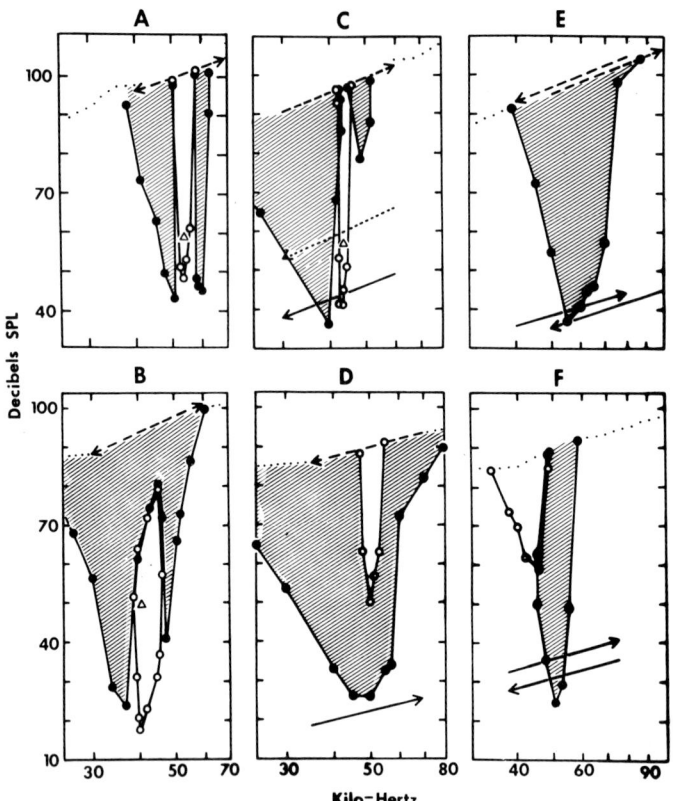

Fig. 6 Excitatory (unshaded) and inhibitory (shaded) areas and thresholds for FM sounds of six I.C. neurons. The ordinates and abscissas respectively represent a stimulus amplitude at threshold in dB SPL and frequency of acoustic stimulus in kHz. A: CF (or pure tone)-specialized neuron, B: Upper-threshold neuron, C: Asymmetrical neuron, D-F: FM-specialized neurons. The symbols are the same as those in Fig. 2 C (Suga, 1965a, 1968, 1969a).

and inhibitory areas was essential to explore neural mechanisms underlying responses of neurons to information-bearing elements. The inhibitory area was easily measured by delivering a single pure tone when a neuron was spontaneously active. When a neuron was spontaneously inactive, a short pure tone was delivered immediately before an excitatory sound in order to measure the inhibitory area, in which the response to the excitatory sound was inhibited by the preceding tone burst. In the T.C. and A.C., most neurons were spontaneously inactive or active at a very low level, so that the inhibitory areas described below were measured with a pair of tone bursts. Unlike peripheral auditory neurons, I.C. and A.C. neurons usually showed no off-response as a rebound from inhibition (Suga, 1965a, b, c, 1968, 1969a).

Unlike the peripheral neurons, more than half of the I.C. and A.C. neurons showed a non-monotonic impulse-count function, which resulted mostly from the interaction between excitation and inhibition. In extreme cases of the non-monotonic function, neurons failed to respond to strong sound. Quantitative studies of impulse-count function, thus, contribute to exploration of not only how stimulus intensity is coded or decoded, but also how excitatory and inhibitory neurons interact to produce a particular type of property of a single neuron.

In cats, various types of response patterns in higher levels are also found, but a phasic on-response appears dominant (Katsuki et al., 1959a, Rose et al., 1963). With ascent from the cochlear nucleus to the I.C. and medial geniculate body, some single neurons show a progressively narrow excitatory area (Katsuki et al., 1958, 1959a), while some others show a wide excitatory area (Rose et al., 1963). Since a broad spectrum in shapes of excitatory areas is found at higher levels of the auditory system of the bats and cats, it is quite reasonable to interpret that both narrowing and widening of excitatory areas occur in the auditory system (Crulkar, 1959, Suga, 1965c).

3.2 Neurons specialized for responding to a particular type of information-bearing element

3.2.1 CF (or pure tone)-specialized neurons

CF-specialized neurons had a very narrow excitatory area sandwiched between large inhibitory areas (Figs. 6 A, 7 C, and 13). The threshold always increased by 60-80 dB for less than 8 % change in frequency of a sound at their best frequencies. In the narrowest excitatory area, a Q-value of 122 was measured. The width of the area was only 5.5 % of the best fre-

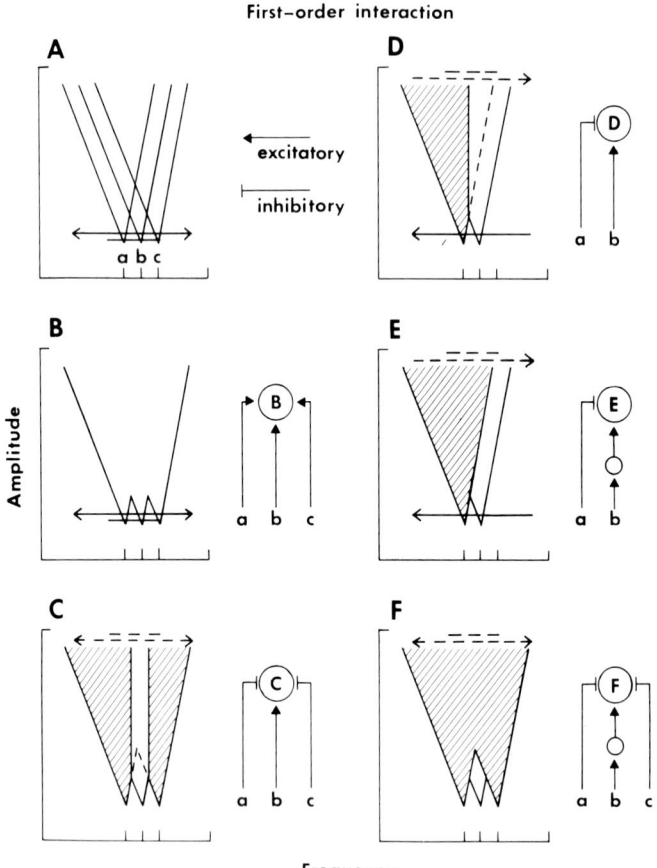

Fig. 7   First-order interactions illustrating fundamental properties of several types of neurons. For simplicity, postsynaptic interactions between two or three primary or primary-like auditory neurons are considered which have different excitatory areas (a, b, and c in A). These neurons respond not only to pure tones, but also to FM sounds and noise bursts, as indicated by a double headed solid arrow and a solid bar, respectively. B: A symmetrical neuron resulting from convergence of excitatory bombardments. C: A CF-specialized neuron resulting from the lateral inhibition mediated by two neurons "a" and   (cont'd)

(Fig. 7, cont'd) "c". D: An asymmetrical neuron resulting from the lateral inhibition mediated by neuron "a". E: An asymmetrical neuron showing upper-thresholds for pure tones. Neuron "a" mediates a lateral inhibition as in D, but its inhibitory bombardment arrives at neuron "E" earlier than an excitatory one does, because excitatory channel "b" has an excitatory interneuron, i.e., delay circuit. F: An upper-threshold neuron. Neurons "a" and "c" mediate the lateral inhibition as in C, but their inhibitory bombardments arrive at neuron "F" earlier than excitatory ones do, because excitatory channel "b" has a delay circuit. The ordinates and abscissas represent stimulus amplitude at threshold and frequency, respectively. Symbols are the same as those in Fig. 2 C. The properties of various types of neurons schematically presented in this figure are based on those described in the previous papers (Suga, 1965a, b, c, 1968, 1969a, Suga and Schlegel, 1973).

quency at 36.6 kHz even at 60 dB above the minimum threshold. The sensitivity of the neuron thus increased at a rate of 2000 dB/octave to the best frequency and decreased at a rate of 1120 dB/octave beyond it. These neurons usually showed a very phasic on-response to tonal stimuli because of inhibition immediately following very rapid excitation.

The CF-specialized neurons did not respond to FM sounds which swept one octave across the excitatory area, because they always stimulated the inhibitory area prior to the excitatory one. These neurons also failed to respond to noise bursts with a 10 kHz bandwidth which simultaneously stimulated both the excitatory and inhibitory areas. Thus, they are called CF-specialized neurons (Suga, 1965a, c, 1969a, Suga and Schlegel, 1973). The properties of this type of neuron are explained by lateral inhibition mediated by two inhibitory neurons with a best frequency either slightly higher or lower than that of an excitatory neuron (Fig. 7, C).

In the neural network models in Figs. 7-9, it is assumed that a neuron is not excited unless EPSP occurs earlier than IPSP and that latencies of both excitatory and inhibitory bombardments monotonically vary with stimulus intensity. At a certain frequency and intensity of a sound stimulus, excitatory and inhibitory bombardments may arrive at a given neuron without any time difference when there is no difference in threshold between excitatory and inhibitory neurons, while an excitatory bombardment may arrive at the neuron later (or earlier) than an inhibitory one when the threshold of an excitatory neuron is higher (or lower) than that of an inhibitory one.

When lateral inhibition occurs on both sides of the excitatory area and an excitatory bombardment delays an inhibitory one, the excitatory area may become a closed area (Figs. 6 B and 7 F). The neuron with such an area is called "upper-threshold unit". The upper-threshold neurons usually showed phasic on-responses to tonal stimuli and they failed to respond to FM sounds and noise bursts, so that they may also be called CF-specialized units. For the excitation of upper-threshold neurons, a stimulus should have a certain frequency and a certain weak intensity. When the stimulus has a strong intensity, it should have a very small rate of intensity increase. The properties of the upper-threshold neurons are also discussed later.

Behavioral and neurophysiological data indicating that the animals use neurons with very narrow excitatory areas for fine frequency discrimination have been obtained in the greater horseshoe bat (Rhinolophus ferrumequinum) and the mustache bat (Chilonycteris p. parnellii and C. rubiginosa). Each of their orientation sounds consists of CF and FM components. The CF component in a predominant harmonic is about 83 kHz in R.f., about 62 kHz in C.p.p. and about 57 kHz in C.r. The threshold curves of their cochlear microphonics and/or neural activities indicate that their auditory system is sharply tuned to the frequencies of the CF components (Grinnell, 1970, Neuweiler, 1970, Airapetianz and Vasilyev, 1971, Pollak et al., 1972). A Q-value is about 25 for R.f. (Neuwiler, 1970) and about 315 for C.p.p. (Pollak et al., 1972). When these bats echolocate a target moving relative to them, echo frequency is shifted by Doppler effect. They then adjust the frequency of the CF component in the orientation sound in order to receive echoes at a preferred frequency 83 kHz in R.f. and 57 kHz in C.r., to which their auditory system is most sharply tuned. When a pendulum is alternately moved toward and away from the greater horseshoe bat hanging down from a perch, the frequency of the CF component of the emitted sound alternately decreases and increases in order to keep echo frequency constant at the preferred frequency (Schnitzler, 1968, 1970, Simmons, 1973b). Under a certain circumstance, Chilonycteris rubiginosa shows a vocal response to an acoustic stimulus. This response is very sharply tuned at a preferred frequency, 62 kHz. A Q-value of the tuning curve of this response is 52. The slope of the tuning curve is about 1,300 and 1,200 dB/octave on both sides of the best frequency (Suga et al., in preparation). Since single neurons do not show any phase-locked responses to such a high frequency pure tone, the above vocal response is undoubtedly mediated by very sharply tuned neurons. This behavioral tuning curve is only slightly wider than the sharpest tuning curve of a single neuron obtained in M.lucifugus (Q-value, 122), so that it appears to be filled by tuning curves of a group of neurons with nearly one and the same best frequency. It is very interesting that the animal utilizes activities of certain auditory neurons and ignores those of almost all neurons tuned to other frequencies.

In cats, the shape of an excitatory area has been systematically studied from the cochlear nerve to the auditory cortex by Katsuki and his co-workers. They have found progressive sharpening of the excitatory area with ascent from the cochlear nucleus to the inferior colliculus and medial geniculate body (Katsuki et al., 1958, 1959a). This sharpening of the area is performed by lateral inhibition (Katsuki et al., 1959b). If they measured inhibitory areas, they probably would have found a narrow excitatory area sandwiched between inhibitory areas. CF-specialized neurons also appear to be in the cat's auditory system.

Upper-threshold neurons have been found in frogs (Potter, 1965) and cats (Greenwood and Maruyama, 1965). If frequency and intensity of a tonal stimulus with an abrupt on-set or a short rise time are changed while searching for single auditory neurons at higher levels, the probability of finding upper-threshold neurons would increase (Suga, 1971).

3.2.2 Asymmetrical and paradoxically asymmetrical neurons[1]

In terms of responses to FM sounds, there were two types of interesting neurons in addition to FM-specialized ones: asymmetrical and paradoxically asymmetrical neurons. Asymmetrical neurons in Figs. 6 C, 7 D, and 7 E, for example, had a narrow excitatory area bounded by a large inhibitory area. Another inhibitory area was often found on the other side of the excitatory area, but it was smaller and the inhibitory effect was usually weak. The stimulation of the inhibitory area caused only inhibition of responses to excitatory stimuli or background activity, if any. Off-responses were usually not evoked as a rebound from the inhibition. When the frequency of an FM sound swept one octave from high frequency to low across the excitatory area, the neurons responded. When the frequency swept in the opposite direction, however, the neurons failed to respond to it, regardless of stimulus intensity. This asymmetry of response was caused by the presence of a large inhibitory area along one side of the excitatory area. That is, the downward-sweeping FM sound first stimulated the excitatory area and then the inhibitory area, so the asymmetrical neurons responded to it, while the upward-sweeping FM sound stimulated the inhibitory area first, so they could not respond to it. This type of neuron is thus called an asymmetrical unit. It should be noted that there were asymmetrical neurons which were sensitive to upward-sweeping FM sounds, but not to downward-sweeping ones. These neurons had an inhibitory area at frequencies higher than their best frequencies (Suga, 1965a, c, 1968).

The properties of asymmetrical neurons are explained by a lateral inhibition mediated by a neuron with a best frequency which is slightly different from that of an excitatory neuron (Fig. 7, D and E). In Fig. 7, neuron "E" shows upper-threshold for sounds in a certain frequency range, unlike neuron "D". The upper-threshold is also a result of a lateral inhibition. When an excitatory bombardment delays an inhibitory

---

[1] Although these two types of neurons belong to the category called generalized units, they are introduced here because the description about their properties takes a role as an introduction for that about FM-specialized neurons.

one, the excitatory area may be completely deleted at the portion where the excitatory area overlaps the inhibitory area. In the neural network model of Fig. 7 E, the delay of the excitatory bombardment is introduced by inserting an excitatory interneuron into the excitatory channel.

There were asymmetrical neurons which responded to FM sounds sweeping across an inhibitory area prior to an excitatory area but not to FM sounds sweeping in the opposite direction (Fig. 8, D). Since the properties of these neurons are not explained by the sequence in which the excitatory and inhibitory areas are stimulated by FM sounds, this type of neuron may be called a paradoxically asymmetrical unit. The basic properties of CF-specialized, asymmetrical and upper-threshold neurons are explained by interaction among primary or primary-like auditory neurons, i.e., by the "first-order interaction", while those of the paradoxically asymmetrical neuron cannot be interpreted by the first-order interaction. One has to consider the "second-order interaction", e.g., an interaction between asymmetrical and primary-like auditory neurons. In Fig. 8, asymmetrical neuron "A" is an inhibitory neuron, and primary-like neuron "B" is an excitatory one (graphs A and B). The excitatory channel has a delay circuit. Neuron "D" receives impulses from these two types of neurons which have best frequencies slightly different from each other. Then, the properties of neuron "D" become paradoxically asymmetrical. When one finds a neuron which responds to FM sounds sweeping from an inhibitory area to an excitatory one or sweeping across the inhibitory area alone, one may consider that its properties are produced by the second or higher order interaction. The asymmetrical and paradoxically asymmetrical neurons can detect the direction of frequency sweep, but their ability to do so is very poor because they also respond to pure tones and noise bursts.

In cats, responses of single neurons to FM sounds had been studied by Nelson et al. (1966), Watanabe and Ohgushi (1968), and Whitfield and Evans (1965). Their experiments indicate that the cat's auditory system contains asymmetrical neurons at the levels above the superior olivary complex. Whitfield and Evans (1965) have found that some phasic cortical auditory neurons

Second-order interaction

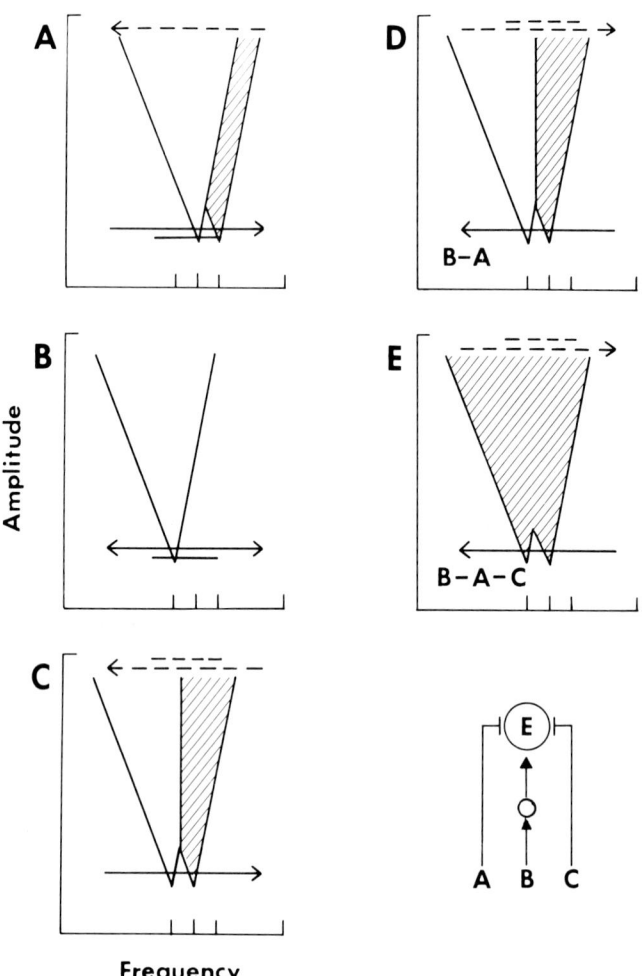

Fig. 8 Second-order interactions illustrating fundamental properties of paradoxically asymmetrical (D) and FM-specialized (E) neurons. In this neural network model both inhibitory neurons "A" and "C" are asymmetrical, while excitatory neuron "B" is symmetrical. Their best frequencies are slightly different from each other as shown in graphs A, (cont'd)

(Fig. 8, cont'd) B, and C. When neurons "A" and "B" interact, paradoxically asymmetrical neuron "D" results (graph D). When neurons "A", "B", and "C" interact, FM-specialized neuron "E" results (graph E). Symbols are the same as those in Fig. 2 C. (See text.)

with an excitatory area responded directionally to FM continuous sounds in which frequency was modulated either sinusoidally or stepwise within the area. In bats, some I.C. or A.C. neurons had a very broad excitatory area (Fig. 4, D). When FM tone bursts sweeping either upward or downward within their excitatory areas were delivered at a low repetition rate, they responded regardless of sweep directions. Since FM signals used as stimuli are different between the experiments with bats and cats, and since response parameters mainly analyzed were also different between these two experiments, it is not yet clear whether there is some difference in properties of asymmetrical neurons between bats and cats. According to my experiments with cats, the auditory cortex contained asymmetrical neurons similar to those of the bats. A few phasic on-responding neurons with a relatively wide excitatory area showed a directionality to FM continuous sounds sweeping within the area, as reported by Whitfield and Evans (1965), but they showed no directionality for 40 msec FM tone bursts sweeping either upward or downward in the same range as swept by the FM continuous sounds (Suga, unpublished data). In order to explore neural mechanisms for the directionality to FM continuous sounds, the recovery cycle of such a neuron should probably be measured as a function of frequency of a pure tone pulse. Paradoxically asymmetrical neurons also appear to be in the cat's auditory system, because some neurons in the I.C. and A.C. responded to FM sounds sweeping just outside their excitatory areas (Nelson et al., 1966, Whitfield and Evans, 1965).

3.2.3 FM-specialized neurons

In the inferior colliculus, about 2 % of the neurons studied responded primarily or exclusively to FM sounds (Fig. 6, D-F; Suga, 1965a, 1968, 1969a). This type of neuron, called the FM-specialized (or -sensitive) unit, comprised not more than 14 % of the neurons studied in the auditory cortex (Suga, 1965c). The neuron in Fig. 8 E, for example, has no excitatory area for CF tones, but it responds to downward-sweeping FM sounds. These neurons do not respond at all to upward-sweeping FM sounds, regardless of stimulus amplitudes. The neuron in Fig. 9 B c, on the other hand, has a tiny excitatory area and responds to FM sounds sweeping the outside of the area. Since

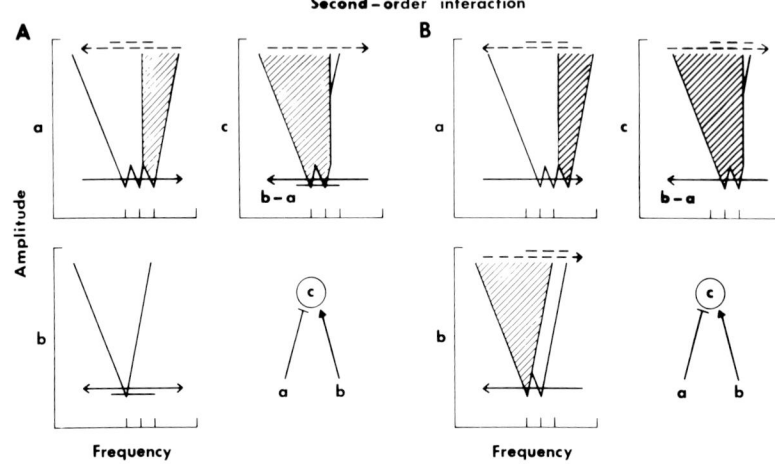

Fig. 9 Second-order interactions illustrating fundamental properties of CF-deaf (Ac) and FM-specialized neurons (Bc). Inhibitory neuron "a" is asymmetrical in both A and B (graph Aa and Ba). Excitatory neuron "b" is symmetrical in A (graph Ab), but it is asymmetrical and shows upper-threshold in B (graph Bb). When these neurons "a" and "b" postsynaptically interact, neuron "c" has CF-deaf properties in A and FM-specialized properties in B. Symbols are the same as those in Fig. 2 C. (See text.)

FM-specialized neurons were not sensitive to noise bursts, they did not respond to a scatter of sound energy which might occur with a rapid frequency sweep, but did respond to the frequency sweep itself. For the excitation of FM-specialized neurons, either direction, range, speed, or functional form of frequency sweep was an important factor (Figs. 10 and 11). Since some FM-specialized neurons showed the best response to FM sounds similar to orientation sounds, the bats obviously have neurons specialized for the

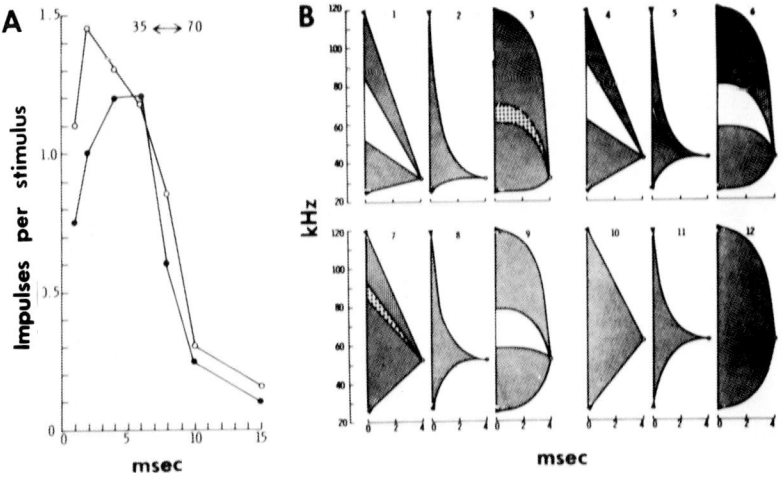

Fig. 10 Responses of FM-specialized neurons to FM sounds sweeping at different rates (A) and functional forms (B).

A: FM sounds of 80 dB SPL always swept over an octave during a specific time period (i.e. the duration of the stimulus), as shown by the abscissa. The ordinate represents the average number of impulses per stimulus. The open circle shows the number of impulses in the response to an upward sweeping FM sound, and the filled circle represents that to a downward sweeping FM sound. The range of frequency sweep is from 35 to 70 kHz. This neuron responded to both upward and downward sweeping FM sounds.

B: The ordinates and abscissas represent frequency in kHz and time in msec, respectively. First, a 4 msec pure tone of 80 dB SPL was delivered (32 kHz in 1-3, 42 kHz in 4-6, 52 kHz in 7-9, and 62 kHz in 10-12). It was then frequency-modulated in different functional forms. The final frequency was kept constant, while the initial frequency of FM was changed in order to measure the range within which responses were obtained. Densely dotted sectors indicate areas within which FM sounds did not excite (cont'd)

(Fig. 10, cont'd) the neuron. FM sounds within the lightly dotted sectors excited the neuron, but the number of impulses per stimulus was slightly lower than that at the threshold. The functional form of frequency sweep is linear in 1, 4, 7 and 10, terminal-frequency-dominantly exponential in 2, 5, 8, and 11, and initial-frequency-dominantly exponential in 3, 6, 9, and 12. This neuron responded only to downward sweeping FM sounds (Suga, 1968).

reception of their species-specific orientation sound. In the bat's brain, there were not only downward-sensitive FM-specialized neurons (Fig. 11 A), but also upward-sensitive ones (Fig. 6, D). Some FM-specialized neurons responded to both upward and downward-sweeping FM sounds(Fig. 6, F). Some others changed their preferred sweep direction with a range of frequency sweep (Fig. 6, E). Properties of FM-specialized neurons studied were not necessarily identical (Suga, 1965a, b, c, 1968, 1969a).

Why do FM-specialized neurons selectively respond to FM sounds in spite of the absence of an excitatory area? The lack of response of the FM-specialized neurons to a pure tone stimulus does not indicate a complete lack of reaction. When a short pure tone pulse was delivered prior to an FM sound excitatory to them, the response to the FM sound was inhibited. By changing the frequency and amplitude of the pure tone, it was possible to measure the area in which the response to the FM sound was inhibited. As shown in Figs. 6 D-F, 8 E, and 9 B c, the FM-specialized neurons always had a large inhibitory area and responded to an FM sound sweeping across this area. In other words, stimulation of the inhibitory area excited the neuron. Although seemingly paradoxical, this result can be explained by the second order interaction, a neural network model similar to that for a paradoxically asymmetrical neuron.

In Fig. 8, primary-like neuron "B" with a delay circuit is excitatory, and asymmetrical neurons "A" and "C" are inhibitory for neuron "E". Then, neuron "E" has an inhibitory area which has the same shape as the excitatory areas of the inhibitory neurons. Since both inhibitory neurons "A" and "C" are sensitive to upward-sweeping FM sounds, but not to downward-sweeping ones, neuron "E" can respond only to downward-sweeping FM sounds. This neural network model predicts that upward-sweeping FM sounds are inhibitory for this FM-specialized neuron. This was found to be true. When an upward-sweeping FM sound was delivered prior to a downward-sweeping FM, the response to the latter was inhibited. In Fig. 9 B, the properties of the FM-specialized neuron are explained by an interaction between two asymmetrical neurons "a" and "b" which are sensitive either to upward or downward-sweeping FM sounds. If neurons "a" and "b" are respectively inhibitory and excitatory, neuron "c" may become downward sensitive as shown in Fig. 9 B.

The neural networks consisting of neurons "a" and "b" which have different properties from those in Fig. 9, also produce properties of FM-specialized neurons which are sensitive only to upward-sweeping FM sounds or sensitive to FM sounds regardless of sweep direction. In these neural network models, the inhibition of the inhibitory neuron by the initial part of the FM sound is essential. The actual neural network existing between primary auditory neurons and a given FM-specialized neuron is obviously more complicated than that in the above model.

As shown by the experimental data and neural network models, no excitatory area for a pure tone indicates the presence of an inhibitory area. This indicates that the statement "a neuron shows no responses to pure tones (or one type of acoustic feature), but to FM sounds (or other type of acoustic feature)" is greatly strengthened by demonstrating that the neuron has an inhibitory area or areas for a pure tone (or that type of acoustic feature).

In the orientation sounds of the greater horseshoe bat (Rhinolophus) and the mustache bat (Chilonycteris) a short FM component follows a long CF component. It is thus very important to study whether the response of an FM-specialized neuron to the FM component is masked by a preceding CF. When a 4 msec long pure tone pulse was delivered immediately prior to a 4 msec FM sound, the response to the latter was inhibited. The frequency range of the pure tone, which caused inhibition, did not, however, include the initial frequencies of the FM sound (Fig. 11, B2). When the noise

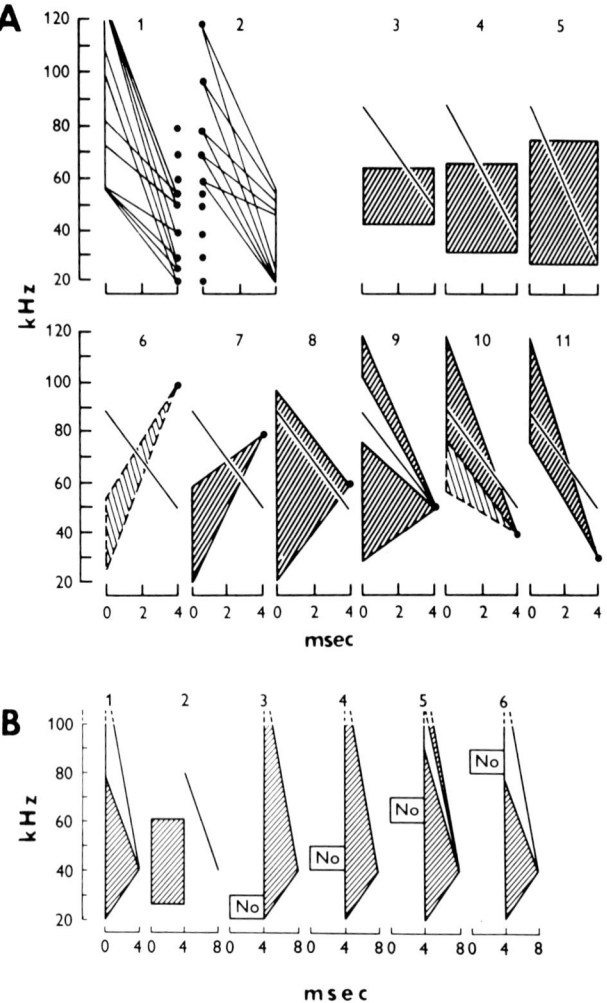

Fig. 11 A: Responses of an FM-specialized neuron to FM sounds (1-2) and inhibitory ranges measured with either pure tones (3-5) or FM sounds (6-11) for the responses to certain FM sounds delivered simultaneously. The ordinates and abscissas, respectively, represent frequency in kHz and time in msec. 1 and 2: By delivering various FM sounds in which linear frequency sweep converged on (1) or diverged from each (cont'd)

(Fig. 11, cont'd) filled circle (2), the ranges of FM sounds which excited the neuron were measured as shown by sectors. The neuron responded only to FM sounds sweeping downward. 3-5: The shaded rectangles indicate the inhibitory ranges in which tone pulse II (80 dB SPL pure tone) inhibited the response to tone pulse I (80 dB SPL FM), which is indicated by an oblique line. 6-11: Ranges of tone pulse II (80 dB SPL FM) are shown by the shaded sectors in which the sound completely (heavily shaded sectors) or incompletely (faintly shaded ones) inhibited the response to tone pulse I sweeping from 90 to 50 kHz at 80 dB SPL. The terminal frequency of tone pulse II is indicated by a filled circle (e.g., 100 kHz in 6)(Suga, 1968).

B: Responses of an FM-specialized neuron to FM sounds sweeping toward 40 kHz (1) and effect of pure tones (2) and noise bursts (3-6) on these responses. The duration and amplitude of these 3 types of sounds were all 4 msec and 80 dB SPL, respectively. The pure tones and noise bursts were delivered immediately prior to the FM sounds. The ordinate and abscissas represent the frequency in kHz and time in msec, respectively. In 1, keeping the final frequency constant, the initial frequency of the FM sound was slowly changed from 20 to 100 kHz in order to measure the range in which the neuron showed response. The open and shaded sectors show that the neuron was and was not excited by FM sounds in the sectors, respectively. In 2, the shaded area shows the range of pure tones which inhibited the response to an FM sound sweeping from 80 to 40 kHz. In 3-6, the range of FM sounds, which excited the neuron, was greatly varied by the preceding delivery of the noise bursts with a 10 kHz bandwidth (open rectangles) which did not excite the neuron (Suga, 1969a).

burst with a 10 kHz bandwidth was delivered instead of the pure tone pulse, the same result as the above was obtained (Fig. 11, B3 - B6). The response of the

FM-specialized neuron to the FM-component of the orientation sound is thus not at all masked by the preceding CF. Such properties of the FM-specialized neuron can be explained by the neural network models in Figs. 8 and 9. In these models, the initial part of an excitatory FM sound inhibits only an inhibitory neuron (or neurons), so that the response of the FM-specialized neuron to the FM component is not masked.

In FM-specialized and asymmetrical neurons, the ratio of downward-sensitive neurons to upward-sensitive ones was approximately two to one (Suga, 1965a). Our recent experiments have indicated that vocal responses of certain species of bats to acoustic stimuli are more sensitive to downward-sweeping FM sounds than to either upward-sweeping ones or pure tones (Suga et al., in preparation). Such a behavior might indicate that the animal utilizes the activity of a particular type of auditory neurons such as downward-sensitive FM-specialized neurons.

In cats, FM-specialized neurons appear to be found in the medial geniculate body (Watanabe and Ohgushi, 1968) and the auditory cortex (Galambos, 1960, Whitfield and Evans, 1965).

3.2.4 Noise-specialized neurons

In the inferior colliculus of bats, only one percent of the neurons studied were either very sensitive to noise bursts or responded only to noise bursts (Suga, 1969a). One of them showed upper-thresholds for noise bursts. When a pure tone pulse was delivered prior to a noise burst, the response to the latter was inhibited, so that these neurons had an inhibitory area.

Since a noise burst consists of many frequencies, the properties of noise-specialized units may be explained by facilitation, i.e., by assuming that neurons to be excited have to have well synchronized excitatory bombardments from more than two neurons. If one of these responds to a pure tone pulse and has a long recovery period, the pure tone pulse may suppress the response to a noise burst following it, because the synchronization of impulses which would be caused by the noise burst is disturbed by the preceding delivery of the pure tone pulse. If this is the case, the inhibitory area described above may not be a "true" inhibitory area. In an alternative explanation, one has to consider some neural network in which excitatory and inhibitory interaction occurs between various types of neurons to erase responses to pure tones and FM sounds of primary or primary-like auditory neurons and to leave only responses to noise bursts. Samples of noise-specialized neurons are too few in bats. Further studies on this type of neuron are required to explore underlying neural mechanisms.

In cats, more than 20 % of the neurons studied in the auditory cortex responded to clicks or noise bursts, but not to pure tones (Galambos, 1960, Evans and Whitfield, 1964, Goldstein et al., 1968). Some of them might not respond to FM sounds. The cat's auditory system appears to have noise-specialized neurons. Neural mechanisms for selective click (or noise burst) responses have, however, not yet been studied at all.

3.3 Neurons non-specialized in terms of responses to information-bearing elements

As described above, neurons specialized for responding to one type of the information-bearing elements were the minority of the auditory system. The majority of neurons responded to all three types of the elements. In other words, the majority would respond to various types of acoustic stimuli. They are thus called "generalized neurons". Asymmetrical neurons may be included in this category. The other major type of generalized neuron may be called "a symmetrical unit", because it has no or just a tiny inhibitory area in contrast to asymmetrical neurons and has a relatively large excitatory area. Some symmetrical neurons had such a broad excitatory area that most of the bat audiogram was covered by it (Fig. 4, D). Since such a broad area had never been found in the auditory nerve and cochlear nucleus, the properties of such symmetrical neurons were apparently produced by convergence of many excitatory neurons with different frequencies on them (Fig. 7, B). Most of the symmetrical neurons showed very phasic on-responses to all pure tones within their broad excitatory areas, so that all excitatory neurons converging upon them appeared to be involved in forward self-inhibition (Suga, 1965a, c). Since these neurons had a large excitatory area, they responded to any pure tones, FM sounds, and noise bursts whenever these sounds had energy falling within the excitatory area (Suga, 1969a).

In cats, some I.C. neurons have excitatory areas broader than those of primary auditory neurons (Erulkar, 1959, Rose et al., 1963). Some cortical auditory neurons also have a very broad excitatory area (Katsuki et al., 1959a, Katsuki, 1966, Goldstein et al., 1968). Interestingly, some cortical auditory neurons with a relatively large excitatory area are directionally sensitive to continuous tones which are frequency-modulated either sinusoidally or stepwise within the area (Whitfield and Evans, 1965). In my experiments, stimuli were always short tone bursts, because the animals emit short tone bursts. When an FM sound swept either upward or downward within broad excitatory areas of cortical auditory neurons of the bat, the neurons always responded to it regardless of sweep directions.

At higher levels, there was a broad continuous spectrum in properties of neurons. Symmetrical and specialized neurons might be considered to be on both ends of this spectrum. There were other types of neurons which were between the above two. That is, there were neurons which responded to two out of the three types of information-bearing elements. Neurons belonging to this category were very rare. "CF (or pure tone) - deaf neurons", which responded to FM sounds and noise bursts, but not to CF tones, have been found in bats. For example, a neuron in Fig. 12 A showed a very low threshold for a downward-sweeping FM sound, but it did not respond to an upward-sweeping FM. Responses to noise bursts showed upper-thresholds. Any tested pure tones higher than 10 kHz failed to excite this neuron. When a pure tone within a shaded area of Fig. 12 A was delivered before a noise burst, the response to the latter was inhibited. This inhibitory area appeared to have some relation with upper-thresholds for noise bursts and directional sensitivity for FM sounds.

In the cat's auditory cortex, a CF-deaf neuron was found, which showed very good responses to FM sounds sweeping between 6 and 12 kHz regardless of sweep directions, and also to noise bursts with a frequency band of 5.5 to 8.5 kHz or wider (Fig. 12, B). For a noise burst with a band of 6 to 8 kHz, the threshold became high (B 1) and an upper-threshold appeared (B 2). A response to a pure tone was absent. The inhibitory area was not measured. The properties

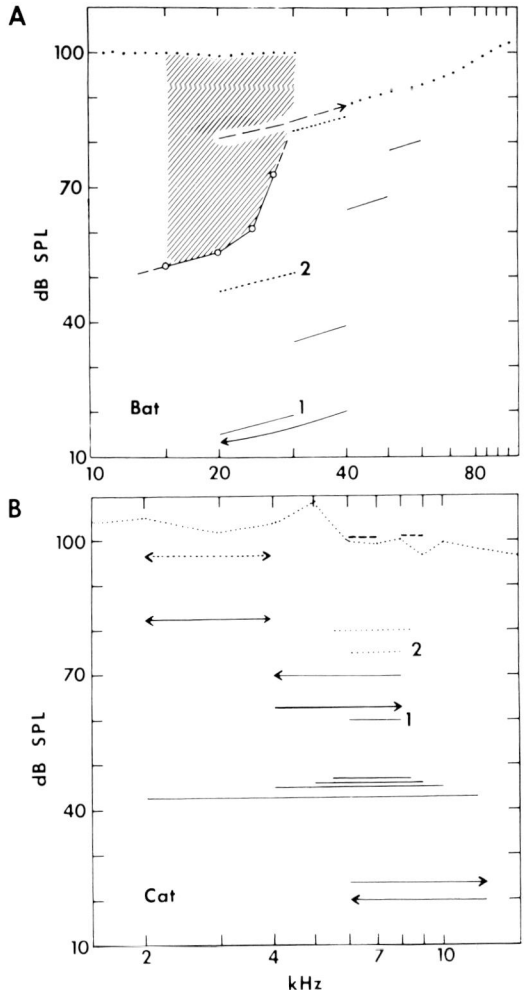

Fig. 12 A: Responses of a CF-deaf neuron in a bat's inferior colliculus to FM sounds and noise bursts. The response to a 40 dB SPL noise burst with a 30-40 kHz frequency band was inhibited by the preceding delivery of a pure tone in the shaded area (Suga, 1969a).

B: Responses of a CF-deaf neuron in a cat's auditory cortex to FM sounds sweeping over an octave and noise bursts with   (cont'd)

(Fig. 12, cont'd) different bandwidths.
Symbols are the same as those explained
in Fig. 2 C.

of a CF-deaf neuron can be explained by the second-order interaction (e.g., Fig. 9, A).

"FM-deaf neurons", which respond to pure tones and noise bursts, but not to FM sounds, have not been found in bats, but a neuron which might be called an FM-deaf unit was found in a cat's auditory cortex (Suga, unpublished data).

"Noise-deaf neurons", which respond to pure tones and FM sounds, but not to noise bursts, have been found. However, these neurons had a small excitatory area and a large inhibitory one. Their thresholds for FM sounds were more than 10 dB lower than those for pure tones at their best frequencies, so they might more appropriately be called FM-specialized neurons (Suga, 1969a).

3.4 Responses of CF- and FM-specialized neurons to sounds with overtones

Sounds produced by animals are usually complex, and often consist of several overtones. This is also true in orientation sounds of some species of bats. For instance, orientation sounds of the mustache bat, Chilonycteris and the naked-backed bat, Pteronotus, consist of several harmonics. If some harmonics stimulate not only the excitatory area of a CF-specialized neuron or excitatory region of an FM-specialized neuron, but also their inhibitory area or areas, the neurons may fail to respond to orientation sounds. In order to study this problem, two sounds with the same envelope were simultaneously delivered. One called "tone pulse I" was either the sound at the best frequency of a given CF-specialized neuron or the best FM sound for a given FM-specialized neuron. The other called "tone pulse II" was either a pure tone pulse or FM sound, the frequency or frequency sweep of which was changed in order to measure inhibitory areas, in which tone pulse II caused inhibition of the response to tone pulse I (e.g., Figs. 11 A and 13). From such experiments, two general rules were found. (1) The weaker tone pulse I, the larger the inhibitory area was. (2) The inhibitory area below the best frequency often included the sound one octave below it, while it was rare that the area above the best frequency included the sound one octave above it. Fig. 13 reveals how the size of the inhibitory areas varied with the amplitude of tone pulse I.

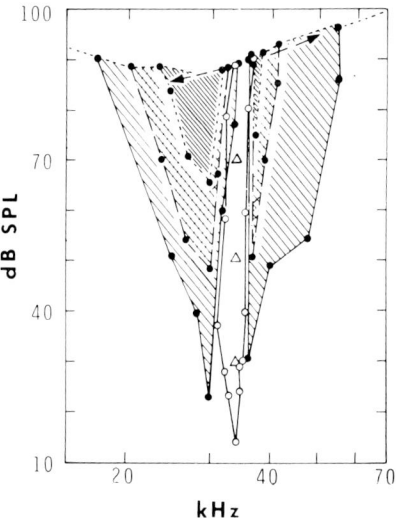

Fig. 13 Excitatory (open) and inhibitory (shaded) areas of a CF-specialized neuron in the inferior colliculus. The inhibitory areas were measured by delivering tone pulse II (pure tone) simultaneously with tone pulse I (pure tone at the best frequency). Three different amplitudes of tone pulse I were used (triangles). With the increase of the excitatory sound in amplitude, the size of the inhibitory area was progressively reduced from the shaded areas enclosed by the solid (cont'd)

(Fig. 13, cont'd) line (obtained with tone pulse I at 30 dB SPL, lower triangle) to the hatched areas enclosed by the broken line (obtained with tone pulse I at 50 dB SPL, center triangle), then to the shaded area enclosed by the dotted line (obtained with tone pulse I at 70 dB SPL, upper triangle) (Suga and Schlegel, 1973).

Let us imagine a complex sound which consists of 3 harmonics, f_1, f_2, and f_3, with f_2 equal to the best frequency. Whether a CF-specialized neuron responds to this complex sound or not depends not only on the frequency of f_2, but also on the frequencies of f_1 and f_3. If the frequencies of f_1 and/or f_3 are inside its inhibitory areas and their intensities are strong relative to that of f_2, the neuron may not respond to this complex sound. The structure of complex sound is therefore very important for the excitation of the CF-specialized neuron. This is also true for other types of neurons which have inhibitory areas.

Asymmetrical neurons commonly have a large inhibitory area at frequencies lower than their excitatory areas, so that the frequency of f_1 is very important in determining whether their responses occur to the complex sound with f_2 equal to their best frequencies. In asymmetrical neurons with a large inhibitory area at frequencies higher than their best frequencies, the frequency of f_3 is very important to determine their excitation. The asymmetrical neurons thus respond to less restricted combinations of components than do CF-specialized units.

Let us look at an example of an FM-specialized neuron which selectively responded to downward sweeping FM sounds (Fig. 11, A1 and A2). When the frequency of a 4 msec tone pulse swept from 90 to 50 kHz at 80 dB SPL, the neuron responded. When a 4 msec pure tone of 80 dB SPL was simultaneously delivered, the response was inhibited. The frequency range of the pure tone for inhibition is shown by the shaded area in Fig. 11, 3. In this case, pure tones between 43 and 65 kHz completely inhibited the response to the FM sound. The inhibition was also evoked by the simultaneous delivery of an FM sound instead of the pure tone. For example, the response to the FM sound sweeping from 90 to 50 kHz was completely inhibited by a sound sweeping from 95 to 60 kHz. The range of an inhibitory FM sound was very broad, as shown by the shaded sector in Fig. 11, A8. The inhibitory range varied when the terminal frequency was changed. Tone pulse II half an octave below tone pulse I partially inhibited the response to the latter, while tone pulse II half an octave above it had no effect on the response (Fig. 11, A, 6-11). These results indicate that not only the parameters of an FM sound or component but also those of other sounds (or components) which simultaneously exist are very important for excitation of the FM-specialized neuron.

In the bullfrog, two components in a croak are indispensable in order to evoke a vocal response (Capranica, 1966). These may be called the first and second CF components. The bullfrog has the amphibian and basilar papillae for sound reception. The amphibian and basilar papillae are respectively tuned for the first and second components in the croak of a mature bullfrog (Frishkopf and Geisler, 1966). When these two papillae are simultaneously excited, the bullfrog shows the vocal response. Interestingly, nerve fibers from the amphibian papillae have not only an excitatory area, but also an inhibitory area which is tuned for frequencies between the two components (Frishkopf and Goldstein, 1963). When an immature bullfrog's croak or a synthetic croak contains a component which stimulates the inhibitory area, the mature bullfrog shows no vocal response to it even if it contains the two CF components at right frequencies (Capranica, 1966). If the inhibitory area were absent, the detection of the species-specific croak of a mature bullfrog would be not exclusive. For instance, the bullfrog would show a vocal response to a white noise stimulus. The bullfrog is thus equipped with the sound receptors for the selective detection of the mature species-specific croak.

In general, the presence of inhibitory areas is essential for the feature extraction from complex sounds. If single neurons had no inhibitory areas, they would respond to any complex sounds whenever a part of the sound energy falls into their excitatory areas. If CF-specialized neurons had no inhibitory areas, for instance, they would not selectively respond to pure tones in spite of their very narrow excitatory areas. The experiments with the bullfrog give direct behavioral evidence indicating the role of the inhibitory area in the recognition of a biologically significant sound.

The I.C. and A.C. of bats contain diverse types of neurons. The presence of these neurons indicates that the auditory system is capable of analyzing not only species-specific orientation sounds and their echoes, but also other sounds. It is to be expected that bats being acoustically specialized, use sounds as the most effective means for communication (Gould, 1971). Furthermore, the bats may hear insects stridulating for communication with either CF tone pulses, noise bursts or click sounds (Blest et al., 1963, Suga, 1966), or may receive warning sounds from insects by touching them (Dunning and Roeder, 1965).

3.5 Neurons responding only to complex sounds

As described above, the higher levels of the auditory system contain neurons which are specialized to respond to one of the three types of sounds: CF tones, FM sounds, and noise bursts. As the next step of neural specialization for acoustic pattern recognition, these specialized neurons may be integrated in various combinations in order to produce neurons which exclusively respond to a particular complex sound. There is, however, no reliable datum indicating the specialization of single neurons to a particular complex sound. Almost no experiments with very vocal mammals have been performed in which acoustic stimuli are suitably programmed to find neurons selectively responding to biologically significant complex sounds. Fortunately, several auditory physiologists are going to attempt to find neurons specialized for responding only to communication sounds. In the near future, neurons may be found which respond only to complex sounds consisting of particular combinations of information-bearing elements, but not to each element. These neurons may be called "complex auditory neurons" for convenience.

The squirrel monkey is very vocal and appears to be suited to studies on neural analysis of communication sounds. Their sounds are classified into eight types (Winter et al., 1966). Recently, Funkenstein et al., (1971) found that three percent of cortical neurons in unanesthetized squirrel monkeys selectively responded to some of their communication sounds. A critical test has, however, not yet been performed as to whether a single component in the complex sound did not excite them or whether a simultaneous presentation of more than one component was essential for their excitation. By the way, the experiments with the squirrel monkeys indicate that neurons which might be complex auditory units are not more than three percent of neurons studied in the auditory cortex. The percentage of complex neurons appears to be surprisingly small. Experiments to demonstrate the presence of complex auditory neurons and to explore neural mechanisms for such a specialization are thus not very efficient, so that two questions arise in the author's mind: (1) is it possible to increase the number of complex auditory neurons by conditioning animals to respond to a particular complex sound? and (2) is the auditory cortex the suitable place to study? Miller (1971) found that single neurons in the auditory cortex of a monkey showed much stronger responses to acoustic stimuli in an animal behaving for a trained task than in a non-behaving one. Strategies for studying complex auditory neurons should probably be reconsidered. In a possible method, for instance, one conditions an animal to press a lever only when a particular complex sound is delivered. Then, one may look for whether there are neurons exclusively responding to this complex sound in the brain. Areas to be studied may not be necessarily in the auditory system, but in the motor system.

In the above, the discussion is forwarded with the assumption that animals have neurons specialized for responding to complex sounds, e.g., "phonemes" in their communication sounds. Since nerve fibers from the amphibian and basilar papillae in the bullfrog must be simultaneously stimulated by acoustic stimuli to initiate a vocal response (Capranica, 1966), it is reasonable to assume that there are neurons which can detect whether the two papillae are simultaneously activated. In other words, there may be "croak-detectors" which receive impulses originating in these two papillae. Frishkopf and Capranica (1966) and Frishkopf et al. (1968) looked for such detectors, but they could not find them. If the bullfrog has no croak-detectors, it appears to suggest that simultaneous activity of higher order neurons of the amphibian and basilar papillae is directly concerned with the recognition of the croak. In short, the experiments with bullfrogs lead us to consider the limitation in neural specialization for pattern recognition. As described in the introduction, one extreme assumption is that complex neurons are necessary to recognize complex acoustic signals. In communication sounds of humans, various phonemes are combined in so different sequences that one may consider that the upper limit of specialization of single neurons for a particular acoustic pattern is probably at most, say, for "words". Recognition of "phrases", and "sentences" may then be directly related to the spatial and temporal patterns of activity of the neurons specialized for "words". Neurons which exclusively respond to the particular spatial and temporal patterns of activities of "word detectors" may be not necessary.

According to Hubel and Wiesel (1965), higher-order hyper-complex neurons appear to be a limit of specialization for pattern recognition in the visual system of cats. The visual cortex, area 18, contains lower-order hyper-complex neurons at 5-10 percent, while area 19 has them at only a few percent. These neurons are apparently specialized to extract particular features from visual signals. If one assumes that hyper-complex neurons are the upper limit of specialization of single neurons for pattern recognition, spatial and temporal patterns of activity of the hyper-complex neurons may be directly related to pattern recognition, without neurons which selectively respond to this particular spatial and temporal pattern.

The problem which can be answered by single-unit studies, is whether there are neurons more specialized for the extraction of complicated features than CF or FM or noise-specialized neurons in the auditory system and higher-order hyper-complex neurons in the visual system. In monkeys, some cortical visual neurons exclusively respond to a specific pattern similar to a monkey's hand (Gross et al., 1972). It is expectable that the brain contains complex auditory neurons which are specialized for exclusively responding to biologically significant complex sounds. For understanding neural mechanisms for pattern recognition, it is essential to determine the limitation of specialization of single neurons for acoustic patterns by studying not only the classical auditory system, but also the vocalization system and/or association areas in the cerebral cortex.

3.6 Responses to AM sounds

Unlike primary auditory and cochlear nuclear neurons, most I.C. and A.C. units did not respond to continuous pure tones, but did respond to tone bursts with particular frequencies (Suga, 1964a, 1965c). This indicates that not only the carrier frequency, but also the change in the amplitude of the carrier sound is an important factor for the excitation of these neurons. In the experiments described above, acoustic stimuli always had a 0.5 msec rise-decay time and 4 msec duration, except for a certain case stated, so the effect of amplitude-modulation was always included in the observation. In order to study the problem of neural analysis of AM sounds, either sinusoidally amplitude-modulated continuous tones or tone bursts with a variable rise-decay time can be used. The type of stimulus should be determined by the type of signal with which animals are naturally concerned. The bats emit short tone bursts for echolocation, so that amplitude-modulated tone bursts appeared to be the most suitable stimuli for experiments with them. Since almost all phasic collicular neurons discharged a few impulses only at the on-set of a tone burst, the rising phase appeared to be particularly important. Accordingly a study was made of the responses of I.C. neurons to tone bursts with different rise times. The duration of a tone burst was 100 msec, unless otherwise stated. The rise time varied from 0.08 to 98 msec. During the rise phase, stimulus amplitude increased roughly linearly with time. The decay time was always 0.5 msec. The carrier sound was at the best frequency of a given neuron (Suga, 1971).

The response patterns of most I.C. neurons which showed phasic on-responses did not change with the rise time, but those of some others changed from inhibitory responses to phasic on-responses (Fig. 14). When the relationship between threshold and rise time was studied by changing the latter from 0.08 to 98 msec, it was found that there were four types of relationships: (1) no change in threshold (Fig. 15 Aa), (2) significant change in threshold (Fig. 15, A c and A d), (3) upper-threshold change but no threshold change (Fig. 15, A b), and (4) both threshold and upper-threshold change (Fig. 14). For instance, single neurons "A" and "B" in Fig. 14 show upper-threshold

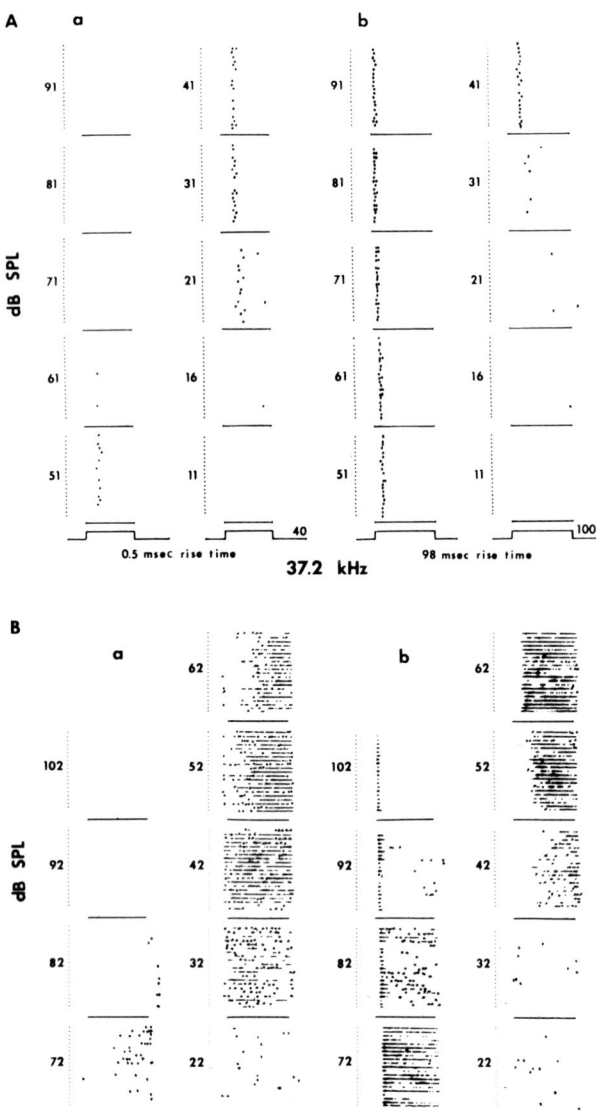

Fig. 14 Responses of two I.C. neurons (A and B) to tone bursts with a rise time of 0.5 (a) or 98 msec (b) are shown by a dotted pattern. One dot corresponds to the peak of one action potential. The sweep of a cathode-ray oscilloscope was displaced vertically before each stimulus. The dots of the left mark the start of the sweep. The sound stimulus is represented by a horizontal bar and square wave at the bottom of each dotted pattern. The duration of the tone (cont'd)

(Fig. 14, cont'd) bursts was 40 msec in Aa and 100 msec in Ab, Ba, and Bb. The repetition rate of the stimulus was 1.5/sec. The plateau amplitude of a stimulus was changed as shown by the numbers to the left of each dotted pattern. The threshold, upper-threshold, and response pattern changed with the rise time. The frequency of the tone burst was set at the best frequency of a neuron which was 37.2 kHz for A and 90.8 kHz for B (Suga, 1971).

for tone bursts with a 0.5 msec rise time. These neurons show no upper-threshold, but do show phasic on-responses to strong tone bursts with a 98 msec rise time. That is, the upper-threshold increases. In these neurons, the threshold also increases with a rise time, but the amount of increase is much smaller than that in the upper-threshold. Fig. 15 A represents threshold-rise time curves of four I.C. neurons. In neuron "c" of Fig. 15 A, the threshold-rise time curve "c" made contact at about 20 msec with the straight dashed line, indicating the minimum rate of amplitude increase necessary for the excitation of the neuron, and changed along the straight dashed line when the rise time was lengthened to more than 20 msec. The threshold-rise time curve indicates that unless the stimulus amplitude increased beyond the threshold of this neuron within 20 msec, the neuron failed to respond to the stimulus. The increase in threshold due to lengthening the rise time from 0.5 to 98 msec was 20 dB (curve c).

It was found that the threshold-rise time curve sometimes deviated from the dashed line after making contact with it. For example, the threshold of neuron "d" for a tone burst with a 98 msec rise time was 17 dB higher than the expected value (curve d in Fig. 15 A). In extreme cases, the deviation from the dashed line appeared at a rise time of 20 msec and increased with a lengthening of rise time. In about 13 % of the neurons studied, the deviation was too large to be an error in the measurement of threshold. Fig. 15 B shows a distribution of the differences in threshold between responses to a 100 msec tone burst with a 0.5 msec rise time and those to a tone burst with a 98 msec rise time. The threshold difference was less than 10 dB in 41 % of the neurons studied,

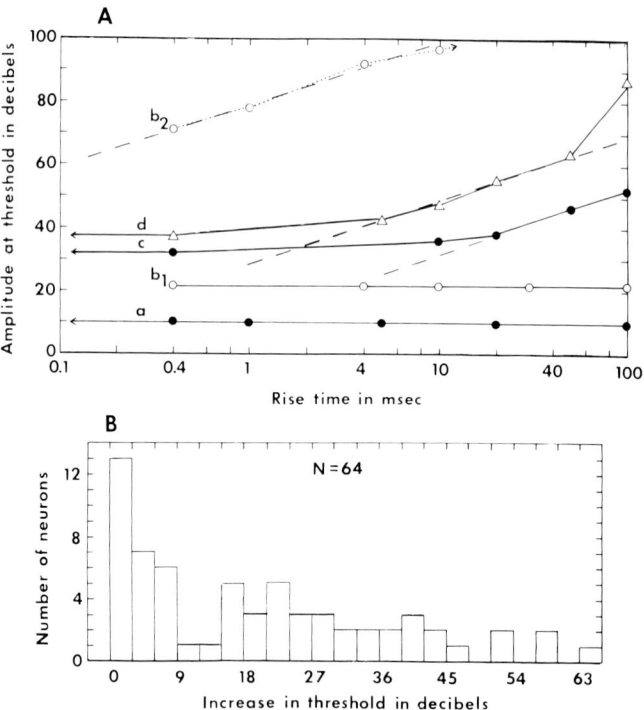

Fig. 15 A: Changes in the threshold (solid line) and upper-threshold (dotted line) of responses of four I.C. neurons (a,b,c, and d) with the rise time of a tone burst set at the best frequency. The duration and the decay time of the tone burst were 100 and 0.5 msec, respectively. The frequency of the tone burst was 29.7 kHz for a, 46.4 kHz for b, 44.9 kHz for c, and 46.0 kHz for d. The dashed lines indicate the minimum (for c and d) or maximum (for b_2) rate of amplitude increase in the stimuli which excited or failed to excite neurons c, d, and b.

B: Distribution of the increase in threshold with a change in the rise time of a tone burst from 0.5 to 98 msec. The total number of I.C. neurons studied was 73. Nine of these showed no response to tone bursts (cont'd)

(Fig. 15, cont'd) with a 98 msec rise time (Suga, 1971).

10-30 dB in 33 %, and more than 30 dB in 26 %.

Those experiments indicate that the rate of amplitude increase is not a very important factor for excitation of about 40 % of phasic neurons, while it is a very important factor for excitation of another 60 % of phasic neurons. For the neurons which showed a large increase in threshold, the rate of amplitude increase did not have to be too small. For the neurons which showed a change in upper-threshold, but not in threshold, the rate had not to be too large. If the rate was large, the amplitude had to be small. For the neurons which showed an increase in both threshold and upper-threshold, the rate had not to be too large or too small. Both the rate and amplitude had to be within a certain range. The rate of rise, as well as plateau amplitude, was thus a very important parameter for the excitation of some phasic I.C. neurons.

Since both the threshold and upper-threshold if any, changed independently with rise time, the excitatory areas of single neurons varied in different ways. For example, neuron "B" of Fig. 16 has a large excitatory area for tone bursts with a 0.5 msec rise time, but a small area for those with a 95 msec rise time. On the other hand, neuron "D" of Fig. 16 has a small closed excitatory area for tone bursts with a 0.5 msec rise time, but a large area for those with a 98 msec rise time. Fig. 16 A shows that the excitatory area of an I.C. neuron (solid line) changes as indicated by a dotted line with lengthening the rise time, while the area of some others (the same solid line) does not change as indicated by a dashed line. Fig. 16 C represents the excitatory area of an I.C. neuron showing upper-threshold changes as indicated by either dotted or dashed line with lengthening the rise time. Inhibitory areas, if any, also changed with rise time. The phasic on-responding neurons appeared to contribute greatly to the analysis of AM sounds, especially to the analysis of the rate of amplitude increase.

The changes in upper-threshold with rise time are easily explained, because upper-threshold neurons always had an inhibitory area engulfing the excitatory

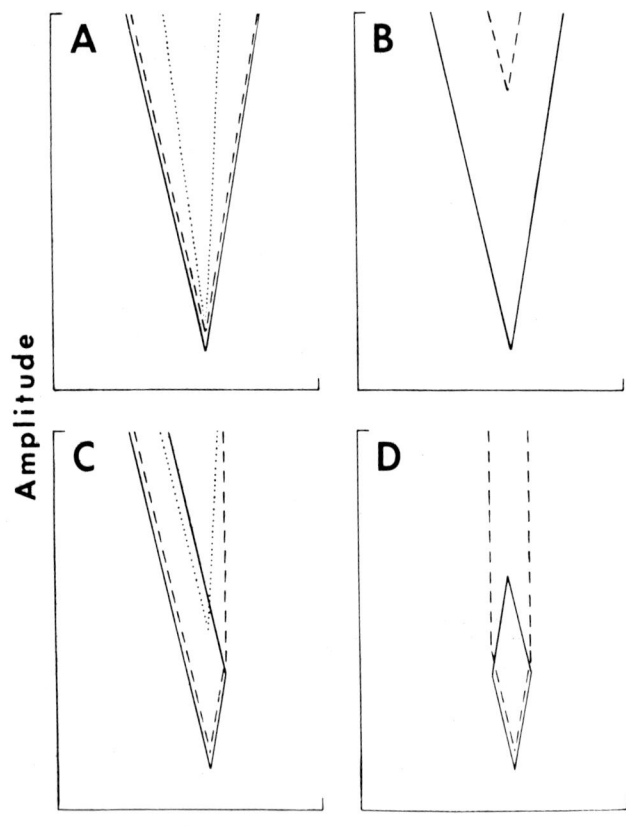

Fig. 16 Changes in the excitatory areas of single I.C. neurons with a lengthening of the rise time of a tone burst from 0.5 to 98 msec. The ordinates and abscissas represent the stimulus amplitude at threshold and the frequency of the stimulus, respectively. In each graph, the solid line represents the excitatory tuning curve measured with a tone burst having a rise time of 0.5 msec. The area above or surrounded by the tuning curve is the excitatory area. When the rise time is lengthened to 98 msec, the tuning curve changes as indicated by either dashed or dotted line. These schematized tuning curves are based on the data obtained by Suga (1971).

area from the top (Figs. 6 B and 7 F). When a strong
sound with a rapid rise time is delivered, both the
excitatory and inhibitory areas are simultaneously
stimulated, so the neuron cannot discharge action potentials. With attenuation of the stimulus, only the
excitatory area is stimulated, so the neuron does respond. When the rise time is long, the excitatory
area is stimulated before the inhibitory area, so the
neuron does not show an upper-threshold and gives a
phasic on-response. This is clearly shown in Fig. 14
B. The changes in threshold with rise time appear to
involve neural inhibition and/or accommodation.

In almost all neurophysiological studies, the tuning
curve or excitatory area has been measured with tone
bursts having an arbitrarily selected rise time. It
should be noted that the shape and size of the tuning
curve or excitatory area of some phasic on-responding
neurons vary greatly with rise time.

4. Epilogue

My experiments performed on the feature extraction
from acoustic signals are still very rudimentary.
Systematic studies on responses to AM sounds and
further quantitative studies on specialized neurons
are needed. Since animals have time-varying acoustic
signals on the left and right ears, binaural interaction and recovery cycles should also be studied in
relation to pattern recognition.

In cats and monkeys, very quantitative data on activity of auditory nerve fibers have been accumulated
and coding of acoustic signals by primary auditory
neurons has been accurately described (see A. R. Møller's review, 1972). Some of the higher order neurons
are obviously concerned with extraction of particular
information from the coded signals. The problem of
decoding, however, has been little discussed, although "responses" of auditory neurons at higher
levels have been described.

Auditory physiologists have been studying the communication system consisting of the auditory and vocalization systems. The echolocation system of a bat
also consists of these two systems, because the bat
emits sounds and listens to echoes coming back from
objects. The auditory system is excited by emitted
sounds, but the amount of excitation is decreased by

contraction of the middle ear muscles (Carmel and Starr, 1963, Henson, 1965) and also by a neural attenuation synchronized with vocalization (Suga and Schlegel, 1972, 1973). On the other hand, activity of the vocalization system is modified by acoustically evoked activity in the auditory system (Suga et al., in preparation). For understanding the neural mechanisms of the communication and echolocation systems, both the auditory and vocalization systems and the coupling between them should be studied.

Acknowledgements

I express my sincere gratitude to Profs. T.H. Bullock, D.R. Griffin, and Y. Katsuki. Without their guidance and support, these experiments could not have been performed. I also wish to thank the following friends of mine, Drs. T.M. Arthur, R.W. Colles, G.D. Lange, J.J.G. McCue, J.A. Simmons, R.A. Suthers and R.R. Pfeiffer for their comments and suggestions and also Ms. J.H. Friend, Mr. T. Gass, Mr. R.H. Hamstra, Ms. G.G. Kennedy, and Mr. W. Bloodwroth for their assistance. The experiments described in the present paper have been supported by the National Science Foundation Research Grants for N. Suga (G B 13904-A1), Bullock, and Griffin. Without such a strong and continuous support by NSF, it would not be possible to carry out these experiments.

References

Adams, L.-J. (1969). Neurophysiologie des Hörens und Bioakustik einer Feldheuschrecke (Locusta migratoria). Z. Vergl. Physiol. 63, 227-289.

Airapetianz, E. Sh., and Vasilyev, A.G. (1971). On neurophysiological mechanisms of the echolocating apparatus in bats (frequency parameters). Int. J. Neurosci. 1, 279-286.

Altes, R.A., and Titlebaum, E.L. (1970). Bat signals as optimally Doppler tolerant waveforms. J. Acoust. Soc. Amer. 48, 1014-1020.

Arthur, R.M., Pfeiffer, R.R., and Suga, N. (1971). Properties of "two-tone inhibition" in primary auditory neurons. J. Physiol. 212, 593-609.

Autrum, A. (1955). L'acoustique des Orthoptéres. Ann. Inst. Nat. Rech. Agron., Paris. (C) Ann. Epiphyt. Fascicule Spécial, pp. 338-355.

Bastian, J. (1967). The transmission of arbitrary environmental information between bottlenose dolphins. In: Animal Sonar Systems (R.G. Busnel, ed.), pp. 803-873. Laboratoire de Physiologie Acoustique, Jouy-en-Josas.

Blest, A., Collett, T., and Pye, J. (1963). The generation of ultrasonic signals by a New World orctiid moth. Proc. Roy. Soc. 158, 196-207.

Busnel, R.R., Busnel, M.C., and Dumortier, B. (1956). Cited by Dumortier, B. In: Acoustic Behavior of Animals (R.G. Busnel, ed.), pp. 583-654. Elsevier, New York.

Cahlander, D.A. (1964). Echolocation with wide-band waveforms: bat sonar signals. Tech. Rep. 271. M.I.T. Lincoln Lab., Cambridge, Mass.

Capranica, R.C. (1966). Vocal response of the bullfrog to natural and synthetic mating calls. J. Acoust. Soc. Amer. 40, 1131-1139.

Carmel, P.W., and Starr, A. (1963). Acoustic and nonacoustic factors modifying middle-ear muscle activity in waking cats. J. Neurophysiol. 26, 598-616.

Denes, P.B., and Pinson, E.N. (1963). The Speech Chain. Bell Tel. Lab. Monogr. Williams & Wilkins Co., Baltimore.

Dumortier, B. (1963). Ethology and physiology studies of sound emissions in arthropoda. In: Acoustic Behavior of Animals (R.G. Busnel, ed.), pp. 583-654. Elsevier, New York.

Dunning, D., and Roeder, K. (1965). Moth sounds and the insect-catching behavior of bats. Science 147, 173-174.

Enger, P.S. (1963). Single unit activity in the peripheral auditory system of a teleost fish. Acta Physiol. Scand. 59, Suppl. 210.

Erulkar, S.D. (1959). The responses of single units of the inferior colliculus of the cat to acoustic stimulation. Proc. Roy. Soc. 150, 336-355.

Evans, E.F., and Whitfield, I.C. (1964). Classification of unit responses in the auditory cortex of the unanesthetized and unrestrained cat. J. Physiol. 171, 476-493.

Fish, M.P., and Mowbray, W.H. (1970). Sounds of Western North Atlantic Fishes. John Hopkins Press, Baltimore.

Friend, J.H., Suga, N., and Suthers, R.A. (1966). Neural responses in the inferior colliculus of echolocating bats to artificial orientation sounds and echoes. J. Cell Physiol. 67, 319-332.

Frishkopf, L.S. (1964). Excitation and inhibition of primary auditory neurons in the little brown bat. J. Acoust. Soc. Amer. 26, 1016.

Frishkopf, L., and Capranica, R. (1966). Auditory responses in the medulla of the bullfrog: comparison with eighth-nerve responses. J. Acoust. Soc. Amer. 40, 1262.

Frishkopf, L., Capranica, R., and Goldstein, M. (1968). Neural coding in the bullfrog's auditory system - a teleological approach. Proc. IEEE 56, 969-980.

Frishkopf, L., and Geisler, C. (1966). Peripheral origin of auditory responses from the eighth nerve of the bullfrog. J. Acoust. Soc. Amer. 40, 469-472.

Frishkopf, L.S., and Goldstein, M.H., Jr. (1963). Responses to acoustic stimuli from single units in the eighth nerve of the bullfrog. J. Acoust. Soc. Amer. 35, 1219-1228.

Funkenstein, H., Nelson, P., Winter, P., Wollberg, Z., and Newman, J. (1971). Unit responses in auditory cortex of awake squirrel monkeys to vocal stimulation. In: Physiology of the Auditory System (M. Sachs, ed.), pp. 307-315. National Educational Consultants, Baltimore.

Furukawa, T., and Ishii, Y. (1967). Neurophysiological studies on hearing in goldfish. J. Neurophysiol. 30, 1377-1403.

Galambos, R. (1960). Studies of the auditory system with implanted electrodes. In: Neural Mechanisms of the Auditory and Vestibular Systems (G.L. Rasmussen and W.F. Windle, eds.), pp. 137-151. C.C. Thomas, Springfield, Ill.

Goldstein, M., Hall, J., and Butterfield, B. (1968). Single-unit activity in the primary auditory cortex of unanesthetized cats. J. Acoust. Soc. Amer. 43, 444-455.

Gould, E. (1971). Studies of maternal-infant communication and development of vocalization in the bat, Myotis and Eptesicus. In: Communications in Behavioral Biology, Academic Press, New York.

Greenwood, D.D., and Maruyama, N. (1965). Excitatory and inhibitory response areas of auditory neurons in the cochlear nucleus. J. Neurophysiol. 28, 863-892.

Griffin, D.R. (1958). Listening in the Dark. Yale Univ. Press, New Haven, Conn.

Griffin, D.R. (1971). The importance of atmospheric attenuation for the echolocation of bats (Chiroptera). Anim. Behav. 19, 55-61.

Grinnell, A.D. (1970). Comparative auditory neurophysiology of neotropical bats employing different echolocation signals. Z. Vergl. Physiol. 68, 117-153.

Grinnell, A.D., and Hagiwara, S. (1972). Studies of auditory neurophysiology in non-echolocating bats, and adaptations for echolocation in one genus, Rousettus, Z. Vergl. Physiol. 76, 82-96.

Grinnell, A.D., and McCue, J.J. (1963). Neurophysiological investigations of the bat Myotis lucifugus stimulated by frequency modulated acoustical pulse. Nature (London) 198, 453-455.

Gross, C.G., Rocha-miranda, C.E., and Bender, D.B. (1972). Visual properties of neurons in inferotemporal cortex of the macaque. J. Neurophysiol. 35, 96-111.

Grozinger, B. (1967). Electrophysiologische Untersuchungen der Hörbahn de Schleie (Tinca Tinca L). Z. Vergl. Physiol. 57, 44-76.

Henson, O.W., Jr. (1965). The activity and function of the middle ear muscles in echolocating bats. J. Physiol. 180, 871-887.

Horridge, G.A. (1961). Pitch discrimination in locusts. Proc. Roy. Soc. (B) 155, 218-231.

Hubel, D.H., and Wiesel, T.N. (1962). Receptive fields, binocular interaction and functional architecture in the cat's visual cortex. J. Physiol. 160, 106-154.

Hubel, D.H., and Wiesel, T.N. (1965). Receptive fields and functional architecture in two non-striate visual areas (18 and 19) of the cat. J. Neurophysiol. 28, 229-289.

Hubel, D.H., and Wiesel, T.N. (1968). Receptive fields and functional architecture of monkey striate cortex. J. Physiol. 195, 215-243.

Jacobs, D.W., and Tavolga, W.N. (1968). Acoustic frequency discrimination in the goldfish. Anim. Behav. 16, 67-71.

Jürgens, U., and Ploog, D. (1970). Cerebral representation of vocalization in the squirrel monkey. Exp. Brain Res. 10, 532-554.

Kalmring, K., Rheinlaender, J., and Rehbein, H. (1972). Akustische Neuronen im Bauchmark der Wanderheuschrecke Locusta migratoria. Z. Vergl. Physiol. 76, 314-332.

Katsuki, Y. (1966). Neural mechanism of hearing in cats and monkeys. Progr. Brain Res. 21A, 71-97.

Katsuki, Y., and Suga, N. (1960). Neural mechanism of hearing in insects. J. Exp. Biol. 37, 279-290.

Katsuki, Y., Suga, N., and Kanno, Y. (1962). Neural mechanism of the peripheral and central auditory system in monkeys. J. Acoust. Soc. Amer. 34, 1396-1410.

Katsuki, Y., Sumi, T., Uchiyama, H., and Watanabe, T. (1958). Electric responses of auditory neurons in cat to sound stimulation. J. Neurophysiol. 21, 569-588.

Katsuki, Y., Watanabe, T., and Maruyama, N. (1959a). Activity of auditory neurons in upper levels of brain of cat. J. Neurophysiol. 22, 343-359.

Katsuki, Y., Watanabe, T., and Suga, N. (1959b). Interaction of auditory neurons in response to two sound stimuli in cat. J. Neurophysiol. 22, 603-623.

Kiang, N.Y.S. (1965). Dischange Patterns of Single Nerve Fibers in the Cat's Auditory Nerve. Res. Monogr. 35. M.I.T. Press, Cambridge, Mass.

Konishi, M. (1963). The role of auditory feedback in the behavior of the domestic fowl. Z. Tierpsychol. 20, 349-367.

Konishi, M. (1965). The role of auditory feedback in the control of vocalization in the white-crowned sparrow. Z. Tierpsychol. 22, 770-783.

Kulzer, E. (1956). Fluzhunde erzeugen Orientierungslaute durch Zungenschlag. Naturwiss. 43, 117-118.

Lettvin, J.Y., Maturana, H.R., Pitts, W.H., and McCulloch, W.S. (1961). Two remarks on the visual system of the frog. In: Sensory Communication (W.A. Rosenblith, ed.), pp. 757-776. M.I.T. Press, Cambridge, Mass.

Michelsen, A. (1966). Pitch discrimination in the locust ear: observations on single sense cells. J. Insect Physiol. 12, 1119-1131.

Michelsen, A. (1971). The physiology of the locust ear. I. Frequency sensitivity of single cells in the isolated ear. Z. Vergl. Physiol. 71, 49-62.

Miller, J. (1971). Single unit discharges in behaving monkeys. In: Physiology of the Auditory System (M. Sachs, ed.), pp. 317-326. National Educational Consultants, Baltimore.

Møller, A.R. (1969). Unit responses in the cochlear nucleus of the rat to sweep tones. Acta Physiol. Scand. 76, 503-512.

Møller, A.R. (1972). Coding of sounds in lower levels of the auditory system. Quart. Rev. Biophys. 5, 59-155.

Nelson, P., Erulkar, S., and Bryan, J. (1966). Responses of units of the inferior colliculus to time-varying acoustic stimuli. J. Neurophysiol. 29, 834-860.

Neuweiler, G. (1970). Neurophysiologische Untersuchungen zum Echoortungssystem der Grossen Hufeisennase Rhinolophus ferrum equinum Schreber, 1774. Z. Vergl. Physiol. 67, 273-306.

Nomoto, M., Suga, N., and Katsuki, Y. (1964). Discharge pattern and inhibition of primary auditory nerve fibers in the monkey. J. Neurophysiol. 27, 768-787.

Norris, K.S., Evans, W.E., and Turner, R.N. (1967). Echolocation in an Atlantic bottlenose porpoise during discrimination. In: Animal Sonar Systems (R.G. Busnel, ed.), pp. 409-436. Laboratoire de Physiologie Acoustique, Jouy-en-Josas.

Nottebohm, F. (1968). Auditory experience and song development in the chaffinch, Fringilla coelebs. Ibis, 110, 549-568.

Nottebohm, F. (1972). In: Auditory Processing of Biologically Significant Sounds (F. Wordan, and R. Galambos, eds.), p. 76. Neurosci. Res. Progr. Bull. 10.

Pfeiffer, R. (1966). Classification of response patterns of spike discharges for units in the cochlear nucleus: tone burst stimulation. Exp. Brain Res. 1, 220-235.

Poljak, S. (1926). Untersuchungen am Oktavussystem der Säugetiere und an den mit diesem koordinier motorischen Apparaten des Hirnstammes. J. Psychol. Neurol. 32, 170-231.

Pollak, G., Henson, O.W., Jr., and Novick, A. (1972). Cochlear microphonic audiograms in the "pure tone" bat Chilonycteris parnellii parnellii. Science 176, 66-88.

Popov, A.V. (1965). Electrophysiological studies on peripheral auditory neurons in the locust. J. Evol. Biochem. Physiol. 1, 239-250.

Potter, D. (1965). Patterns of acoustically evoked discharges of neurons in the mesencephalon of the bullfrog. J. Neurophysiol. 28, 1155-1184.

Potter, R.K., Kopp, G.A., and Kopp, H.G. (1966). Visible Speech. Dover, New York.

Rose, J., Greenwood, D., Goldberg, J., and Hind, J. (1963). Some discharge characteristics of single neurons in the inferior colliculus of the cat. I. Tonotopical organization relation of spike-counts to tone intensity and firing patterns of single elements. J. Neurophysiol. 26, 294-320.

Sachs, M.B., and Kiang, N.Y.S. (1968). Two-tone inhibition in auditory nerve fibers. J. Acoust. Soc. Amer. 43, 1120-1128.

Schnitzler, H-U. (1968). Die Ultraschall-Ortungslaute der Hufeisen-Fledermäuse (Chiroptera-Rhinolophidae) in verschiedenen Orientierungssituationen. Z. Vergl. Physiol. 57, 376-408.

Schnitzler, H-U. (1970). Echoortung bei der Fledermaus Chilonycteris rubiginosa. Z. Vergl. Physiol. 68, 25-38.

Simmons, J.A. (1971a). Echolocation in bats: signal processing of echoes for target range. Science 171, 925-928.

Simmons, J.A. (1971b). The sonar receiver of the bat. Ann. N.Y. Acad. Sci. 188, 161-174.

Simmons, J.A. (1973a). The resolution of target range by echolocating bats. J. Acoust. Soc. Amer. (In press).

Simmons, J.A. (1973b). Response of the Doppler sonar system in the bat. Rhinolophus ferrumequinum. J. Acoust. Soc. Amer. (Submitted).

Suga, N. (1964a). Single unit activity in cochlear nucleus and inferior colliculus of echo-locating bats. J. Physiol. 172, 449-474.

Suga, N. (1964b). Recovery cycles and responses to frequency modulated tone pulses in auditory neurones of echolocating bats. J. Physiol. 175, 50-80.

Suga, N. (1965a). Analysis of frequency modulated sounds by auditory neurones of echolocating bats. J. Physiol. 179, 26-53.

Suga, N. (1965b). Responses of cortical auditory neurones to frequency modulated sounds in echo-locating bats. Nature (London) 206, 890-891.

Suga, N. (1965c). Functional properties of auditory neurones in the cortex of echolocating bats. J. Physiol. 181, 671-700.

Suga, N. (1966). Ultrasonic production and its reception on some neotropical tettigoniidae. J. Insect. Physiol. 12, 1039-1050.

Suga, N. (1968). Analysis of frequency-modulated and complex sounds by single auditory neurones of bats. J. Physiol. 198, 51-80.

Suga, N. (1969a). Classification of inferior collicular neurones of bats in terms of responses to pure tones, FM sounds and noise bursts. J. Physiol. 200, 555-574.

Suga, N. (1969b). Echolocation and evoked potentials of bats after ablation of inferior colliculus. J. Physiol. 203, 707-728.

Suga, N. (1969c). Echolocation of bats after ablation of auditory cortex. J. Physiol. 203, 729-739.

Suga, N. (1970). Echo-ranging neurons in the inferior colliculus of bats. Science 170, 449-452.

Suga, N. (1971). Responses of inferior collicular neurones of bats to tone bursts with different rise times. J. Physiol. 217, 159-177.

Suga, N., and Katsuki, Y. (1961). Central mechanism of hearing in insects. J. Exp. Biol. 38, 545-558.

Suga, N., and Schlegel, P. (1972) Neural attenuation of responses to emitted sounds in echolocating bats. Science 177, 82-84.

Suga, N., and Schlegel, P. (1973) Coding and processing in the nervous system of FM signal producing bats. J. Acoust. Soc. Amer. (In press).

Tavolga, W.N. (1960). Sound production and underwater communication in fishes. In: Animal Sounds and Communication, (W.E. Lanyon and W.N. Tavolga, eds.), pp. 93-136. Am. Inst. Biol. Sci. Press, Washington, D.C.

Walker, T.J. (1958). Cited by Dumortier, B. In: Acoustic Behavior of Animals, (R.G. Busnel, ed.), pp. 583-654. Elsevier, New York.

Watanabe, T., and Ohgushi, K. (1968). FM sensitive auditory neuron. Proc. Jap. Acad. 44, 968-973.

Whitfield, I.C., and Evans, E.F. (1965). Responses of auditory cortical neurons to stimuli of changing frequency. J. Neurophysiol. 28, 655-672.

Winter, P., Ploog, D., and Latta, J. (1966). Vocal repertoire of the squirrel monkey (Saimiri sciureus), its analysis and significance. Exp. Brain Res. 1, 359-384.

Yanagisawa, K., Hashimoto, T., and Katsuki, Y. (1967). Frequency discrimination in the central nerve cords of locusts. J. Insect Physiol. 13, 635-643.

Figures 2, 6, 10, 11, 12, 14, 15 reproduced by permission of the Journal of Physiology.

DISCUSSION

DALLOS: If I understand you correctly you refer to one of your plots as an N_1 "audiogram". How can that be obtained? My understanding of the N_1 is that it is a response to the onset transient in the signal, and especially in the frequency range where you are operating, the actual carrier frequency of the burst has a rather small effect on the transient content.

SUGA: Yes, N_1 represents the summation of action potentials first evoked by an acoustic stimulus. When a stimulus rise time is shortened, the amplitude of N_1 becomes large because of a simultaneous excitation of primary auditory neurons and an increase in the number of activated neurons due to scattering of sound energy over neighboring frequencies. The rise time of the tone burst used was 0.5 msec, which is apparently too short. However, the frequency of the sound delivered was very high, so that there were many waves within a rising phase and there was not much spreading of sound energy. We can obtain a reliable audiogram of a bat with such a stimulus. N_1 audiograms measured with the same setup were different from species to species and were related to acoustic behavior of the animals. This is not explained by acoustic transients.

KOHLLÖFFEL: You work with very high frequencies, and you record very sharp tuning curves. Can you be certain that in this frequency range the acoustic system preceding the cochlea, e.g. the middle ear, does not introduce rather sharp resonance?

SUGA: In bats of the genus _Myotis_, the tuning curve with regard to summated neural activity is not very sharp, but some single neurons are. In this case, the sharp tuning curve is obviously not due to the resonance in the middle ear. In _Pteronotus suaprensis_ which was previously called _Chilonycteris_, a sharp tuning curve was obtained for the cochlear microphonic. In this case the sharp curve is probably due to some non-neural events. We do not know the mechanisms for this sharp tuning. Since there is a nice correlation between this sharp tuning and acoustic signals used by the bat for echolocation, this sharp tuning for a specific frequency appears to be essential for echolocation, regardless of its mechanisms.

MICHELSEN: You showed that the hearing is suppressed by the animal's own sound emission. There could also be a central mechanism for enhancing the response to an echo?

SUGA: If the time course of the neural attenuation is very short, the response to an echo may not be suppressed although the response to the outgoing sound is. Then, echo-detection may be improved. However, we do not know whether this neural attenuation actually improves echo-detection. In the lateral lemniscus, there are neurons which show facilitation of responses to the second sound in a paired stimuli. This kind of facilitation may also improve echo-detection.

MICHELSEN: You could also have a gate which was triggered by the emission of a sound and opened at the time when you are anticipating an echo.

SUGA: The contraction of the middle ear muscles and neural attenuation, which occur synchronously with vocalization, may correspond to such a gate. Since efferent fibers in the lateral line system become active immediately before and during an animal's movements (Russell, 1971) the olivo-cochlear bundle of mammals may become active synchronously with vocalization, and may attenuate self-stimulation.

Reference

Russell, I.J. (1971). The role of the lateral-line efferent system in Xenopus laevis. J. Exp. Biol. 54, 621-641.

PATTERNS OF ACTIVITY OF SINGLE NEURONS OF THE AUDITORY CORTEX IN MONKEY

John F. Brugge and Michael M. Merzenich[1]

University of Wisconsin
Madison, Wisconsin
USA

1. Introduction

The location and extent of auditory cortex on the superior temporal gyrus of primates have been studied repeatedly over the past half century. Results from evoked potential studies especially, have shown us some of the topographic organization of this region and have laid much of the ground work for more detailed mapping studies using microelectrode recording methods. The results of these experiments, as illuminating as they often are, alone give few clues as to the functional properties of single elements making up a cortical field. However, they do provide a frame of reference within which functional properties of single neurons can be studied. In this paper we summarize some of our major findings both as regards the organization of cortical fields and the properties of single neurons within them.

2. Results

2.1 Representation of the Cochlear Partition on the Superior Temporal Plane

Methods

We have employed microelectrode recording methods to study in detail the topographic organization of the auditory projection area of the superior temporal

---

[1] Present Address: University of California, School of Medicine, Coleman Memorial Laboratory, HSE-863, San Francisco Medical Center, San Francisco, California 94122.

plane in macaque monkeys (M. arctoides and M. mulatta). Details of our study are published elsewhere (Merzenich and Brugge, 1973) and we only briefly describe here major features of the experiments. Action potentials from single neurons or neuron clusters are recorded with tungsten microelectrodes in the superior temporal plane of monkeys under barbiturate anesthesia. The supratemporal plane is exposed by removing overlying parietal cortex making it possible to systematically explore a wide area, to accurately determine the recording sites and to later construct a map of the distribution of the penetrations. Pure tones are delivered to the ears via tubes sealed into the external auditory canals and the best frequency of neurons or neuron clusters is determined at several depths within each penetration. Since the majority of neurons in any given electrode penetration have similar best frequencies it is possible to assign an average best frequency value to each recording site. With few exceptions best frequencies of neurons within any given penetration departed from this average value by less than 0.1 octave. After the experiment the brain is perfused and embedded in celloidin. Serial sections are stained with thionin. Electrode penetrations are identified in these sections and the distribution of recording sites thereby related to the cytoarchitecture of the superior temporal plane.

Primary Auditory Cortex

There is on the superior temporal plane a prominent elevation that is bounded rostromedially by the inferior limiting sulcus and often caudally and rostrally by a shallow dimple (Fig. 1A). A major portion of this elevation comprises a relatively distinct field of cortex that can easily be discerned in Nissl stained material (especially in sections cut in the sagittal plane). This cortical field is often referred to as "koniocortex". The major features of its cellular structure, which when taken together distinguish it from surrounding cortex, are (1) a dense population of small cells and blurring of the laminar pattern in layers II-IV, (2) a broad layer V sparsely populated with small and medium size pyramidal cells and (3) a well defined dense layer VI. Over the crown of the elevation, where the outer strata are most densely packed and layer V is particularly broad, one

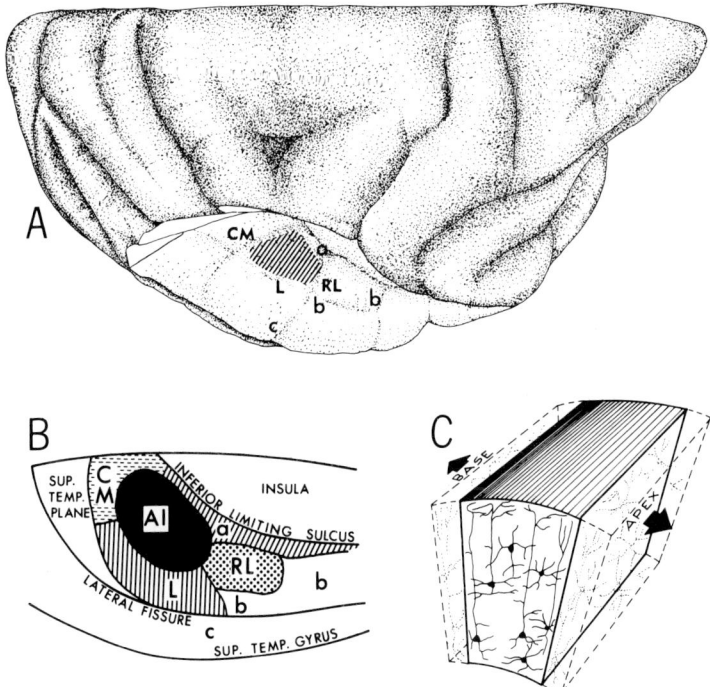

Fig. 1 A. Dorsal view of the monkey brain with parietal cortex removed to show the position and extent of primary auditory cortex (cross hatching) on the superior temporal plane. AI = primary auditory field; RL= rostrolateral field; L = lateral field; CM = caudomedial field; a = field bordering AI medially and rostrally mostly buried in the inferior limiting sulcus; b = wide area of cortex rostral and lateral to other defined fields; c = lateral surface of the superior temporal plane.

B. Schematic drawing of the superior temporal plane showing major subdivisions based upon cytoarchitectonic and physiological observations. Abbreviations same as those used in A.

C. Drawing to illustrate the manner in which a small region of the cochlear partition is represented in a segment of auditory cerebral cortex.

most easily recognizes the vertical alignment of cells
that von Economo and Koskinas (1925) describe in man
as the "rainshower formation". This entire field is
considered to be the primary receiving area of afferent fibers from the medial geniculate body. It can
be considered the homologue of area AI in cat (Rose,
1949, Rose and Woolsey, 1949) and comprises a portion
of the primary field desribed by Woolsey and Walzl
(1944) and Kennedy (1955) on the basis of evoked potential experiments. It is likely homologous to area
TC as described by von Economo in man (1927). In macaque monkeys it has been described by Bonin and Bailey (1947) and more recently by Sanides (1972). Within this cortical field there is a complete and orderly representation of the cochlear partition.

Surface maps from four experiments are shown in Fig.
2. In each experiment only a portion of the supratemporal plane was explored in detail. Each number on
the map is the center frequency value (in kHz) for
neurons isolated in a vertical penetration at that
site. The dotted lines are the approximate cytoarchitectonic boundaries of the primary auditory field.
These experiments taken together illustrate that the
frequency range over which a monkey is known to hear
is represented within the bounds of the primary field,
defined cytoarchitectonically. Lowest best frequencies
are represented rostrolaterally in the primary field;
they increase systematically at successively more
caudal and medial penetration sites. Highest octaves
are represented in the caudomedial aspect of the
field. Furthermore, points having the same or nearly
the same best frequency are arranged along a line.
Such isofrequency lines can be easily drawn, for
example, for the 1.0 and 2.0 kHz points in Fig. 2A.

Since neurons with very similar best frequencies are
also arrayed vertically with respect to one another
(Hind et al., 1960, Gerstein and Kiang, 1964, Abeles
and Goldstein, 1970) we can suggest that at sound
pressure levels near threshold the resultant motion
of a small region on the basilar membrane ultimately
leads to excitation of a relatively small population
of neurons that can be viewed as being arranged in a
band having dimensions of length, depth and width
(Fig. 1C). When frequency of a tone changes, the
position of the band shifts accordingly. When sound
pressure levels are raised the contour of the band

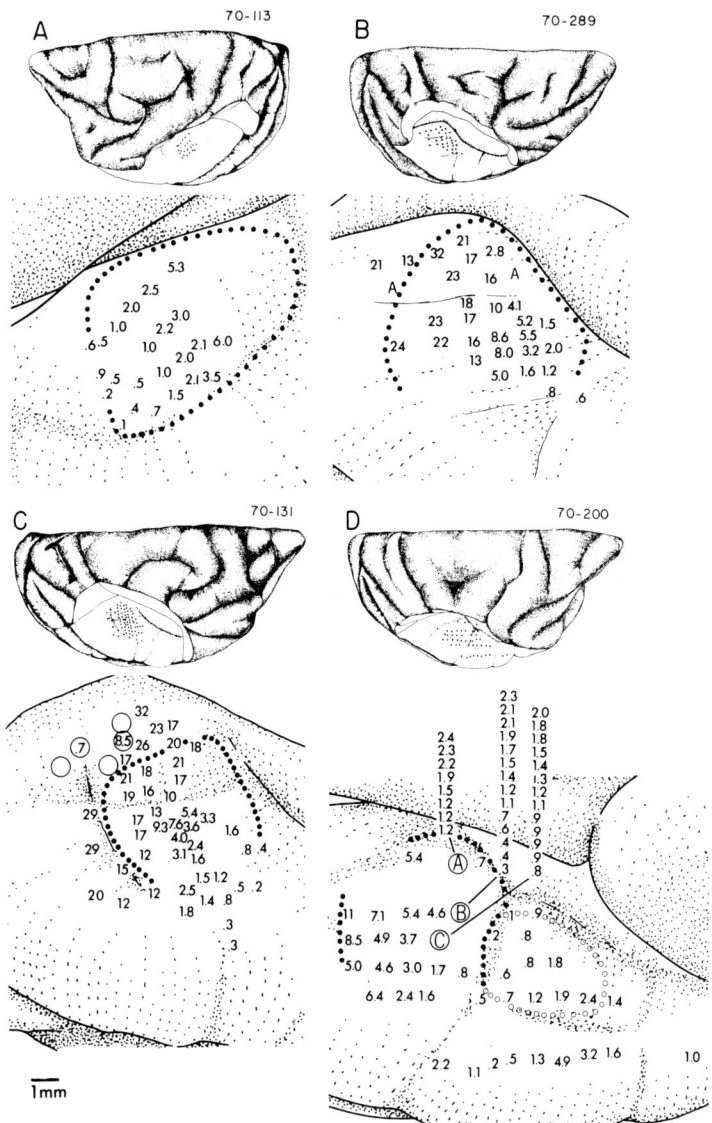

Fig. 2 Surface maps from four experiments showing the distribution of best frequencies obtained in microelectrode penetrations into the superior temporal plane. The drawing above each map shows the exposed superior temporal plane with the pattern of electrode penetrations established in the experiment repre- (cont'd)

(Fig. 2, cont'd) sented by an array of dots. Number on the map corresponds to a dot on the drawing and is the average best frequency (in kHz) of neurons encountered in a penetration at that site. The approximate boundaries of the primary field are outlined by a dotted line. Field RL is enclosed by a line of open circles in D. Large open circles in C indicate sites where neurons were found that responded to tones but for which best frequencies could not be determined. The letter A on a map indicates that best frequency was determined at only one cortical depth.

will change as nearby neurons with different best frequencies and with response areas of different profiles are successively recruited into the active population. More than 20 years ago Tunturi (1950, 1952) drew attention to isofrequency strips of auditory cortex in the dog and from strychnine evoked potential experiments presented data to show that a gradient in responsiveness may exist along them. Later in this paper we describe some of the properties of cortical neurons that suggest that frequency organization may be just one part of an organizing principle that may include the dimension of sound intensity and the location of a sound source in space.

Even though the topographical pattern of best frequencies can be seen on surface maps, the highly contoured surface of the superior temporal plane introduces errors into such a two-dimensional representation. On the other hand, an electrode that penetrates some distance within the most active cortical layers gives a far more accurate picture of the tonotopical organization that exists there. Results of three such penetrations which passed down the anterior wall of the elevation within middle cortical layers are shown in Fig. 2D. The columns of numbers are best frequencies of neurons obtained at regular intervals over a distance of 1 to 2 mm. Best frequencies make up regular high to low progressions, in one case covering three octaves, as the elctrode approaches the rostral border of AI.

Cortical Fields Surrounding AI

Boundaries between cortical fields are often not sharply defined anatomically and thus, when a penetration is made in the boundary region, there is always a question as to what field it should be assigned. The boundaries between fields can be made to stand out more clearly if best frequency determinations are made across cytoarchitectural border regions and the boundaries assigned on the basis of anatomical and physiological data taken together. On this basis the primary auditory field can be separated from the rest of auditory cortex around it. This surrounding belt is itself not uniform in cellular structure and the electrophysiological data have suggested a way that it can be parcelled into several divisions (Fig. 1B).

Contiguous with AI rostrolaterally is a small cortical field (RL) that can be separated from the primary field largely on the basis of physiological data. In approaching this field within AI best frequency declines in a regular way reaching a minimum value in the boundary region between the fields then rises again systematically in the rostrolateral field (Fig. 2D). This field has been described by Sanides (his field paAr; 1972). It occupies a position that would correspond to area EP in new-world monkeys and cat (Woolsey, 1972).

Laterally, AI merges with the lateral field (L). The progression of best frequencies parallels that in the primary field, i.e. low frequencies are represented rostrally and high frequencies caudally. The boundary is difficult to discern cytoarchitectonically in sections cut in the sagittal plane but there is little doubt that some of the most lateral penetrations in Figs. 2C and 2D can be assigned to this field. It probably comprises a portion of the region referred to in man as field TB by von Economo (1927) and in the macaque monkey as field TA by Bonin and Bailey (1947) and field paAH by Sanides (1972).

A caudomedial field (CM) stands in contrast to AI cytoarchitectonically. Its position on the superior temporal plane relative to AI suggests that it be considered the homologue of area AII (Woolsey, 1972). If this is so then the field has probably not been mapped completely and likely extends onto the overlying parietal cortex. The field appears to be homologous with a portion of area TD of von Economo (1927) and with at least a portion of field paAC of

Sanides (1972) in macaque monkey.

Medial to AI, and in the inferior limiting sulcus is an auditory field (labelled a in Fig. 1B). This field, along with those labelled b and c, are activated by acoustic stimulation but have not been studied in any detail.

2.2 Response Properties of Single Neurons in Unanesthetized Monkeys

Methods

Young monkeys (M. mulatta) weighing between five and eight pounds are used. They are handled on a leash and trained to sit quietly in a primate chair in a soundproof room for several hours each day with their heads rigidly held by stainless steel sockets that have been previously implanted into their skulls. Between these daily training sessions they are usually returned to their individual home cages. The monkeys are fed in the restraining chair and after a few weeks most of them require little coaxing into it. Once the animal has learned to sit quietly for several hours daily a plastic chamber is implanted to support a microdrive which guides a glass-insulated platinum-iridium electrode through dura mater and overlying parietal cortex into the superior temporal plane.

Sounds are delivered through plastic tubes that are sealed into soft molds which in turn fit snuggly into the outer ear and canal. The other end of each plastic tube is connected to shallow metal cavities over the front surfaces of the dynamic earphones. The advantages of this system are that it is comfortable for the animal and that sounds can be routed to each ear independently.

Data from isolated neurons are recorded on analogue tape, then later reduced to digital form and analyzed using a LINC computer.

We watch the animals closely on a televison monitor.

Excitability of single neurons

While the monkeys' heads are rigidly held the animals are, within limits, free to move their limbs, torso and mouth. Thus, it is not uncommon for them to stretch, groom, shake, yawn and chew during recording sessions. These movements, as small as they often appear to be, many times have a profound effect upon the excitability of isolated neurons (Fig. 3). Middle ear muscles are known to be active during body movements and it is possible that this action contributes to the apparent reduction of effectiveness of a tonal stimulus. (Galambos and Rupert, 1959, Carmel and Starr, 1963).

Under these experimental conditions monkeys very often become drowsy and sleep soundly after several hours of sitting in a quiet room. The effect of sleep on the discharge of a neuron is often dramatic. One example is shown in Fig. 3. In this neuron the spike count during slow-wave sleep is reduced by 60 % below that obtained in the waking state. In several experiments in which EEG recordings were made simultaneously with single unit recordings the decrease in excitability during epochs of slow-wave sleep continued as the animal drifted in and out of periods of REM sleep characterized by low-voltage fast activity and rapid eye movements.

Relation between spike-count and SPL

It is a common finding in our experiments that as the SPL at one ear (usually the contralateral one) is raised the number of spikes evoked by the tone increases to a maximum value and then decreases. The functions obtained can be sharply peaked and a change of 10 dB on either side of the most effective SPL can reduce the count by as much as 90 % of its maximum value (Fig. 9 inset). Raising or lowering SPL further, results in spike-counts that approach the number obtained when no stimulus is delivered to the ear. On the other hand, there are cells that give nearly maximal responses over a broad range of SPL and while the count drops at high intensity we usually are un-

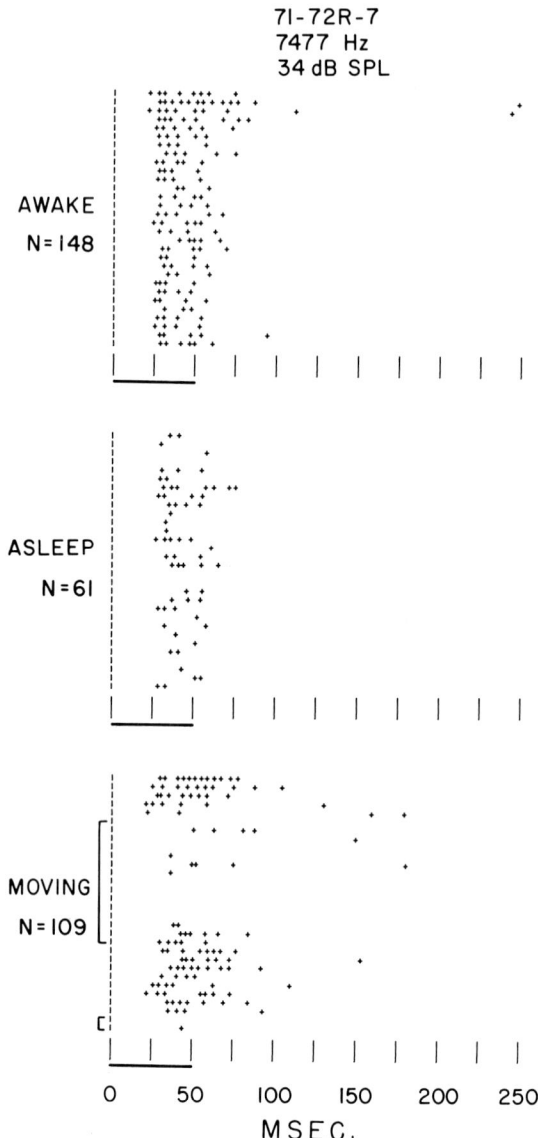

Fig. 3 Firing patterns of a single cortical neuron during periods when the monkey was (a) awake but sitting quietly, (b) sleeping, and (c) awake but making small body movements. N = number of spikes during the first 100 msec. of the discharge. Contralateral ear (cont'd)

(Fig. 3, cont'd) was stimulated alone at 34 dB SPL. Tone duration: 50 msec. Repetition rate: 1/sec. In these dot displays and all others the short vertical bars to the left indicate the onset of the stimulus. The occurrence of an action potential is indicated by a dot. Horizontal bar below each display indicates the tone length. SPL in this and all other figures re: .0002 dyne/cm^2.

able to reduce it to the level of spontaneous activity. Spike-count functions from the same animal actually form what appears to be a continuum and the ones mentioned above seem to form the extremes. Thus, in any given animal there is a population of neurons which, at best frequency, are very sensitive to changes in SPL; another population is relatively insensitive to these changes and between them is a population with intermediate sensitivity.

We studied the responses to changes in SPL in 41 neurons and in 36 of them could determine the most effective SPL. Fig. 4A shows normalized spike-count functions for four units in one monkey. The most effective SPLs range from about 20 to 85 dB. The distribution of most effective SPLs for the entire sample population is shown in Fig. 4B. As is seen there the range of most effective SPLs is from 15 to 94 dB SPL. It probably extends to higher levels. However, these levels have not been explored systematically since the range of our earphones did not extend beyond 90 dB SPL at most stimulus frequencies. Thus, the intensity functions for four units included in Fig. 4B never reached a maximum value. These data would suggest that regardless of where the stimulus lies within the dynamic range of the ear there exists a population of cortical neurons that is firing maximally. Other pools of cells will be firing at submaximal rates; still others will be virtually silent or at spontaneous level because the SPL is either too high or too low. Changing SPL results in a shift in the active neuron pool and many neurons once most active become less so and many of those once marginally active are brought to maximal response. Whether the most effective SPL at best frequency will also be most effective at other frequencies within the response area will be known only when the full profile of a cortical neuron can be obtained. Neverthe-

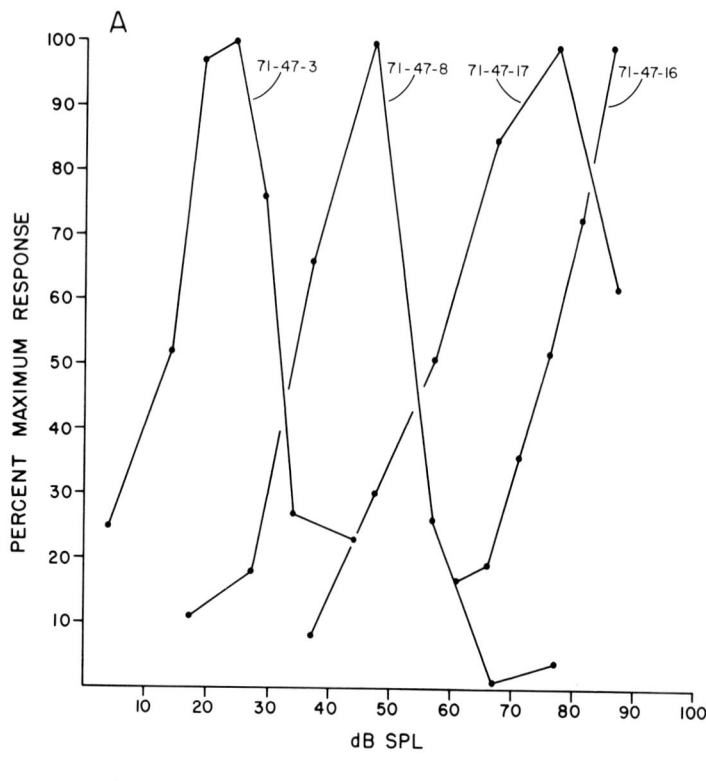
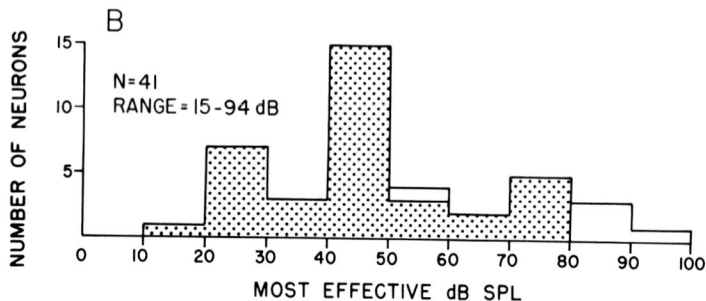

Fig. 4 A. Normalized spike-count functions for four neurons in the same animal at best frequency. B. Distribution of the most effective SPL at best frequency for 41 neurons in 9 hemispheres in 8 monkeys. Peak response covers a range of nearly 80 dB. Open bars indicate five neurons whose spike-count function had not reached maximum values at those SPLs. Abscissa: SPL at contralateral ear alone.

less it is intriguing to us to consider a neuron as being sensitive to a narrow range of SPL since it implies that SPL may be represented by a "place" in central auditory structures.

Firing Patterns of Single Neurons

Neurons in auditory cortex may develop very complex response areas that reflect converging excitatory and inhibitory inputs from various sources that interact both temporally and spacially. Fig. 5 presents data

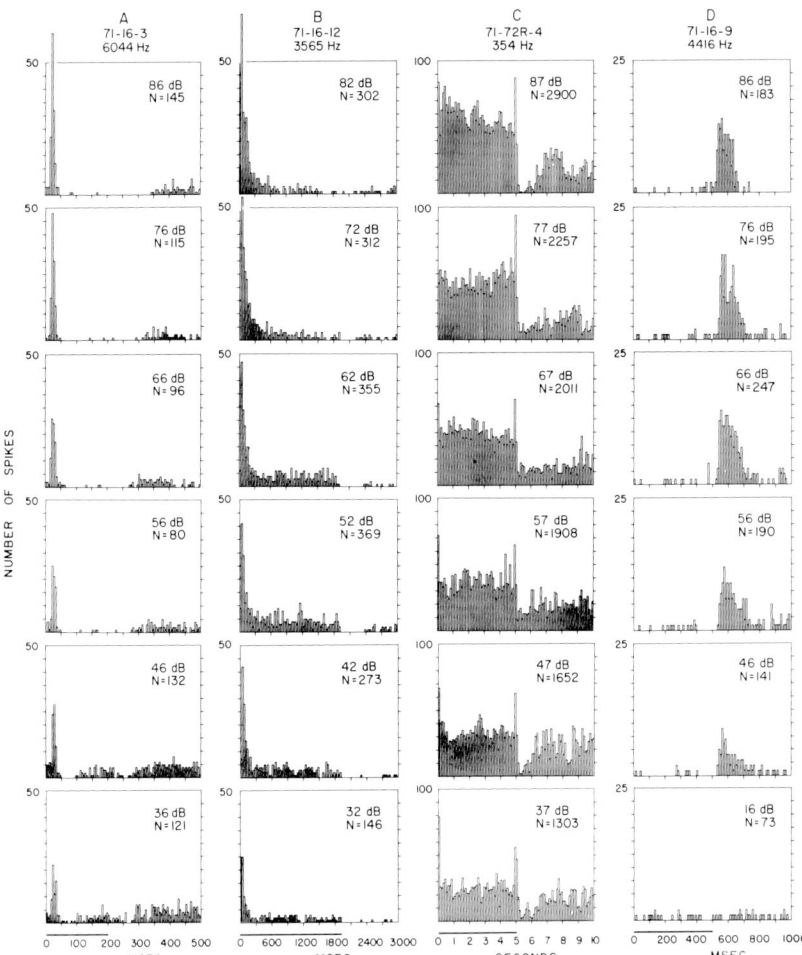

Fig. 5 Response histograms showing the firing patterns of four cortical neurons at different SPLs at best frequency. Horizontal bar represents the tone duration for all histograms in that column. N= total number of spikes during the tone. Number of stimulus repetitions: A:100, B:20, C:5, D:20.

from four neurons at best frequency showing the kinds of response profiles that can be recorded. There are, of course, variants of these and many intermediate patterns can be obtained even within the response area of a single neuron. Gerstein and Kiang (1964) earlier recognized the variety of firing patterns that can be obtained from a single cortical neuron when sounds such as clicks and noise are employed. In our experiments it is rare to find a neuron that generates only one or two spikes in response to a tonal stimulus although this is a common response in animals under anesthesia. Occasionally a unit is found that fires a brief burst of spikes followed by a silent period and resumption of spontaneous activity (Fig. 5A). Commonly, however, the cell responds at best frequency with a high discharge rate that adapts to a low level over a period of less than one second (Fig. 5B). A few cells have relatively high rates (about 40/sec) at favorable frequencies and SPLs and these rates can be sustained for relatively long periods of time (Fig. 5C). Fig. 5D shows a response frequently seen although the details of the pattern differ from one cell to the next. A tone of best frequency may be ineffective, or may reduce spontaneous activity. This is followed by a fairly vigorous response when the tone is turned off. The "off" response can be transient in nature or can be sustained for several hundred milliseconds.

Some cortical mechanisms involved in binaural hearing

A human listener can normally locate with considerable accuracy the source of the sound he hears. He may utilize a number of cues, some of them quite subtle, to determine both its direction and distance. Among those cues are the difference in sound pressure at the two ears caused by the acoustic shadow of the head and the difference in time of arrival of the stimulus at the two ears. The former depends upon the azimuth at higher frequencies and, in man, can amount to nearly 20 dB (Stevens and Davis, 1938). The mechanisms of interaction of inputs from the two ears have been studied at lower levels of the auditory system in areas where neurons are likely receiving convergent input (Rose et al., 1966, Goldberg and Brown, 1969, Brugge et al., 1970). Thus, while cells in auditory cerebral cortex do not appear to be primary sites of convergent input from the two ears their integrity in man and in animals appears essential for normal binaural hearing (Neff et al., 1956, Masterton and Diamond, 1964, Jerger et al., 1969, Cranford et al., 1971).

When a cortical neuron is excited by a pure tone delivered to just one ear it is usual, but by no means the rule, that stimulation of the contralateral ear is more effective than stimulation of the ipsilateral ear in evoking a discharge. Frequently, stimulation of the ipsilateral ear alone appears to be without effect especially when the level of spontaneous activity is low. However, when the stimulus is routed to the two ears, a tone that appears to be ineffective when delivered to one ear alone, is often shown to have a very powerful influence on the discharge of the neuron. The degree to which converging inputs evoked by stimulation of the two ears interact depends critically upon the sound pressure level at the two ears and when low frequency tones are employed upon the relative times at which the tones arrive at the two ears (Brugge et al., 1969).

Figs. 6 and 7 present data from a neuron studied at its best frequency of about 350 Hz. It had a moderate level of spontaneous activity and the effect of stimulating each ear alone was hardly impressive, especially at low SPL. When the tone was delivered to both ears in phase the discharge rate increased markedly even at SPLs where monaural stimulation appeared to be ineffective. Thus, the apparent threshold of this cell was at least 10 dB lower when the two ears were stimulated in phase than when each ear was stimulated alone. Furthermore, the effect was seen over a range of some 60 dB. Switching the tones 180° out of phase resulted in a spike-count function midway between the functions obtained when each ear was stimulated alone.

At low frequencies cortical neurons can be extraordinarily sensitive to small changes in the time of arrival of the stimulus at the two ears. Fig. 8 shows data from one neuron obtained at two frequencies and several sound pressure levels. The spike count is a periodic function of interaural time delay. The period of the function is equal to the period of the stimulating tone. The functions each reach a maximum value when the ipsilateral ear stimulus is delayed

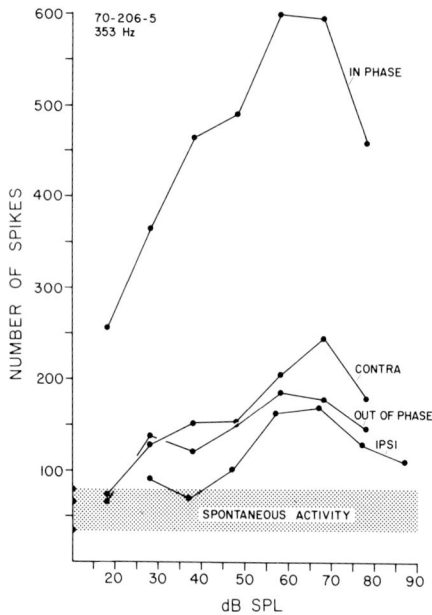

Fig. 6 Spike-count functions for a cortical neuron at best frequency of 353 Hz. Tone was delivered to each ear individually and to both ears in and out of phase. Tone duration: 320 msec. Repetition rate: 1/sec. Ordinate: total number of spikes during tone in 20 stimulus repetitions. For binaural stimulation the SPL at the ipsilateral ear was 9 dB greater than at the contralateral ear. Abscissa for binaural curves is for the ipsilateral ear SPL.

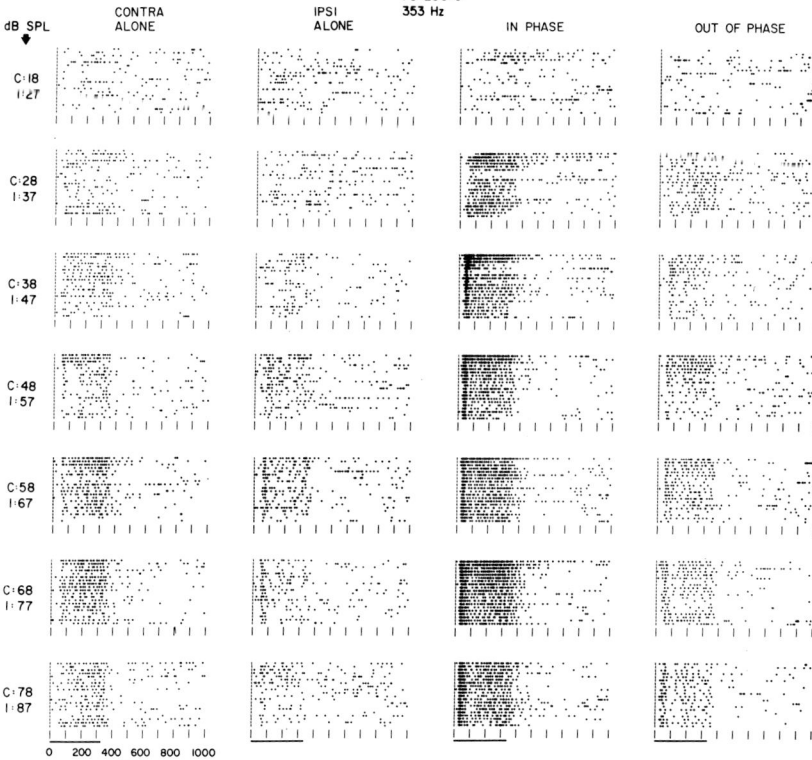

Fig. 7 Firing patterns of cortical neuron whose spike-count functions are shown in Fig. 6.

by 0 to 200 μsec and this remains relatively constant over a wide range of SPLs. Neurons exhibiting this behavior detect absolute interaural time delays and are said to have a "characteristic delay" (Rose et al., 1966).

The existence of neurons capable of detecting an absolute time delay suggests that the direction of a sound source may be represented in the auditory system by a place. However, the exact locus of the source is ambiguous if only time cues are employed and, indeed, complete localization of low-frequency tones is very difficult. Since most sounds in nature are complex there are usually available to the listener additional cues, and cells in auditory cortex are known to be sensitive to one of them (Brugge et al., 1969).

Fig. 9 presents data from two neurons that were extremely sensitive to small interaural shifts of

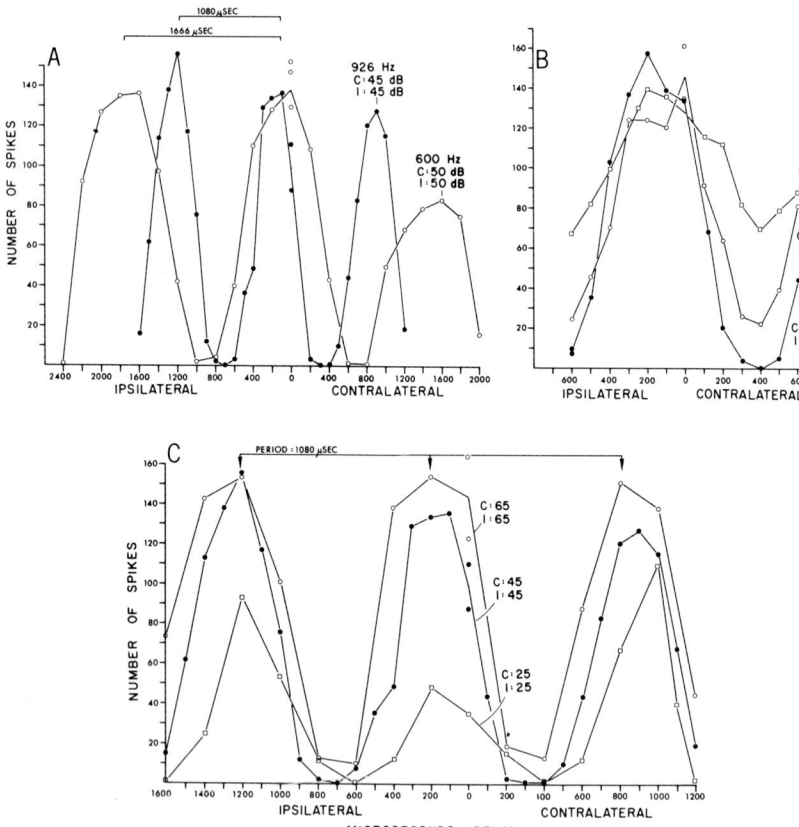

Fig. 8 Periodic spike-count functions for a single cortical neuron when low frequency tones are delivered to both ears and the time of arrival of one tone is delayed. Tone duration: 100 msec. Repetition rate: 1/sec. SPL of contralateral tone (C) and ipsilateral tone (I) given on figure along with frequency and period of stimulating tones. Ordinate: total number of spikes during tone in 20 stimulus repetitions. Abscissa: Interaural time delay.

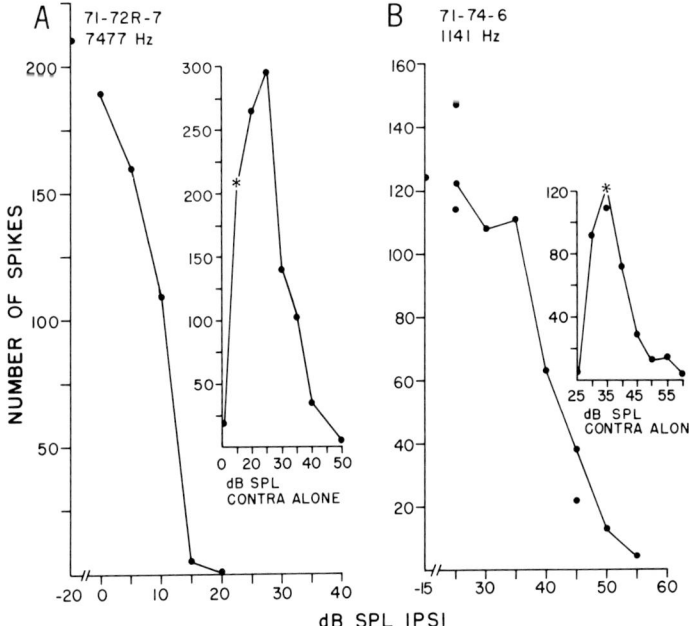

Fig. 9 Spike-count functions for two cortical neurons at best frequency obtained when the contralateral ear was stimulated alone (insets) and when the contralateral ear was stimulated at a constant SPL (star on inset graph) and the SPL at the ipsilateral ear was varied (large graph). Ordinate: total number of spikes during tone in 30 stimulus repetitions. Tone duration: 300 msec. Repetition rate: 1/sec.

SPL. The inset shows the spike-count functions obtained when the contralateral ear was stimulated alone. When sounded alone the ipsilateral stimulus was without observable effect. The larger graph plots the number of spikes evoked when the contralateral ear was held at a constant SPL and the intensity at the ipsilateral ear was raised. The effect is to reduce the number of spikes evoked by 5 % for every 1 dB increase in SPL. The dynamic range is about 20 dB, corresponding to the interaural difference in SPL that could be expected at higher frequencies. It is of interest that such a response is seen at low frequency where in man a small interaural difference may still exist.

Acknowledgments

We express our thanks to JoAnn Eckleberry and Isabel Lucey for preparing histological material, T.P. Stewart for photographic work, Dee Urban for her art work and Michele Mosher for typing the manuscript.

This research was supported by NIH Program Project Grant NS-06225 and NIH Neurophysiology Training Grant NS-05236.

References

Abeles, M., and Goldstein, M.H. (1970). Functional architecture in cat primary auditory cortex: columnar organization and organization according to depth. J. Neurophysiol. 3, 172-187.

Bonin, G.v., and Bailey, P. (1947). The neocortex of Macaca mulatta, in Ill. Monogr. Med. Sci. 4, no. 4, Univ. of Illinois Press, Urbana.

Brugge, J.F., Dubrovsky, N.A., Aitkin, L.M., and Anderson, D.J. (1969). Sensitivity of single neurons in auditory cortex of cat to binaural tonal stimulation; effects of varying intraural time and intensity. J. Neurophysiol., 32, 1005-1024.

Brugge, J.F., Anderson, D.J., and Aitkin, L.M. (1970). Responses of neurons in the dorsal nucleus of the lateral lemniscus of the cat to binaural tonal stimulation. J. Neurophysiol. 33, 441-458.

Carmel, P.W., and Starr, A. (1963). Acoustic and non-acoustic factors modifying middle-ear muscle activity in waking cats. J. Neurophysiol. 26, 598-616.

Cranford, J., Ravizza, R., Diamond, I.T., and Whitfield, I.C. (1971). Unilateral ablation of the auditory cortex in the cat impairs complex sound localization. Science 172, 286-288.

Economo, C.v. (1927). L'Architecture cellulaire normale de l'écorce cérébrale. Masson, Paris.

Economo, C.v., and Koskinas, G.N. (1925). Die Cytoarchitectonik der Hirnrinde des erwachsenen Menschen. Springer-Verlag, Berlin.

Galambos, R., and Rupert, A. (1959). Action of middle ear muscles in normal cats. J. Acoust. Soc. Amer. 31, 349-355.

Gerstein, G.L., and Kiang, N.Y.S. (1964). Responses of single units in the auditory cortex. Exp. Neurol. 10, 1-18.

Goldberg, J.M., and Brown, P.B. (1969). Response of binaural neurons of dog superior olivary complex to dichotic tonal stimuli: some physiological mechanisms of sound localization. J. Neurophysiol. 32, 613-636.

Hind, J.E., Rose, J.E., Davies, P.W., Woolsey, C.N., Benjamin, R.M., Welker, W.I., and Thompson, R.F. (1960). Unit activity in the auditory cortex. In: Neural Mechanisms of the Auditory and Vestibular Systems (G.L. Rasmussen and W. Windle, eds.) C.C. Thomas, Springfield, Ill.

Jerger, J., Weikers, N.J., Sharbrough, F.W., and Jerger, S. (1969). Bilateral lesions of the temporal lobe. A case study. Acta Oto-Laryngol, Suppl. 258.

Kennedy, T.T.K. (1955). An electrophysiological study of the auditory projection areas of the cortex in monkey (Macaca mulatta). Thesis. Univ. of Chicago.

Merzenich, M.M., and Brugge, J.F. (1973). Representation of the cochlear partition on the superior temporal plane of the macaque monkey. Brain Res. (In press).

Masterton, R.B., and Diamond, I.T. (1964). Effects of auditory cortex ablation on discrimination of small binaural time differences. J. Neurophysiol. 27, 15-36.

Neff, D., Fisher, J.F., Diamond, I.T., and Yela, M. (1956). Role of auditory cortex in a discrimination requiring localization of sound in space. J. Neurophysiol. 19, 500-512.

Rose, J.E. (1949). The cellular structure of the auditory region of the cat. J. Comp. Neurol. 91, 409-440.

Rose, J.E., and Woolsey, C.N. (1949). The relations of thalamic connections, cellular structure and evokable electrical activity in the auditory region of the cat. J. Comp. Neurol. 91, 441-466.

Rose, J.E., Gross, N.B., Geisler, C.D., and Hind, J.E. (1966). Some neural mechanisms in the inferior colliculus of the cat which may be relevant to localization of a sound source. J. Neurophysiol. 29, 288-314.

Sanides, F. (1972). Representation in the cerebral cortex of its areal lamination patterns. In: Structure and Function of Nervous Tissue, Vol. 5. Academic Press, New York.

Stevens, S.S., and Davis, H. (1938). Hearing. Its Psychology and Physiology. Wiley, London.

Tunturi, A.R. (1950). Physiological determination of the arrangement of the afferent connections to the middle ectosylvian auditory area in the dog. Amer. J. Physiol. 162, 489-502.

Tunturi, A.R. (1952). A difference in the representation of auditory signals for the left and right ears in the iso-frequency contours of the right middle ectosylvian auditory cortex of the dog. Amer. J. Physiol. 168, 712-727.

Woolsey, C.N., and Walzl, E.M. (1944). Topical projection of the cochlea to the cerebral cortex of the monkey. Amer. J. Med. Sci. 207, 685-686.

Woolsey, C.N. (1972). Tonotopic organization of the auditory cortex. In: Physiology of the Auditory System, A Workshop (M.B. Sachs, ed.). National Educational Consultants, Baltimore.

DISCUSSION

KATSUKI: How many neurons did you get in one single penetration?

BRUGGE: It would vary. In a good experiment we should have one cell and hold it for a long time. In another we could have as many as 7 or 8 units.

KATSUKI: How long did you hold the response?

BRUGGE: The record is about 3 or 4 hours. We perhaps have a handful of cells out of the 90 that we have studied that we could hold for more than an hour or so. It is not unusual to hold one for half an hour.

DAVIS: I was very much impressed by the precision of the anatomical locations, the tonotopic orderliness of the best frequencies, and in general the close relation between the positivity that you observe and the parameters of the stimulus. You have alluded to the difference between waking and sleeping. Can you tell us about effects of different types of anesthesia? We are all well aware of how important a parameter this has been in the earlier corresponding animal experiments and the mapping of cortical fields. Please also say something about the relation to the slow cortical responses such as we are using in audiometry.

BRUGGE: I can not give you any insights on slow cortical responses. I can only tell a little bit about anesthesia. On one occasion we studied a unit in the unanesthetized animal and then later, gave barbiturate anesthetic. The effect was a very dramatic one. The unit became virtually unresponsive. We have looked at cortical neurons under anesthesia in the past. Generally speaking we find cells in the auditory cortex far more active in the awake than in the anesthetized animal.

As far as the question of the origin of the various waves in the scalp evoked potential is concerned, we have not really directed our attention to this problem. The later waves that Dr. Davis has been studying, seem not to have an obvious counterpart in our data, but that may be simply because we have not studied cortical responses under conditions most favorable for revealing them.

DAVIS: The human slow wave that I am asking about is scalp-negative at 100, positive at 200 msec, roughly. It has a strangely long refractory period with the halftime recovery of amplitude at about 2 sec. You could miss it completely unless you look for it. I am not sure that animals give an analogous response.

BRUGGE: The organization of auditory cortex in man is likely to be similar to that in the rhesus monkey. Those interested in EEG audiometry might find the monkey to be a very useful model for experimental work. I would be very interested to know whether anyone has recorded evoked potentials from the scalp of monkey or if this is something you think should be followed up.

DAVIS: It would be extremely helpful to many people if you could determine whether these slow evoked potentials are there in this kind of preparation and to find out whether they come specifically from the auditory cortex or not. The earlier waves that we can also record from the same electrode positions have quite different dynamic properties. You can repeat the stimuli ten times a second without much adaptation of a wave which has a 40 msec peak latency. I think we pass in the cortex a very interesting boundary line here to the totally different slow response. The latter is an on-effect and off-effect; it is not a continuing effect. There is also the dc activity that Keidel and his group have recently described. It persists during continued tonal stimulation.

ZWISLOCKI: You spoke of effects of long time motion on your recordings. Did you find these effects at high frequencies also, or just at low frequencies? This would have something to do with the muscle reflex in the middle ear, I believe.

BRUGGE: What I showed was probably the most dramatic example of the effect by body movement. We have not studied the effect systematically although we have seen it both at high and low frequencies. In our experiments it has been a confounding effect and we have worked hard to get around it.

ZWISLOCKI: Were these intensity functions obtained with short bursts or long duration tones?

BRUGGE: These functions are usually obtained using tone bursts of several hundred msec duration. I did not show the temporal patterns of the spikes. Some were transient responses which may have been to onset of stimulation. Others responded during the full duration of the tone. The counts are taken throughout the tone regardless of the discharge pattern.

ZWISLOCKI: But the normal tonic functions were obtained among others with short, reasonably short bursts?

BRUGGE: Yes, they would be anywhere from 100-500 msec in duration.

PFALZ: You showed that not only frequencies have a certain space on the surface of the cortex, but also the intensity ranges have their certain spaces. Could you tell me something about whether perhaps the neighboring intensity ranges also are neighbors in the cortex, and secondly perhaps whether they are organized in a level paralleling the surface or perhaps in a level vertically arranged to the surface?

BRUGGE: I meant to put that more into the realm of

speculation. First of all, the curves that I showed were taken only at the characteristic frequency. Whether or not a cell responds in this way to changes of sound pressure level at all frequencies to which it is sensitive is right now not known. There are some cells in which the most effective SPL can shift when frequency is changed. I would not want to state at this point that a neuron really has a specific most effective sound pressure level at all of its frequencies. However, if that turned out to be the case, it would be very interesting to know how those SPL's were distributed.

PFALZ: Have you any idea whether a certain layer of the cortex is especially engaged with the intensity problems?

BRUGGE: The neurons that I showed you were recorded at virtually all levels and we have not at this point segregated them.

GREEN: First I would like to ask a short question concerning this phase effect. Could you tell us something about its frequency limit?

BRUGGE: In our experiments we have only seen the effect at frequencies up to about 1500 Hz. It is known from Dr. Rose's experiments that the frequency can go close to 3000 Hz. In experiments that we did a number of years ago (Brugge et al., 1969) we showed that cortical neurons were sensitive to interaural time delays at 2400 Hz.

GREEN: In that respect I would say it parallels more the masking level difference phenomenon. The cutoff frequency would be about 1000 to 2000 Hz. The second question concerns this intensity function and the fact that it is non-monotonic. It seems to me that this raises the question as to what is the best frequency. I guess one way to phrase the question is, are you sure that the best frequency is the same at all intensities? You have an intensity and frequency of the signal as two co-ordinates and then rate as

the third dimension and you must have some idea as
to the general configuration at that space.

BRUGGE: I am simply referring now to best frequency
at threshold SPL. That would be equivalent to the tip
of the tuning curve. It is true of other auditory
synaptic stations that if you look at the whole profile of a cell in its intensity-frequency domain,
the most effective frequency can shift considerably.
It may shift by an octave or more. We have not studied neurons here in sufficient detail to show this.
Perhaps Dr. Rose could comment on it since he perhaps
has seen it too in the cochlear nucleus.

ROSE: Indeed in the dorsal cochlear nucleus, for instance, a dramatic and orderly shift in the most effective frequencies may occur as a function of sound
pressure level. This shift may be either towards
lower of higher frequencies in comparison with the
best frequency at threshold.

EVANS: I want to ask whether you have noticed any
systematic difference between the anesthetized and
unanesthetized preparations in respect to the difficulty of defining a characteristic frequency to
the cells. I ask this because you are aware of the
discrepancy which still exists between your own very
beautiful demonstration of mapping in the cortex,
the primary cortex of the monkey, and these two series of experiments which have been done in the cat.
The main difference besides species is anesthesia.

BRUGGE: In the awake animal normally all of those
cells that we encounter in a single penetration have
very similar best frequencies. It is known that one
can often jump out of that arrangement of best frequencies to a best frequency several octaves away and
then jump back in again. This has not been our experience, so that what we see in the awake animal is
consistent with what we see under anesthesia. I just
would like to comment on the way we did the experiment. I think perhaps it contributes partly to what
appears to be a discrepancy between the sets of data
you refer to. In order to see the overall picture of

the cochlear map, we find that we must do a large part of the work in one animal in a very fine grain. It is not sufficient to get a few points in one animal and then superimpose the results from several experiments. Neither the surface landmarks nor the boundaries of cytoarchitectonic fields themselves are very constant.

SUGA: Do you think there is a possibility that the intensity of the stimulus is expressed by the activity of a certain type of neuron at higher levels, rather than by a discharge rate, because many cortical neurons showed a nonmonotonic impulse-count function.

BRUGGE: It is intriguing to us to think that it might be possible. I do not know how strong the evidence for it is and I do not think that ours is particularly strong. I simply put that out as something that we suggested by our observations.

References

Brugge, J.F., Dubrovsky, N.A., Aitkin, L.M., and Anderson, D.J. (1969). Sensitivity of single neurons in auditory cortex of cat to binaural tonal stimulation; effects of varying intraural time and intensity. J. Neurophysiol. 32, 1005-1024.

Keidel, W.D. (1971). D.C.-potentials in the auditory evoked response in man. Acta Otolaryngol. 71, 242-248.

Rose, J.E., Gross, N.B., Geisler, C.D., and Hind, J.E. (1966). Some neural mechanisms in the inferior colliculus of the cat which may be relevant to localization of a sound source. J. Neurophysiol. 29, 288-314.

EFFERENT CROSSED INHIBITION IN THE VENTRAL COCHLEAR NUCLEI

R. Pfalz

Hals-Nasen-Ohrenklinik der Universität
7900 ULM
Germany

Inhibition of the cochlear nucleus after electrical stimulation of the cortex was shown by Jouvet and Desmedt (1956). This finding stressed the old opinion, that the descending auditory pathways, described as early as 1909 by Cajal may well have a feed-back function. As we know from Cajal (1909) and Lorente de Nó (1933) the ratio of afferent to efferent neurons is promising for more communication between the two systems in the cochlear nuclei than in the cochlea. In 1961 inhibition of single afferent units in the cochlear nucleus by acoustical stimulation of the opposite ear was demonstrated (Pfalz, 1961). Later experiments extended and confirmed these findings (Pirsig and Pfalz, 1967). Meanwhile in 1965, Dunker, et al. were able to show that this crossed efferent inhibition of the cochlear nuclei is partly abolished after cutting of the crossing fibers in the trapezoid body, a finding in harmony with Cajal's (1909) anatomical knowledge. On the basis of these facts the experiments to be reported here were started.

Thirty-nine guinea pigs out of a total of 65 animals yielded reliable results. General anesthesia was induced by a sodium-barbiturate (EVIPAN Bayer), and complete immobilization by curare (HAF). The left cochlea had one of its four turns fenestrated as shown in Fig. 2. In the region of fenestration the organ of Corti was removed. The perilymph was drained. A bipolar electrode grasped the spiral osseous lamina. Single rectangular shocks of a length of 0.05 msec and a strength of 2.0 to 5.0 V stimulated an area of 500-1000 of the primary afferents under the electrode. The width of the stimulated area corre-

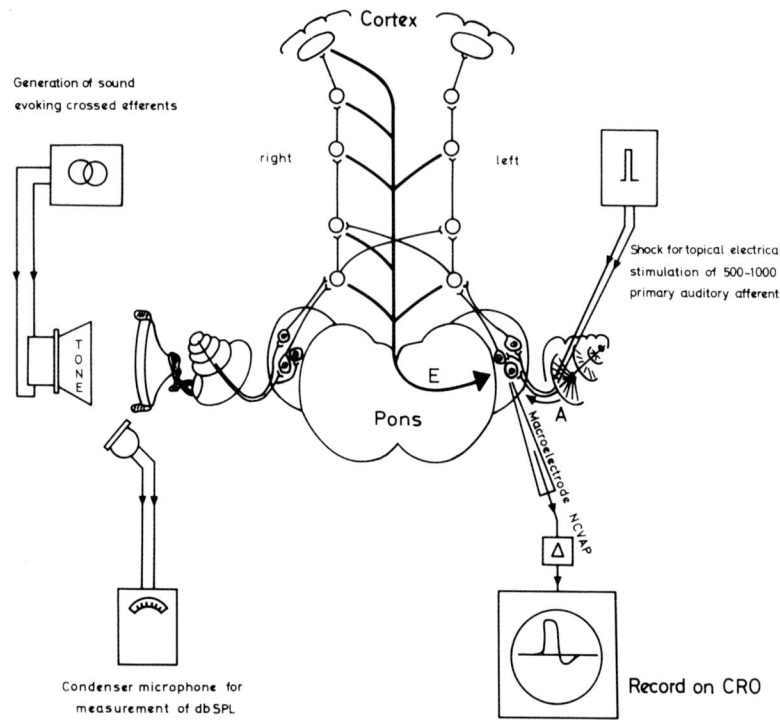

Fig. 1 Experimental arrangement. Three ganglion cells on either side represent the ventral cochlear nucleus (NCV) of the guinea pig. Single shocks to the left spiral osseous lamina will evoke a compound afferent action potential in the left nucleus (NCVAP). The NCVAP can be allocated to pitch for the place of electrical stimulations is known at the lamina. The left cochlea no longer responds to sound because it is prepared as shown in Fig. 2. Pure tones to the right intact ear, therefore, will stimulate exclusively the right ear. No afferent pathways from the right ear to the left NCV are known. Nevertheless, sound at the right inhibited the afferent NCVAP at the left. The inhibition was completely abolished by ear wax in the right meatus and recurred after removal of the wax. This inhibition, therefore, is assumed to have been transmitted by crossed auditory efferent fibers (E) to the ventral cochlear nucleus. (From Pfalz, 1969).

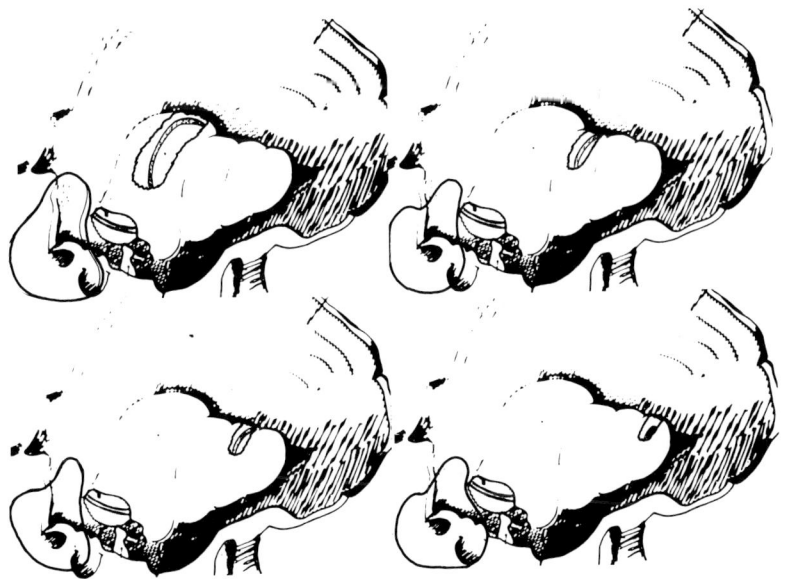

Fig. 2 Left cochlea of guinea pig as exposed and prepared in the present experiments. The animal is on its back. The four types of fenestration of the cochlea in the different turns are drawn using a diagram of von Békésy (1944). At the lower left of each picture the place has been indicated from where the ventral cochlear nucleus (NCV) was reached by drilling.(From Pfalz, 1969).

sponded to approximately the musical interval of a quint. The evoked compound action potential (AP) was picked up from the left ventral cochlear nucleus (VCN). The position of the tip of the 100-micron steel wire electrode was traced in 12 out of the 39 guinea pigs by serial histology. The AP of the ventral cochlear nucleus (VCNAP) could be correlated to a certain frequency range because the place of stimulation was known in the cochlea. This was defined on the basis of the data given by von Békésy (1944), Fernandez (1952) and Tasaki et al. (1952).

The experimental situation could be kept constant for ten to twenty hours. During this time pure tones were applied to the intact right eardrum. Pure tones of more than 40 dB SPL on the right would, as a rule, strongly inhibit the shock-evoked AP in the left ventral cochlear nucleus. The crossed inhibition disappeared after obstruction of the right external auditory meatus by artificial ear wax. Inhibition also disappeared 20 to 90 sec after i.v. injection of 0.35-1.00 ml of a 0.1 % solution of strychnine nitrate (Pirsig and Pfalz, 1967).

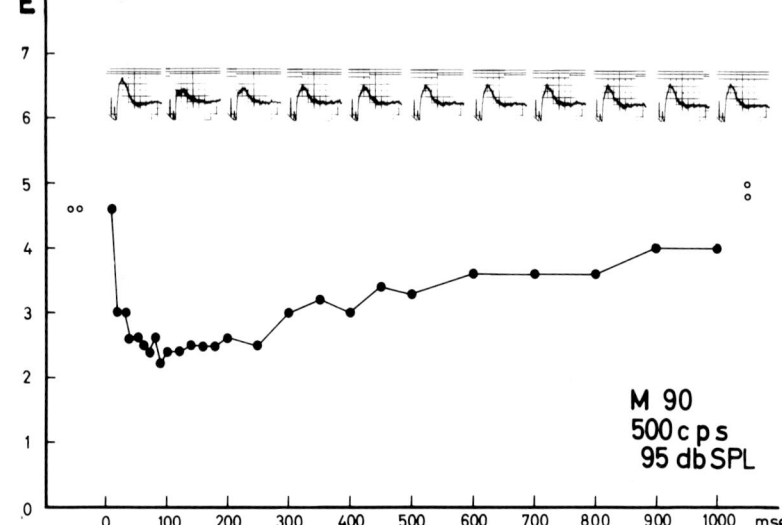

Fig. 3 Time course of the crossed auditory efferent inhibition in the ventral cochlear nucleus (NCV) <u>during</u> continued sound stimulation by 500 Hz/95 dB SPL. Ordinate: amplitude of the negative compound afferent action potential in the left NCV in relative units of the CRO-screen, of which ten photographs were included in the diagram at the moment of their registration above the curve. For each of the 30 dots of the curve a corresponding photograph had to be taken. Empty circles represent the amplitude of the afferent NCVAP without contralateral exposure to sound, i.e. without crossed efferent inhibitory interaction. (From Pfalz, 1969).

Some data on the crossed efferent inhibition may be interesting: latency was 5-15 msec at medium and high sound intensities; inhibition was less than 50 % in 13 guinea pigs, more than 50 % in 11 guinea pigs and 100 % in 15 guinea pigs; time course of inhibition was slow, inhibition after latency climbing up only within 80-100 msec to its maximum; phasic exponential decline after the inhibitory maximum brought inhibition to a steady state after 300-1000 msec, although the tone at the opposite ear was still present. After offset of tone, inhibition needed 30-80 msec to fall to zero. Oxygen-sensitivity of the efferent mechanism was less critical than that of the afferent pathway including the hair cells at the right.

The frequency function of the crossed inhibitory system was checked in 27 out of the 39 guinea pigs. Twenty of these animals showed a clear minimum of threshold at that very frequency range of tone at the right ear, that corresponded to the frequency range of the place of shock stimulation at the left spiral osseous lamina. Thus, the second order afferents communicate with their efferent mates of the opposite side, which have the same frequency range. This was true not only with the shock-electrode in the first (basal) turn, but also when the shock was applied to the second, third or fourth turn. This has been summarized in Fig. 4. Above the threshold inhibition will increase from zero up to its maximum if the sound intensity increases by 60 dB. The interanimal variation was $\pm$ 5 dB. Thus the intensity function of the crossed inhibition turned out to be a nearly linear curve with a rather constant gradient of 15 % of inhibition per 10 dB.

It is interesting to note that as a result of the inhibition, not only the amplitude of the AP in the ventral cochlear nucleus was reduced, but also the latency of the afferent AP was clearly augmented by, at the most, 0.2-0.6 msec as a function of contralateral sound intensity. This was found in 20 out of 25 guinea pigs, investigated in this regard.

Some speculations may be offered for discussion. Basic information on the location of a sound source is buried in the physical parameters of interaural time difference and interaural intensity difference. In view of the fact that it is crossed as well as being a continuous function of sound intensity, the efferent inhibition will amplify neurally the physical intensity difference and time differences at the two ears. The amplification factor as calculated from our data appears to be approximately doubling the discrimination acuity. Because this neural amplifica-

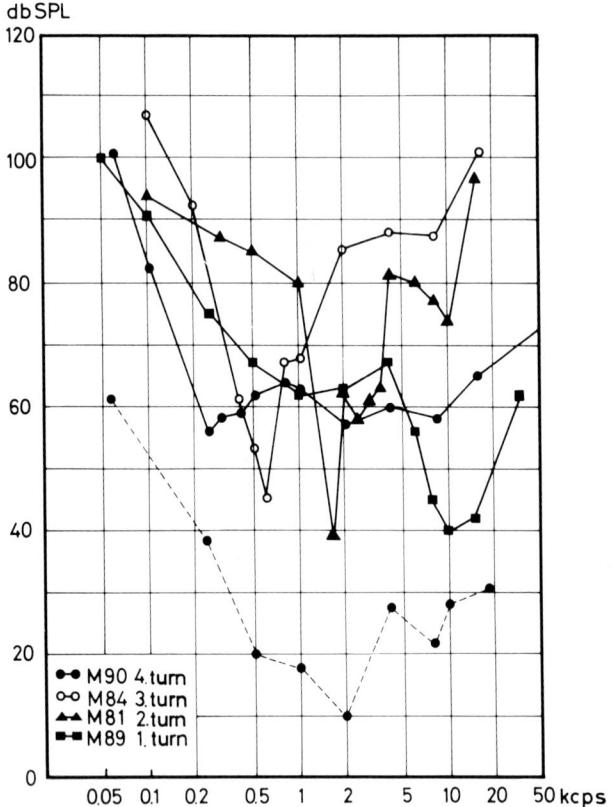

Fig. 4 Tonotopographical attribution of the crossed efferent inhibition to the secondary afferent system in the ventral cochlear nucleus.

Ordinate: efference-evoking sound intensity at the right ear in dB SPL; abscissa: sound frequency at the right ear in kcps. In the left lower corner beside the symbols the number of guinea pig is given; furthermore, the cochlear turn at the left, where a small area of the spiral lamina was stimulated electrically, is recorded in the lower left corner. The lowest dotted line is the normal auditory threshold of guinea pig drawn from the data of Stevens et al. (1935). Above that, four threshold curves of crossed efferent auditory inhibition in the NCV are drawn with (cont'd)

(Fig. 4, cont'd) the afference-evoking shock (see Fig. 1) in the first, second, third or fourth turn respectively. It is discernible that each of the four thresholds shows clearly a minimum, i.e. a "best frequency" of crossed efferent inhibition. This minimum for the individual curve (efferent threshold) coincides with the very frequency range of the afferents stimulated at the other side by the electrical shock (see Fig. 1). Connecting the four minima by another line would lead to a curve parallelling approximately a line of "equal loudness of 25 phons", reflecting the threshold of the compound crossed efferent system as a whole. (From Pfalz, 1969).

tion would depend on interaural intensity differences, the mechanism would have its significance mainly at frequencies higher than 1000 Hz.

The slow time course of the efferent crossed system, with maximum inhibition after 80-100 msec, is in good accord with the durations needed in man to achieve the best possible directional discrimination (Tobias and Schubert, 1959). Clinicians are familiar with the way in which lesions on one side of the pons widen the zone of midline sensation by the factor of two and at the same time deviate the midline sensation towards the side of the lesion (Matzker, 1957). This might be explained by destruction of the crossed efferent inhibition of the ventral cochlear nucleus of one side, i.e. the side of the lesion. Also the results of experimental commissurotomies at all levels in the brain stem and the brain are in full harmony with this view: only at the level of the pons will cutting of the crossing fibers result in a reduction of the directional discrimination acuity from 4^0 to 8.8^0 (Naumann, 1958, Neff, 1961).

Probably the cochlear nucleus complex is the first level of binaural neural interaction, mediated via efferent slow, crossing pathways. The functional meaning still remains an unsolved question.

References

Békésy, G. v. (1944). Über die mechanische Frequenzanalyse in der Schnecke verschiedener Tiere. Akust. Z. 9, 3.

Cajal, R.y. (1909). In: Histologie du système nerveux de l'homme et des vertèbres, Vol. I., Maloine, Paris.

Dunker, E., Grubel, G., and von Rehren, D. (1965). Zur Funktionsweise des efferenten auditorischen Systems. II. Änderung von Variabilität der Spike-Intervalle und Hemmungsempfindlichkeit nach Durchschneidung ventral im Bruckenhirn kreuzender Bahnen (Hund). Pfügers Arch. Gesamte Physiol. 283, 270.

Fernandez, C.J. (1952). Dimensions of the cochlea (guinea pig). J. Acoust. Soc. Amer. 24, 519.

Jouvet, M., and Desmedt, J.D. (1956). Contrôle central des messages acoustiques afférents. Compt. Rend. Hebd. Seances Acad. Sci. 243, 1916-1917.

Lorente de No, R. (1933). Anatomy of the eight nerve. III. General plan of structure of the primary cochlear nuclei. Laryngoscope. 43, 327.

Matzker, J. (1957). Ein neuer Weg zur otologischen Diagnostik zerebraler Erkrankungen. Z. Laryngol. Rhinol. 36, 177.

Nauman, G.C. (1958). Sound localization: The role of the commissural pathways of the auditory system of cat. Thesis. Univ., of Chicago, Chicago.

Neff, W.D. (1961). Neural mechanisms of auditory discrimination. In: Sensory Communication (W. Rosenblith, ed.), p. 259. M.I.T. Press, Cambridge, Mass.

Pfalz, R. (1961). Hemmung spontan aktiver Einzelneurone des Nucleus cochlearis bei adaequater Reizung des Kontralateralen Ohres (Meerschweinchen). Pfügers Arch. Gesamte Physiol. 274, 38.

Pfalz, R.K.J. (1969). The ventral cochlear nucleus: The significance of the crossed, inhibitory pathways towards the nucleus for directional hearing. In: Advan. Oto-Rhino-Laryng., Vol. 16, pp. 1-94. Karger, Basel/New York.

Pirsig, W., and Pfalz, R. (1967). Neurone im Nucleus cochlearis ventralis die von homolateral durch elektrischen Reiz an der Schneckenbasiswindung erregt wurden: Entladungsmuster, Latenzzeit und Adaptationsverhalten (Meerschweinchen). Arch. Klin. Exp. Ohr.- Nas.- Kehlk. Heilk. 189, 71.

Stevens, S.S., Davis, H., and Lurie, M.E. (1935). The localization of pitch perception on the basilar membrane. J. Genet. Psychol. 13, 297.

Tasaki, I., Davis, H., and Legouix, J.P. (1952). The space-time pattern of cochlear microphonics (guinea pig), as recorded by differential electrodes. J. Acoust. Soc. Amer. 24, 502.

Tobias, J.V., and Schubert, E.D. (1959). Effective onset duration of auditory stimuli. J. Acoust. Soc. Amer. 31, 1595.

Figures 1, 2, 3, and 4 reproduced from ADVANCES IN OTOLOGY, RHINOLOGY AND LARYNGOLOGY Vol. 16 by permission of Karger.

DISCUSSION

PFEIFFER: What is the location, within the cochlear nucleus, of the units that are affected by the contralateral stimulation?

PFALZ: Because we used gross electrodes we were unable to locate these units precisely and we can only say that in the majority of cases, we have been in the ventral cochlear nucleus.

KIANG: Truman Mast has reported on binaurally sensitive units in the dorsal cochlear nucleus. One also finds binaural effects for some units in the anteroventral cochlear nucleus. Since the characteristics of units in different parts of the cochlear nucleus are very different, it would be very important to establish the location of the units from which you record.

PFALZ: I think one limiting point was that so many people have been studying the olivary cochlear bundle and nobody has really been engaged with efferents to other nuclei.

MICHELSEN: What are the relative strengths of the efferent effects on the cochlea and the cochlear nucleus? As far as I understand you have excluded the efferent effect on the cochlea itself by stimulating the cochlea.

PFALZ: Yes. There might be a possibility that the shock electrode not only brought about this input to the cochlear nucleus, making the compound action potential but also other spikes might have come to the olivary cochlear bundle reducing the response of the opposite cochlea where we applied sound. I did not check the effect because according to Fex's data, the inhibitory effect by the OCB to the opposite cochlea would be very small.

EVANS: I just had a small comment in relation to the earlier discussion. I think that the work of Koerber et al. (1966) has given us a clue to the answer to Pfeiffer's question. You showed that the units you were recording from were spontaneously active in spite of having destroyed the cochlea. They showed that under these conditions, only units in the dorsal division of the cochlear retained their spontaneous activity. So it is probable in your experiments that you are recording from the dorsal nucleus.

PFALZ: In my microelectrode studies, I had no possibility to localize the electrode tip so this is a good indication that we have been in the dorsal cochlear nucleus. I am not sure whether the gross electrode located in the ventral cochlear nucleus really recorded from the ventral cochlear nucleus alone. Maybe the potentials also came from the dorsal nucleus.

KIANG: How can you be sure that you were in the ventral cochlear nucleus? What are your criteria?

PFALZ: I only have serial histology in twelve guinea pigs to rely on. In the example I presented, my calculations showed that I was rather near the dorsal part of the nucleus but in other experiments I am very sure that the recordings are made from the middle of the ventral cochlear nucleus.

KIANG: In the anteroventral cochlear nucleus or the posteroventral cochlear nucleus?

PFALZ: In the guinea pig the distinction between AVCN and PVCN is not yet clear as in cat. We can therefore not decide upon the location from our fixed brain stem preparations.

Reference

Koerber, K.C., Pfeiffer, R.R., Warr, W.B., and Kiang, N.Y.S. (1966). Spontaneous spike discharges from single units in the cochlear nucleus after destruction of the cochlea. Exp. Neurol. 16, 119-130.

VI
PSYCHOACOUSTICS

IN SEARCH OF PHYSIOLOGICAL CORRELATES OF PSYCHOACOUSTIC CHARACTERISTICS

Jozef J. Zwislocki

Syracuse University
Syracuse, New York
USA

Introduction

Sensory research is generally pursued on two separate channels, one psychological and one physiological. The dichotomy probably results from the vastness of the accumulated knowledge on the one hand and from its incompleteness on the other. We simply do not understand the fundamental relationship between physiological events and conscious behavior.

Von Békésy (1960) once wrote that, when a system is complicated and not well known, one is relegated to the study of its parts in isolation. This fate, he complained, befell many of his experiments. But, he added hopefully, "When considered in connection with other experiments carried out subsequently by the author and many other workers in this field they take on a broader meaning and perhaps now may be woven into a more general structure." I believe this may be true.

If explanation of a set of phenomena means an accounting in terms of other, more elementary phenomena, the most obvious explanation in sensory research must consist of a physiological accounting for sensory behavior. Of course, such accounting must be rudimentary at present since many pieces of information are still missing, and one cannot hope to see more than some fragmentary pictures of the huge jig-saw puzzle before us. Even these pictures are not quite clear because the pieces of the puzzle are not cut precisely. But perhaps enough can be seen to make a look worthwhile.

The available time allows me to discuss only one of the fragmentary pictures, one with an apparently simple design. However, it covers a substantial area, relating some fundamental physiological and psychoacoustic characteristics in time, frequency, and intensity domains. The picture concerns central masking, a subject I have already discussed in the past (Zwislocki et al., 1967, 1968; Zwislocki, 1969, 1970, 1971, 1972), but which has gained in scope and definition since my last discussion.

Central masking manifests itself as a threshold elevation of a test sound presented to one ear in the presence of a masking sound in the contralateral ear, when a direct acoustic interaction between the two sounds is precluded. Such an isolation can be achieved by means of appropriate insert phones. Our routinely used system provides an interaural acoustic insulation of more than 80 dB. Thus, central masking results from a purely neural interaction between the two ears, a circumstance of considerable advantage in the analysis of the auditory system. Cochlear nonlinear interactions that complicate monaural masking are avoided.

Central masking produces only a small threshold change, as compared to monaural masking. This means a great experimental disadvantage but also a decisive analytical advantage, as I shall endeavor to demonstrate.

Our experiments on central masking concern both steady-state and transient conditions. In the first, the masker consisted of continuous tones or broadband random noise, and the test stimulus, of tones presented in 250-msec bursts at a repetition rate of about one per second. In the second, the masker consisted of 250-msec bursts of tones or random noise repeated not more often than once per second, and the test stimulus, of 10-msec tone bursts with a Gaussian envelope. Whenever possible, a forced choice psychophysical method was used to minimize the effect of decision criteria.

Experimental Results

The following figures show some of our results.

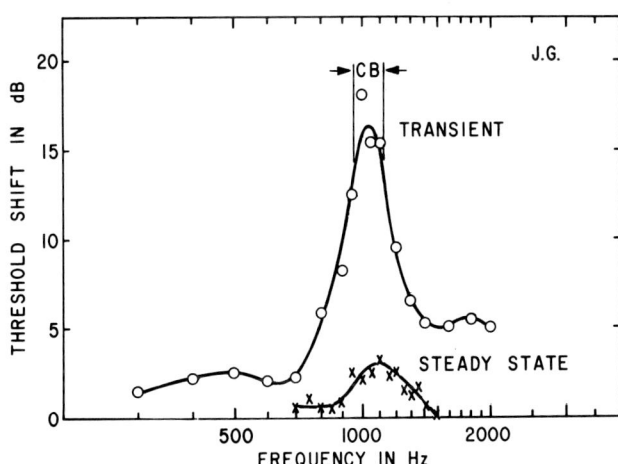

Fig.1 Individual transient and steady-state frequency distributions of central masking obtained with a 1000 Hz, 60 dB SL pure-tone masker and variable test-tone frequency. CB means critical band width. (From Zwislocki et al., 1968).

Figure 1 (Zwislocki et al., 1968) compares individual steady-state and transient frequency distributions of central masking for a 1000 Hz masker at 60 dB SL. The transient distribution was obtained with test bursts delayed by 20 msec from the masker onset. Several characteristic features are apparent. The transient masking component is much greater than the steady-state component, although it is small compared to monaural masking which would have exceeded 40 dB for a 60-dB masker. The transient masking effect has a rather sharp maximum near the masker frequency, and the width of the peak is consistent with Zwicker's critical band (Zwicker et al., 1957). The peak of the steady-state masking effect is relatively flat and is shifted somewhat toward higher frequencies.

The sharp frequency distribution of the transient masking component indicates that the test tone acts as a scanning device with a reasonably sharp resolu-

tion. This is not entirely surprising since, at the
required low intensities, the test tone excites a
small group of nerve fibers with a narrow spatial
distribution. As the test frequency changes, this
excitation must coincide with different groups of
fibers excited by the masker. In this way, the excitation distribution produced by the masker is scanned
along a tonotopic surface. The small test intensities
produce neural excitations that are nearly directly
proportional to sound intensity, as will be shown
later on. Consequently, the masking patterns may be
expected to closely resemble the corresponding neural
excitation patterns.

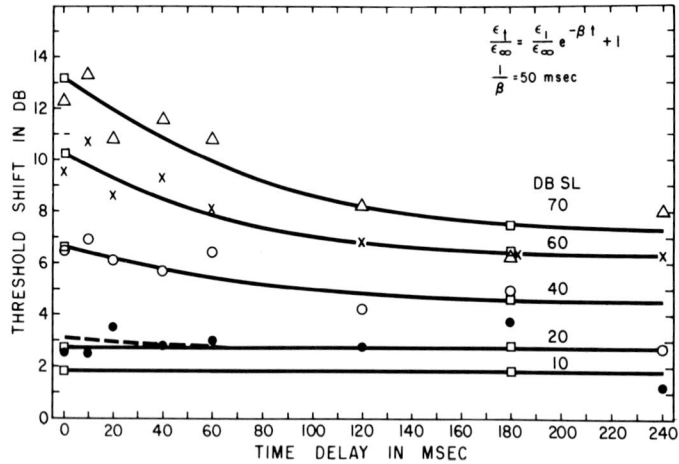

Fig.2   Fast temporal decay of central masking at
various masker SLs. Medians of 6 listeners.
The curves follow the equation shown in the
upper right corner. Masker and test frequencies at 1000 Hz.

The curves of Fig. 1 imply that central masking decreases with masker duration, and Fig. 2 (Zwislocki,
1970) shows a fast component of the decay. It was
measured by gradually delaying the 10-msec test tone
with respect to the masker onset. The frequency of
both the masking and test tones was at 1000 Hz, and
the masker SL varied in steps from 10 to 70 dB. The
curves approximating the median data obey the exponential equation shown in the upper right corner.
The decay time constant amounts to approximately

50 msec. As can be seen, the fast decay is practically completed within 100 msec; it increases with the masker SL. The fast decay is followed by a slow decay that lasts for about 1 minutes and appears to be rather unstable.

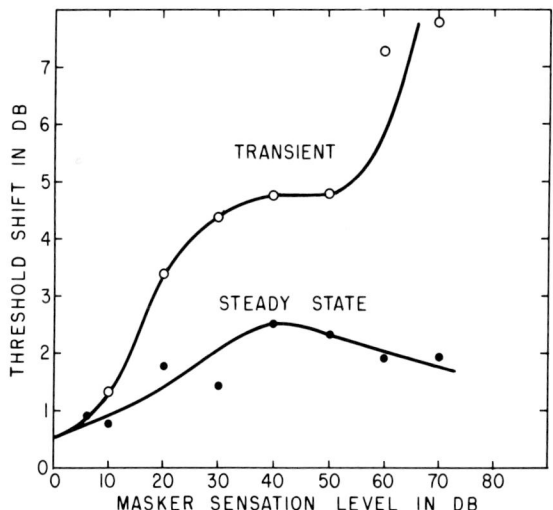

Fig.3 Median transient and steady-state intensity characteristics of central masking determined on 5 and 4 listeners, respectively. Masker and test frequencies at 1000 Hz. Transient curve determined at 20-msec delay from masker onset.

The threshold shift produced by central masking grows much less with masker intensity than does the threshold shift produced by monaural masking. The numerical relationship is nonlinear and may even be nonmonotonic. Corresponding median intensity data for transient and steady-state conditions are shown in Fig. 3. They are based on groups of 5 and 4 listeners, respectively. The transient masking data were obtained with a delay of 20 msec from the masker onset. In both situations, the masking and test stimuli consisted of sinusoids at a frequency of 1000 Hz. Note the plateau in the transient curve between 40 and 50 dB SL, and the maximum in the steady-state curve in about the same intensity range. Most individual data showed the same pattern. Only one listener out of five did not show the plateau in transient masking results, and one listener out of four had a plateau instead of a maximum in the steady-state results.

Many more data on central masking were gathered, but time does not permit me to show them. Instead, I now would like to discuss the simple numerical relationship we found between central masking characteristics and single-unit recordings obtained at low neural levels of the auditory system.

A Psychophysiological Theory of Central Masking

A functionally simple psychophysiological relationship was found with the help of an elementary mathematical theory based on three postulates. All the postulates could be derived from empirical data independent of central masking. They are as follows:

1. Signal detectability is determined by the signal-to-noise ratio in the neural domain.
2. Neural inputs from the two ears are arithmetically added in a binaural integrating stage.
3. The <u>driven</u> neural firing rate is directly proportional to sound intensity at low intensity levels.

The first postulate should be interpreted to the effect that, under given experimental conditions, detectability remains constant when the signal-to-noise ratio is constant. It is consistent with the theory of signal detection (Green and Swets, 1966) and with data on monaural masking (for instance, Hawkins and Stevens, 1950). The data show a constant signal-to-noise ratio in the stimulus domain. Since the detection process operates on neural events rather than on acoustic waves, it is reasonable to assume that the constant signal-to-noise ratio is preserved in the neural domain. Such an assumption is consistent with S.S. Stevens's (1955) power law. Power function transformation preserves ratio constancy. If detection is controlled by a constant signal-to-noise ratio in the neural domain, the ratio constancy may or may not be reflected in the stimulus domain, depending on the transformation between the stimulus intensity and neural excitation. But it is difficult to see how a constant signal-to-noise ratio could arise in the stimulus domain unless it were preserved in the neural domain.

The monaural masking curve deviates from a constant ratio between the signal and masker intensities at low masker levels (Miller, 1947). This deviation can be corrected by including in the masking stimulus the intrinsic noise of the organism. That such noise exists, is beyond any reasonable doubt. Accordingly, the threshold in quiet may be regarded as a masked threshold (Miller, 1947).

The second postulate results from known synaptic processes. The postsynaptic output tends to be directly proportional to the weighted algebraic sum of presynaptic inputs (Katz, 1949; Eccles, 1964; Darian-Smith et al., 1968). Results of experiments on binaural summation in units of the medial superior olive are roughly consistent with the more general observations (Goldberg and Brown, 1969). The medial superior olive could be the site of binaural interaction responsible for central masking.

The third postulate results from a reasonably recent and not yet formally published analysis of single-unit recordings which shows that the driven firing rate is directly proportional to stimulus intensity at low stimulation levels. The relationship seems to hold for all primary units with spontaneous activity and for many units without it. It appears to be preserved in the cochlear nucleus and in the superior olive. Figure 4 shows corresponding data for two 8th nerve units. They were obtained by Wiederhold (1967) by means of 40-msec bursts of sinusoids at the units' CFs. The original data are indicated by crosses and triangles. The filled circles show the driven firing rates derived from the original data by subtracting the spontaneous activity. The lower curve approximating the derived data tends toward a slope of one at low intensity levels, as indicated by the straight line. This means a direct proportionality between the firing rate and stimulus intensity.

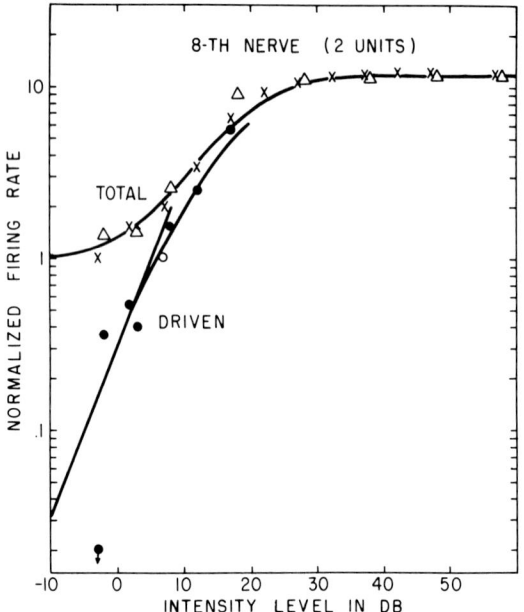

Fig. 4 Firing rates of two 8th nerve units in response to 40 msec tone bursts at their CFs. Data normalized with respect to spontaneous activities. Unfilled symbols indicate total firing rates, filled circles, driven activity. Curves approximate data. Lower curve approaches slope of one indicated by straight line. (Original data from Wiederhold, 1967, Units: W 248-4 and W 236-19.)

Demonstration of a quantitative psychophysiological relationship requires a mathematical formulation. On the basis of the postulate on linear summation, the output of the binaural integrating stage can be expressed by the equation

$$E_Q = K(E_{SQ} + E_I + ME_I), \qquad (1)$$

in the absence of the extrinsic noise, and by the equation

$$E_M = K(E_{SM} + E_I + M(E_N + E_I)), \qquad (2)$$

in its presence. In these equations, K is a proportionality constant; E_{SQ} and E_{SM} are the neural excitations produced by the signal in the absence and presence of the masking noise, respectively; E_I is the excitation produced by the intrinsic noise; E_N, that produced by the extrinsic noise; and M indicates the proportion of the excitation in the masking pathway, which interacts with the excitation in the test pathway. The terms E_{SQ} and E_{SM} have the significance of a signal; the rest of the terms on the right side of Eqs. (1) and (2) have the significance of noise. According to the postulate on constant signal-to-noise ratio, we can write

$$\frac{E_{SM}}{E_I + M(E_N + E_I)} = \frac{E_{SQ}}{E_I + ME_I} , \qquad (3)$$

or, after simple transformation,

$$\frac{E_{SM}}{E_{SQ}} = 1 + \frac{M}{1 + M} \cdot \frac{E_N}{E_I} . \qquad (4)$$

Because of the assumed direct proportionality between neural firing rate and stimulus intensity, we have

$$\frac{E_{SM}}{E_{SQ}} = \frac{S_M}{S_Q} , \qquad (5)$$

where S_Q and S_M are the signal intensities in the absence and presence of extrinsic masking noise, respectively. Substituting from Eq. (5) in Eq. (4), we obtain

$$\frac{S_M}{S_Q} = 1 + \frac{M}{1 + M} \cdot \frac{E_N}{E_I} , \qquad (6)$$

the desired mathematical expression relating the psychophysical threshold intensities to neural activities. Since we want to predict neural firing rates from psychophysical thresholds, we turn Eq. (6) around:

$$\frac{E_N}{E_I} = \frac{1 + M}{M} \left(\frac{S_M}{S_Q} - 1\right) . \qquad (7)$$

The resulting equation is very simple, but has the flaw that the constants E_I and M are not well known. They introduce an ill-defined amount of arbitrariness into the numerical relationships. The constants can be eliminated if we are willing to limit our calculations to ratios among firing rates. Let us accept a reference masked threshold S_O and a corresponding neural excitation E_O. Then,

$$\frac{E_O}{E_I} = \frac{1+M}{M} \left(\frac{S_O}{S_Q} - 1\right) . \qquad (8)$$

Division of Eq. (7) by Eq. (8) produces

$$\frac{E_N}{E_O} = \frac{S_M/S_Q - 1}{S_O/S_Q - 1} , \qquad (9)$$

a theoretical psychophysiological relationship that has no free constants.

It now becomes possible to calculate ratios of firing rates from ratios of psychophysical threshold intensities and to compare them to empirical data.

Comparison of Calculated and Empirical Data

We may begin by determining neural tuning curves that relate the stimulus intensity and frequency for a constant firing rate. The required psychophysical data are shown in Fig. 5 for one listener (Zwislocki et al., 1968). They were obtained by means of 250-msec masking bursts and 10-msec test bursts with simultaneous onsets. The masker sensation level was increased in 10-dB steps. To achieve compatability with neural data, the test frequency was kept constant at 1000 Hz and the masker frequency varied. As the microelectrode location determines the unit under investigation, the test-tone frequency does the same for a group of fibers with similar CFs. According to the theory of this paper, equal threshold shifts correspond to equal neural excitations produced by the masker. As a consequence, horizontal lines intersecting the masking curves determine pairs of frequency and intensity values producing equal theoretical firing rates. The locus of these pairs constitutes theoretical tuning curves.

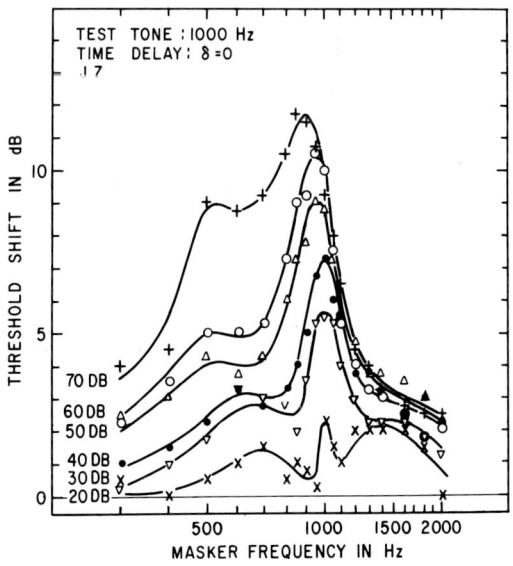

Fig.5 Individual transient frequency distributions of central masking obtained with a 1000 Hz test tone and a masker of variable frequency and SL. The time delay between the masking- and test-tone onsets was zero. (From Zwislocki et al., 1968).

Two such tuning curves resulting from data of two listeners are plotted in Fig. 6 by means of thin lines. They are normalized so that their tip corresponds to a masker sensation level of 20 dB. As was shown previously (Zwislocki, 1972), the reference level has little effect on the shape of the theoretical tuning curves. For comparison, crosses and closed circles indicate corresponding empirical data for an 8th nerve unit (Kiang et al., 1970) and a unit of the anteroventral cochlear nucleus (Kiang et al., 1965), respectively. The units had their best frequencies in close vicinity of 1000 Hz, and were normalized to 1000 Hz by means of a parallel shift along the log frequency scale. Such a small shift could not introduce any appreciable error. As can be seen, the theoretical and empirical curves agree along all dimensions. The deviations are within

the scatter of physiological data that can be found
in the literature. Somewhat more extensive comparisons were shown elsewhere (Zwislocki, 1972). Unfortunately, no comparisons of theoretical and empirical tuning curves could be made for the MSO because
of insufficient data. However, there are indications
that the tuning curves remain reasonably invariant
up to the superior olive and beyond.

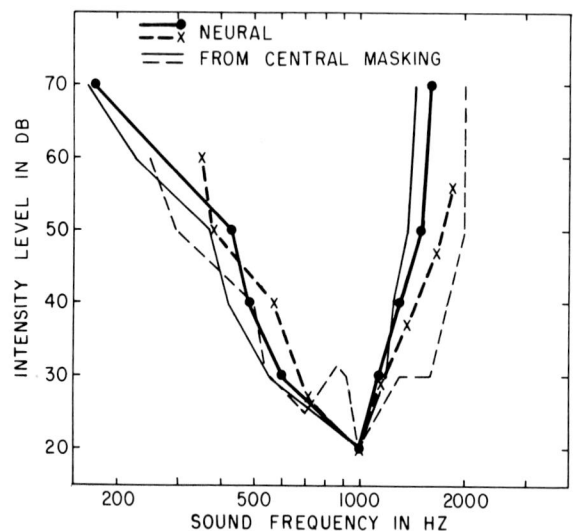

Fig.6 Empirical neural tuning curves and tuning
curves derived from individual central masking
data. Crosses -- 8th nerve data (Kiang et al.,
1970, animal K 491, CF ≃ 1.15 kHz); circles
— AVCN data (Kiang et al., 1965, CF ≃ 1.0
kHz). The neural data were obtained by means
of 25-msec tone bursts. All data are normalized with respect to 1000 Hz and 20 dB IL.

Another characteristic that appears to remain substantially stable in large populations of units in
several low-level nuclear complexes is the fast decay of firing rate. It proceeds nearly exponentially
with a time constant of ≈50 msec. The amount of decay
seems to depend on the initial firing rate, i.e.
once the unit reaches its saturation level, further
increases in stimulus intensity do not affect it.
The same qualitative features are exhibited by the
temporal decay of central masking. Figure 7 shows

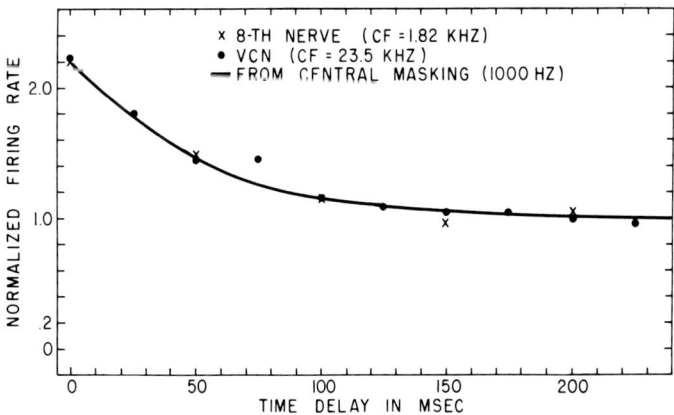

Fig. 7 Fast temporal decay of firing rate: empirical and theoretical data normalized with respect to asymptotic values. Crosses -- 8th nerve data (Kiang, 1965, unit K 297-43); circles -- VCN data (Pfeiffer, 1966, unit P 21-2).

a quantitative comparison between the temporal decay of normalized firing rate calculated from median central masking data and that measured on two units, one in the 8th nerve and one in the VCN. Again, no appropriate data were found for the MSO. More extensive comparisons were shown elsewhere (Zwislocki, 1971, 1972). To assure maximum correspondence between the theoretical and empirical data, Fig. 7 refers to saturation levels which are reached at about 40 dB above a unit's threshold and at 40 dB SL of the masker. The crosses indicate the 8th nerve data, the filled circles those of the VCN, and the curve is theoretical. As can be seen, both sets of empirical data closely follow the theoretical curve. It should be pointed out that the decay seems to be independent of sound frequency in both neural firing and central masking. The 8th nerve data were recorded on a unit with a CF = 1.82 kHz, the VCN data, on a unit with a CF = 23.5 kHz, and the central masking data were obtained at 1 kHz.

Firing rate as a function of stimulus activity is perhaps the most fundamental neural characteristic. A corresponding theoretical characteristic derived from the transient central masking data of Fig. 3 is shown by a solid line in Fig. 8. It is compared to normalized single unit data recorded in the 8th nerve, the VCN, and the MSO by means of short tone bursts. The data are typical of primary-like neural characteristics. Note their uniformity, which is due in part to normalization. The theoretical and empirical data appear to be mutually consistent over an intensity range of 50 dB. At higher levels, a systematic difference arises. The theoretical curve resumes its ascent, whereas the empirical firing rates remain at a plateau. This is the only systematic difference found thus far between the central-masking and neural data recorded from primary-like units. Its meaning is obscure. At the high levels, central masking could be produced by a different neural population, or a component of neural activity could be escaping the current neurophysiological recording techniques. The discrepancy is the more curious since it does not appear in the steady state intensity characteristic.[1]

---

[1] Just before my departure for the meeting, a plausible explanation of the discrepancy occurred to me. The theory assumes that the output of the binaural interaction stage is directly proportional to the sum of the binaural inputs. Such proportionality cannot extend over an infinite range, and saturation effects should make themselves felt at sufficiently high inputs. This means that binaural units exposed to a high input from the masker ear would become insensitive to the input from the test ear. Accordingly, the signal intensity would have to be increased in order to achieve criterion detection. The upturn of the transient masking curve in Fig. 3 at high masker levels probably reflects the required signal increment. Interestingly, the steady-state curve does not show a secondary ascent. This could indicate that peripheral adaptation prevents the input to the binaural units from reaching their saturation. In any event, the departure of the theoretical curve in Fig. 8 from the trend of the empirical data seems to indicate that the bounds of the theory have been exceeded rather than some mysterious physiological processes.

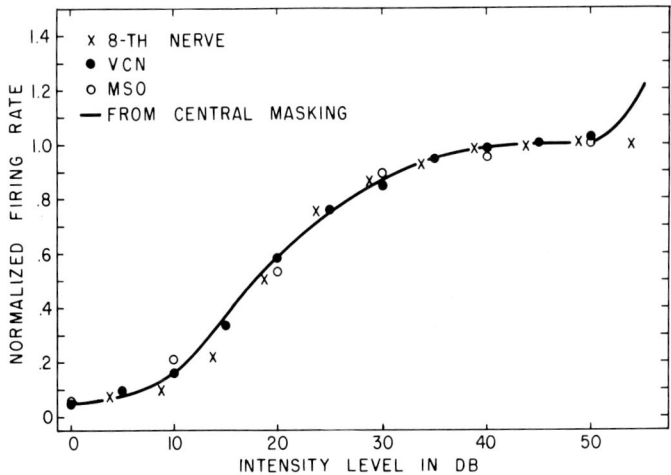

Fig. 8 Transient neural intensity characteristic: empirical and theoretical data normalized with respect to the plateau at medium intensity levels. Crosses -- 8th nerve data (Wiederhold, 1967, unit W 248-4); filled circles -- VCN data (Møller, 1968, unit 65-18); unfilled circles -- MSO data (Goldberg and Brown, 1969, unit 66-42-3).

Examples of steady state theoretical and empirical intensity characteristics are shown in Fig. 9. The theoretical values are derived from individual results determined on two listeners, the empirical data stem from two 8th nerve units (Kiang, 1965, units: 305-18 and 308-53) and may be considered typical. It is apparent that both sets of results belong numerically to the same population. To be sure, the unfilled symbols mark the theoretical, the filled symbols, the empirical values.

A restriction must be mentioned with respect to Fig. 9. Not all neural characteristics have a negative

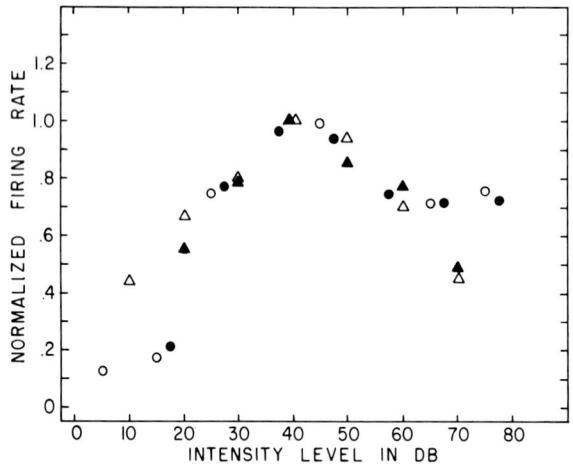

Fig. 9 Steady-state neural intensity characteristic: empirical data and theoretical data derived from 2 individual listeners. All the data are normalized with respect to the maximum firing rate. Empirical data from Kiang, 1965, units: 305-16 and 308-53 . Further explanation in text.

slope at high intensity levels, and the same is true of individual central masking results. The slope seems to be produced by a shift in CF, which increases with stimulus intensity. It is possible that the shift depends on stimulus duration, and that stimuli that last for minutes are more likely to produce it than stimuli that last for seconds. At least, central masking results point in this direction.

Intensity characteristics with a negative slope are often encountered at higher neural levels. Since such characteristics are found under both the steady state as well as transient conditions, their correspondence to central masking characteristics is not clear. Consequently, they are omitted in our psychophysiological considerations.

Conclusions

More comparisons between central masking results and neural data are possible than I have been able to include in this presentation. Additional instances have been pointed out in a recent article (Zwislocki, 1972). The agreement between the theoretical neural characteristics and single unit data from the 8th nerve, the cochlear nucleus, and the superior olive is too general to be considered fortuitous. This is particularly so since the underlying mathematical equation does not contain any explicit free constants. Only the reference intensity level in Figs. 8 and 9 could be adjusted, which means a parallel shift along the abscissa axis, without any modification of the curve shape. Such an adjustment is trivial from the pont of view of the questions under consideration.

If the agreement between the neural responses derived from central masking and the empirical data is not fortuitous, significant consequences ensue. Some of them are listed below.

1) The postulates of constant signal-to-noise ratio in the neural domain, of arithmetic additivity in the binaural integrating stage, and of direct proportionality between low level neural excitation and stimulus intensity hold within a sufficient approximation.

2) The constancy of the signal-to-noise ratio must be preserved between the relevant stage of binaural interaction and the detection stage. Consequently, only power-function transformations are allowed.

3) The threshold effects of central masking, when expressed in terms of intensity ratios, are linearly related to neural activity at the relevant stage of binaural interaction.

4) The agreement between neural characteristics derived from central masking and single-unit recordings from the 8th nerve indicate that fundamental neural characteristics in the frequency, time, and intensity domains are preserved from the periphery up to at least the first stage of binaural interaction. This is consistent with direct empirical evidence.

5) Since central masking must be controlled by groups of neurons, its linear relationship with characteristics of single units indicates that these characteristics, including the absolute sensitivity, are uniform.

6) Since the central masking effects involved in our psychophysiological comparisons were measured on humans, and the neural data were obtained on anesthetized animals, we must infer that the latter were a valid representation of relevant neural activity in awake humans.

As interesting as all these specific consequences may be, none seems to me as perplexing as the fact that a behavioral response can reflect linearly fundamental characteristics of individual neurons located in sensory periphery.

References

Békésy, G. v. (1960). Experiments in Hearing. McGraw-Hill, New York.

Darian-Smith, I., Rowe, M.J., and Sessle, B.J. (1968). "Tactile" stimulus intensity: information transmission by relay neurons in different trigeminal nuclei. Science 160, 791-794.

Eccles, J.C. (1964). The Physiology of Synapses. Academic Press, New York.

Goldberg, J.M., and Brown, P.B. (1969). Response of binaural neurons of dog superior olivary complex to dichotic tonal stimuli: some physiological mechanisms of sound localization. J. Neurophysiol. 32, 613-628.

Green, D.M., and Swets, J.A. (1966). Signal Detection Theory and Psychophysics. John Wiley and Sons, New York.

Hawkins, J.E., Jr. and Stevens, S.S. (1950). The masking of pure tones and of speech by white noise. J. Acoust. Soc. Amer. 22, 6-13.

Katz, B. (1949). Depolarization of sensory terminals and the initiation of impulses in the muscle spindle. J. Physiol. 111, 261-282.

Kiang, N.Y.S. (1965). Discharge Patterns of Single Fibers in the Cat's Auditory Nerve. Res. Monogr. 35. M.I.T. Press, Cambridge, Mass.

Kiang, N.Y.S., Pfeiffer, R.R., Warr, W.B., and Backus, A.S.N. (1965). Stimulus coding in the cochlear nucleus. Ann. Otol. Rhinol. Laryngol. 74, 463-485.

Kiang, N.Y.S., Moxon, E.C., and Levine, R.A. (1970). Auditory-nerve activity in cats with normal and abnormal cochleas. In: Sensorineural Hearing Loss. (G.E.W. Wolstenholme and J. Knight, eds.), pp. 241-268. J. and A. Churchill, London.

Miller, G.A. (1947). Sensitivity to changes in the intensity of white noise and its relation to masking and loudness. J. Acoust. Soc. Amer. 19, 609-619.

Møller, A.R. (1968). Unit responses in the cochlear nucleus of the rat to pure tones. Acta Physiol. Scand. 75, 530-541.

Pfeiffer, R.R. (1966). Classification of response patterns of spike discharges for units in the cochlear nucleus: tone-burst stimulation. Exp. Brain Res. 1, 220-235.

Stevens, S.S. (1955). The measurement of loudness. J. Acoust. Soc. Amer. 27, 815-829.

Wiederhold, M.J. (1967). A study of efferent inhibition of auditory nerve activity. Thesis. M.I.T. Cambridge, Mass.

Zwicker, E., Flottorp, G., and Stevens, S.S. (1957). Critical band width in loudness summation. J. Acoust. Soc. Amer. 29, 548-557.

Zwislocki, J.J. (1969). Central auditory masking. Archiwum Akustyki 4, 359-373.

Zwislocki, J.J. (1970). Central masking and auditory frequency selectivity. In: Frequency Analysis and Periodicity Detection in Hearing (R. Plomp and G.F. Smoorenburg, eds.), pp. 445-454. Sijthoff, Leiden, The Netherlands.

Zwislocki, J.J. (1971). Central masking and neural activity in the cochlear nucleus. Audiology 10, 48-59.

Zwislocki, J.J. (1972). A theory of central auditory masking and its partial validation. J. Acoust. Soc. Amer. 52, 644-659.

Zwislocki, J.J., Damianopoulos, E.N., Buining, E., and Glantz, J. (1967). Central masking: some steady-state and transient effects. Percep. and Psychophys. 2, 59-64.

Zwislocki, J.J., Buining, E. and Glantz, J. (1968). Frequency distribution of central masking. J. Acoust. Soc. Amer. 43, 1267-1271.

Figures 1 and 5 reproduced by permission of Journal of the Acoustical Society of America.

DISCUSSION

BRUGGE: I wonder if you could tell us what features of the discharge pattern would not agree with your model.

ZWISLOCKI: You could see that the characteristics of all units that are not primary-like cannot agree because of the agreement of the model with the 8th nerve units.

BRUGGE: I see. So if they deviate from that pattern, they would disagree with your model.

ZWISLOCKI: Yes.

BRUGGE: Do they disagree in any orderly way?

ZWISLOCKI: Well, for one thing, some of the units in the 8th nerve have intensity characteristics that are non-monotonic for long-duration stimuli but not for short bursts. The same is true for the characteristics derived from central masking. On the other hand, some units in the cochlear nucleus have non-monotonic intensity characteristics for short bursts. In the dorsal cochlear nucleus, there are units whose PST histograms do not show the nice exponential decay, as I showed in my paper, but a distinctly different time pattern. These are just two examples of units that do not agree with the model.

KOHLLÖFFEL: Could we imagine that essentially the same model approach can be used for the second population of units as for the first population and that you just stack these two mechanisms on top of each other?

ZWISLOCKI: I do not think that there is any other population. I think that the theoretical curve of Fig. 8 resumes its ascent because, as I said, one of the theoretical assumptions has been exceeded more specifically, the assumption according to which the output of the binaural stage is directly proportional to the input.

EVANS: In your paper you demonstrated two radically different sets of psychophysical results, depending on whether transient or continuous stimuli were used. What parameters of your model have to be adjusted to account for this?

ZWISLOCKI: Well, one thing I showed is a decay of masking and of neural firing rate as a function of duration. If you have a post-stimulus time histogram, let us say for a burst that lasts 200 msec, and you plot the number of spikes per bin, you see such a decay. Now, this is only one decay, which I showed. There is a slow decay of central masking, which has a time constant on the order of 4 minutes. This decay agrees with that of at least two neurons we find in Kiang's monograph (1965). The psychophysically measured decay is not very stable, by the way.

Reference

Kiang, N.Y.S. (1965). Discharge Patterns of Single Fibers in the Cat's Auditory Nerve. Res. Monogr. 35. M.I.T. Press, Cambridge, Mass.

TEMPORAL EFFECTS IN PSYCHOACOUSTICAL EXCITATION

E. Zwicker

Technische Universität München
8 München 2, Arcisstr. 21
Germany

The psychoacoustical excitation is a second approximation of the ear's frequency selectivity whereas the critical band concept - using rectangular shaped filters - is the first approximation. Psychoacoustical excitation is measured by masking pure tones by sounds. The term "psychoacoustical excitation" is abbreviated in this paper to "excitation". Excitation E is a value comparable to sound intensity, not to sound pressure. Mostly the logarithmic value, the excitation level

$$L_E = 10 \lg \frac{E(Z)}{E_0} dB \qquad (1)$$

is more useful because of the large dynamic range of

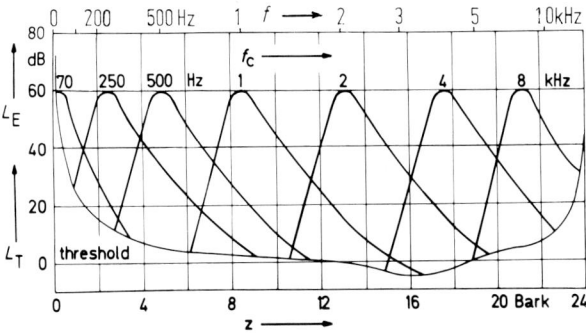

Fig. 1 Threshold level L_T in quiet and excitation level L_E for 7 narrow bands of noise, one critical band wide, with different centre frequencies f_c but equal SPL of 60dB, as function of the critical band rate z (lower abscissa) or as function of the corresponding frequency f (upper abscissa) (from Zwicker, 1970).

the ear (see Zwicker, 1958, Zwicker and Feldtkeller, 1967, Zwicker, 1971). Most used are the excitation patterns. In these E or L_E are plotted as function of the critical band rate z which is correlated to frequency f as shown in Fig. 1 and 5 on the two abscissas. To discuss temporal effects in excitation we have to begin with the steady state condition. Further on the effects produced by slow changes, quick changes, periodical changes and statistical changes will be discussed. Comparing the effects produced by steady state and changes, respectively, it may be possible to find some critical durations, time constants or repetition rates by means of which the temporal behavior of the ear can be characterized at least in a very first approximation.

1. Steady state condition

For long duration of the masker or even continuous masker and for long duration (>200 ms) of the signal, the ear reaches a condition, in which the sensation is independent of temporal effects. This is the steady state condition for which the excitation patterns produced by narrow band noises (similar to tones) have been measured for different center frequencies (Fig. 1) and different sound pressure levels (Fig. 2). This behavior of the ear has been measured

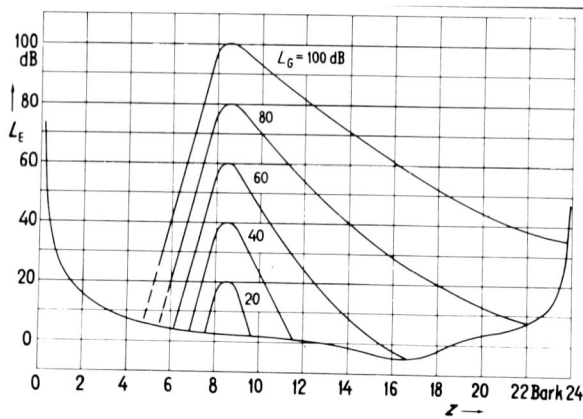

Fig. 2 Excitation level L_E for a one critical band wide noise, centered at 1 kHz, with different SPL_S L_G, as function of the critical band rate z (from Zwicker and Feldtkeller, 1967).

in much detail (Zwicker, 1958, Zwicker, 1963) and is

very fundamental, although individual observers show differences in second order effects. It had been demonstrated that the frequency selectivity of the hearing system becomes independent of the center frequency if the frequency f is transformed into the critical band rate z on a linear scale (Fig. 1). The frequency difference between the two 3 dB-points corresponds to the critical band width. The slopes of the patterns towards lower frequencies are independent of center frequency and level and have a steepness of about 27 dB/Bark which is 27 dB per critical band (Fig. 1 and 2). On the other hand the slopes of the patterns towards higher frequencies depend clearly on level (Fig. 2); the slope becomes more flat for increasing level of the masking narrow band noise.

2. Slow changes

Before talking about changes of the time pattern of the masker, a small paragraph about the influence of the duration of the signal on its threshold should be inserted. The threshold of narrow band signals like tones depends on signal duration in a simple way (Feldtkeller and Oetinger, 1956, Zwislocki, 1960). For long durations (T_S > 200 ms) the threshold is independent of duration while for durations shorter than 200 ms the product of duration T_S and sound intensity I_S has to be constant to reach threshold. This means that for T_S = 20 ms the intensity must be magnified by a factor of 10 or the level must be increased 10 dB in relation to the long duration signal. 20 dB increase is necessary for a 2 ms signal impulse (see Fig. 8a). Since in studies of temporal effects in excitation the duration of the signal is kept short but constant, this dependence of the signal's threshold on duration is not important but should be known to understand the absolute value of the masked threshold. The critical duration of 200 ms for the signal will be discussed later (summary) in connection with other critical durations.

Slow changes are understood as those for which the excitation pattern can be composed out of the steady state pattern: The hearing system is able to follow the change of the stimulation completely. Sinusoidal changes have the advantage that the spectrum produced by the changes can be calculated and controlled. The dependence of the threshold on amplitude and frequency modulation (Zwicker, 1952) and the threshold of roughness for amplitude modulation (Terhardt, 1970) as function of the frequency of modulation were studied. Fig. 3 shows the threshold of modulation and of

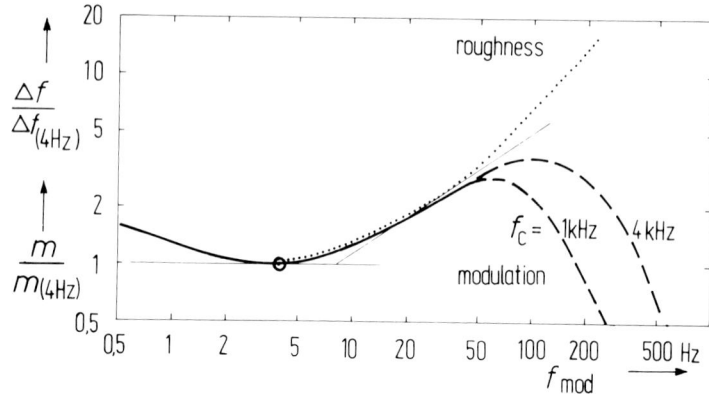

Fig. 3 Just audible sinusoidal modulation (frequency shift Δf for frequency modulation and modulation factor m for amplitude modulation) as function of the frequency f_{mod} of modulation. The values related to the values at a frequency of modulation of 4 Hz

$$(\frac{\Delta f}{\Delta f_{(4Hz)}} \text{ and } \frac{m}{m_{(4Hz)}})$$

are used as ordinate (solid and dashed). The relative factor $m/m_{(4Hz)}$ of amplitude modulation is also shown for the threshold of roughness (dotted). The two thin lines indicate a useful approximation.

roughness as function of the frequency f_{mod} of modulation relative to the threshold at f_{mod} = 4 Hz. At 4 Hz the thresholds reach a minimum. For lower frequencies of modulation the thresholds rise, and the ear becomes less sensitive, although it can follow the changes easily. For those very slow changes the memory seems to be not good enough to store the preceding situation for comparison. Frequencies of modulation larger than 5 Hz produce temporal patterns of stimulation which the ear - expressed by excitation pattern - cannot follow completely: a larger factor m of modulation or a larger frequency shift Δf is necessary to reach threshold. The higher the frequency of modulation, the higher rises the threshold. At

very high frequencies of modulation the threshold of
modulation decreases again because of the audibility
of side tones - dependent on the carrier frequency f_c
as indicated in Fig. 3 - while the threshold of
roughness increases further.

This behavior of the hearing system shows up not only
for threshold of roughness but also for the roughness
itself - strength of roughness - (Terhardt, 1968) and
is almost independent of level.

The shape of the curves shown in Fig. 3 can be idealized by the thin straight lines with an edge at about
8 Hz. This value belongs to a time constant τ of
about 20 ms. This seems to be a second critical duration, which is characteristic for the ability of the
ear to follow temporal changes slower than that
value.

3. Quick change

The excitation in transient conditions is measured
by masking experiments in which the masker is switched on and off as shown in Fig. 4. The results of the
experiments can be divided into 3 different groups.
Backward-masking takes place before the masker
starts. Then a range of simultaneous masking follows
in which masker and signal are present at the same
time. Finally a range of forward masking is notified
in which - similar to backward masking - the masker
influences the threshold of the signal at time intervals in which the masker is absent physically. Forward masking is more pronounced than backward
masking. As indicated in Fig. 4, the masking effect
depends somewhat on the spectrum of masker and signal, respectively.

In all such experiments, the signal has to be a very
short impulse in order to get the wanted fine time
resolution. Since time resolution and necessary bandwidth are strongly related, the short duration of the
signal elicits a larger bandwidth. Thus, it is most
essential to avoid a situation in which the ear may
be able to pick up spectral parts of the signal,
which have been thought to be inaudible. Some months
ago a letter to the editor (Zwicker and Fastl, 1972
b) was published on that problem, and the reader may
be referred to that article.

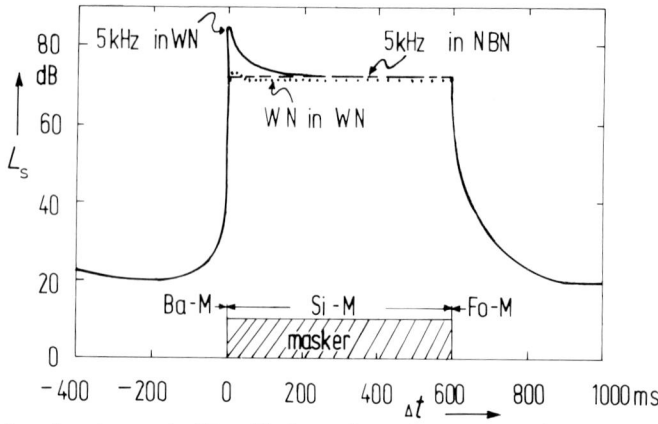

Fig. 4 Backward (Ba.M.), simultaneous (Si.M.) and forward masking (Fo.M.) produced by a sequence of 600 ms long maskers followed by a pause of 600 ms. The level of the signal at threshold is plotted as function of the delay time Δt between onset of the masker and onset of the signal.

As signals 2 ms long impulses of 5 kHz-tones (5kHz) or of white noise (WN), as maskers white noise (WN) or narrow band noise (NBN) centered at 5 kHz are used. The levels of the maskers are chosen in such a way that steady state thresholds coincide.

Broad band sounds used as masker and as signal produce spectral conditions which are easy to handle. The results of different authors agree quite well (Stein, 1960, Raab, 1963, Elliott, 1967) and show backward, simultaneous and forward masking as indicated in Fig. 4. Narrow band signal and masker have to be used to proceed to masking results which may be useful in solving the question as to whether the critical band and the frequency selectivity of the ear develop during excitation or exist permanently with fixed steep filter slopes. The results of different authors in such a masker-signal condition do not agree (Scholl, 1962, Elliott, 1965, 1967, Zwicker, 1965a, 1965b, Green, 1969, Zwicker and Fastl, 1972a, 1972b, Fastl, 1972). Our opinion of this problem is given in the letter to the editor mentioned above and can be summarized: The critical band and the frequency selectivity of the ear as measured by masking effects

seem to act in such a way that they can be
thought of as being installed like a permanently
available filter system.

This statement was documented again by Fastl (1972)
comparing simultaneous masking effects produced by a

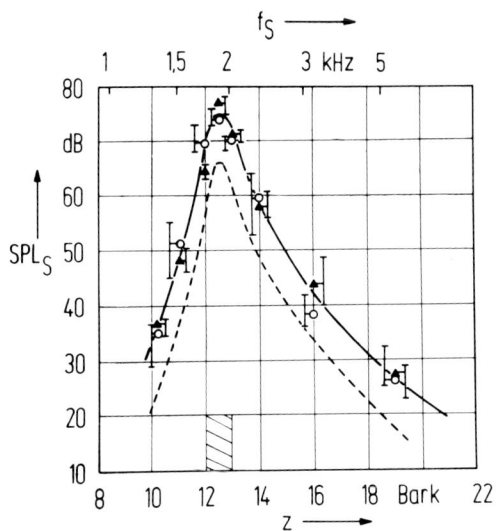

Fig. 5 Simultaneous masking of a critical band
noise (SPL = 70 dB) centered at 12.5 Bark
(hatched area). SPL_S of signal is plotted as
function of its frequency f_S and critical
band rate z, respectively. For continuous
masker: signal duration T_S = 500 ms (dashed
curve) and T_S = 10 ms (filled triangles).
For 10 ms masker duration and T_S = 10 ms the
open circles represent the central values
with interquartile ranges (from Fastl, 1972).

critical band wide noise with durations of 500 ms and 10 ms while the signals were 10 ms long tone impulses of different frequencies but carefully narrowed spectral width (Fig. 5). The results show no difference for the two mentioned conditions, while the masked threshold produced by continuous masker and 500 ms-signals, i.e. the steady state excitation pattern, shows exactly the same frequency characteristic. This means again that no increase of the selectivity during the stimulation by the masker takes place.

4. Periodical change

Only a few measurements were undertaken to study backward, simultaneous and forward masking during periodical changes of the sound like amplitude or frequency modulation. However, a result (Zwicker, 1970) with octave band noise centered at 4 kHz used for masker as well as for signal is available. There, the threshold L_T of a signal burst composed of 0.5 ms impulses was measured as function of the delay t_v between offset of the masker and onset of the signal as indicated in the schematic drawings in Fig. 6. The masker was presented in series of impulses of the duration T/2, where T is the period containing impulse and pause correlated with the pulse rate f_p by

$$T = \frac{1}{f_p}. \qquad (2)$$

For very low pulse rate and long duration of impulse and pause, the masked threshold of the signal reaches the steady state masking condition and the threshold in quiet, respectively. At a pulse rate f_p = 10 Hz (see Fig. 6a) the steady state condition is still reached, but the threshold in the gap lies above the threshold in quiet so that the value ΔL - as used in Fig. 6 - becomes smaller. In Fig. 6b the pulse rate is increased to f_p = 50 Hz resulting in a further decrement of ΔL, while in Fig. 6c with f_p = 200 Hz the value ΔL is very small and just measurable only. At pulse rates of 500 Hz the masker sounds not only like a steady sound, but the value ΔL decreases towards an unmeasurable amount, indicating that the excitation cannot follow at all such quick periodical changes.

Summarizing and approximating this result in simple numbers we may conclude that the ear is able to pick

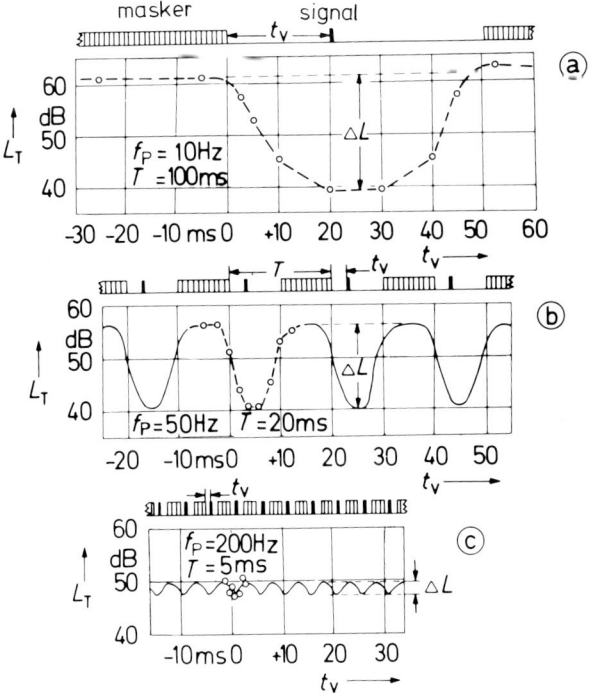

Fig. 6 Masked threshold L_T of a burst of 0.5 ms long signal impulses as function of the delay time t_v between the offset of the masker and the onset of the signal. The masker bursts are composed of impulses and pauses of identical length

$$\frac{T}{2} = \frac{1}{2 f_p}.$$

Signal and masker are produced of octave bands of noise at 4 kHz center frequency. The level of the masker is 50 dB. The schematic drawings illustrate the time sequence of the stimuli (from Zwicker, 1971).

up the time structure of a sound only if its period (duty cycle 50 %) is longer than 4 ms or in other words, if the pauses are larger than 2 ms. Pauses shorter than that duration cannot be detected. Sounds with a pulse rate of more than 500 Hz produce sensations without time structure. This result agrees not only with other psychoacoustical results of forward masking (Stein, 1960), roughness (Terhardt, 1968) and the limits of periodicity pitch (Ritsma, 1962, Walliser, 1969) but also with the physiological results produced by stimulation with amplitude modulated tones (Møller, 1972).

5. Statistical change

Many sounds have a strong periodicity and also last so long that they can be regarded as periodical steady state sounds. On the other hand, sounds with no periodicity but with strong temporal changes are quite common, too. Such sounds change statistically in amplitude or/and in frequency and spectrum shape, respectively. The reason for studying effects produced by statistical changes becomes clear, if it is assumed that the ear may behave differently for periodical changes producing some kind of temporal rhythm which does not appear in sounds changing statistically.

The first measurements to study these effects were undertaken with computerproduced white noise-like sounds which have a period the length of which produces no special sensation of rhythm. With a period longer than 1 to 2 s the rhythm of the sounds is almost undetectable. The advantage of such artificial sounds is the possibility of triggering a short signal which can be presented again and again at a certain time of the total temporal pattern of the artificial sound.

Artificial white noise filtered by a narrow band filter with a bandwidth of 12 Hz at a center frequency of 4 kHz was used as masker exciting the ear similar to a 4 kHz tone with approximately statistical changes in amplitude. The rate of the amplitude changes is restricted up to a maximum value which is related to the bandwidth of 12 Hz. The instantaneous sound pressure level L_{NBN} of the narrow band noise is shown in Fig. 7 as solid line for a certain timerange of the total period of the noise. A 5 ms-4 kHz-tone impulse was used as signal. To avoid artifacts produced by spectral effects, the signal was switched on and off with a Gaussian shaped gating signal with a rise time of 2 ms and then fed additionally through a third octave band filter.

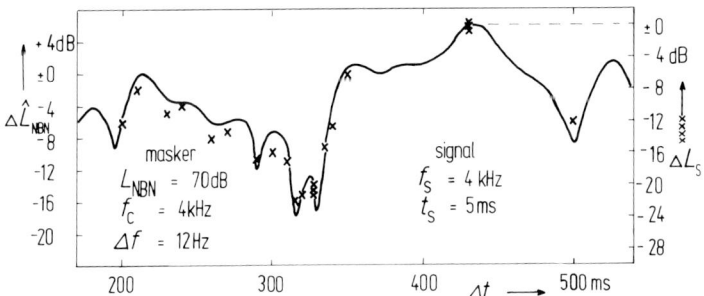

Fig. 7 Instantaneous sound pressure level $\hat{L}_{NBN}$ of an artificial noise of 12 Hz bandwidth centered at 4 kHz as function of time Δt after the "begin" of the noise with very low repetition rate (almost undetectable). The crosses indicate the threshold L_S of a 5 ms long 4 kHz-tone signal as function of the delay time Δt between "begin" of the noise and onset of the signal.

The threshold of such a signal was measured in a preliminary experiment by only one observer several times as function of the delay time Δt between the "start" of the artificial noise and the onset of the signal. The averaged thresholds are marked as crosses in Fig. 7. The 3 crosses at the same delay-time indicate the variability in threshold if certain points are reproduced. A comparison between the instantaneous level $\hat{L}_{NBN}$ and the masked thresholds indicates that the threshold follows L_{NBN} very closely. Most of the peaks and valleys of $\hat{L}_{NBN}$ show up in the threshold of the signal.

Although these are only the very first results of a larger series of measurements, it looks as though the ear reacts against statistical changes in a way very similar to that we have found when using periodical changes, at least for bandwidths of smaller size. This may be interpreted as indication that the ear's psychoacoustical excitation follows the temporal functions regardless of statistical or periodical stimulations, the latter of which produce a sensation of rhythm.

Summary

Three different critical durations can be extrapo-

lated out of the mentioned results if only the very
first order effects are taken into account. Two of
them belong to the temporal behavior of the excitation, while the longest and first seems to belong to
the time needed to create a sensation limit like

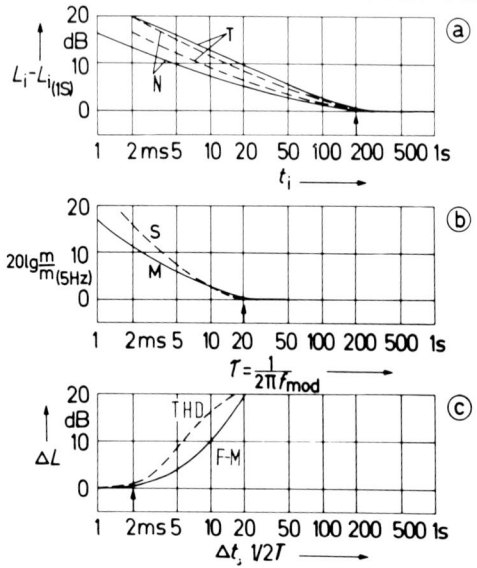

Fig. 8   The 3 critical durations of 200 ms, 20 ms
and 2 ms.

(a) Equal loudness contours as function of
duration (loudness: dashed; threshold:
solid). N for noises, T for tones.

(b) Equal strength (S) of roughness contour
and threshold of amplitude modulation
(M) as function of the time constant τ
related to the frequency f_{mod} of modulation.

(c) Threshold difference (THD) ΔL from Fig.6
and difference ΔL between simultaneous
and forward masking (F-M) as function of
$\frac{1}{2}$ T and the delay time Δt, respectively
(from Zwicker, 1971).

threshold or a sensation itself like loudness. If
equal loudness contours (threshold included) are
drawn in such a way that the level increment ΔL =
$L_i - L_{i(1s)}$ necessary to produce equal loudness is

plotted as function of the duration of the sound, the curves in Fig. 8a are produced. The ear behaves differently for durations longer than 200 ms in relation to durations shorter than 200 ms.

The second, next smaller critical duration is in the vicinity of about 20 ms. It becomes clear, if the threshold of modulation or the strength of roughness is shown as function of the time constant τ which is correlated to the frequency of modulation f_{mod}

$$\text{by } \tau = \frac{1}{2\pi f_{mod}}. \qquad (3)$$

This is shown in Fig. 8b where a logarithmic ordinate scale is used. The critical duration again divides two ranges in which the ear behaves differently. This critical duration may indicate the range in which temporal effects related to the temporal shift of the excitation pattern are most effective.

The shortest and last critical duration belongs to a value of about 2 ms and indicates the shortest temporal structure of the stimulus which can influence the excitation-time pattern. Shorter temporal structures do not show up in the excitation-time pattern. The threshold differences ΔL shown in Fig. 6 are plotted in Fig. 8c (THD) as function of the duration $\frac{1}{2} T$ of the impulse or the pause. Also the difference ΔL between simultaneous masking and forward masking (F-M) using white noise as masker and as signal is shown. Both curves point to the abscissa at 2 ms, indicating the shortest critical duration important for excitation.

It may be necessary to point out that this short critical duration belongs to one and the same pathway. In other words, time patterns in a certain pathway can be indicated only if they have a time structure with intervals longer than 2 ms. This does not mean that the ear may be unable to detect very short time differences - as in localization. For such sensations the ear makes use of the time differences between the two pathways - a completely different situation. On the other hand the three critical durations 200 ms, 20 ms and 2 ms seem to play an important role in psychoacoustics.

References

Elliott, L.L. (1965). Changes in the simultaneous masked threshold of brief tones. J. Acoust. Soc. Amer. 38, 738.

Elliott, L.L. (1967). Development of auditory narrow-band frequency contours. J. Acoust. Soc. Amer. 42, 143.

Fastl, H. (1972). Temporal effects in masking. Symposium on Hearing Theory 1972. IPO Eindhoven, Holland.

Feldtkeller, R., and Oetinger, R. (1956). Die Hörbarkeitsgrenzen von Impulsen verschiedener Dauer. Akust. Beih. (Acustica) H. 2, 489-493.

Green, D.M. (1969). Masking with continuous and pulsed sinusoids. J. Acoust. Soc. Amer. 46, 939.

Møller, A. (1972). Coding of amplitude and frequency modulated sounds in the cochlear nucleus of the rat. Acta Physiol. Scand. 86, 223-238.

Raab, D.H. (1963). Backward masking. Psychol. Bull. 60, 118.

Ritsma, R.J. (1962). Existence region of the tonal residue I. J. Acoust. Soc. Amer. 34, 1224.

Scholl, H. (1962). Das dynamische Verhalten des Gehörs bei der Unterteilung des Schallspektrums in Frequenzgruppen. Acustica 12, 101-107.

Stein, H.J. (1960). Das Absinken der Mithörschwelle nach dem Abschalten von Weißem Rauschen. Acustica 10, 116-119.

Terhardt, E. (1968). Über akustische Rauhigkeit und Schwankungsstärke. Acustica 20, 215-224.

Terhardt, E. (1970). Frequency analysis and periodicity detection in the sensations of roughness and periodicity pitch. In: Frequency Analysis and Periodicity Detection in Hearing (R. Plomp and G.F. Smoorenburg, eds.), pp. 376-394. Sijthoff, Leiden, The Netherlands.

Walliser, K. (1969). Zusammenhänge zwischen dem Schallreiz und der Periodentonhöhe. Acustica 21, 329-336.

Zwicker, E. (1952). Die Grenzen der Hörbarkeit der Amplitudenmodulation und der Frequenzmodulation eines Tones. Akust. Beih. (Acustica) H.3, 125-133.

Zwicker, E. (1958). Über psychologische und methodische Grundlagen der Lautheit. Akust. Beih. (Acustica) H.1, 237-258.

Zwicker, E. (1963). Über die Lautheit von ungedrosselten und gedrosselten Schallen. Akust. Beih. (Acustica) 194-211.

Zwicker, E. (1965a). Temporal effects in simultaneous masking by white-noise bursts. J. Acoust. Soc. Amer. 37, 653-663.

Zwicker, E. (1965b). Temporal effects in simultaneous masking and loudness. J. Acoust. Soc. Amer. 38, 132-141.

Zwicker, E. (1970). Masking and psychological excitation, as consequences of the ear's frequency analysis. In: Frequency Analysis and Periodicity Detection in Hearing (G.F. Smoorenburg and R. Plomp, eds.), pp. 376-394. Sijthoff, Leiden, The Netherlands.

Zwicker, E. (1971). Zusammenhänge zwischen neueren Ergebnissen der Psychoakustik. In: Akustik und Schwingungstechnik, pp. 9-21. VDI-Verlag, Düsseldorf.

Zwicker, E., and Fastl, H. (1972a). Zur Abhängigkeit der Nachverdeckung von der Störimpulsdauer. Acustica 26, 78-82.

Zwicker, E., and Fastl, H. (1972b). On the Development of the critical band. J. Acoust. Soc. Amer. 52, 699-702.

Zwicker, E. and Feldtkeller, R. (1967). Das Ohr als Nachrichtenempfänger. 2. erw. Aufl., Hirzel-Verlag, Stuttgart.

Zwislocki, J. (1960). Theory of temporal auditory summation. J. Acoust. Soc. Amer. 32, 1046.

Figure 1 reproduced from FREQUENCY ANALYSIS AND PERIODICITY DETECTION IN HEARING edited by R. Plomp and F.G. Smoorenburg, 1969, by permission of Sijthoff, Leiden, The Netherlands.

Figure 2 reproduced from DAS OHR ALS NACHRICHTENEM-PFÄNGER by E. Zwicker and R. Feldtkeller, 1967, by permission of Hirzel-Verlag, Stuttgart.

Figures 6 and 8 reproduced from AKUSTIK UND SCHWINGUNGSTEKNIK, 1971, by permission of VDI-Verlag, Düsseldorf.

DISCUSSION

ZWISLOCKI: I just wanted to remind you that there are other time constants which you may have missed. It is an intriguing phenomenon that several things seem to increase with a time constant of 200 msec but why does not masking increase with the masker duration? If you increase the duration of the tone, then its threshold improves and the loudness grows. From this you would conclude that excitation increases somehow with duration. Why does the masking then not increase when the delay between the test tone and the onset of the masker increases?

ZWICKER: The model I presented is a very simplified one. There are many special temporal effects in masking which are not included. In addition, lots of nonlinear effects are involved in masking and I completely agree on your finding that even a quite short masker sound can give a strong masking effect. On the other hand the excitation time pattern does not go down much during stimulation pauses of 2 msec.

GREEN: Well, perhaps I had better say something about these stationary time-invariant filters since Dr. Zwicker and I have argued about this at some length. I would agree that for functional analysis of the system you can assume a stationary filter as Dr. Zwicker has described it. However, I think that if any sharpening is neural in nature, that is, if there really is a need to sharpen the cochlear mechanical tuning to predict the 8th nerve tuning curves, then you can expect that to take time. Since the excitation and the inhibition processes may indeed have different time constants, it seems to me that you really are interested in very fine details of the time course of these things. I think, however, that a very good starting assumption for a functional description is a stationary time-invariant filter.

ZWICKER: We have the feeling that what we measure by excitation-critical band rate-time pattern (including this quick rise and slower decay) gives us something similar to that information which is transferred from low levels to higher levels. This idea is still a speculation right now but it may be interesting to discuss it. It means that at higher levels something else may be produced out of that information coming from low levels but what I would like to make quite clear is that nothing can be produced at higher levels which was not already available at the lower levels. On the other hand the filter system I talked about is not completely linear. If you raise the level of the upper slope of the excitation-critical band, the rate pattern becomes flatter; this is a kind of a non-linearity. But all measurements have shown that (1) the hearing system reacts in such a way and (2) that this filter system can be thought of as always available, quite in agreement with the physiological data available now.

SCHWARTZKOPFF: Well, I wonder if you know the work of the late Dr. Batteau who studied monaural auditory localization?

ZWICKER: Well, I do not know his work but I may say that we have not found any result, at least in a frequency range above 500 Hz, in which phase is involved for monaural perception.

EVANS: I think that one need not necessarily take that as an explanation, because the time differences Batteau (1968) referred to were in the context of echoes generated by the pinna. Such echoes produce changes in the spectrum of ambient sounds in the same way that mixing delayed with undelayed noise generates the acoustic gratings that I referred to in my paper. The spectral composition of Batteau's echo signals will be a function of the delay. It seems therefore quite reasonable that the effect that Dr. Batteau was observing could be simply explained in spectral terms.

GREEN: I think that that is exactly the explanation

of Batteau's result and I would like to agree with
Dr. Evans that the effect amounts to detecting a
change in the spectrum over about 10 kHz region. I
think those results are probably due to spectral
changes and not temporal.

ZWISLOCKI: May I come back to my question to you?
From the point of view of signal detection theory,
it seems that detection of a signal in noise may
depend on the variance of what you call excitation,
rather than excitation itself. So, if you assume
that, on the other hand, detection of the signal
depends on the integral of the signal taken over a
certain time period and, on the other hand, on the
variance of the noise, you can very well put together
the fact that masking does not increase with the
duration of the masker but does increase with the
duration of the signal.

ZWICKER: Yes, thank you for that comment. The only
problem is that you have to have both masker and
signal very short in order to measure this effect.
I do not see any other possibility.

References

Batteau, D.W. (1967). The role of the pinna in human
    localization. Proc. Roy. Soc. B. 168, 158-180.

Batteau, D.W. (1968). Role of the pinna in localiza-
    tion: theoretical and physiological consequences.
    In: Hearing Mechanisms in Vertebrates (A.V.S. de
    Reuck and J. Knight, eds.), pp. 234-239. J. & A.
    Churchill, London.

MINIMUM INTEGRATION TIME

David M. Green

University of California, San Diego
La Jolla, California
USA

1. Introduction

The integration of sensory information can be likened to the process of taking a running average. The instantaneous input of the sensory system is convolved with a temporal weighting function or time window to produce an output that is a smoothed or averaged version of the input (Munson, 1947, Zwislocki, 1960, 1969). In many experiments the subject should average or integrate for as long a period of time as possible. Consider, for example, the task of detecting a signal of various duration partially masked by continuous noise. For long duration signals the longer the integration time the better the signal-to-noise ratio, and hence the better the detection performance. Thus the results of such studies can be used to estimate the longest averaging time that the subject can achieve. The estimates of integration time derived from this kind of study range between 100 to 300 msec (Plomp and Bouman, 1959, Scholl, 1962). Such long integration times are effective in dealing with the requirements of this particular psychophysical task. The results imply that somewhere in the nervous system the information is combined over these relatively long periods of time. One task for which a shorter integration time would be advantageous is the detection of a click centered in a continuous noise. Assuming that the integration time is longer than the duration of the click, the shorter the integration time the better the signal-to-noise ratio. A brief integration time would also be desirable if one is trying to distinguish between two transients that differ only in their phase spectrum, that is, transients that have identical power spectra but different fine structure. In this case a shorter integration time would preserve more of the variation in input than a longer integration time. The duration of these short temporal windows we call <u>minimum integration times</u>. These minimum integration times probably reflect the operation of an early stage of auditory processing which is likely to be located more peripherally than the stage responsible for the longer integration periods.

A minimum integration time obviously establishes certain limits in both recognition and masking experiments. A systematic study of these limits will then provide us with estimates of the minimum integration time. The central theme of this paper is to describe a number of different procedures used to estimate the minimum integration time. Unfortunately all of the estimates are not the same and it is clear that our understanding of this aspect of auditory processing is still incomplete. We begin by considering the problem of discriminating between two brief signals that differ only in their phase spectrum.

2. Discrimination among Huffman Sequences

A Huffman sequence is a specially constructed digital signal. It is a signal of finite duration and is constructed of n digital samples, where n is a power of two. Once n is fixed, one can construct $n/2!$ signals; each having the same energy spectrum but a different phase spectrum. Thus, the wave shapes of all these signals are different but their energy spectra and durations are identical. If an observer can distinguish between two Huffman sequences of the same class (same n), then one is sure that the basis of the distinction is something other than the energy spectrum of the signal.[1] One simple hypothesis is that the

---

[1] An important feature of this work is the control of the energy spectrum. Slight changes in the timing of pulses are detectable at incredibly small values. For example, Leshowitz (1971) has shown that a gap of 6 μsec between brief pulses can be reliably detected. The basis of this discrimination, as he demonstrates in a series of controlled experiments, is undoubtedly slight differences in energy spectrum above 4 kHz. These kinds of changes are also probably responsible for the perception of temporal "jitter", Pollack (1968).

observer can distinguish temporal events within the
waveform, and hence that his integration period is
shorter than the total duration of the Huffman sequence.
Studies of how discrimination depends upon
the duration of the Huffman sequence can therefore be
used to estimate the minimum integration time of the
ear. James Patterson (1970) was the first to use this
technique in the systematic study of this problem.

To understand Patterson's work we must understand a
little more about Huffman sequences. A Huffman sequence
can be viewed as the response of a special
filter to a pair of impulses. The first excites the
filter, and, if the response is not over at the end
of T seconds, another impulse of appropriate amplitude
and of opposite polarity is applied to terminate
the filter's response. Thus the duration of the signal
is exactly T seconds. The special filter is an all-
pass filter composed of overlapping a high-pass and
low-pass section. The amplitude response of the filter
is flat, but there is a 360° phase change in the
frequency region where the sections overlap. We call
this frequency region the center frequency of the all-
pass filter. The rate of phase change as a function
of frequency, or, equivalently, the amount of time
delay introduced in this frequency region, is determined
by the degree of tuning of the two filter sections.
We refer to this parameter as the Q of the all-
pass filter. We can cascade at most n/2 such filters
and therefore produce n/2! distinct signals. The regions
of frequency delay can be compounded in n/2!
ways. All these signals have the same energy spectrum,
the same Q, and the same duration. Patterson measured
how a number of these parameters affected the observer's
ability to discriminate pairs of signals selected
from the same class. While all the parameters have a
slight effect on the ability to discriminate among
pairs he found, as a general rule, that discrimination
was possible as long as the total duration of the signals
was 1 or 2 msec. Discrimination among the Huffman
sequences is always somewhat subtle and at times
requires considerable practice on the part of the observer.
Despite the subtlety of the judgement, discrimination
does not improve appreciably once the
Huffman signals are as little as 5 dB above their
masked threshold. It is also of interest to note that
when a Huffman sequence is masked by white Gaussian
noise, the threshold value is essentially the same

for all members of the same class. That is, Huffman sequences having the same duration have essentially the same threshold value in white Gaussian noise.

The latter finding is perhaps not too surprising when one realizes that Huffman sequences have essentially a flat power spectrum. The spectral level is probably the only important parameter when the sequences are used as signals to be detected against a white noise background. If, however, Huffman sequences are used as maskers of sinusoidal signals having the same duration, then the amount of masking depends heavily upon the particular sequence employed. For 10 ms sequences, differences in masking as large as 25 dB are obtained depending upon the particular Huffman sequence that we employ as a masker. In general a Huffman sequence having most of its energy concentrated at a particular time within the total duration of the sequence is a poor masker. Such a masker is, in effect, an impulse in the time domain. A much better masker, and one that nearly resembles the masking produced by white Gaussian noise, is a Huffman sequence composed of a number of cascaded all-pass filters with center frequencies chosen haphazardly so that the energy is distributed relatively uniformly over the entire interval.

If the energy is not uniformly distributed over the entire interval then the observer can apparently utilize an integration time shorter than the duration of the entire sequence. He thereby improves the signal-to-noise ratio at some time within the interval, and achieves better detection results. This result also suggests that the minimum integration time of the ear is less than the total duration of the Huffman sequence, in this case 10 msec. It would be interesting to pursue Patterson's result using a variety of different durations to determine at what point the masking is largely independent of the particular sequence chosen. This value should occur around 1 to 2 msec since this is the point at which discrimination among different Huffman sequences begins to fail.

3. The Minimum Integration Time as the Function of Frequency

While Patterson's experiments have probed a number of features of the minimum integration time many questions remain unanswered. One important issue is whether or not the minimum time depends upon frequency. One hypothesis is that these brief integration times simply reflect the first stage filtering involved in the process of frequency analysis. At mid to high frequencies, the width of the critical band is of the order of 200 to 1000 Hz and this corresponds to a time constant of 2 msec or less. According to this hypothesis, the minimum integration time is simply the limit set by the bandwidth of the frequency analysis system. Since the critical bandwidth is heavily dependent upon frequency, the minimum integration time should vary with frequency. The change should be as much as an order of magnitude as one moves from the low frequency region, say 600 Hz, to a relatively high frequency region, say 4000 Hz. To test this hypothesis we need to measure the temporal limits of discrimination using signals in which the information is contained in a single frequency region. The only change among the signals would be how that information is packaged in time; that is, we must change the phase spectrum of the signals at a fixed frequency locus.

Recall that the Huffman sequence can be viewed as a signal generated by passing an impulse through an all-pass filter composed of two overlapping sections. The frequency at which this overlap occurs determines the frequency region in which energy is delayed. The attenuation rates of the high and low-pass sections determine the rate of phase change, and hence the amount of the delay at that frequency. We, therefore, generated a set of signals with the same center frequency but different bandwidths for the all-pass filter. We asked whether the subjects were able to discriminate between any two of these signals. Specifically we measured how much difference in delay is required to achieve 75 % discrimination in a two-alternative force-choice task.

Fig. 1 shows a sequence of such signals. They are arranged from left to right in order of increasing delay. The pressure waveforms associated with these signals are shown in the second and bottom row of the graph. Above each waveform we display a rough sound spectogram analysis. We computed the spectogram for each waveform by simply cutting it into four equal slices and computing the energy spectrum in each time slice. Time is represented on the abscissa, linear

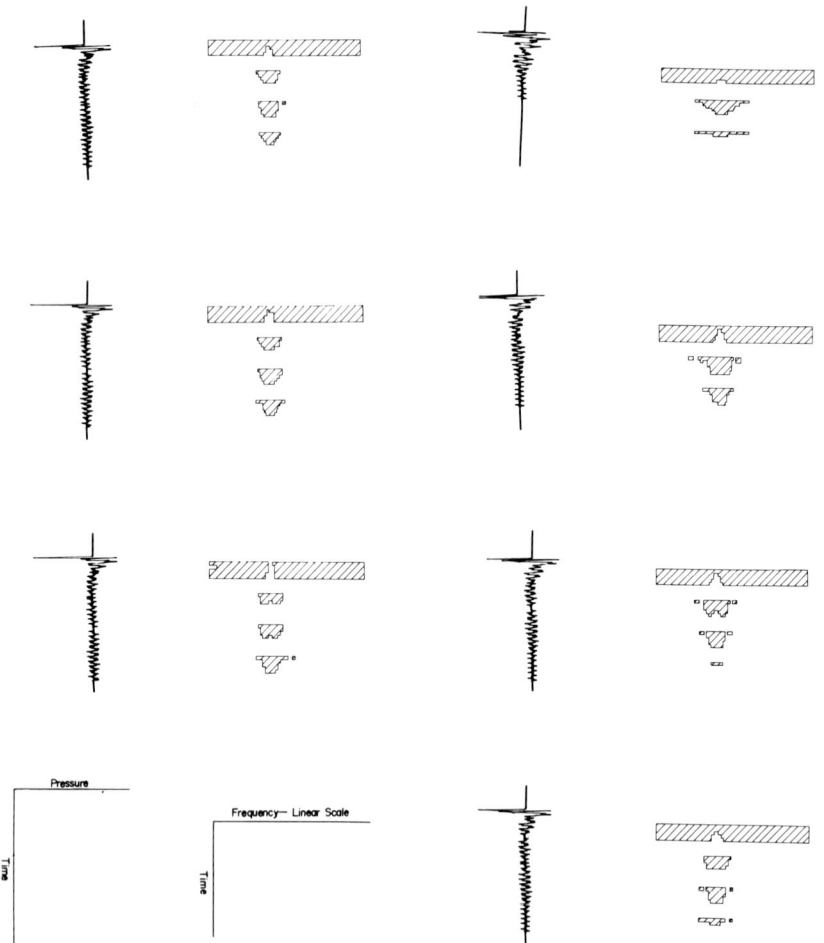

Fig. 1 Waveforms and short term energy spectra of signals used in the Huffman sequence experiment. The "center frequency" of the all-pass filter is 1875 Hz. The number of sample points is 128, so the duration is 12.8 msec. The delay caused by the filtering increases from left to right in the figure. The standard for the paired comparison judgements is a medium delay (6.4 msec approximately). This waveform appears in the upper right panel.

frequency along the ordinate. The thickness of the rectangles codes the amount of energy at that time-frequency coordinate. As one can see, the bulk of the energy in the waveform is concentrated at the beginning of the interval. This corresponds to the initial impulse in the time waveform. At the center frequency of the filter namely 1875 Hz, the energy is progressively delayed in the successive signals by changing the bandwidth of the all-pass filter. Thus, for the bottom-right side of the drawing, we have used a very narrowly tuned filter. This introduces a considerable delay in the energy occurring at 1875 Hz. At the top-left of the figure the bandwidth of the filter is much broader and hence less delay is introduced.

Our tests were run by selecting a signal with medium delay, and using that as a standard in a discrimination test. We systematically measured the observer's ability to discriminate the standard from some other signal in the set. As the delay is increased or decreased progressively from the standard, the discrimination becomes easier. For example, one can achieve about 100 % discrimination if one is attempting to distinguish the standard from either extreme shown in Fig. 1. The change in delay needed to achieve about 75 % correct was measured by interpolation. Three center frequencies were used and three durations for the signals were employed as parameters, 3.2, 6.4, and 12.8 msec. The general results were much the same for all conditions of the experiment. The change in delay, Δt, needed to discriminate among the signals was 2.2 ms at 625 Hz, 2.4 ms at 1875 Hz, and 2.1 ms at 4062 Hz. Thus the minimum integration time appears to be essentially the same at all frequencies.

These series of experiments were run at an overall level of 90 dB SPL, (measured when the sequence is played repetitively). That is, the sequence would generate the same energy as a 90 dB sinusoid gated for 3.2, 6.4 or 12.8 msec. An additional short series of experiments were conducted in which the level was varied over a 40 dB range; from 100 dB to 70 dB. Discrimination became progressively worse as the level was lowered. The values of Δt were almost twice as large at the lowest level compared with the highest level, but the value of Δt changed only about 20 % at the three highest levels. In terms of sensation level, the lowest level was about 25 dB above the threshold for detection.

4. Temporal Modulation Transfer Function

A rather different way to investigate the minimum

time constant of the auditory system has been pursued by Dr. Neal Viemeister in our laboratory. This approach stems from the system analysis point of view and involves the detection of a brief signal, a click, presented at various times during a temporally varying noise masker. Specifically, the amplitude of wide band noise was modulated, about 90 %, by a sinusoidal signal. The average overall level of the noise (with no modulation) was about 65 dB. The detection threshold of a brief pulse was measured as the click was presented at several different phases of the modulation cycles. The resulting measurements could be well fitted by a sinusoid of a certain amplitude and phase. This amplitude and phase value, determined for several modulation frequencies, was used to estimate the temporal transfer characteristic of the auditory processor used by the observer in this experiment.

Fig. 2 shows some typical threshold measurements fit-

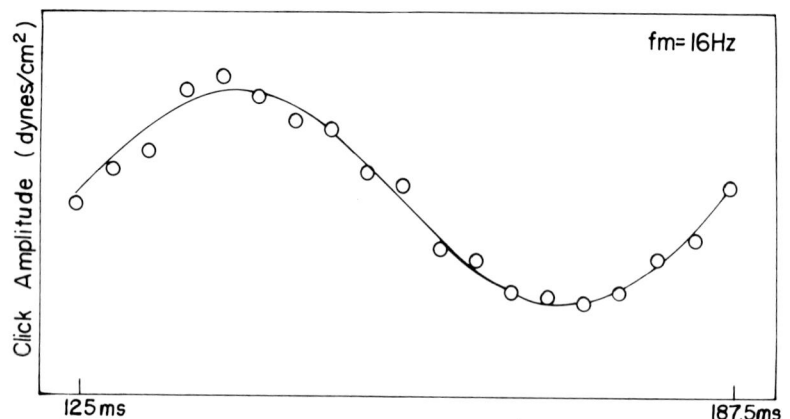

Delay T(msec) from Onset
of Sinewave Modulation

Fig. 2   The threshold amplitude of a click presented at various phases of a noise the amplitude of which is sinusoidally modulated. The frequency of modulation is 16 Hz so data from an entire period of the modulation are shown on the figure. The solid line fit to the data provides an estimate of the amplitude (used in Fig. 3a) and phase (used in Fig. 3b) of the internal representation of the masker.

ted by a sinusoid. A continuous noise was modulated for 500 ms. The click was inserted on the first zero crossing of the sinusoidal modulation voltage at least 125 ms after the onset of the modulation. In the present case the modulation frequency was 16 Hz so the graph shows the amplitude threshold for the click during an entire period or 62.5 ms. As one can see from the graph, the threshold for the click was elevated when the signal is presented near the peak of the modulation sinusoid and is considerably lower when the click is presented during a valley of the modulation cycle. At this low modulation frequency, there is practically no phase shift. The click threshold very nearly tracks the instantaneous power of the noise. A set of such threshold measurements performed at a variety of modulation frequencies is shown in Fig. 3a and 3b. The peak-valley difference

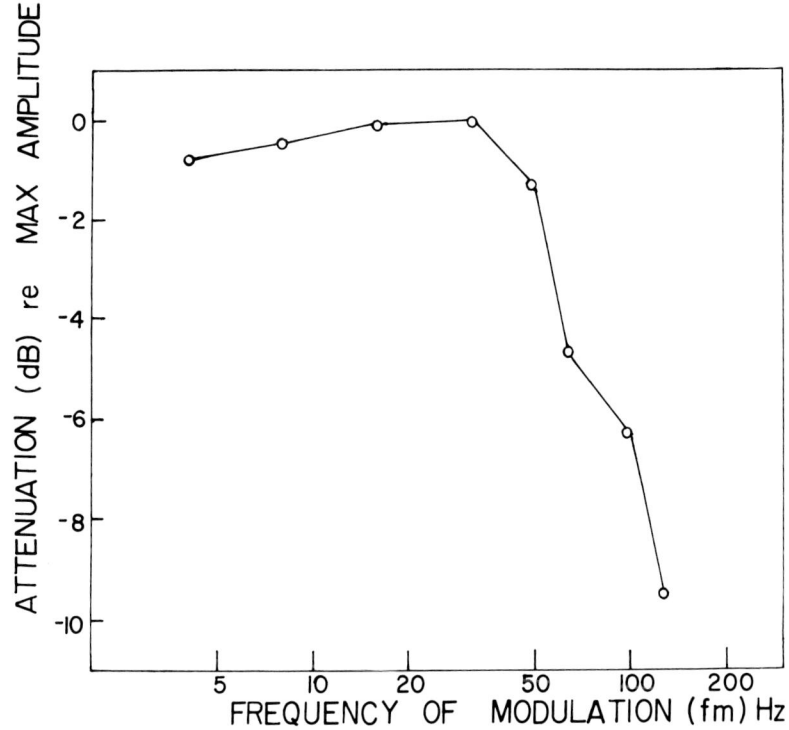

Fig. 3a The relative variation in click threshold, in dB, as a function of the frequency of modulation of the noise. The   (cont'd)

(Fig. 3a, cont'd) ordinate is scaled so that the maximum variation is set at 0 dB. The ordinate is proportional to 20 log of the peak to trough ratio derived from Fig. 2.

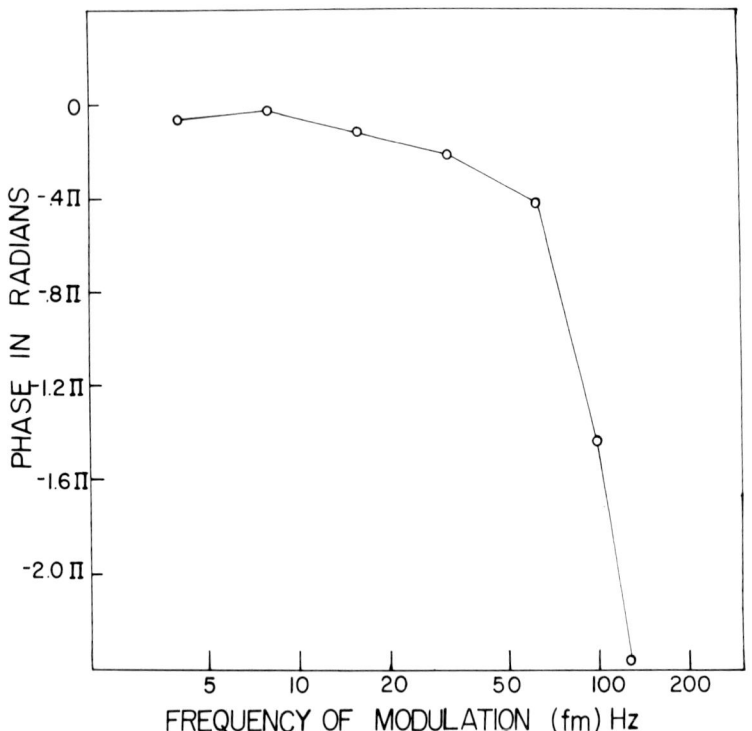

Fig. 3b The phase of the sinusoid fit to the masking data (such as that shown in Fig. 2) as a function of the frequency of modulation.

in the threshold of the click is maximum at low modulation frequencies, and diminishes as the modulation frequency increases. In Fig. 3a we have simply plotted the amplitude of the click threshold, as it is fit to the data, re the maximum amplitude. The phase measurements show practically no phase shift at low frequency and progressively more phase shift at the higher frequency. Both the decline in the amplitude function with modulation frequency and the change in estimated phase which exceeds π radians, indicate that the temporal integrator is a third or fourth-order system. The 3 dB point of the amplitude thresh-

old is approximately 60 - 100 Hz, depending upon the
observer. This corresponds to a time constant of approximately 1 - 3 msec. The preliminary nature of
these measurements should be emphasized. They were
started by Dr. Viemeister during the past six months
and there are a number of parameters that remain to
be explored. Nevertheless, the early results are encouraging and it is hoped that considerably more insight into the nature of the integration process can
be obtained from this technique. One important experimental question will involve filtering the noise
so that it occupies only certain regions of the
spectrum and repeating these measurements for each
region separately. Whether the results will be largely independent of frequency region, similar to the
Huffman sequence results, is not yet known.

5. The Critical Masking Interval

A third method of estimating the minimum integration
time was tried about a year ago in our laboratory by
Drs. Penner, Robinson and myself. We measured the
masked threshold of a click placed in the center of
a burst of noise. Both the click and the noise were
low-pass filtered at about 5 kHz. The click had a
nominal duration of 100 μsec. The noise burst used
to mask the click was varied from 100 μsec to 300
msec and two different noise levels were used. Let
me emphasize once again that the click was always
presented in the center of the noise masker.

As the duration of the noise masker is diminished,
we certainly expect that the detectability of the
click would be initially unaffected because the minimum integration time of the ear is probably much less
than 300 msec. In fact we might expect from our previous results that the threshold of the click would
be largely independent of the duration of the noise
down to a duration of approximately 1 - 3 msec. At
that point, the click threshold should decrease since
the noise effective in masking the signal will diminish once we have passed this minimum integration
time. The basis for this inference is exactly the
same as the corresponding inference made in the original critical band study. In fact our procedure is
nothing more than the temporal analog of Fletcher's
original experiment (Fletcher, 1940).

The results of our measurements for two different

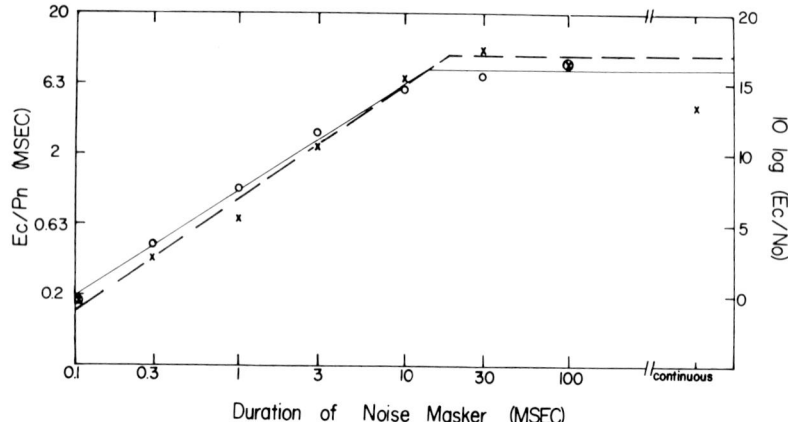

Fig. 4 Effect of masker duration on the click threshold. The nominal masker bandwidth is 5175 Hz and the click duration is 100 μsec. The noise spectrum level is either 57 dB (circles) or 37 dB (x's). On the right hand ordinate is the ratio of click energy to the noise energy in a one cycle band, in dB. On the left hand ordinate is the ratio of click energy to noise power, in msec.

noise levels are shown in Fig. 4. As one can see, the breakpoint in the function occurs at somewhat longer durations than we had expected. The breakpoint appears to be in the neighborhood of 10 to 20 msec and slightly dependent on noise level.

Actually we expected to find the breakpoint to be somewhat larger than the measurements derived from other techniques for the following reasons. Suppose the minimum integration window is roughly rectangular in shape. To detect a signal placed in the mid-point of a noise burst, the optimum location for the window is just overlapping either the leading or the trailing edge of the click. This is better than centering the window on the click since the effective noise can be reduced by half in this way. Thus, if one assumes the minimum integration time is of the order of 2 - 3 msec, then the breakpoint should occur between 4 and 6 msec in Fig. 4. Unhappily the results are probably 2 to 3 times that number and we feel this inconsistency is well beyond the range of experimental error.

In an attempt to resolve this inconsistency we have
explored a variety of shapes for the time window in
addition to the rectangular one. A rectangular time
window is clearly unrealistic. Moreover, a more realistic time window would allow one to enlarge the
theory to account for both forward and backward
masking. However, none of these assumptions could
explain the difference between the 2 msec value found
in the earlier experiments and the 20 msec value
measured in the present experiment.

We cannot explain this discrepancy. However, there
are several features of the last experiment that are
troubling. One is shown in Fig. 4. It is the threshold for the click when masked by continuous noise. As
one can see the threshold for continuous noise is
about 3 dB lower than the threshold for even the
longest gated condition. Admittedly this difference
is small, but it was observed in the data of all
three subjects. Moreover it replicates a previous
finding by Green and Sewall (1962). One plausible
hypothesis is that the auditory temporal parameters
are somewhat influenced by whether or not the ear is
in steady state conditions. The integration times are
perhaps somewhat different under transient and steady
state conditions. On the other hand this hypothesis
does not seem likely since the Huffman sequences are
transient signals and the minimum time constant estimated with these signals appears to be much smaller.
Furthermore Viemeister's modulation technique estimates the integration filter under steady state conditions. At present we are unable to provide satisfactory explanation of this discrepancy or to suggest the factors responsible for it.

We do not know if the breakpoint in Fig. 4 depends on
the frequency composition of the signal; Dr. Penner
is pursuing this topic at present. We might expect
that it is not because this task is similar to one
studied by Miller and Garner (1948). They measured
the threshold of a pure tone as a function of the
interruption rate of a noise masker. The improvement
in threshold as a function of the rate of interruption was nearly independent of frequency of the signal, for frequencies from 250 to 4000 Hz.

6. Summary

The shortest averaging time that the auditory system

can use to detect or recognize differences among brief signals is called the minimum integration time. Three different experimental procedures have been used in an attempt to measure this minimum integration time. Two of the procedures, discrimination of phase changes in Huffman sequences, and the detection of a click in sinusoidally modulated noise, yield an estimate of about 2 ms. Moreover one of these procedures suggests that the minimum integration time is independent of frequency. In contrast, the detectability of a click centered in a rectangular burst of noise improves as the duration of the noise burst is reduced to less than 20 ms. Thus, with this procedure our estimate of the minimum integration time is about ten times larger than the other estimate. No hypothesis can be advanced at this time to explain the discrepancy.

Finally, we should note that the basis of the observer's judgements is slight differences in the quality of these brief sounds. These qualitative differences are usually subtle and could not be made unless the standard and the test stimuli were compared in close temporal continguity. The processes responsible for these judgements may be quite different from those involved in the judgement of temporal order, (Hirsh, 1959; Hirsh and Sherrick, 1961). Experiments on the judgement of temporal order suggest, for example, that 20 to 30 ms is needed before it is clear that the onset of a high-frequency tone occurred before the onset of a low-frequency tone. More work, both of a theoretical and empirical nature, is needed in this area. The essential problem is to understand the processes responsible for the different estimates of the auditory system's time-constants and to clarify the diverse estimates obtained with the different experimental procedures.

Acknowledgement

This research was supported by the National Institutes of Health, Public Health Service, U.S. Department of Health, Education, and Welfare. I would like to also thank Dr. Neal Viemeister, Dr. James H. Patterson, for their comments on various aspects of this research, and to Dr. Frederic L. Wightman, for reading and commenting on several drafts of this paper.

References

Fletcher, H. (1940). Auditory patterns. Rev. Mod. Phys. 12, 47-65.

Green, D.M., and Sewall, S.T. (1962). Effects of background noise on auditory detection of noise bursts. J. Acoust. Soc. Amer. 34, 1207-1216.

Hirsh, I.J. (1959). Auditory perception of temporal order. J. Acoust. Soc. Amer. 31, 759-767.

Hirsh, I.J., and Sherrick, Jr., C. E. (1961). Perceived order in different sense modalities. J. Exp. Psychol. 62, 423-432.

Leshowitz. B. (1971). The measurement of the two-click threshold. J. Acoust. Soc. Amer. 49, 462-466.

Miller, G.A., and Garner, W.R. (1948). The masking of tones by repeated bursts of noise. J. Acoust. Soc. Amer. 20, 691-696.

Munson, W.A. (1947). The growth of auditory sensation. J. Acoust. Soc. Amer. 19, 584-591.

Patterson, J.H., Jr. (1970). Perception of transient signals having identical energy spectra. Thesis. University of California, San Diego.

Plomp, R., and Bouman, M.A. (1959). Relation between hearing threshold and duration for tone pulses. J. Acoust. Soc. Amer. 31, 749-758.

Pollack, I. (1968). Can the binaural system preserve temporal information for jitter? J. Acoust. Soc. Amer. 44, 968-972.

Scholl, H. (1962). Über die Bildung der Hörshwellen und Mithörschwellen von Impulsen. Acustica. 12, 91-101.

Zwislocki, J.J. (1960). Theory of temporal auditory summation. J. Acoust. Soc. Amer. 32, 1046-1060.

Zwislocki, J.J. (1969). Temporal summation of loudness: An analysis. J. Acoust. Soc. Amer. 46, 431-441.

DAVID. M. GREEN

DISCUSSION

ZWICKER: What was the repetition rate in your last experiment?

GREEN: It was 2-interval forced choice task. There were two noise bursts separated by one second and then three or four seconds were allowed for an answer and the trial would be repeated.

ZWICKER: Do you have in mind to measure this a little bit as a function of the repetition rate, too, because if you have it at 10 msec you can measure this, or at 20 msec you can increase the repetition rate too.

GREEN: This would be very similar, as I understand it, to the experiment that you did, except that you used a signal between the noise bursts. The problem I see with that, and I wanted to talk to you later about it, is that as you increase the repetition rate you present the signal more often so there will be a confounding with the fact that you can also integrate over a longer period of time. This longer integration boosts the signal-to-noise ratio. This may lead to a loss of precision in your estimate of the breakpoint since the increasing portion of the curve may have a slope of $1\frac{1}{2}$ dB/double rather than 3 dB/double because of the long term integration effects.

ZWICKER: How long was the duration of the signal?

GREEN: It was a 100 μsec click; that is, the electrical pulse to the transducer was 100 μsec.

PFEIFFER: What was the noise structure?

GREEN: The noise was wide-band gaussian noise. Both signal and noise were filtered through about a 5,000 Hz low pass filter, for the data shown in Fig. 4.

PFEIFFER: You did not look at anything where there were instances of high pass noise? I am asking this because of some work of Bell Telephone Laboratories. They used high pass noise in efforts to have only the very lowest end of the threshold curve functioning. They were looking at some click interactions. The experiment acutally deals with two-click stimulation rather than one.

GREEN: This would concern the question of periodicity. As Dr. Zwicker pointed out, there is obviously a close relation between these investigations and such questions as the limit of residue pitch. It may well be that if you cannot resolve the time structure of the wave form then you cannot achieve a residue pitch. I have not pursued those comparisons in any detail; some of them are fairly close but others are difficult to understand.

PFEIFFER: What would happen if you tried to use your two pulses, which in essence sound like clicks, in the presence of noise?

GREEN: Despite the fact that you can think of them as two pulses, each of these brief waveforms sounds like a single click. If you add noise the result is really incredible. The recognition of two Huffman sequences is nearly perfect once the pair are 5 dB above their masked threshold. The qualitative differences between the two Huffman sequences are very subtle and you would think that a small amount of noise would just destroy the discrimination. If I played these sequences at 2 msec duration, I doubt that anybody in the room would believe that they were different. There are very slight qualitative changes in the sound. Of course this may simply mean that we do not have a very rich vocabulary describing these brief events and normally do not make subtle distinctions among them. In any case they are remarkably unaffected by masking noise.

DAVID M. GREEN

DALLOS: Would it be possible to improve the last experiment and go toward the 2 msec time constant by making the noise burst and the click coincident at the onset instead of placing the click in the middle?

GREEN: Yes, potentially, you can move the click on both sides, as Dr. Zwicker explained, and trace out the whole shape of this temporal window. If things were linear, that would work and you would have a potentially powerful method of analysis. In fact, you ought to be able to take the transform of that function and get Vimeister's results with the modulation of the noise and so on. The problem is, a variety of other things happens. Our thought was that by placing it in the center we would have at least a very simple condition and we would come very close to the 2 msec number and if that was successful we would proceed. But right now we are faced with 20 instead of 2 and I doubt you can get an order of magnitude by moving the click around within the noise burst.

DALLOS: But do you really have the simplest condition? With your paradigm you have both forward and backward masking acting on that click, whereas in the other case (coincident onsets) you would have eliminated at least one of those effects.

GREEN: My hunch is you would pick up more problems than you would solve but you might be right.

KIANG: One would like to know what happens in the auditory nerve when this stimulus is used. What happens as you shorten the duration of the noise bursts? Would you like to know that or do you think you can predict that already?

GREEN: I was hoping that I would get a simple answer so that I could avoid further complications, but obviously I did not. It may well be that the next step is to vary the frequency content of that click and see what happens to this 20 msec number.

VII
SPECIALIZED HEARING IN ANIMALS

ECHOLOCATION

Donald R. Griffin

The Rockefeller University
New York, N.Y.
U.S.A.

1. Introduction

Echolocation is an active perceptual process requiring both generation of sounds and sensory analysis of the resulting echoes. It can provide a fruitful bridge between the physiological and behavioral levels of scientific inquiry, because it is rapidly coming to be understood with increasing clarity by new physiological discoveries. The data and ideas that I can contribute are primarily concerned with behavior rather than with mechanisms at the cellular or molecular levels. Hence for a time I felt some doubt whether I could contribute anything appropriate for a symposium on Basic Mechanisms in Hearing. But a little reflection reaffirmed my conviction that behavior is both significant and basic. Because the component organs, cells, and even macromolecules of living organisms are so precisely adapted for their roles in physiology and behavior, we cannot hope to understand the parts without full appreciation of the whole. It is in this sense that behavior is as basic as biophysics and biochemistry. Scientists are enthusiastic about what each group considers truly basic mechanisms. But problems that appear basic to one discipline are often disdainfully dismissed as "mere phenomenology" by colleagues whose attention is focussed at another level of organization.

Dr. Suga has already presented the results of analytical studies of auditory neurophysiology in which he and his colleagues have been so successful during the past several years. I will therefore attempt to sketch the biology of echolocation from a perspective that will encompass both physiology and behavior, and I will also outline the variety of specialized forms of echolocation that animals present for our scrutiny. To appreciate the physiology of echolocation it is necessary to avoid what I have come to call "simplicity filters" that restrict our attention to an excessively narrow portion of either of the two important spectra - the spectrum of organizational levels and the phylogenetic spectrum of animal diversity. One form of simplicity filter is the widespread tendency to think in terms of the neuron, the mammal, or even the organism, with the implication that only a single system of each kind is significant. Unless we are truly confident of complete homogeneity, as we are for a given kind of atom or molecule, this "simplicity filter" can lead to overlooking highly significant data. It is desirable to strive for a happy mean between the belief that every subspecies is a totally different universe, and the highly focussed attitude of the molecular biologist who confidently expects in the near future to account for all the complexities of biology as neatly predictable reaction products.

2. The phylogenetic range of echolocation

2.1 Bats

While bats were the first animals in which echolocation was postulated (Hartridge, 1920) and clearly demonstrated (Griffin and Galambos, 1941), it is also practiced by a few terrestrial mammals, many marine mammals, and certain cave dwelling birds. Even among bats where echolocation is highly developed, it is almost wholly limited to one of the two suborders. Most of the suborder Megachiroptera (fruit eating bats of the African and Eurasian tropics) are visual animals with relatively large eyes and external ears that do not differ greatly from those of non-flying mammals. The single exception is the genus Rousettus, a fruit eating bat intermediate in size between the large flying foxes of the genus Pteropus and the mouse-sized nectar feeding members of the suborder Megachiroptera. While Rousettus does not differ appreciably in external appearance from other megachiropterans, it is the only member of this suborder that can fly successfully in totally dark caves. When flying in the dark it emits audible clicks that serve as orientation sounds. One captive individual was able, after considerable practice, to detect wires as small as about one millimeter in diameter by echolocation (Griffin et al., 1958).

All bats of the suborder Microchiroptera generate their orientation sounds in the larynx. Rousettus, on the other hand, uses the tongue to produce sharp clicks. In the two groups of echolocating birds the orientation sounds almost certainly originate in the syrinx, although no directly applicable experiments have yet been carried out. Despite the difference between a mammalian tongue and an avian syrinx, the resulting sounds are very similar. All consist of very brief clicks containing primarily frequencies between 5 and 10 kHz. Because of the low frequency and short duration (ordinarily about 1 to 3 msec), there are only a few complex sound waves, so that the clicks have a broad frequency spectrum. But we have no useful information about what portion of this spectrum is actually utilized for echolocation, and in the case of Steatornis and Collocalia we do not even have any direct measurements of the frequency range of auditory sensitivity.

Grinnell and Hagiwara (1972b) studied the auditory sensitivity of Rousettus and four other genera of Megachiroptera by means of evoked potentials. Auditory thresholds were lowest around 50 kHz and did not differ appreciably between the echolocating and non-echolocating species. These experiments together with others such as those of Ralls (1967) on mice indicate that in mammals sensitivity to ultrasonic frequencies is more closely correlated with small size than with use of echolocation.

2.2 Birds

Echolocation has been convincingly demonstrated in two distantly related groups of cave dwelling birds, the oil bird of tropical America (Steatornis caripensis) (Griffin, 1953a), and several (but not all) species of the genus Collocalia, the swiftlets of Southeast Asia (Novick, 1959). In both these avian examples, echolocation is used only for obstacle avoidance in dark caves, to the best of our knowledge, but it can nevertheless reach a respectable level of acuity. Collocalia vanikornesis can dodge obstacles as small as rods 6.3 millimeters in diameter even when flying in rather cramped quarters. But plastic covered wires 3 millimeters in diameter were not avoided above the chance level (Griffin and Suthers, 1970). The auditory system in Steatornis, as in owls, shows specializations suggestive of improved sensitivity or at least greater emphasis on hearing as compared with vision (Schwartzkopff, 1968). In several species of Collocalia Hollander (1971) has shown that those making greatest use of echolocation tend to have somewhat larger auditory portions of the brain.

2.3 Cetacea

Echolocation as practiced underwater by whales and porpoises is in some respects more difficult to study than that of bats or cave dwelling birds. Most cetaceans are large; the largest ones cannot yet practicably be brought into captivity at all. Sound waves travel for long distances in water, which has the advantage that orientation sounds can be detected farther from the animal than is ordinarily the case in air. But there is a corresponding disadvantage that often the observer cannot see, and hence cannot identify, the echolocating cetacean. Hence we have more information about the nature of emitted orientation sounds than about the perceptual capabilities of underwater echolocators. Schevill and Lawrence (1953a, 1953b, 1956) first demonstrated convincingly that porpoises (Turicops truncatus) could echolocate small objects in turbid water that effectively precluded vision. Kellogg (1953, 1961) and Kellogg et al. (1953) performed significant experiments with captive porpoises of the same species showing that they could discriminate between similar objects and could avoid even complex and multiple obstacles. Norris et al. (1961) first confirmed the fact of echolocation with blindfolded captive porpoises, and many investigators have shown by experiments basically similar to those just cited that many other species of cetaceans make use of echolocation. Especially interesting are the virtually blind river dolphins, Plantanista gangetica (Herald et al., 1969, Pilleri, 1970, 1971). These animals are so nearly blind and inhabit such murky water that echolocation plays a very major role in their lives, but adequate behavioral studies remain to be carried out. The available information about cetacean echolocation has been reviewed recently by Evans (in preparation).

As already emphasized by Dr. Suga, bats employ orientation sounds that last only a few msec but contain sufficiontly high frequencies that considerable numbers of sound waves are included - ordinarily on the order of 100 waves. The orientation sounds of bats have moderately complex frequency patterns and the clicks used for echolocation by cave dwelling birds and by <u>Rousettus</u> seem crude and primitive by comparison. But before jumping to what might seem a logical conclusion (aided perhaps by a sort of simplicity filter) that an orderly frequency pattern is correlated with highly refined and effective echolocation, we are brought up short by the inescapable fact that every cetacean so far studied uses for echolocation nothing but very brief clicks. These may vary in intensity and repetition rate but they invariably have durations of less than one msec and frequency spectra that extend virtually over the entire range of sensitivity of the animals concerned. Echolocating bats and birds have brains no larger than one or a very few grams in weight, whereas most echolocating cetaceans have brains comparable in size to our own. Even the smallest echolocating dolphins have brains weighing several hundred grams and the world's largest brains are found in the heads of whales, not of men. Perhaps with a kg of brain one can accomplish superb echolocation based solely upon broad band clicks, whereas if one is limited to a gram or two, more elaborate frequency patterns are required for effective orientation sounds.

Regardless of such considerations it has been abundantly demonstrated that relatively small cetaceans, with brains limited in size to roughly 1500 grams, can make remarkably precise and complex discriminations between very similar objects by echolocation. These pairs of successfully discriminated echolocation targets have included geometrically identical targets constructed of slightly different metal alloys. Our admiration should be tempered, however, by recognition of the fact that the acoustic impedance of water and metals differs much less than the contrast between air and almost any object that serves as an echolocation target for bats. This in turns means that relatively small differences in acoustic properties of underwater targets produce large differences in the echoes they return. Nevertheless, since such relatively simple clicks are being used as orientation sounds, the differences between echoes necessarily become subtle and difficult to analyze. They may include phase relationships as well as differences in Fourier spectrum.

2.4 Terrestrial mammals

Turning briefly at this point to terrestrial animals, we know only enough about the echolocation of shrews (Gould et al., 1964, Buchler, 1972) and rats (Rosenzweig and Riley, 1955) to recognize that it exists. The orientation sounds are extremely faint and can be detected by the best available microphones only at distances of a few centimeters. The experiments so far carried out demonstrate only that when shrews are obliged to jump a few centimeters in the dark from a circular platform they can echolocate another platform a few centimeters distant and avoid jumping into empty space. It may well be that echolocation is only a marginal mode of perception in these animals and used to a limited extent as they occasionally must make short leaps in darkness. Only after more thorough study will it be possible to say with any confidence whether or not echolocation has a larger role than this.

Of more immediate human concern, Supa et al. (1944) resolved a controversy of long standing by conclusively establishing that so-called facial vision of blind men is in large measure (although perhaps not totally) echolocation. Subsequent work by Kellogg (1962) and Rice (1967a, 1967b) has improved upon older experiments and demonstrated that, at least under favorable laboratory conditions, blind or blindfolded human subjects can detect by echolocation objects as small as disks of a few centimeters in diameter. In the case of our own species, however, echolocation may have practically no normal function, but only be called into play in the special case of blindness. The practical, humanitarian importance of human echolocation is sufficient to justify much more intensive investigation than has yet been devoted to the subject. We tend to reach for gadgets, figuratively speaking, and most research on aids for the orientation of the blind has followed the path of developing miniature portable instruments for echolocation rather than seeking ways to improve the natural capability of purely auditory echolocation

which blind men possess to varying degrees. A curtain
of implicit pessimism seems to block attempts to analyze human echolocation or develop means for improving its effectiveness. Yet when one contemplates the
spectacular feats of the auditory analysis and dic-
crimination performed routinely by the human brain
when dealing with speech or music, it is difficult to
justify the prevailing view that blind men cannot extract more than the most limited sort of information
from audible echoes.

3. The relationship of echolocation to other sensory channels

It is important to recognize that specialized as
bats are for echolocation it is not the only way in
which they gather information from their surround-
ings. In our first flush of enthusiasm over the discovery of echolocation in bats it seemed as though
vision was completely expendable. But later experiments have shown that even in bats such as the family Vespertilionidae that are highly specialized for
echolocation, vision is important under many circumstances (Suthers et al., 1969, Suthers, 1970). Even
those fruit eating bats that are capable of echolocation use olfaction to locate some of their food.
Especially in homing and migrations over considerable distances (Cochrum, 1969), vision appears to be
of primary importance (Griffin, 1970, Williams and
Williams, 1970a).

Another important type of orientation behavior exhibited by many bats under a variety of circumstances can be designated for convenience as spatial
memory. After they have become quite familiar with a
particular area, which may be a cave, a laboratory
room, or even perhaps an outdoor feeding area, bats
are often astonishingly prone to collide with newly
erected obstacles. In laboratory situations they also show convincing evidence of turning back from
the former location of obstacles such as moveable
partitions, and they may even go through moderately
complex flight maneuvers appropriate for entering a
home cage and may execute complex landing maneuvers
at a landing place that has just been removed
(Moehres and Oettingen-Spielberg, 1949, Griffin,
1958, Neuweiler and Moehres, 1967). Under natural
conditions many kinds of bats can be captured in

nets or traps consisting of closely spaced arrays of
threads or of wires even though in a laboratory experiment the same species can avoid smaller wires or
threads by echolocation. I have sometimes called
bats behaving in this way "Andrea Doria bats" or
perhaps at this symposium I should call them "Stockholm bats", with reference to the tragic collision
between these two ocean liners off the coast of the
United States several years ago despite the fact
that both ships were equipped with normally functioning radar. It has been suggested that "Andrea
Doria behavior" in bats means that they have ceased
to emit orientation sounds, but whenever an adequate
microphone has been available, this has not been the
case (Griffin, 1958), so it seems far more likely
that echoes are being ignored even though they are
reaching the bat's ears. Skepticism about the importance of echolocation is often based on this type of
behavior, but I believe this reflects a basic reluctance to credit a small mammal with a skill that resembles advanced human technologies. When birds are
captured in nets, no one suggests that they are
blind.

Students of whales and porpoises do not often report
behavior analogous to that of the bats that ignore
the echoes returning to their ears and crash into
newly erected obstacles or turn back from recently
removed walls of an experimental chamber. Many aspects of the behavior of bats can best be understood
by recognizing the important role of spatial memory,
and this may well be one aspect of orientation behavior where the cetaceans are far superior to bats,
although strictly comparable experiments have not
been carried out.

4. Adaptations of pulse repetition rate

It is a universal property of echolocation systems
that relatively short pulses are used for the emitted orientation sounds. In some bats these may be as
long as roughly 50 msec, but more often durations
are on the order of 1 or 2 msec. In a few bats pulse
duration is long enough to produce extensive overlap
in time between outgoing signal and returning echo,
but no animal has been found to employ for echolocation anything approaching a continuous signal. This
limitation is not found in artificial radar and sonar systems, although most of these also employ

brief pulses with relatively low duty cycle. But in
CW-FM radar or sonar the emitted frequency varies
progressively, and this allows echoes to be discriminated from the outgoing signal on the basis of frequency differences, the magnitude of which is a convenient measure of target range. It is pertinent to
inquire why no animals have apparently developed a
system of this type, even though the analogy has
been suggested on theoretical grounds (Pye, 1962).
A clue may be the increase in pulse repetition rate
that occurs in all echolocating animals yet studied
whenever they face difficult orientation problems.
It is as though brief pulses were essential for animal echolocation, and further that better information is obtained when many separate pulses are emitted per unit time. Repetition rates characteristically change over a range of one to two orders of
magnitude, with the highest occurring just when some
difficult target is being closely approached and
when it is necessary for the animal to make the most
precise reactions to it. The increase in pulse repetition rate as bats approached wire obstacles was
one of the first properties noted by Galambos and
Griffin (1942) and by Dijkgraaf (1946). It has also
been observed in all other echolocating bats, in the
two cave dwelling birds discussed above, and in all
echolocating cetaceans. The evidence for it is only
suggestive in shrews and blind men, but in the latter case it is complicated by uncertainties about
what constitutes a truly effective orientation sound
for human echolocation (Rice, 1967a, 1967b).

5. Echolocation of flying insects

Because the first investigators of echolocation in
bats lived in temperate latitudes our knowledge was
limited for many years to the rather small fraction
of the order Chiroptera that is available in Western
Europe and North America. I can recall many respected colleagues reinforcing one of my own simplicity
filters shortly after almost everyone was satisfied
that "the" bat avoided obstacles by echolocation
based pulses of high frequency sound. It seemed
rather foolish to indulge in further investigations
of the minutiae that might be disclosed by studying
the same bat out-of-doors or other species of bats
than conveniently available members of the family
Vespertilionidae. Data available up to approximately
1950 indicated that the orientation sounds were re-

markably uniform, all having a downward sweep in frequency of approximately an octave. To be sure there were slight differences in the range of frequencies employed, with larger species such as Eptesicus fuscus using somewhat lower frequencies or longer wavelengths than the best studied small bats of the genus Myotis.

It was almost by accident and for a completely different, unimportant reason that I happened in 1951 to go to the trouble of taking what then was inconveniently bulky apparatus out-of-doors to listen to the same species of bats pursuing insects rather than flying through a laboratory room dodging obstacles. The first evening of such observation shattered the simplicity filter of uniformity in the orientation sounds (Griffin, 1953b). Not only did pulse repetition rates increase over a much greater range when insects were pursued than when wires were dodged, the frequency patterns also turned out to be different. During the cruising or searching phase of insect hunting the pulses had a longer duration than we had ever observed before. In Eptesicus fuscus and Lasiurus borealis there were often periods of at least a few msec in which the frequency varied rather slightly, although in other parts of the pulse the same octave downward frequency sweep was evident. These early field studies immediately suggested that, contrary to previous opinion, echolocation was employed not only for avoiding stationary obstacles but in the active pursuit of flying insects.

It was necessary to bring this behavioral phenomenon into the laboratory, however, to obtain conclusive evidence that at least under some conditions echolocation was the sole method by which flying insects were detected and intercepted (Griffin et al., 1960). Fairly high densities of small insects such as mosquitos or fruit flies were needed to elicit active insect hunting, but under optimal conditions the rate of insect catching could be measured simply by weighing a bat before and after a few minutes of hunting. The estimated rate of capture agreed fairly well with the number of rapid increases in pulse repetition rate or "buzzes", indicating that the great majority of pursuits were successful. Passive detection of insects through sounds generated by their flight still remained a possibility, but other experiments seemed to rule this out rather conclusively. Weight gain and frequency of buzzes were not affected by darkness, and artificial targets such as mealworms tossed gently into the air were pursued with virtually identical patterns of orientation sound. Loud noise at 100-10,000 Hz had no effect on rate of insect capture, although the flight sounds of Drosophila were thoroughly masked. But even quite weak and non-uniform ultrasonic noise caused the bats to give up the pursuit of flying insects. In other situations bats do catch insects by passive homing toward sounds generated by the insects (Moehres, 1950, Kolb, 1961). There is not a single mode of insect interception, although neither visual nor olfactory pursuit of insects has yet been observed. Recognition that small moving insects are intercepted by echolocation by some species should not preclude awareness that the zoological spectrum of bats and their behavior is not limited to this impressive auditory accomplishment.

In recent years an active group of Russian investigators, particularly Airapetjantz and Konstantinov, have reported extensive investigations of echolocation in both bats and marine mammals. Much of this work has been well summarized by Airapetjantz and Konstantinov (1970). My inability to read Russian, and the incomplete nature of available translations have unfortunately limited my ability to review this extensive work. I will therefore comment only on one small portion, where a conclusion significantly different from that of comparable studies in Western Europe and North America has been reached.

Airapetjantz et al. (1969) conducted experiments on the insect catching behavior of bats of the families Vespertilionidae and Rhinolophidae in a large outdoor flight cage. Bats of both families are reported to detect insect prey by hearing sounds generated by the wing motions of the insects. The vespertilionid species Myotis oxygnathus showed the same changes in its orientation sound described above - great shortening of the pulse duration and increased pulse repetition rate during the approach to an interception of a flying insect. Rhinolophus ferrum-equinum are not reported to use echolocation at all but to catch flying insects by passive location. In other experiments Konstantinov (pers. comm.) reports the use of echolocation by Rhinolophus as long as the insect is stationary, but the cessation of sound emission when a moth moves its wings. These reports are entirely inconsistent with all other studies of insect catching behavior, and obviously further work will be necessary to determine whether some methodological difference is responsible (such as inadequately sensitive microphones that fail to detect all but the most intense orientation sounds) or whether the Russian investigators have discovered a different type of insect catching behavior.

6. Comparative morphology of orientation sounds

Field observations disspelled the mistaken impression that the orientation sounds of bats were fixed and invariable. Even an individual bat such as Myotis lucifugus or Eptesicus fuscus adapts the duration and frequency pattern of its orientation sounds according to the behavior in which it is engaged. There is a tendency for the duration to shorten as the pulse repetition rate is increased, and in most insectivorous bats overlap between outgoing sound and echo is avoided in almost all cases (Cahlander et al., 1964). I would have predicted in advance that if there were any change at all when a bat approached its small moving insect prey, the wavelengths would shorten. But in fact exactly the opposite occurs in all species on which adequate data are available. In the shorter pulses emitted during the terminal phase of insect pursuit the frequency is lowered, so that the wavelengths are longer. No fully adequate explanation has become available, although one may hypothesize that limitations of laryngeal physiology are involved and that at close range it is more important for the bat to make many separate pulses than to obtain more precise information or detect small targets with shorter wavelengths. The physiological acoustics of bat larynges is still a neglected area, to which very little has been added since our initial investigations (Novick and Griffin, 1961). This situation will probably change in the near future with new experimental methods being brought to bear by physiologists such as Roberts (1972) and Thomas (1972).

At nearly the same time as our first observations of bats hunting insects under natural conditions Moehres (1951, 1953) discovered that the horseshoe bats of Western Europe (family Rhinolophidae) used a drastically different type of orientation sound. These are also insectivorous bats, differing externally from the Vespertilionidae principally in having around the nostrils a peculiar fleshy nose leaf superficially resembling a horseshoe. The orientation sounds are emitted through the nostrils, and they consist of pure tones having a single frequency which was held constant within a given species, although this frequency tends to vary inversely with body weight. The nostrils are spaced about a half wavelength apart which probably aids the formation of a narrow beam in the horizontal plane (Moehres, 1953, Grinnell and Hagiwara, 1972a). These constant frequency orientation sounds while substantially longer than those previously known from the family Vespertilionidae are still relatively short, never exceeding 50-100 msec. They are conveniently designated "CW pulses" in contrast to the frequency modulated or "FM pulses" of the Vespertilionidae. Other bats employ constant frequencies for part of each orientation sound. Ordinarily this component is briefer and less precisely constant. Many species show a wide range of variation from sounds that are predominantly constant frequency to those showing nothing but the octave of downward frequency sweep characteristic of the family Vespertilionidae. A good example is Noctilio leporinus which catches both flying insects and small fish. The fish catching behavior is guided by echolocation, but it is small disturbances at or above the water surface that are detected rather than underwater echoes (Suthers, 1965). In the course of scanning a water surface for echoes from small objects that may indicate food available for snatching with the specialized hind claws, N. leporinus employ a range of orientation sounds that include some with almost nothing but a constant frequency and others, especially in the terminal phase or buzz, that are basically indistinguishable from those of Myotis lucifugus.

Further investigation showed that in addition to the prominent CW portion, bats of the family Rhinolophidae also have at the end of the pulse a downward sweeping FM portion, and sometimes also a short portion with rising frequency just preceding the CW signal (Griffin, 1962). Although these orientation sounds are so long that considerable overlap between

outgoing sound and echo ordinarily occurs, they too
are shortened in duration and increased in repetition rate as the horseshoe bat approaches an obstacle
or engages in other patterns of flight that require
especially accurate information for successful orientation.

Thus by 1953 the simpleminded picture of "the bat"
and its invariant FM orientation sounds was broken
apart along both the behavioral and phylogenetic
cleavage planes. The suborder Microchiroptera includes many morphologically diverse groups of bats,
the great majority of which are confined to tropical
regions. The pinna and associated structures such as
the tragus are often of complicated shapes and many,
but not all, of these tropical bats have elaborate
nose leaves. These vary from relatively simple leaf-
like shapes to the more complicated structures characteristic of the family Rhinolophidae which includes many tropical species as well as the few that
extend into Western Europe. In the 1950's students
of echolocation in bats began a series of expeditionary studies around the world, this being necessary at least initially because many species are
very difficult to maintain in good health in captivity (Griffin and Novick, 1955, Kulzer, 1956, Moehres
and Kulzer, 1955a, 1955b, 1956, 1957, Novick, 1958a,
1958b, Griffin, 1958). Gradually improving instrumentation has been required to build up a reasonably
complete and balanced picture. In this, the work of
Novick (1962, 1963a, in preparation), Schnitzler
(1968, 1970, in preparation) and Suthers (1965) has
played an important role.

All members of the suborder Microchiroptera have
been found to employ echolocation to some extent,
but there are wide variations in its relative importance. There is a rough spectrum with the families
Vespertilionidae and Rhinolophidae at one end with
great emphasis on echolocation and the family Phyllostomatidae at the other end, including many species that use vision or olfaction in finding fruit
or nectar and pollen of flowers. They apparently use
echolocation only to a limited extent for detecting
stationary objects. The vampire bats of the family
Desmodontidae fall into this group (Suthers, 1970).
The family Phyllostomatidae is a large one containing a great range of species adapted for different

ways of life. Some are almost exclusively fruit or
nectar feeding, although even these probably take
insects from time to time along with nectar and pollen, but do not, as far as we know, hunt flying insects on the wing. Others are largely insectivorous,
though we do not yet know under just what conditions
they catch their insect prey.

Bats which hunt flying insects or other moving prey
emit much more intense orientation sounds. This generalization appears valid for a considerable variety
of species, although it is prudent to keep an open
mind until more data are available before erecting
it into another rigid simplicity filter. The differences are often on the order of 30 dB, and in the
more specialized fruit eating bats or vampire bats
the orientation sounds are only marginally detectable by our best apparatus. Intensities at 10 cm
from the mouth are commonly on the order of 1 dyne
per cm^2 and frequencies often are above 70, and in
a few cases as high as 150 kHz. With the apparatus
available when these "whispering bats" were first
studied, we could not detect any orientation sounds
at all! The improved plastic dielectric microphones
first described by Kuhl et al. (1954) constituted a
real breakthrough in instrumentation, and enabled
these faint orientation sounds to be detected reliably for the first time, at least at close range.

There are smaller variations in emitted intensity
among insectivorous bats depending upon whether flying insects are pursued on the wing or stationary
insects are taken from large surfaces or from vegatation. For instance the long-eared bats of the genus Plecotus are said to feed on stationary insects,
and their orientation sounds are distinctly lower in
intensity (Griffin, 1958), but the available evidence is not yet adequate for firm conclusions.

Another pattern that appears to simplify the otherwise bewildering variety of orientation sounds is
the tendency for active hunters of flying insects to
use almost exclusively FM pulses with a downward
frequency sweep of an octave or more and with one or
at most two harmonically related frequencies containing the bulk of the energy. When, as in the best
studied members of the family Vespertilionidae, the
observed FM signals sweep from roughly 100 to about

50 kHz, second harmonics usually become discernible only in the later portions of the signal. But it must be recognized that available microphones are so limited in sensitivity above 100 kHz that higher harmonics might have escaped our notice. The whispering bats that feed primarily on fruit, on the blood of much larger animals, or to an unknown extent on non-flying insects, show a strong tendency to use orientation sounds with three or more prominent frequencies all sweeping downward at the same time. Some but not all of these components are clearly harmonically related. These signals seemed at first to be so complex as to suggest that they were bursts of noise, but more careful analysis with sound spectrographs showed that the pattern of downward frequency sweeps was almost invariably present. The picture is complicated by the fact that in many bats of this group the fundamental or even second harmonic may be present at a much lower intensity level than some of the higher harmonics. This in turn suggests that the basic laryngeal mechanisms for production of the orientation sounds may well include a fundamental frequency of membrane vibration in the low ultrasonic range with acoustic filters in the respiratory system that selectively modulate the harmonics (Pye, 1967, Roberts, 1972). The durations of the individual pulses in this group of whispering bats tend to be only one or a few msec and occasionally even less than one msec.

The family Emballonuridae have been considered on morphological grounds to be primitive, but they show in their echolocation as many specializations and refinements as any other group of bats. Furthermore they seem to be well equipped both visually and acoustically. Many species are active by day at least in the dim light under a forest canopy, such as the abundant neotropical genus Saccopteryx which is often seen hunting insects in daytime, although in relatively dense shade for the most part. These bats roost in exposed locations where they are visible, but their eyes are relatively large and they see an approaching predator or investigator quite easily so that they are difficult to capture at rest. Even when hunting in daylight they emit orientation sounds in a pattern strikingly similar to that of the Vespertilionidae. It seems likely, although conclusive evidence is not available, that when they hunt small insects in dense shade they detect them by echolocation and yet have retained in their evolution more effective vision than other families specialized to a superficially similar degree for insect hunting by echolocation.

A more clear-cut example of significant specialization of orientation sounds is the occurrence of long constant frequency pulses strikingly similar to those of the family Rhinolophidae in a common insectivorous bat of the New World tropics. This species has usually been called Chilonycteris rubiginosa in papers dealing with echolocation. Unfortunately the systematics of bats is still not fully worked out, and this species and its close relatives have been in an especially confusing state until the recent taxonomic revision by Smith (1972). Impatient as we experimental biologists tend to be with what seems like endless shuffling of tongue twisting scientific names, this example shows how necessary the tedious work of systematists can be. These bats were until recently considered part of the large family Phyllostomatidae, but several lines of evidence (including studies of echolocation) have led to their separation into a distinct family Mormoopidae in Smith's revision. All are insectivorous, and none has the simple spear-shaped nose leaf of the other bats with which they were formally associated. Like other insectivorous bats that pursue flying insects on the wing their orientation sounds are intense, and the former Chilonycteris rubiginosa (now renamed Pteronotus parnellii) is a remarkable convergence in its echolocation on the distantly related bats of the family Rhinolophidae which are confined to Africa, Eurasia, and Australasia. Like the Rhinolophus first studied by Moehres, Pteronotus parnellii keeps a remarkably constant frequency within its 10-20 msec CW portion, and this is sometimes preceded and always followed by rising and falling frequencies respectively. Another convergence is the rapid back and forth movements of the external ears correlated with the emission of CW orientation sounds described by Moehres (1953) for the European horseshoe bats and equally prominent in the neotropical P. parnellii (Griffin et al., 1962, Pye et al., 1962, Schnitzler, 1970). The possible significance and physiological correlates of these features of echolocation behavior will be discussed below.

This comparative survey, while not by any means complete, has probably already exceeded the limits many would consider appropriate for this symposium. But I hope to show in the following section that there are important and significant specializations, among at least the major groups of bats mentioned above, that are worthy of the attention of auditory physiologists. If I can do no more than attentuate the illusion that there is such a thing as "the bat" or even "the echolocating bat", this section will have served an important function.

7. Neurophysiological adaptations for echolocation

Dr. Suga has reviewed elsewhere in this symposium the thorough and highly significant experiments that he and his colleagues have carried out on the auditory system of echolocating bats. These have been confined for the most part to bats of the family Vespertilionidae, and indeed to closely related members of the genus Myotis. These are the same bats in which echolocation was discovered and with which, for the convenience of investigators in North America and Western Europe, most lines of experimentation have been begun. In this section I will attempt to review comparative neurophysiological studies of various other bats that throw some light upon the different or at least modified mechanisms that appear to be adaptations to various patterns of echolocation behavior.

Despite the difficulties of neurophysiological experiments with cetaceans, Bullock and his colleagues have analyzed responses of the large and specialized auditory system with implanted electrodes, and significant differences have been found between the comparable responses of porpoises and sea lions that may help explain the neural mechanisms of echolocation (Bullock et al., 1968, 1971, Bullock and Ridgway, 1972). Recovery of sensitivity after a brief sound is much more rapid in the cetaceans, as in bats, an apparent adaptation to avoid masking by an emitted orientation sound.

8. Audiograms

To consider first the range of frequencies to which the auditory system responds, recordings of evoked potentials have shown that all bats studied to date, including non-echolocating members of the suborder Megachiroptera, have good sensitivity well above the range of human hearing. Most of the data have been from what Grinnell (1963) originally designated as N_4 evoked potentials, which were interpreted as arising in the posterior colliculus, but as we now know from the work of Suga and his colleagues primarily consisting of synchronized neuronal discharges in the lateral lemniscus (Suga et al., 1966). Whether one wishes to call these "LL" with Suga and Schlegel (1972) or "N_4" as seems best because of wide prior usage, these evoked potentials clearly represent synchronized activity of large numbers of neurons constituting an input to the posterior colliculus. Like all evoked potentials recorded with relatively large electrodes, they provide only a generalized view of the performance of the system concerned. But while they do not preclude the existence of cells having different properties, they reflect functions for which a large fraction of the system is specialized.

As reviewed by Grinnell (1970) and by Grinnell and Hagiwara (1972a, 1972b), all bats studied to date show good sensitivity at or near the frequencies prominent in their orientation sounds. A note of caution concerning methodology is important in this connection. As first demonstrated by Grinnell (1963) and Harrison (1965) anesthetized bats allowed their body temperatures to fall to room temperature. Both at the level of cochlear microphonics and, even more prominently at the levels of N_1 and N_4, cooling has a disproportionately great effect on responses to higher frequencies. Similar results were obtained by Grinnell and Hagiwara (1972a). These differential temperature effects may be of interest and importance in connection with theories of auditory physiology.

9. Reduction of sensitivity during emission of orientation sounds

Hartridge (1945) suggested that bats might have mechanisms analogous to the "transmit-receive" circuits of radar and sonar systems to protect the delicate auditory mechanism from the very intense emitted sounds. Although this suggestion did not seem convincing at the time, any more than did Hartridge's original suggestion (1920) that bats might orient themselves by means of high frequency sound, Henson (1965, 1967, 1970) has found that Hartridge was indeed correct. At least in certain species (Tadarida brasiliensis and Pteronotus parnellii), and presumably in other bats as well, contraction of the middle ear muscles reduces sensitivity by 10-30 dB, at least under laboratory conditions. Furthermore, and in many ways even more surprising, relaxation occurs rapidly enough so that maximum sensitivity is available for echoes returning within a very few msec. These quantitative specializations of the protective middle ear muscle reflex known in other mammals demonstrate the degree to which bats are adapted not only for hearing in general but for echolocation in particular. These middle ear reflexes presumably operate together with the "neural attenuation" discussed by Suga and Schlegel (1972). It is also important to recognize that this mechanism operates to a far more limited extent in anesthetized bats than in those that are fully awake (Henson, 1970).

10. Doppler compensation

An especially prominent case of correspondence between emitted frequencies and maximum sensitivities is found in the family Rhinolophidae and in Pteronotus parnellii, both of which employ relatively long CW portions in their orientation sounds. The earlier surmise that these long constant frequency signals were used by bats to detect and take advantage of Doppler shifts in echo frequency has been confirmed in a series of ingenious experiments by Schnitzler (1968, 1970). In both Rhinolophus and Pteronotus parnellii the emitted frequency is adjusted over a range of a few hundred Hz so as to hold the Doppler shifted echo at a value constant within one hundred or two hundred Hz when relative movement occurs between bat and target. This was especially striking in one of Schnitzler's experiments with a target that moved back and forth as a pendulum. The bat (Rhinolophus ferrum-equinum) followed the movements of the pendulum to a good approximation by raising and lowering its emitted frequency in a cyclic fashion. Recordings of evoked potentials have shown that the auditory system of these bats is narrowly tuned to a frequency almost, but not quite, equal to the frequency emitted when the bat is at rest. Neuweiler (1970) found the minimum thresholds for evoked potentials in Nembutal anesthetized R. ferrum-equinum at exactly the frequency of the emitted sounds. Other experiments indicate that the maximum sensitivity may be slightly above the frequencies emitted by a bat at rest. Similar audiograms have been recorded by Grinnell (1967, 1970), Grinnell and Hagiwara (1972a), Henson (1967, 1970), Neuweiler et al. (1971), Schuller (1972), and Pollak et al. (1972).

Recognizing the limitations of evoked potential audiograms, it is nevertheless clear that a large portion of the auditory system in these "CW" bats is tuned to a narrow frequency band which is close, if not precisely equal, to the emitted frequency during the major portion of the orientation sound. Furthermore laryngeal mechanisms not yet investigated in detail adjust the emitted frequency with great precision to hold Doppler shifted echoes within the narrow band of maximal sensitivity. Recordings from single units confirm this picture by showing that some neurons at least have similar spectral sensitivity to that indicated by the evoked potential audiograms.

The recent work of Pollak et al. (1972) shows that much of the sharp tuning occurs at the peripheral level. This development appears to be a radical departure from our previous understanding of tuning in the auditory system of mammals, although recent developments have shown strong tendency for more and more of the tuning to be assigned to the peripheral portions of the system (Møller, 1972). Further work may be necessary to clarify the situation completely, but if this report of Pollak et al. is confirmed, it will represent a clear example of the importance to an area of basic physiology of considering a reasonably broad and representative phylogenetic spectrum of experimental animals. Møller concludes that "with regard to mammals commonly used in auditory neurophysiological studies (cat, guinea-pig, monkey, bat and rat), evidence has not shown as yet that a significant difference exists in the response patterns of single cells in the lower auditory pathway except for the fact that the tone frequency range of response varies among species." It is heartening to a student of bats to find at least "the" bat included among mammals commonly used in auditory neurophysiological studies, and perhaps the findings of Pollak et al. will provide a significant and intriguing exception to Møller's generalization. The degree of sharpness of tuning found in these experiments is truly remarkable. And the thresholds are reported to increase with slopes of 150-210 dB per kHz. If the cochlea of any mammal can achieve such remarkably sharp tuning, our basic ideas about the physiology of frequency discrimination must take this seriously into consideration. Further developments in this area will obviously be of the greatest importance.

11. Off responses of CW bats

Interesting differences between CW and FM bats have been reported by Grinnell (1970; in preparation) and Grinnell and Hagiwara (1972a) with respect to on and off responses at the levels of N_1 and N_4. These investigations have strongly indicated a significant difference between bats that emit relatively long CW signals (10-20 msec or longer) and those that have only a short CW component (less than about 8 msec). These short CW bats include some close relatives of Pteronotus parnellii such as P. suapurensis from Panama and also several bats of the genus Hipposideros and the closely related genus Aselliscus studied in New Guinea by Grinell and Hagiwara (1972a). Hipposideros and Aselliscus are closely related to Rhinolophus, but they fall clearly into the category of short CW bats with only one species H. diadema somewhat intermediate in length of the CW portion of the orientation sounds.

This classification on the basis of length of CW component seems in itself of limited significance, but studies of N_1 and N_4 evoked potentials have shown a highly suggestive correlation. In FM bats there is seldom if ever a clear off response and the audiogram is rather broad with a more gradual rise in threshold at low frequencies and a steep rise above the frequency with lowest threshold. In the long CW bats, the genus Rhinolophus and P. parnellii, the off responses are prominent and when each is used as criterion for an audiogram the resulting curves are different. The off response has a minimum threshold very close to the frequency emitted at rest, while the on response shows two minima, one slightly above and the other a few kHz below the emitted frequency. Finally in the short CW bats the off response has its minimum at or close to the emitted frequency, but the on response shows only one minimum and that at slightly lower frequencies (Grinnell, in preparation).

Neurophysiologists who lack confidence in anything other than unitary spikes from single units will doubtlessly find this somewhat complex picture confusing and be tempted to remove it from their thinking with some sort of simplicity filter. But I suggest that just as Grinnell's original studies of evoked potentials opened the way for more refined and penetrating analyses with microelectrodes, we may expect that when experiments similar to those described by Suga with bats of the family Vespertilionidae are extended to these two other types of bats a highly significant picture will emerge of excitatory and inhibitory excitation interacting in new patterns to provide the mechanism for a modified form of echolocation.

As far as we now know only the long CW bats exhibit compensation for Doppler shifts of the type discovered by Schnitzler (1968, 1970). The short CW bats appear not to adjust the CW frequency, and not to hold it so precisely constant. Grinnell postulates that in these bats the function of the CW portion is to provide improved signal to noise ratio by concentrating the emitted signal into a narrow band and permitting parts of the auditory system to be tuned to the same frequencies. Where Grinnell tends to think in terms of enhancement of response to the terminal FM portion of echoes, Simmons (1973b) suggests that the short CW components serve as a sort of early warning mechanism to alert the bat that a target is present at greater range than would be detectable by means of the FM component alone.

12. Future prospects

We are clearly now passing into an area where the data do not yet permit clear resolution of the types of questions discussed above. The line of attack in the realm of neurophysiology is fairly straightforward: single units should be studied by methods similar to those employed so successfully by Suga with other bats. As Suga's recent experiments have shown

it will probably also be important to evaluate the
effects of anesthesia on the more complex interactions, and we can no longer assume that the technically easier procedures of working with anesthetized
animals will reveal the full picture. Behavioral investigations will also be important, because it is
difficult to see how any other approach can reveal
as clearly just what use bats make of the echoes
they receive. Schnitzler's experiments should be extended to other species that employ constant frequency components, but Doppler compensation may not
be the only function of such signals. Simmons' suggestion can presumably be tested by determining the
maximum range at which a given target is detectable
by bats employing both short CW and pure FM signals.
Since all CW bats also employ FM components, and
since these tend to become more prominent when orientation problems are difficult (Griffin, 1962,
Schnitzler, 1968), differential masking experiments
may be helpful to determine the relative importance
of CW and FM components. Bats may complicate such
experiments by shifting the frequency composition of
the orientation sounds when tested with masking or
jamming noises, but sufficient experimental ingenuity can probably suffice to keep the experimenter
in control of the situation, provided that he does
not underestimate the complexity of the living mechanisms with which he is dealing.

13. Sensitivity and acuity

It is the behavioral performance of an echolocating
animal, in the final analysis, which is the primary
criterion by which the system must be evaluated.
Neuroanatomical hypertrophy of auditory portions of
the brains of the suborder Microchiroptera had attracted the attention of neuroanatomists for many
years before echolocation was discovered. (For example Polyak, 1925, 1926). But even Polyak (1946) found
it inconceivable that echolocation could be used to
detect small flying insects. In this context it is
appropriate to inquire how much information about the
nature of objects bats actually obtain by echolocation.

A first step has been taken to measure the success
of various bats at detecting vertical wires as a
function of the size of the wires (Griffin and

Novick, 1955, Griffin, 1958, Schnitzler, 1967, 1968). The bats highly specialized for echolocation under favorable conditions show thresholds of wire diameter well below 1 mm, even down to 0.2 or 0.1 mm. Grinnell and Griffin (1958) also measured the distance at which an approaching bat first reacted to wires of various sizes by beginning to increase its pulse repetition rate. The average distance of detection, or at least of reaction, ranged from 90 cm for 0.18 mm wires up to 215 cm for obstacles 3 mm in diameter. Long CW bats such as Rhinolophus ferrum equinum detect objects of similar size at considerably greater distances, perhaps even up to 8-10 m (Moehres, 1953).

Atmospheric absorption of high frequency sound sets severe limits on the effective range of echolocation (Griffin, 1971, Evans et al., 1972, Bass et al., 1972). But we have very little evidence concerning the distance at which large objects are actually detected. Casual observation suggests that when insectivorous bats fly at altitudes from roughly 20 to 100 m their minimal pulse repetition rates are approximately what one would expect if the bat waited after the emission of one orientation sound until it had heard an echo from the ground before emitting another pulse. On the other hand bats of the genus Tadarida in the Southwestern United States commonly fly to very great altitudes (1000 - 2000 m) where atmospheric absorption must preclude any possibility of hearing echoes from the ground (Williams and Williams, 1970b).

The ability of many bats to fly close to one another without apparent difficulty has often raised the question of mutual interference or jamming. Preliminary experiments suggested that even ultrasonic noises which superficially appeared to approximate the level of the emitted orientation sounds had virtually no jamming effect. When quantitative experiments were attempted (Griffin et al., 1963) we found that available loudspeakers set severe limits on our ability to fill a flight space with broad band noise sufficiently intense to cause any detectable increase in the threshold of detectable obstacle size. We therefore selected the long-eared bats Plecotus rafinesquii which emit relatively faint and relatively low frequency orientation sounds, and with considerable effort were able to produce a limited sort of jamming. Wires of roughly one mm diameter could be detected only at the chance level in our maximum noise intensity, but obstacle avoidance performance increased as the noise was reduced in intensity. While the fundamental frequencies in the orientation sounds swept from about 40 to 25 kHz, we found that the bats could detect small wires with echoes of the second harmonics if only the fundamental frequency range was occupied by jamming noise. In broad band jamming noise the bats were reluctant to fly and had to be dropped into the air to obtain adequate numbers of trials. Yet in any but the highest noise levels the most skillful individuals could fly through four successive rows of staggered wires dodging at far above the chance level. It is important to bear in mind the distinction between such a forced flight jamming experiment in which the bat is obliged to do the best it can in a difficult situation and experiments in which noise causes bats to cease efforts to catch insects or make other behavioral discriminations based on echolocation (Griffin et al., 1960).

These jamming experiments employed a rectangular flight chamber with the broad band ultrasonic noise impinging from two banks of loudspeakers at opposite ends. The signal to noise ratio of echoes detected by bats in these jamming experiments allowed comparison of their performance with signal detection theory. Since the echo intensity varies inversely as the cube of distance from cylindrical obstacles (assuming that spherical waves are emitted from the bat's mouth) it was necessary to estimate the distance at which the wires were detected. This we did by the same method employed in the quiet by Grinnell and Griffin (1958), basing our estimate on the distance at which the pulse repetition rate first increased. The resulting data were then compared with the predictions based on the classical equations of Shannon and Weaver assuming that the air between wire and bat could be considered a single communication channel. To our great surprise, the resulting data indicated that the bats performed significantly better than the ideal detector of signal detection theory. (E/N_o well below unity).

The explanation (I am tempted to say the rescue of signal detection theory) depends on the fact that bats have two ears. When the noise was not of maximum intensity or frequency coverage the bats flew relatively straight with only minor dodging maneuvers from end to end of the chamber. But with a truly challenging noise they shifted to flight paths that approached the rows of wires obliquely, so that echoes and noise reached their ears from different directions. Neurophysiological experiments showed that thresholds for N_4 evoked potentials were strongly affected by directional differences between test signals and masking noise (Grinnell, 1963).

14. Discrimination between similar targets

Another aspect of echolocation that must be of considerable importance to bats is their ability to discriminate between echoes from different classes of objects. Selective responses to faint echoes are essential; it would be highly maladaptive for a bat to pursue every faint echo. We therefore asked to what extent bats could discriminate between the echoes from various targets (Griffin et al., 1965). At the start of such an experiment hungry bats may fail to show any discrimination at all. Pebbles or similar inedible objects approximating the size of insects can be tossed up to wild bats and they will often be pursued with what appears to be the same vocal emission and flight manuevers as those directed against edible insect prey. The customary simplicity filter suggests no capability of discrimination. But we found that Myotis lucifugus learned in the course of several days to discriminate between edible mealworms and many types of small objects of roughly comparable size. If a dozen mealworms plus several inedible objects were tossed up in front of a bat well adjusted to life in Webster's flight chamber, it often succeeded in selecting one mealworm from the cloud of similar targets. Once it had learned the nature of the problem, a bat would only occasionally catch one of the inedible targets. In an attempt to quantify such experiments and determine what acoustic criteria were employed, we conducted many experiments in which one target at a time was tossed up into the air in front of an approaching bat. The nature of the target was randomly varied; it might be an edible mealworm or a small disk of roughly comparable dimensions. We used disks because, like mealworms, their echoes varied considerably as the target tumbled and twisted during its irregular trajectory. It seemed likely that bats could distinguish targets by overall echo intensity, but we wondered whether more complex echo patterns would be discriminable. The more successful and experienced bats did learn to achieve a high level of discrimination, catching roughly 90% of the mealworms and attacking only 10-20% of the inedible targets. Controls showed that the choices were made by echolocation.

The actual echoes generated by both disks and mealworms showed wide and overlapping ranges of variation in spectral intensities of echoes, so that it was difficult to understand what property of the echoes allowed as reliable discrimations as the bats in fact achieved. Certainly the overall intensity must have been a wholly inadequate criterion, since both classes of targets varied 20 dB or more as they moved through the air. We could not find evidence that any single band of frequencies within the octave frequency sweep provided a more reliable criterion, and it seems likely that some more complex "fine structure" of echo spectrum was employed. Other criteria such as the temporal pattern of echo variation are plausible alternatives (Griffin, 1967). Bradbury (1970) carried out similar experiments in which some of the pertinent variables were better controlled, and at least one of his experimental animals appeared to be utilizing differences in echo spectrum. At the very least these experiments demonstrate an impressive ability to make discriminations between classes of targets on the basis of moderately complex echo patterns.

15. Discriminative training

A long step forward has been taken by Simmons (1970, 1971a, 1971b) who has perfected a powerful new method for testing the acuity of echolocation in bats. This method is similar in some respects to the Lashley jumping stand, but modified into a "Simmons flying stand" in which a bat is trained to fly from one starting platform to either of two landing platforms depending upon echoes they return. In many experiments Simmons uses bats that are blinded by bilateral enucleation. Positive reinforcement in the form of mealworms is provided by the experimenter when the bat makes the correct choice, and after each error it is picked up by hand and returned to the starting place. The method has proved most effective, and bats have been trained to discriminate according to size and shape of triangular plastic targets, according to the angular position of the two landing platforms relative to a third object (Peff and Simmons, 1972) and according to target distance. In the shape discrimination experiments of Simmons and Vernon (1971) Eptesicus fuscus learned to detect differences as small as 17% in the surface area of triangular targets several wavelengths in size. They also discriminated between triangles of the same area differing in shape. The actual differences in echoes returned by these classes of targets have not yet been analyzed in detail. Peff and Simmons (1972) have demonstrated that bats can determine angular position of a target by echolocation within ±6 to 8°.

The most informative experiments have involved discrimination of target range (Simmons, 1971a, 1973a). The nearer or farther targets were varied randomly between right and left to avoid position habits. Eptesius fuscus proved able to discriminate with better than 90% success the nearer or the farther target when the difference in distance was as small as 3 cm. Range resolution was the same whether the fixed target was at 30, 60, or other longer distances. The orientation sounds employed by E. fuscus in these experiments had a duration of approximately 2.5 msec (pulse length about 85 cm) and swept in frequency from about 50 to 25 kHz. (Wavelengths 0.7 to 1.4 cm.) The envelope patterns of these orientation sounds and their echoes are complex and variable due in part to shifting phase relations. There is no abrupt onset or other prominent change in amplitude to serve as a prominent time marker. Yet by focussing their attention first at one and then the other of two targets, bats can determine relative distance with the accuracy stated above.

Simmons compares the observed performance of his bats with the predictions of signal detection theory for the range resolving capabilities of an ideal detector, which is assumed to take advantage of all mathematically conceivable information contained in the echoes. According to well established theory the curve relating percent correct responses to difference in target range should correspond to the envelope of the autocorrelation function representing the ambiguity in echo arrival time. This function depends upon the detailed frequency and envelope pattern of the orientation sound and its echoes. The correspondence between theoretical and observed curves appears to be so close as to demonstrate that the brains of these bats are acting as ideal detectors in the sense the term is used in signal detection theory. When there are shifting mixtures of fundamental and second harmonic the theory predicts that the performance curve should have an inflection, and in experiments with Phyllostomus hastatus such kinks do in fact appear, providing even more remarkable agreement between theory and observation than in the case of Eptesicus fuscus.

Simmons (1973a) has further refined this training method by arranging for the electronic generation of echoes rather than relying upon differences in actual distance. Variable delay circuits are inserted between a microphone close to the starting platform and small loudspeakers located on the landing platforms. In this way a sort of phantom echo is generated which would appear to come from some point in the same direction as the landing platform but at a distance where no physical object is in fact present. With appropriate training bats learn to make equally accurate discriminations on the basis of echo delay time even though the actual targets and loudspeakers were not shifted in distance. These beautiful experiments not only confirm and extend the quantitative measurement of bats' ability to make precise discriminations based on the differences in echo delay; they demonstrate rigorously for the first time that echo delay is in fact the criterion used by bats for determining distance to targets. Although this had always seemed the most likely possibility, other criteria such as echo intensity, beat notes postulated to exist between outgoing sound and echo, and possible differences in spectral composition of echoes due to varying amounts of atmospheric absorption, had previously remained alternative possibilities.

Simmons has elaborated these experiments to compare bats employing different types of orientation sounds and has shown a most satisfying correspondence between the predictions of signal detection theory and the performance actually exhibited by various kinds of bats. He has also repeated Schnitzler's experiment with electronically simulated Doppler shifts and has shown that the emitted frequency is adjusted precisely to maintain a constant received echo frequency even when there is no physical motion of bat or target (Simmons, 1973b). Schnitzler (in preparation) has also demonstrated by experiments in flight chambers containing helium - oxygen mixtures that Doppler compensation occurs when the difference between the originally emitted frequency and the echo is due to an "unexpected" change in the speed of sound rather than to relative motion of bat and target.

In this area of behavioral discrimination experiments, as in the comparative neurophysiological experiments reviewed above, space has not permitted mention of all of the important experiments that have been reported, and the papers cited above will be rewarding to readers interested in appreciating the full capabilities of echolocation as it has evolved in bats. The history of research on echolocation has included a long series of surprises in which the discovery of a new behavioral capability has opened our eyes to the probable existence of an unanticipated neural mechanism. Given the enthusiastic momentum of so much new talent that has been attracted to these problems, I am confident that we are far from having reached the end of the road.

References

Airapetjantz, E. Sh., and Konstantinov, A.I. (1970). Echolocation in nature. Nauka, Leningrad.

Airapetjantz, E. Sh., Konstantinov, A.I., and Matjushkin, D.P. (1969). Brain echolocation mechanisms and bionics. Acta Physiol. Acad. Sci. Hungar. 35, 1-17.

Bass, H.E., Bauer, J., and Evans, L.B. (1972). Atmospheric absorption of sound: analytical expressions. J. Acoust. Soc. Amer. 52, 821-825.

Bradbury, J.W. (1970). Target discrimination by the echolocating bat Vampyrum spectrum. J. Exp. Zool. 173, 23-46.

Buchler, E. (1972). The use of echolocation by the wandering shrew, Sorex vagrans Baird. Thesis. Univ. Montana. Missoula, Montana.

Bullock, T.H., Grinnell, A.D., Ikezono, E., Kameda, K., Katsuki, Y., Nomoto, M., Sata, O., Suga, N., and Tanagisawa, K. (1968). Electrophysiological studies of central auditory mechanisms in cetaceans. Z. Vergl. Physiol. 59, 117-156.

Bullock, T.H., Ridgway, S.H., and Suga, N. (1971). Acoustically evoked potentials in midbrain auditory structures in sea lions (Pinnipedia). Z. Vergl. Physiol. 74, 372-387.

Bullock, T.H., and Ridgway, S.H. (1972). Evoked potentials in the central auditory system of alert porpoises to their own and artificial sounds. J. Neurobiol. 3, 79-99.

Cahlander, D.A., McCue, J.J.G., and Webster, F.A. (1964). The determination of distance by echolocating bats. Nature (London) 201, 544-546.

Cochrum, E.L. (1969). Migration of the guano bat Tadarida brasiliensis. In: Contributions to mammalogy. (J.K. Jones, Jr., ed), pp. 303-336. Museum of Natural History, Univ. Kansas, Lawrence, Kansas.

Dijkgraaf, S. (1946). Die Sinneswelt der Fledermäuse. Experientia. 2, 438-448.

Evans, W.E. (1973). Echolocation of cetaceans based on experiments with fresh water and marine delphinids. (In preparation).

Evans, L.B., Bass, H.E., and Sutherland, L.C. (1972). Atmospheric absorption of sound: theoretical predictions. J. Acoust. Soc. Amer. 51, 1565-1575.

Galambos, R., and Griffin, D.R. (1942). Obstacle avoidance by flying bats; the cries of bats. J. Exp. Zool. 89, 475-490.

Gould, E., Negus, A., and Novick, A. (1964). Evidence for echolocation in shrews. J. Exp. Zool. 154, 19-38.

Griffin, D.R. (1953a). Acoustic orientation in the oil bird, Steatornis. Proc. Nat. Acad. Sci. 39, 884-893.

Griffin, D.R. (1953b). Bat sounds under natural conditions, with evidence for the echolocation of insect prey. J. Exp. Zool. 123, 435-466.

Griffin, D.R. (1958). Listening in the dark. Yale Univ. Press. New Haven, Conn.

Griffin, D.R. (1962). Comparative studies of the orientation sounds of bats. Symp. Zool. Soc. London. 7, 61-72.

Griffin, D.R. (1967). Discriminative echolocation by bats. In: Animal sonar systems. (R.-G. Busnel, ed.), pp. 273-306. Laboratoire de Physiologie Acoustique, Jouy-en-Josas.

Griffin, D.R. (1970). Migrations and homing of bats. In: Biology of bats. (W.A. Wimsatt, ed.), pp. 233-264. Academic Press, New York.

Griffin, D.R. (1971). The importance of atmospheric attenuation for the echolocation of bats (Chiroptera). Anim. Behav. 19, 55-61.

Griffin, D.R., and Galambos, R. (1941). The sensory basis of obstacle avoidance by flying bats. J. Exp. Zool. 86, 481-506.

Griffin, D.R., and Novick, A. (1955). Acoustic orientation of neotropical bats. J. Exp. Zool. 130, 251-300.

Griffin, D.R., Novick, A., and Kornfield, M. (1958). The sensitivity of echolocation in the fruit bat Rousettus. Biol. Bull. 115, 107-113.

Griffin, D.R., and Suthers, R. (1970). Sensitivity of echolocation in the cave swiftlet. Biol. Bull. 139, 495-501.

Griffin, D.R., Webster, F.A., and Michael, C. (1960). The echolocation of flying insects by bats. Anim. Behav. 8, 141-154.

Griffin, D.R., Dunning, D.C., Cahlander, D.A., Webster, F.A., Pye, J.D., Flinn, M., and Pye, A. (1962). Correlated orientation sounds and ear movements of horseshoe bats. Nature (London), 196, 1185-1188.

Griffin, D.R., McCue, J.J.G., and Grinnell, A.D. (1963). The resistance of bats to jamming. J. Exp. Zool. 152, 229-250.

Griffin, D.R., Friend, J.H., and Webster, F.A. (1965). Target discrimination by the echolocation of bats. J. Exp. Zool. 158, 155-168.

Grinnell, A.D. (1963). The neurophysiology of audition in bats. J. Physiol. 167, 38-127.

Grinnell, A.D. (1967). Mechanisms of overcoming interference in echolocating animals. In: Animal sonar systems. (R.-G. Busnel, ed.), pp. 451-505. Laboratoire de Physiologie Acoustique, Jouy-en-Josas.

Grinnell, A.D. (1970). Comparative auditory neurophysiology of neotropical bats employing different echolocation signals. Z. Vergl. Physiol. 68, 117-153.

Grinnell, A.D. (1973). Neural processing mechanisms in echolocating bats correlated with differences in emitted sounds. (In preparation).

Grinnell, A.D., and Griffin, D.R. (1958). The sensitivity of echolocation in bats. Biol. Bull. 114, 10-22.

Grinnell, A.D., and Hagiwara, S. (1972a). Adaptations of the auditory nervous system for echolocation, studies of New Guinea bats. Z. Vergl. Physiol. 76, 41-81.

Grinnell, A.D., and Hagiwara, S. (1972b). Studies of auditory neurophysiology in non-echolocating bats, and adaptations for echolocation in one genus, Rousettus. Z. Vergl. Physiol. 76, 82-96.

Harrison, J.B. (1965). Temperature effects on responses in the auditory system of the little brown bat Myotis 1. lucifugus. Physiol. Zool. 38, 34-48.

Hartridge, H. (1920). The avoidance of objects by bats in their flight. J. Physiol. 54, 54-57.

Hartridge, H. (1945). Avoidance of obstacles by bats. Nature (London) 156, 55.

Henson, O.W. (1965). The activity and function of the middle ear muscles in echolocating bats. J. Physiol. 180, 871-887.

Henson, O.W., Jr. (1967). The perception and analysis of bio-sonar signals by bats. In: Animal sonar systems. (R.-G. Busnel, ed.), Vol. II, pp. 949-1003. Laboratoire de Physiologie Acoustique, Jouy-en-Josas.

Henson, O.W., Jr. (1970). The ear and audition. In: Biology of Bats. (W.A. Wimsatt, ed.), Vol. II, pp. 181-263. Academic Press, New York.

Herald, E.S., Brownell, R.L. Jr., Frye, F.L., Morris, E.J., Evans, W.E., and Scott, A.B. (1969). Blind river dolphin: first side-swimming cetacean. Science 166, 1408-1410.

Hollander, P. (1971). Adaptations for echolocation in cave swiftlets (Collocalia). Thesis. Yale Univ. New Haven, Conn.

Kellogg, W.N. (1953). Ultrasonic hearing in the porpoise, Tursiops truncatus. J. Comp. Physiol. Psychol. 46, 446-450.

Kellogg, W.N. (1961). Porpoises and sonar. Univ. of Chicago Press, Chicago.

Kellogg, W.N. (1962). Sonar system of the blind. Science 137, 399-404.

Kellogg, W.N., Kohler, R., and Morriss, H.N. (1953). Porpoise sounds as sonar signals. Science 117, 239-243.

Kolb, A. (1961). Sinnesleistungen einheimischer Fledermäuse bei der Nahrungssuche und Nahrungswahl auf dem Boden und in der Luft. Z. Vergl. Physiol. 44, 550-564.

Kuhl, W., Schodder, G.R., and Schröder, F.K. (1954). Condenser transmitters and microphones with solid dielectric for airborne ultrasonics. Acustica 4, 519-532.

Kulzer, E. (1956). Flughunde erzeugen Orientierungslaute durch Zungenschlag. Naturwissenschaften 43, 117-118.

Moehres, F.P. (1950). Zur Orientierung der Fledermäuse. Natur Volk 80, 153-161.

Moehres, F.P. (1951). Über eine neue Art von Ultraschall-Orientierung bei Fledermäusen. Verh. Deut. Zool. Ges. Wilhelmshaven, pp. 179-186.

Moehres, F.P. (1953). Über die Ultraschallorientierung der Hufeisennasen (Chiroptera-Rhinolophidae). Z. Vergl. Physiol. 34, 547-588.

Moehres, F.P., and Kulzer, E. (1955a). Ein neuer, kombinierter Typ der Ultraschallorientierung bei Fledermäusen. Naturwissenschaften 42, 131-132.

Moehres, F.P., and Kulzer, E. (1955b). Untersuchungen über die Ultraschallorientierung von vier afrikanischen Fledermausfamilien. Verh. Deuts. Zool. Ges. Erlangen, pp. 59-65.

Moehres, F.P., and Kulzer, E. (1956). Über die Orientierung der Flughunde (Chiroptera-Pteropodidae). Z. Vergl. Physiol. 38, 1-29.

Moehres, F.P., and Kulzer, E. (1957). Megaderma-ein konvergenter Zwischentyp der Ultraschallpeilung bei Fledermäusen. Naturwissenschaften 44, 21-22.

Moehres, F.P., and Neuweiler, G. (1966). Die Ultraschallorientierung der Grossblatt-Fledermäuse (Chiroptera-Megadermatidae). Z. Vergl. Physiol. 53, 195-227.

Moehres, F.P., and Oettingen-Spielberg, T. (1949). Versuche über die Nahorientierung und das Heimfindevermögen der Fledermäuse. Verh. Deuts. Zool. Ges. Mainz. pp. 248-252.

Møller, A.R. (1972). Coding of sounds in lower levels of the auditory system. Quart. Rev. Biophys. 5, 59-155.

Neuweiler, G. (1970). Neurophysiologische Untersuchungen zum Echoortungssystem der Grossen Hufeisennase Rhinolophus ferrum-equinum Schreber, 1774. Z. Vergl. Physiol. 67, 273-306.

Neuweiler, G., and Moehres, F.P. (1967). The role of spatial memory in the orientation. In: Animal sonar systems. (R.-G. Busnel, ed.), pp. 129-140. Laboratoire de Physiologie Acoustique, Jouy-en-Josas.

Neuweiler, G., Schuller, G., and Schnitzler, H.-U. (1971). On- and off-responses in the inferior colliculus of the greater horseshoe bat to pure tones. Z. Vergl. Physiol. 74, 57-63.

Norris, K.S., Prescott, J.H., Asa-Dorian, P.V., and Perkins, P. (1961). An experimental demonstration of echo-location behavior in the porpoise, Tursiops truncatus (Montagu). Biol. Bull. 120, 163-176. Univ. Kansas, Lawrence, Kansas.

Novick, A. (1958a). Orientation in palaeotropical bats. I. Microchiroptera. J. Exp. Zool. 138, 81-154.

Novick, A. (1958b). Orientation in palaeotropical bats. II. Megachiroptera. J. Exp. Zool. 137, 443-462.

Novick, A. (1959). Acoustic orientation in the cave swiftlet. Biol. Bull. 117, 497-503.

Novick, A. (1962). Orientation in neotropical bats. I. Natalidae and Emballonuridae. J. Mammal. 43, 449-455.

Novick, A. (1963a). Orientation in neotropical bats. II. Phyllostomatidae and Desmodontidae. J. Mammal. 44, 44-56.

Novick, A. (1963b). Pulse duration in the echolocation of insects by the bat, Pteronotus. Ergeb. Biol. 26, 21-26.

Novick, A. (1965). Echolocation of flying insects by the bat, Chilonycteris psilotis. Biol. Bull. 128, 297-314.

Novick, A. (1973). Echolocation in bats: a Zoologists' view. (In preparation).

Novick, A., and Griffin, D.R. (1961). Laryngeal mechanisms in bats for the production of orientation sounds. J. Exp. Zool. 148, 125-146.

Peff, T.C., and Simmons, J.A. (1972). Horizontal-angle resolution by echolocating bats. J. Acoust. Soc. Amer. 51, 2063-2065.

Pilleri, G. (1970). Platanista gangetica, a dolphin that swims on its side. Rev. Suisse Zool. 77, 305-307.

Pilleri, G. (1971). Beobachtung über das Paarungsverhalten des Gangesdelphins, Platanista gangetica. Rev. Suisse Zool. 78, 231-234.

Pollak, G., Henson, O.W. Jr., and Novick, A. (1972). Cochlear microphonic audiograms in the "pure tone" bat Chilonycteris parnellii parnellii. Science. 176, 66-88.

Polyak, S. (1925). Untersuchungen am Octavussystem der Säugetiere und dem mit diesem koordinierten motorischen Apparate des Hirnstammes. J. Psychol. Neurol. 32, 170-231.

Polyak, S. (1926). The connections of the acoustic nerve. J. Anat. 60, 465-469.

Polyak, S. (1946). The human ear in anatomical transparencies. Sonotone Corp., Elmsford, New York. (distributed by T.H. McKenna, New York).

Pye, J.D. (1962). Mechanisms of echolocation. Ergeb. Biol. 26, 12-20.

Pye, J.D. (1967). Synthesizing the waveforms of bat's pulses. In: Animal sonar systems. (R.-G. Busnel, ed.), pp. 43-67. Laboratoire de Physiologie Acoustique, Jouy-en-Josas.

Pye, J.D., Flinn, M., and Pye, A.D. (1962). Correlated orientation sounds and ear movements of horseshoe bats. Nature (London) 196, 1186-1188.

Ralls, K. (1967). Auditory sensitivity in mice: Peromyscus and Mus musculus. Anim. Behav. 15, 123-128.

Rice, C.E. (1967a). Human echo perception. Science 155, 656-664.

Rice, C.E. (1967b). The human sonar system. In: Animal sonar systems. (R.-G. Busnel, ed.), pp. 719-755. Laboratoire de Physiologie Acoustique, Jouy-en-Josas.

Roberts, L.H. (1972). Variable resonance in constant frequency bats. J. Zool. 166, 337-348.

Rosenzweig, M.R., and Riley, D.A. (1955). Evidence for echolocation in the rat. Science 121, 600.

Schevill, W.E., and Lawrence, B. (1953a). High-frequency auditory response of a bottle-nosed porpoise, Tursiops truncatus (Montagu). J. Acoust. Soc. Amer. 25, 1016-1017.

Schevill, W.E., and Lawrence, B. (1953b). Auditory response of a bottle-nosed porpoise to frequencies above 100 kc. J. Exp. Zool. 124, 147-165.

Schevill, W.E., and Lawrence, B. (1956). Food-finding by a captive porpoise (Tursiops truncatus). Breviora, Mus. Comp. Zool., Harvard Univ. 53, 1-15.

Schnitzler, H.-U. (1967). Discrimination of thin wires by flying horseshoe bats (Rhinolophidae). In: Animal sonar systems. (R.-G. Busnel, ed.), pp. 69-87. Laboratoire de Physiologie Acoustique, Jouy-en-Josas.

Schnitzler, H.-U. (1968). Die Ultraschallortungslaute der Hufesienfledermäuse (Chiroptera-Rhinolophidae) in verschiedenen Orientierungssituationen. Z. Vergl. Physiol. 57, 376-408.

Schnitzler, H.-U. (1970). Echoortung bei der Fledermaus Chilonycteris rubiginosa. Z. Vergl. Physiol. 68, 25-38.

Schnitzler, H.-U. (1973). Control of Doppler shift compensation in the greater horseshoe bat, Rhinolophus ferrum-equinum. (In preparation).

Schuller, G. (1972). Echoortung bei Rhinolophus ferrum-equinum mit frequenzmodulierten Lauten, evoked potentials im colliculus inferior. Z. Vergl. Physiol. 77, 306-331.

Schwartzkopff, J. (1968). Structure and function of the ear and of the auditory brain areas in birds. In: Hearing mechanisms in vertebrates. (A.V.S. de Reuck and J. Knight, eds.), Churchill, London.

Simmons, J.A. (1970). Distance perception by echolocation: the nature of echo signal-processing in the bat. Proc. Int. Bat Res. Conf. 2nd. Bijdragen tot de Dierkunde 40, 87-90.

Simmons, J.A. (1971a). Echolocation in bats: signal processing of echoes for target range. Science 171, 925-928.

Simmons, J.A. (1971b). The sonar receiver of the bat. Ann. N. Y. Acad. Sci. 188, 161-174.

Simmons, J.A. (1973a). The resolution of target range by echolocating bats. J. Acoust. Soc. Amer. (In press).

Simmons, J.A. (1973b). Response of the Doppler sonar system in the bat, Rhinolophus ferrum-equinum. J. Acoust. Soc. Amer. (Submitted).

Simmons, J.A., and Vernon, J.A. (1971). Echolocation: discrimination of targets by the bat, Eptesicus fuscus. J. Exp. Zool, 176, 315-328.

Smith, J.D. (1972). Systematics of the Chiropteran family Mormoopidae. Univ. Kansas Mus. of Natural History Miscellaneous Publ. 56. Lawrence, Kansas.

Suga, N., Friend, J.H., and Suthers, R.A. (1966). Neural responses in the inferior colliculus of echolocating bats to artificial orientation sounds and echoes. J. Cell. Comp. Physiol. 67, 319-332.

Suga, N., and Schlegel, P. (1972). Neural attenuation of responses to emitted sounds in echolocating bats. Science. 177, 82-84.

Supa, M., Cotzin, M., and Dallenbach, K.M. (1944). "Facial vision". The perception of obstacles by the blind. Amer. J. Psychol. 57, 133-183.

Suthers, R.A. (1965). Acoustic orientation by fish-catching bats. J. Exp. Zool. 158, 319-348.

Suthers, R.A. (1970). Vision, olfaction, taste. In: Biology of Bats. (W.A. Wimsatt, ed.), Vol. II, pp. 265-309. Academic Press, New York.

Suthers, R.A., Chase, J., and Braford, B. (1969). Visual form discrimination by echolocating bats. Biol. Bull. 137, 535-546.

Thomas, S.P. (1972). Flight physiology and energetics of the echolocating bat Phyllostomus hastatus. Thesis. Indiana Univ. Bloomington, Indiana.

Williams, T.C., and Williams, J. (1970a). Radio tracking of homing and feeding flights of a neotropical bat, Phyllostomus hastatus. Anim. Behav. 18, 302-309.

Williams, T.C., and Williams, J.M. (1970b). Bat hazards to aircraft: detection by radar. In: Proc. World Conf. on bird hazards to aircraft. Ottawa, Nat. Res. Counc. Can., pp. 307-319.

DONALD R. GRIFFIN

DISCUSSION

DAVIS: Am I correct that certain parts of the midbrain are highly developed in the bat? The inferior colliculus, for example: could you give us a little more detail on this?

GRIFFIN: The auditory portions of the brain up to about the level of the inferior colliculus are all very large. Polyak (1925, 1926) made this point in some long papers. In the more anterior regions this hypertrophy is much less. Furthermore the visual areas are correspondingly small. This correlates well with the reliance on echolocation. There are bats that do not echolocate (suborder Megachiroptera except for Rousettus), and they have much less hypertrophy of the auditory mid-brain areas.

EVANS: Could you give us some idea why some bats find it useful to use frequency modulated tones for echolocation while others use steady tones?

GRIFFIN: The constant frequency bats are obviously well adapted for dealing with Doppler shifts. This is shown behaviorally. The others pretty clearly get a broad band out of their FM sweep. Whether they get any other advantages compared to say a noise band or an upward sweeping is more difficult to judge, because there just do not happen to be any bats using those patterns for comparative studies. My own feeling is that FM bats probably can discriminate spectral differences in the echoes and that this gives them the ability to distinguish between different kinds of targets. But the evidence for this (Griffin, 1967, Bradbury, 1970), I will admit, is equivocal. Probably Simmons' experiments will eventually clarify the situation.

EVANS: Is Simmons saying that it is the duration of the signal or the fact that it changes in frequency which is crucial?

GRIFFIN: I think the theory simply says that if you have a wide band you transmit more information. There are people in this room who are far more competent than I to discuss signal detection theory, but I believe the ideal detector is assumed to do everything you can possibly do with a given signal. Since you make such a generous assumption it does not matter how the frequencies are arranged. But the bandwidth is important, and in this sense the FM bats do seem to have an advantage. This downward frequency sweep is a very widespread pattern, particularly in insect catching bats. Furthermore it is a suitable signal for range discrimination.

SCHWARTZKOPFF: What do you think of the older idea of Möhres (Möhres, 1953) who was pointing at the fact that these bats with such a long duration constant frequency cry are turning their heads during crying and getting by that some kind what he called acoustical image formation?

GRIFFIN: I think Simmons' experiments have in a way made that sort of theory a little obsolete. Möhres said that these bats have a narrow beam of sound which they sweep around in different directions. Unfortunately there are practically no behavioral observations of actual insect catching under natural conditions by any of these constant frequency bats, so we really know very little about their tactics. We also have inadequate evidence about the shape of the emitted sound pattern; while it is somewhat beamed it does not seem to be an extremely narrow pencil-beam. I suspect that even horseshoe bats hear useful echoes from a cone of at least $60°$. In short, I think they have some sort of acoustic image, but I do not know whether this is achieved by scanning. Bats can catch insects among vegetation where they must be getting strong echoes from other objects at only slightly different range and angle.

ZWISLOCKI: You brought up a somewhat philosophical question of the simplicity filter and I feel I have to say something in defence of those of us who use simplicity filters, like myself. I suggest that you use, instead of one simplicity filter, a bank of simplicity filters. You could then at least see the spectrum. I would like to caution, on the other side, against completely wide filters.

GRIFFIN: Good. I agree that ideally one should have a quiver full of different simplicity filters rather than relying on any one.

References

Bradbury, J.W. (1970). Target discrimination by the echolocating bat Vampyrum spectrum. J. Exp. Zool. 173, 23-46.

Griffin, D.R. (1967). Discriminative echolocation by bats. In:Animal Sonor Systems (R.-G. Busnel, ed.), pp. 273-306. Laboratoire de Physiologie, Jouy-en-Josas.

Möhres, F.P. (1953). Über die Ultraschallorientierungen der Hufeisennasen (Chiroptera-Rhinolophidae). Z. Vergl. Physiol. 34, 547-588.

Polyak, S. (1925). Untersuchungen am Octavussystem der Säugetiere und dem mit diesem koordinierten motorischen Apparate der Hirnstammes. J. Psychol. Neurol. 32, 170-231.

Polyak, S. (1926). The connections of the acoustic nerve. J. Anat. 60, 465-469.

Simmons, J.A. (1970). Distance perception by echolocation: the nature of echo signal-processing in the bat. Proc. Int. Bat Res. Conf., 2nd. Bijdragen tot de Dierkunde 40, 87-90.

FUNCTION OF THE SWIMBLADDER IN FISH HEARING

Olav Sand and Per Stockfelth Enger

University of Oslo
Oslo
Norway

1. Introduction

The sensory cells in the acoustico-lateralis system in vertebrates are hair cells, and the proper stimulus for these cells is the shear movement of the sensory hairs. By virtue of this, the fish ear is a detector of the kinetic sound component, particle velocity or particle displacement, rather than of sound pressure. Essentially transparent to waterborne sound (Griffin, 1950, 1955, Pumphrey, 1950), a fish will vibrate at the same phase and amplitude as the surrounding water particles when exposed to sound. The denser otoliths, in close contact with the sensory epithelium in the ear, will lag behind these movements, thereby stimulating the hair cells.

A gas bubble in water pulsates when exposed to sound, and because of the high compressibility of gas relative to water, the radial displacement amplitude of the bubble surface is much greater than the displacements of water particles in the absence of a bubble. A gas filled swimbladder in fish may improve hearing, provided that the swimbladder pulsations are transferred into an amplified movement of the otoliths. The swimbladder will then function as a pressure-displacement transformer in a sound field, and the auditory system will respond to sound pressure, though the end organ is still sensitive to particle motion.

Close to the sound source, in the acoustical near-field, the ratio between particle displacement and sound pressure increases with decreasing sound source distance, whereas this ratio is constant far from the sound source, in the acoustical far-field (Harris, 1964). The hearing in fish without a swimbladder may then be reasonably efficient in the near-field, where the particle displacements are large compared to the sound pressure. In the far-field the hearing in these fish will be less efficient.

2. Evidence for an auditory function of the swimbladder in fish with a specialized bladder-ear connection

In the ostariophysi the swimbladder is linked to the sacculi through a chain of small bones, the Weberian ossicles. Already Weber (1820) assumed an auditory function of these ossicles, and the possible mechanism of this apparatus was studied in detail by von Frisch (1938), and later reviewed by Alexander (1966). Poggendorf (1952) found that removing this mechanical link between the bladder and the ear reduced the hearing sensitivity of Ictalurus (=Amiurus) nebulosus with 30-40 dB at some frequencies, and he also demonstrated that this fish was sensitive to sound pressure.

Ostariophysi fish generally have lower auditory thresholds and higher upper frequency cut-off than non-ostariophysi fish (see Tavolga, 1971). This is shown in Fig. 1, which compares audiograms for goldfish (Carassius auratus), a typical Ostariophysi, and cod (Gadus morhua) a typical con-Ostariophysi. However, it is seen that herring (Clupea harrengus), which also is a non-Ostariophysi, has an upper frequency cut-off comparable to that of goldfish. Wohlfart (1936) showed that the swimbladder in clupeids has long anterior extensions, which terminate in gas filled capsules coupled to the perilymph of the ear. Other non-ostariophysi families which also have a close connection between the swimbladder and the ear are Anabantidae, Balistidae, Engraulidae, Holocentridae, Moridae, Mormyridae, Notopteridae, Ophiocephalidae, Sciaenidae and Sparidae (Jones and Marshall, 1953, Alexander, 1966, van Bergeijk, 1967, Tavolga, 1971). Anatomical considerations make it likely that the swimbladder has a positive effect on hearing also in these families.

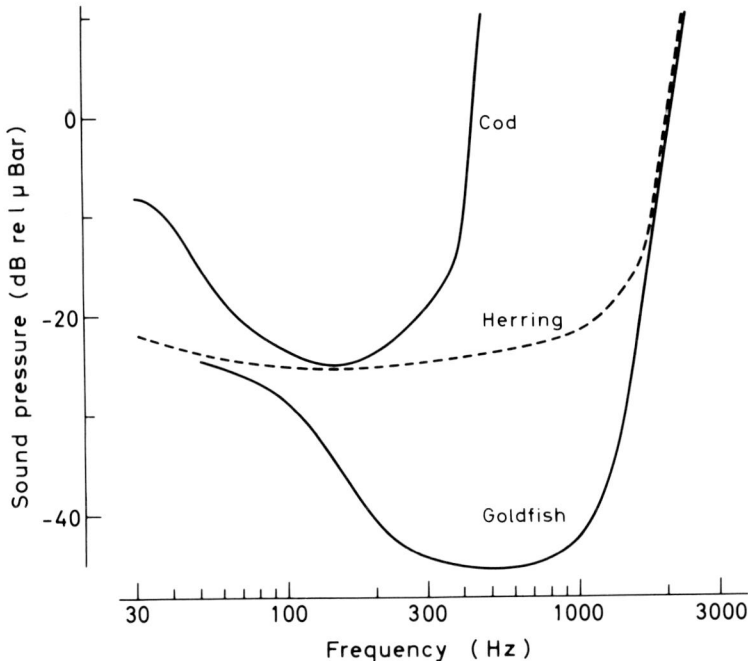

Fig. 1 Comparison between audiograms for cod (Chapman and Hawkins, 1973), herring (Enger, 1967) and goldfish (Jacobs and Tavolga, 1967).

3. Evidence for an auditory function of the swimbladder in fish without a specialized bladder-ear connection

For fish lacking a mechanical linkage between the swimbladder and the ear, the situation has, until recently, been rather confusing. Poggendorf (1952) was the first to suggest a possible auditory function of the swimbladder even in these fish. This assumption was based on his finding that Ictalurus remained sensitive to sound pressure even with the Weberian ossicles destroyed. Van Bergeijk (1964) and Alexander (1966) hypothesized that the swimbladder might improve hearing in fish without a specialized bladder ear connection. Sound-induced swimbladder pulsations would then be transmitted to the ear through the ordinary body tissues, which have nearly the same acoustical properties as water. The mechanical loss would of course be greater than within the more specialized groups, but provided the distance between the bladder and the ear was not too great, the swimbladder could be of considerable advantage.

It has been difficult to provide experimental evidence for this hypothesis. The reason is that most work on hearing in fish has been confined to laboratory conditions, where only small tanks and pools have been used. The acoustics of such small tanks are extremely complicated and not at all comparable to the situation in the open sea (Parvulescu, 1967). If the dimensions of the tank are smaller than one wavelength, large particle displacements may be generated throughout the entire water volume by only small sound pressures. Under such conditions the significance of the swimbladder in hearing will be slight. Actually, data obtained by Enger (1966) indicate that the ratio of displacement to sound pressure in a small tank may be so large that the displacement amplification provided by the swimbladder in the ostariophysi goldfish is of no auditory importance.

Experiments intending to clarify the role of the swimbladder in hearing must be conducted under more natural acoustical conditions. Enger and Andersen (1967) therefore substituted the laboratory tank with the sea itself. These authors, recording microphonic potentials from cod and sculpin (Cottus scorpius), varied the ratio between sound pressure and particle displacement at the fish by changing the distance to the sound source. Saccular microphonic potentials from the sculpin, which lacks a swimbladder, were only recorded in the near-field, where the displacements are relatively large. This fish was evidently sensitive to particle motion. However, microphonic potentials were obtained from cod even in the far-field, where the displacements are relatively small. The authors suggested that this difference in sensitivity between the two species was due to the existence of a swimbladder in cod. On the other hand, their data from cod did not show that this species was sensitive to sound pressure, rather than particle motion, and no direct evidence of a pressure displacement transforming function of the swimbladder was given (Chapman and Hawkins, 1973).

Chapman and Hawkins (1973) also worked under field conditions and varied the sound source distance to

obtain different sound pressure/displacement ratios.
Measuring acoustic thresholds in cod, they found that
the relevant auditory stimulus was sound pressure for
frequencies above about 50 Hz. Their data indirectly
indicate that the swimbladder in cod is utilized in
hearing from 50 Hz up to the upper frequency limit.
Studies on sharks (Banner, 1967) just as those on the
sculpin (Enger and Andersen, 1967) have indicated
that fish without a swimbladder are sensitive to particle motion, and not sound pressure. This evidence
was questioned by Offutt (1970), who suggested that
the otolith hair cell system is directly pressure
sensitive due to a proposed piezoelectric effect of
the otoliths. This theory was refuted by Chapman and
Sand (1973), who clearly showed that flatfish, which
lack a swimbladder, are sensitive to particle motion.
Working in the sea, they measured auditory thresholds,
and Fig. 2 gives their data from one dab (Limanda
limanda).

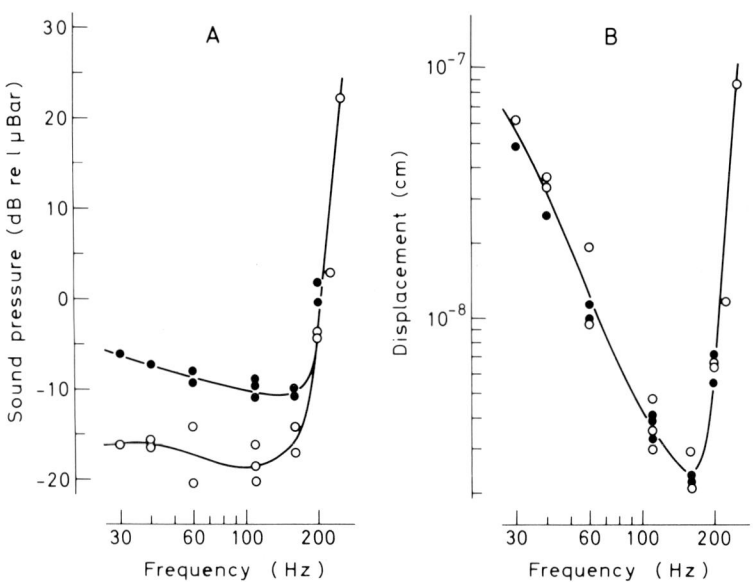

Fig. 2   Auditory thresholds from a dab, given as
         sound pressure (A) and displacement (B)
         audiograms. Values for two different sound
         source distances (o: 70 cm; ●: 300 cm) are
         included. Note that the sound pressure thresh-
         olds are independent of sound source (cont'd)

(Fig. 2, cont'd) distance, whereas the displacement thresholds are not. (After Chapman and Sand, 1973).

It is seen that whereas the sound pressure thresholds are a function of sound source distance, the displacement thresholds are not. Furthermore, the flatfish had both a lower upper frequency cut-off and generally higher thresholds than cod which were examined under similar experimental conditions (Chapman and Hawkins, 1973). The authors attributed these differences between cod and flatfish, both in respect to the relevant stimulus parameter and the threshold values, to the functioning of the swimbladder as a pressure displacement transformer in cod. This was even more convincingly shown by supplying the flatfish with an artificial swimbladder, a small toy balloon placed just beneath the head of the fish. Fig. 3

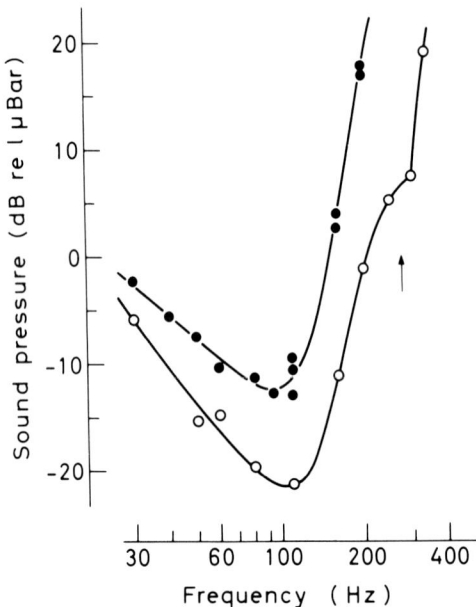

Fig. 3 The normal sound pressure audiogram (●) for a dab compared with the thresholds obtained after supplying the fish with an artificial swimbladder (o). Note that introducing this bladder causes both an extension of the audible frequency range and a general (cont'd)

(Fig. 3, cont'd) lowering of the threshold
values. The arrow indicates the balloon resonance frequency (After Chapman and Sand,
1973).

compares sound pressure audiograms for a dab with and
without such an artificial bladder, and the difference is quite striking. The upper frequency cut-off
was extended about 3/4 octave, and the artificial
swimbladder improved the sensitivity of flatfish
close to that of cod for frequencies below about 110
Hz.

It thus had been clearly demonstrated that the swimbladder may serve as a displacement amplifier which
might be utilized in hearing. However, evidence that
the natural swimbladder does function as an accessory
auditory organ in unspecialized fish was so far indirect. As van Bergeijk (1964) has pointed out, the
existence of an auditory active swimbladder will complicate the directional hearing in fish. It was not
improbable that the fish might refrain from utilizing
the swimbladder in hearing, for instance through an
orientation of the hair cells, which would make these
cells insensitive to displacements radially from the
swimbladder.

Wersäll et al. (1967) studied the morphological polarization of the sensory cells in the labyrinth of
the burbot (Lota vulgaris), and the sensitive axis of
the saccular sensory epithelium was in a dorsoventral
direction, supporting the above mentioned hypothesis.
However, the suspension of the otolith might cause
complicated otolith movements when the fish was exposed to sound, and experimental evidence was needed
to establish whether or not the fish was sensitive to
displacements radiated from the swimbladder.

Enger et al. (1973), working on haddock (Melanogrammus aeglefinus), measured saccular microphonic potentials as a function of the vibration direction. The
fish was clamped to a rotatable vibrating table, and
the microphonic potentials were recorded by implanted
electrodes. The microphonic potentials were found to
exhibit directional sensitivity, and the axis of
maximal sensitivity seemed to be along the long axis
of the fish in most cases. Fig. 4 shows data for 200
Hz from one haddock, evidently sensitive to displacements radially directed from the swimbladder. The

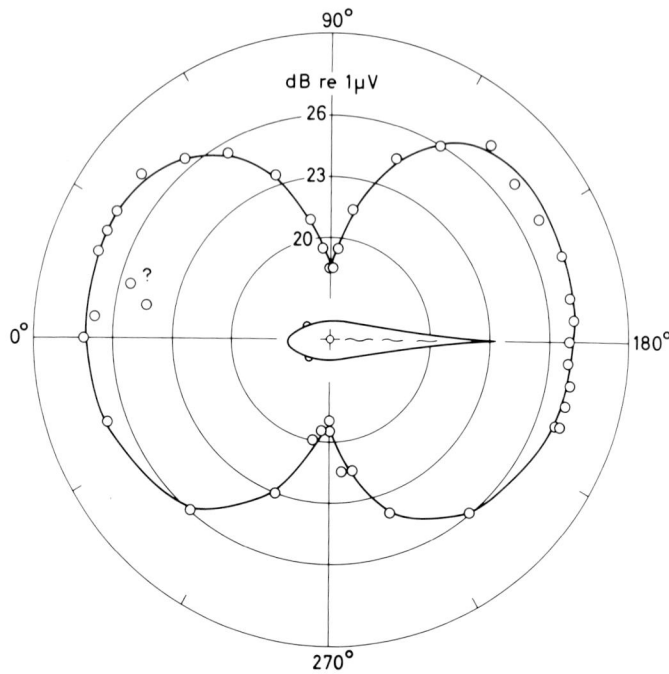

Fig. 4 Amplitude of saccular microphonic potentials from a haddock as a function of vibration direction. The horizontal vibration amplitude was kept constant at 6.10^{-6} cm and the frequency was 200 Hz. Note the directional sensitivity of the microphonic potentials (After Enger et al., 1973).

orientation of hair cells and the suspension of the sacculi allow the swimbladder to act as an accessory hearing organ.

These reports on cod (Chapman and Hawkins, 1973), flatfish (Chapman and Sand, 1973) and haddock (Enger et al., 1973) point towards an auditory function of the swimbladder, and an additional piece of direct evidence for this has been supplied by Sand and Enger (1973) in a study on cod. They worked at 6 m depth in the sea and recorded microphonic potentials from the sacculus with implanted electrodes. The microphonic potentials are caused by the summed extracellular current from several hair cells, due to their receptor

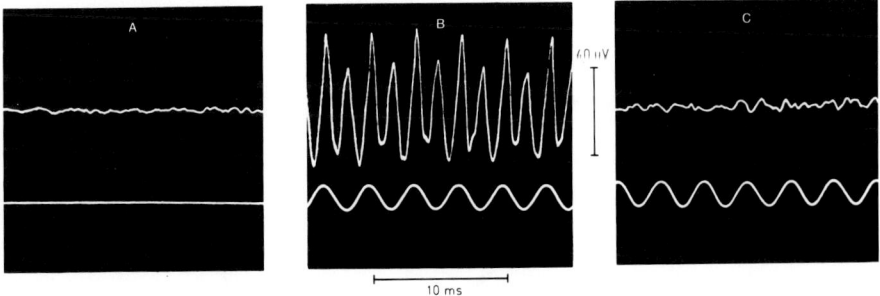

Fig. 5 Oscillographic recordings of the saccular microphonic potentials (upper trace) in a cod evoked by background noise (A) compared to the microphonic potentials generated by 300 Hz tone of 22 dB with (B) and without (C) gas in the swimbladder. Sound recordings on lower beam. Note the pronounced decrease in the microphonic potentials caused by emptying the bladder. (From Sand and Enger, 1973).

potentials (Flock, 1971). The microphonic potentials are ultimately linked to the excitation of auditory nerve fibers, and comparison of microphonic potentials at different swimbladder volumes could therefore directly indicate an influence of the swimbladder on hearing ability. Fig. 5 compares the microphonic potentials evoked by background noise only (A) with the microphonics generated by a 300 Hz tone of 22 dB with (B) and without (C) gas in the swimbladder. It is evident that emptying the swimbladder has a dramatic effect on the saccular microphonics, which decrease to a level close to the electric background noise. Fig. 6 gives the sound pressure generating microphonic potentials just above the electric noise level as a function of frequency in another fish. Values for three different swimbladder volumes are included and it is seen that for all frequencies above about 100 Hz the existence of gas in the swimbladder has a positive effect on the microphonic potentials. These data are not difficult to interpret: The swimbladder in cod is utilized in hearing for all

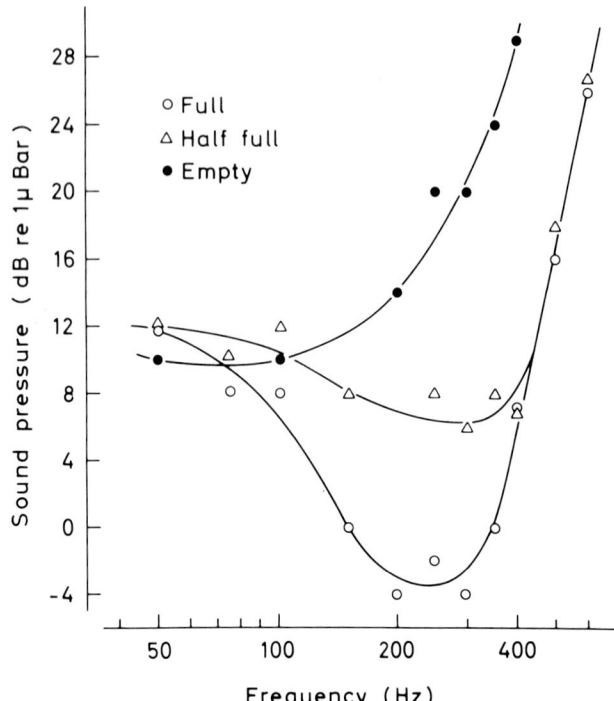

Fig. 6 Microphonic "audiograms" showing the sound pressure necessary to evoke microphonic potentials just above the noise level as a function of frequency. Values for three different swimbladder volumes are included. Note that for all frequencies above 100 Hz the existence of gas in the swimbladder has a positive effect on the microphonic potentials. (From Sand and Enger, 1973).

frequencies from a lower transient frequency to the upper frequency cut-off. This lower transient frequency is a function of several parameters and will vary under natural conditions (see Chapman and Hawkins, 1973; Sand and Hawkins, 1973).

4. Acoustical properties of the cod swimbladder

Since the swimbladder has an auditory function in an unspecialized fish like the cod, it seems likely that a swimbladder has a positive auditory effect in all fish, whether they have a specialized bladder-ear connection or not. Unfortunately, the majority of acoustical measurements on fish have been performed by using frequencies far above the auditory range, in connection with the development of fish searching equipment. However, McCartney and Stubbs (1971) developed a technique for measuring the resononce frequency and degree of damping of the swimbladder at low frequencies. This technique was adopted by Sand and Hawkins (1973), who have provided a detailed study of the resonant behavior of the cod swimbladder. Their data are surprising. All previous authors working on problems regarding swimbladder resonance had assumed the bladder to behave like a passive, damped bubble (Pumphrey 1950, Poggendorf, 1952, de Vries, 1956, Harris, 1964, Alexander, 1966, van Bergeijk, 1967), but this turned out to be completely wrong for the cod swimbladder. With fish adapted to different depths the resonance frequency and degree of damping were measured while the fish was rapidly lowered and raised in the water, without allowing time for gas to be secreted or absorbed. Fig. 7 A, gives the results from one of these experiments,

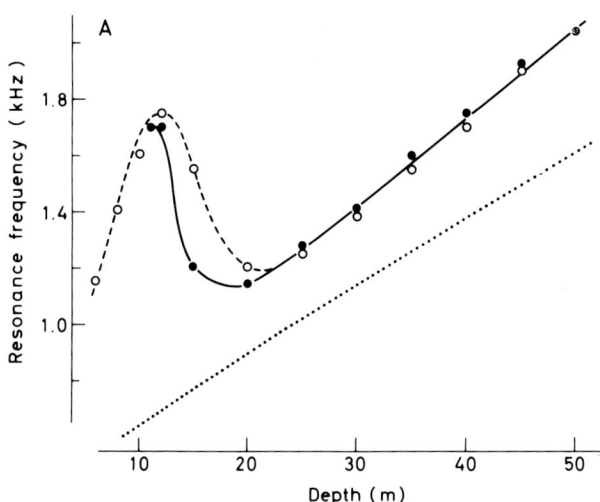

Fig. 7 (A) Resonance frequency of the cod swimbladder as a function of depth. The 16 cm fish was adapted to 11 m. Filled and open symbols indicate lowering and raising the fish, respectively. The dotted line gives the theoretical values for a free gas bubble of the same volume as the swimbladder: Note (cont'd)

(Fig. 7 (A), cont'd) the elevated resonance frequency around the adaptation depth.

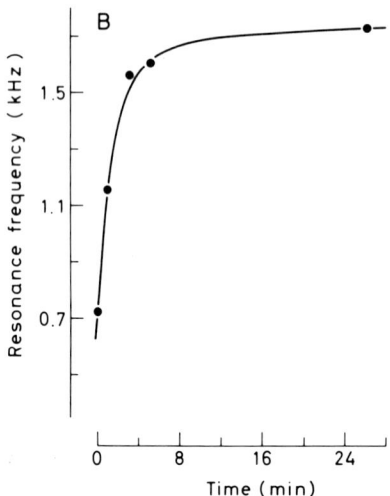

(B) Re-elevation of the resonance frequency after raising a 14 cm cod from its adaptation depth of 15 m to 8 m. Note the very rapid initial increase in resonance frequency. (After Sand and Hawkins, 1973).

and shows the resonance frequency as a function of depth for a cod initially adapted to 11 m. The theoretical curve for a free bubble of the same volume as the swimbladder is given for comparison. For hydrostatic pressures more than about twice the adaptation pressure, the resonance frequency of the swimbladder increases with depth in the manner of a free gas bubble, although the measured values were about 25 percent above those of a comparable bubble. Near the adaptation depth, however, the resonance frequency of the bladder showed a steep increase, reaching values ranging from 200 to 600 percent of the expected values for different fish. Around the adaptation depth the swimbladder was heavily damped, showing Q values close to 1.

It is seen from Fig. 7 A that the resonance frequency is different for the downward and upward movement of the fish, indicating that some kind of adaptation to the new depths had occurred during the experimental

period of about 30 minutes. This regain of the
elevated resonance frequencies, after moving the fish
away from the adaptation depth, was studied in more
detail. Fig. 7 B gives the resonance frequency as a
function of time after raising a fish to 8 m from its
adaptation depth of 15 m. Following the initial decline caused by the transfer to the new depth, the
resonance frequency changed very rapidly, and a 100
percent increase was observed in less than four minutes. This adaptation is too fast to be accounted for
by a change of the mass of swimbladder gas, which is
a rather slow process (see Alexander, 1966). Whereas
the slightly elevated resonance frequencies at depths
far from the adaptation depth could be explained by a
combined effect of the elongated swimbladder shape
and a certain stiffness of the tissues surrounding
the swimbladder, a heavy increase of this stiffness
of the tissues in the adapted fish was postulated to
explain the high resonance frequencies observed
around the adaptation depth. This phenomenon has
speculatively been attributed to a muscular mechanism.

As pointed out by Sand and Hawkins (1973), this elevated resonance frequency of the adapted fish is interesting from an auditory point of view. If the
swimbladder were resonating within the audible frequency range, the relative frequency sensitivity of
the fish would be expected to alter with depth, since
the resonance frequency both for a bubble of constant
mass and a bubble of constant volume increases with
depth. However, well below the resonance frequency
the pulsation amplitude of a gas bubble in water is
nearly constant for constant sound pressure, and is
thus independent of frequency (see Sand and Hawkins,
1973). By maintaining a resonance frequency well
above the upper frequency limit of hearing, the fish
will obtain a relative frequency sensitivity which
is independent of depth. These workers also observed
that the relative elevation of the resonance frequency in adapted fish increases with fish size,
which fits well with the hypothesis of an auditory
function of this elevation. Larger fish, with a greater swimbladder volume than smaller fish, would of
course need to increase their resonance frequency
more to reach above the upper frequency limit of
hearing. In no cases did the authors observe the resonance frequency in adapted fish to fall below this
limit, which is 400-500 Hz in cod. In addition to

these elevated resonance frequencies, the heavy damping of the swimbladder will also tend to minimize the auditory effect of different resonance frequencies at different depths and fish sizes.

Poggendorf (1952) measured the resonance frequency of the isolated swimbladder in Phoxinus laevis, using an optical technique. He found that this frequency corresponded fairly well to the optimal auditory frequency range in Ictalurus, and concluded that the extra gain that the swimbladder will provide at resonance was utilized in this fish. However, since these resonance measurements were performed on isolated swimbladders, the situation for the living fish is difficult to predict. Nevertheless, it cannot be ruled out that the swimbladder resonance may be of auditory importance in the Ostariophysi and possibly other groups.

References

Alexander, R.M. (1966). Physical aspects of swimbladder function. Biol. Rev. 41, 141-176.

Banner, A. (1967). Evidence of sensitivity to acoustic displacements in the lemon shark, Negaprion brevirostris (Poey). In: Lateral Line Detectors (P.H. Cahn, ed.), pp. 265-273. Indiana Univ. Press, Bloomington, Indiana.

van Bergeijk, W.A. (1964). Directional and nondirectional hearing in fish. In: Marine Bio-Acoustics (W.N. Tavolga, ed.), pp. 281-299. Pergamon Press, Oxford.

van Bergeijk, W.A. (1967). The evolution of vertebrate hearing. In: Contributions to Sensory Physiology (W.D. Neff, ed.), Vol. 2, pp. 1-49. Academic Press, New York.

Chapman, C.J., and Hawkins, A.D. (1973). A field study of hearing in the cod, Gadus morhua L. (In preparation).

Chapman, C.J., and Sand, O. (1973). Field studies of hearing in two species of flatfish Pleuronectes platessa (L) and Limanda limanda (L)(Family Pleuronectidae). Comp. Biochem. Physiol. (In press).

de Vries, H. (1956). Physical aspects of the sense organs. Progr. Biophys. Biophys. Chem. 6, 207-264.

Enger, P.S. (1966). Acoustic threshold in goldfish and its relation to the sound source distance. Comp. Biochem. Physiol. 18, 859-868.

Enger, P.S. (1967). Hearing in herring. Comp. Biochem. Physiol. 22, 527-538.

Enger, P.S., and Andersen, R. (1967). An electrophysiological field study of hearing in fish. Comp. Biochem. Physiol. 22, 517-525.

Enger, P.S., Hawkins, A.D., Sand, O., and Chapman, C.J. (1973). Directional sensitivity of saccular microphonic potentials in the haddock. (In preparation).

Flock, Å. (1971). The lateral line organ mechanoreceptors. In: Fish Physiology (W.S. Hoar and D.J. Randall, eds.), Vol. V, pp. 241-263. Academic Press, New York.

von Frisch, K. (1938). Über die Bedeutung des Sacculus und der Lagena für den Gehörsinn der Fische. Z. Vergl. Physiol. 25, 703-747.

Griffin, D.R. (1950). Underwater sounds and the orientation of marine animals - a preliminary survey. Tech. Rep. No. 3, Proj. NR 162-429. ONR and Cornell Univ.

Griffin, D.R. (1955). Hearing and acoustical orientation in marine animals. Deep-Sea Res. 3, Suppl., 406-417.

Harris, G.G. (1964). Considerations on the physics of sound production by fishes. In: Marine Bio-Acoustics (W.N. Tavolga, ed.), pp. 233-247. Pergamon Press, Oxford.

Jacobs, D.W., and Tavolga, W.N. (1967). Acoustic intensity limens in the goldfish. Anim. Behav. 15, 324-335.

Jones, F.R.H., and Marshall, N.B. (1953). The swimbladder. Biol. Rev. 28, 16-83.

McCartney, B.S., and Stubbs, A.R. (1971). Measurements of the acoustic target strengths of fish in dorsal aspect, including swimbladder resonance. J. Sound Vib. 15, 397-420.

Offutt, G.C. (1970). A proposed mechanism for the perception of acoustic stimuli near threshold. J. Aud. Res. 10, 226-228.

Parvulescu, A. (1967). Acoustics of small tanks. In: Marine Bio-Acoustics (W.N. Tavolga, ed.), Vol. 2, pp. 7-13. Pergamon Press, Oxford.

Poggendorf, D. (1952). Die absoluten Hörschwellen des Zwergwelses (Amiurus nebulosus) und Beiträge zur Physik des Weberschen Apparates der Ostariophysen. Z. Vergl. Physiol. 34, 222-257.

Pumphrey, R.J. (1950). Hearing. Symp. Soc. Exp. Biol. 4, 3-18.

Sand, O., and Enger, P.S. (1973). Evidence of an auditory function of the swimbladder in the cod. (In preparation).

Sand. O., and Hawkins, A.D. (1973). Acoustic properties of the cod swimbladder. J. Exp. Biol. (In press).

Tavolga, W.N. (1971). Sound production and detection. In: Fish Physiology (W.S. Hoar and D.J. Randall eds.), Vol. V, pp. 135-205. Academic Press, New York.

Weber, E.H. (1820). De aure et auditu hominis et animalium. Pars I. De aure animalium aquatilium. Leipzig.

Wersäll, J., Gleisner, L., and Lundquist, P.-G. (1967). Ultrastructure of the vestibular end organs. In: Myotatic and Vestibular Mechanisms (A.V.S. de Reuck and J. Knight, eds.), pp. 105-120. Churchill, London.

Wohlfahrt, T.A. (1936). Das Ohrlabyrinth der Sardine (Clupea pilchardus Walb.) und seine Beziehungen zur Schwimmblase und Seitenlinie. Z. Morphol. Oekol. Tiere 31, 371-410.

DISCUSSION

BRUGGE: I wonder if you would clarify the source of the saccular microphonic. Is there any reason to believe that the maccula of the utricle and for that matter, the cristae of the semi-circular canal are not activated by the movements of the endolymph?

ENGER: I think there are other people in this room who are much better qualified to clarify the source of saccular microphonics. All I can say is that I can record saccular microphonics from my fish by placing the electrodes in proximity to the sensory cells in the sacculus.

BRUGGE: Does that mean that the utricle and the semi-circular canals are not contributing to the microphonic?

ENGER: I do not think that they contribute to the microphonic I showed you because of the small distance (considerably less than a millimeter) between the saccular sensory epithelium and my electrodes, whereas the distance to the utricle is about a centimeter and a half. They could be from the lagena which is located just behind the sacculus. The hearing sense in fish, as determined from elimination experiments, is localized to the sacculus and the lagena, not so much to the utricle and semi-circular canals.

MICHELSEN: You said that the effective parameter of the sound wave is the displacement. I suppose that this is only true, when the swim-bladder is intact? The rest of the system looks like a pressure receiver?

ENGER: The hair cells are sensitive to displacement, but since the swim-bladder acts as a pressure/displacement transformer, the complete auditory system of the fish will be sensitive to sound pressure.

MICHELSEN: Well, in the far-field you still have the diffraction caused by the body of the fish.

SCHWARTZKOPFF: I should like to come back to your question, Dr. Brugge. I think Furukawa (Furukawa and Ishii, 1967) and Matsuura (Matsuura et al., 1971) have studied conditions for the generation of microphonics within the sacculus of the goldfish. Flock knows of course better about this than I do.

FLOCK: I noticed on your record of the microphonic potential that it was the second harmonic of the driving frequency. This fits very well with the double orientation that you see in the sacculus. The fundamentals cancel out and you are left with the harmonic component.

ENGER: Yes, in the usual pattern of the saccular microphonics, in fish the frequency is the double of the stimulating sound.

References

Furukawa, T., and Ishii, Y. (1967). Effects of static bending of sensory hairs on sound reception in the goldfish. Jap. J. Physiol. 17, 572-588.

Matsuura, S., Ikeda, K., and Furukawa, T. (1971). Effects of Na^+, K^+, and ouabain on microphonic potentials of the goldfish inner ear. Jap. J. Physiol. 21, 563-578.

THE MECHANICS OF THE LOCUST EAR: AN
INVERTEBRATE FREQUENCY ANALYZER

Axel Michelsen

Institute of Biology
Odense University
Denmark

1. Introduction

We shall now turn to the ear of the desert locust, an invertebrate hearing organ which has a much simpler anatomy than the complex ear of the vertebrates. Still simpler insect ears are known (e.g. the ear of the noctuid moth), but the locust ear combines a fairly simple anatomy with a reasonably complex function. Until recently, the locust ear was the only invertebrate hearing organ known to discriminate sound frequencies (Popov, 1965, Michelsen, 1966).

Frequency analysis takes place in an organ consisting of a membrane and four groups of receptor cells. One can remove the membrane and its receptor cells with a pair of scissors and mount it on a small platform of wax. The preparation is ready for experiments in less than five minutes (Fig. 1). The operation is started by decapitating the animal, so no artificial respiration or anesthesia is necessary. When this isolated ear preparation is placed in a sound field, the vibrations of the membrane and receptor cells may be measured with laser light or capacitance probes. The results can then be compared with the sensory response of the receptor cells. This article deals with the physical basis of the frequency discrimination shown by the four groups of receptor cells in such an isolated ear preparation.[1]

---

[1] Most aspects of this problem have been discussed earlier (Michelsen, 1971a, b, c), but some new observations are also presented.

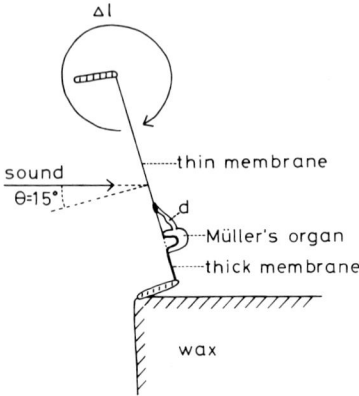

Fig. 1 The tympanal organ mounted for investigation with a vertical microelectrode.

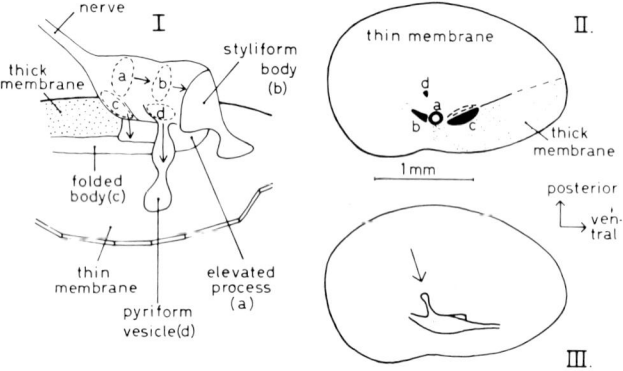

Fig. 2 The anatomy of the tympanal organ. I, Müller's organ (right ear). The position of the receptor cells (a-d) and the attachment parts of the membrane are shown. Arrows indicate the direction of the dendrites. II, The left ear seen from outside the animal. The dark areas indicate the areas of attachment of the receptor cells. III, The right ear seen from the inside. The arrow indicates the visual angle of I.

2. Anatomy

The locust has a tympanal organ (ear) on each side of the first abdominal segment. It consists of a sclerotized ring forming a recess in the abdomen and encircling a membrane, the tympanum. The tympanum is bean-shaped and about 2.5 × 1.5 mm at its widest (Fig. 2). The dorsal end is somewhat wider than the ventral end. The total area is about 3 mm^2. Most of the tympanal membrane consists of cuticle (2-3 µm thick), which is covered on the inside by a layer of cells (1-2 µm thick) and by the wall of an air sac. This thin part of the membrane has an area of about 2.4 mm^2. In the ventral-anterior corner, however, the membrane is about 8-10 µm thick. The area of this thick part of the membrane is about 0.5-0.6 mm^2.

Four specialized regions with much thicker cuticle are situated between the middle of the tympanum and the anterior edge. They are the elevated process, the styliform body, the folded body, and the pyriform vesicle. The four anatomical groups of receptor cells (called a, b, c, and d by Gray, 1960, who described the fine structure of the ear) are attached to these bodies (Fig. 2). The total arrangement of receptor cells and attachment bodies is called the Müller organ. The receptor cells of the a-, c-, and d-groups are orientated in three almost mutually perpendicular planes. The fourth group (b) is orientated in the same plane as the a-group. The a-group comprises about half of the total number of receptor cells, and the three other groups about 8-12 cells each.

3. Frequency discrimination

Information about the frequency of a sound may be signalled by auditory receptors in two different ways. The anatomical groups of receptor cells may differ as to characteristic frequency, thus providing the CNS with information about frequency (the place principle). At low frequencies the receptor cells may also send trains of nerve impulses to the CNS, each corresponding to a certain phase of the sound wave (the telephone principle).

The telephone principle is illustrated by the response of several hair sense organs in insects to low frequency sound (some hundred Hz). It is doubtful, however, that the insect CNS extracts the information about frequency coming from these hairs. The receptor cells of the locust ear are also able to

signal the frequency when stimulated with mechanical vibrations below some hundred Hz. At frequencies around one hundred Hz they respond once per sine wave.
At very low frequencies (around 20 Hz) the entire tympanal organ responds twice per sine wave (Storm and Michelsen, unpublished data). These frequencies are so far below the resonance frequencies of the ear that the membrane will hardly move when acted upon by sound waves. The tympanal organ is sensitive to sound between one and forty kHz, and in this range the nerve impulses from the receptor cells are not phase-locked with the sound waves.
The four anatomical groups of receptor cells in the locust ear (Fig. 2) differ as to frequency sensitivity (the place principle). Fig. 3 shows the threshold

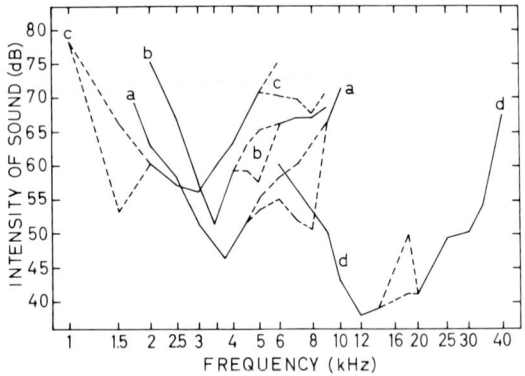

Fig. 3 The threshold curves for the four groups of receptor cells in the isolated locust ear. Broken lines indicate variations in threshold curves for different cells within each group.

curves of the four groups. The maximum sensitivity of each group of receptor cells is limited to a small number of discrete frequency bands. In most cases the frequencies of maximum sensitivity are around 3.7 kHz for the a-cells, 3.5 kHz for the b-cells, and 12 kHz for the d-cells. In some cells a second sensitivity maximum was observed around 8 kHz (a), 5 kHz (b), and 19 kHz (d)). The response of the c-cells is more complex, but the preferred frequencies are 1.5 kHz, 2-3 kHz (all cells), and 8 kHz.
So, in a large number of cells there is a tendency for a second (and sometimes a third) maximum sensitivity at another frequency than the "characteristic

frequency". The "CF" is not easy to define here, because the response at the second maximum may sometimes be as large or even larger than the response to the "CF" itself. In some cells, on the other hand, the second maximum was very small or entirely lacking. It is not possible to say whether there is a real variation in the properties of the individual receptor cells within a group in a certain ear. Almost all recordings are from different preparations, so the variation may just be a reflection of this. In spite of these variations, the difference in frequency response between the groups is highly significant. This is even true for the a- and b-cells, which are very similar. Their characteristic frequencies differ by about 300 Hz, but the tuning (Q-value) of the b-cells is about two times larger than that of the a-cells.

4. The expected vibrations

The compliance of the tympanal membrane is mainly determined by its tension, so the tympanum is physically speaking a membrane (in contrast to a plate, in which stiffness is an important factor). The compliance is constant (about 0.14 m/Newton) for displacements up to 50-100 µm, i.e. in this range Hooke's law is obeyed (a linear relationship between displacement and force).

The compliance is about the same for most parts of the tympanum. The mass, however, is rather unevenly distributed. About two-thirds of the total weight (about 45 µg) is in the Müller organ (the receptor cells and the cuticular bodies, see Fig. 2). The thin membrane, on the other hand, takes 5/6 of the total area, but only 1/5 of the total weight.

So, the tympanal membrane is far from homogeneous. Furthermore, the presence of the four cuticular bodies in the tympanum is likely to affect its vibration. These bodies are stiff, and together with a cuticular rod they cover most of the boundary between the thin and thick parts of the tympanum. The presence of this boundary at the edge of the thin membrane appears to allow it to vibrate independently of the entire tympanal membrane (see below).

Membranes acted upon by a harmonic driving force may vibrate in many different ways (Fig. 4). If the membrane is circular, homogeneous, and acted upon by an evenly distributed force (sound wave), only the circularly symmetrical modes of vibrations are to be expected (Fig. 4, a-c; Fig. 5). If one of these conditions is not fulfilled, the vibrations may be con-

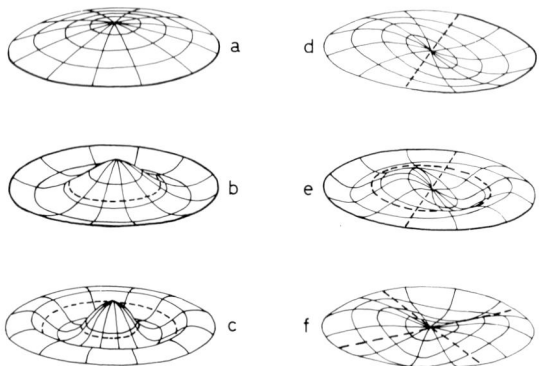

Fig. 4   The first three circularly symmetrical modes of vibration in a circular membrane (a-c), and some other possible modes (d-f). The nodal lines are indicated by dotted lines. Further explanation in the text. (Redrawn from P.M. Morse: Vibration and sound. Copyright 1936, 1948 by the McGraw-Hill Book Company, Inc. Used with permission of McGraw-Hill Book Company).

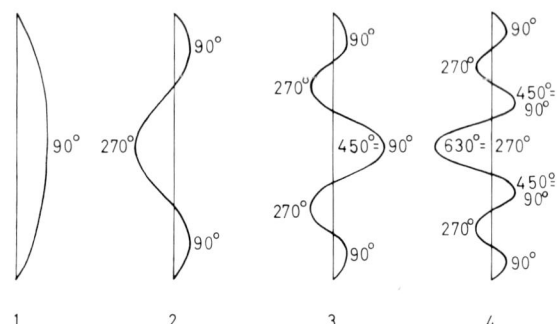

Fig. 5   The first four circularly symmetrical modes of vibration in a membrane. The approximate phase lags (between driving force and membrane displacement) are indicated at resonance for the different parts of the membrane. (1-3 are identical to a-c on Fig. 4).

siderably more complex (Fig. 4, d-f).

The circularly symmetrical modes of vibration are the most simple, and the experiments show that such vibrations dominate the behavior of the tympanal membrane (see below). At low frequencies the membrane will tend to move as a whole (Fig. 4, a), and its behavior very much resembles that of a simple driven oscillator. At very low frequencies the maximum displacement of the membrane will be almost in phase with the driving force, but as the frequency approaches the first resonance, the displacement will be delayed relative to the force. At the first resonance frequency this delay is 90° (Fig. 5, 1), and somewhat above the first resonance the instantaneous displacement of the membrane is nearly opposed to the driving force (i.e. the phase lag is about 180°).

If the frequency is increased, a circular nodal line appears at the edge and moves towards the center. The part of the membrane around the center has remained out of phase with the force, but the part outside the nodal circle is almost in phase with the force. The amplitude of the overall motion now increases, and a second resonance is reached (Fig. 4, b and 5, 2). At a higher frequency a new nodal line will be formed, and so on. It is apparent that the vibration of the center of the membrane will be delayed more and more relative to the driving force. The variation in the amplitude of vibration will be rather smooth for the center: it will be a maximum at the resonance frequencies and a minimum at other frequencies. But obviously this is not true for parts of the membrane which are at or near to a nodal circle at resonance. Since the receptor cells attach to small areas on the membrane, this problem had to be considered in detail (see Michelsen, 1971 b).

The tympanal membrane is far from homogeneous, and it is not circular. Nevertheless, the calculated resonance frequencies for the circularly symmetrical vibrations of the thin membrane and the entire membrane are fairly close to the observed characteristic frequencies of the receptor cells (Fig. 6).

Most of the observed best frequencies are fairly close to one of the expected resonance frequencies. On the other hand, the number of expected resonances

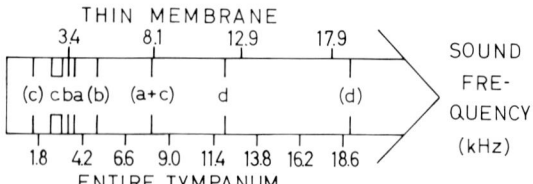

Fig. 6 The expected resonance frequencies for the thin membrane (above) and for the entire tympanum (below), compared with the preferred frequencies of the four groups (a-d) of receptor cells (center). Letters in brackets indicate frequencies not preferred by all cells in a group.

is so large in the frequency range 1-20 kHz that a wide variety of explanations may be given for several of the observed best frequencies. The problem also arises as to how the receptor cells can be so selective: each group of receptor cells prefers only two or three bands of frequencies. Obviously, direct observations are necessary.

5. The observed vibrations

Two different methods were used to study the vibration patterns of the tympanal membrane. Time average holograms were produced (for details see Michelsen, 1971 b), and the real image of the ear was photographed with a camera. Equal amplitudes of vibration can be seen as fringes (light and dark lines, Figs. 7-9). With the angles of incidence and reflection used, the distance between two dark lines (or between two light lines) will normally correspond to a difference of 0.40 μm in peak-to-peak amplitude. When the fundamental vibration is observed, one can determine the displacement of the center simply by counting the number of rings. This is, however, not the case when higher, circularly symmetrical modes of vibration are observed. The concentric "bubbles" of the membrane, vibrating 180° out of phase (see Fig. 5), may each give rise to one or more rings. The position of the nodal lines could not be determined directly, so the phase relationships of the vibrations had to be measured before the nature of the observed vibrations could be determined.

The phase of the membrane vibration relative to the

driving force (Fig. 5) was measured with a capacitance electrode. It made it possible to measure the phase and relative amplitude of vibration of 0.01 mm^2 areas of the membrane (for details see Michelsen, 1971 b). The absolute amplitude of vibration could not be estimated with this method. In order to interpret the results it is necessary to know the magnitude and phase of the driving force relative to that of the sound wave. These figures can be calculated if the "effective distance" ($\Delta 1$ of Fig. 1) is known; and this figure can be estimated by experiments (see Michelsen, 1971 c).

In the preceding paragraph the expected vibrations have been discussed. They were calculated on the assumption that the tympanal membrane behaves as an ideal membrane. It is obvious that the entire tympanum is very far from homogeneous, and that the thin part of the membrane, although fairly homogeneous, is not circular. The most surprising feature of the vibrations, as observed by means of laser holography and the capacitance electrode, is how well they follow the predicted behavior. There are, of course, several minor deviations, but the overall impression is that of a general agreement.

The best correlation with theory is found for the resonance frequencies, which normally deviate less than 10 % from the expected values. The most surprising deviation from theory is that the spatial position of the center of vibration is not constant. An ideal membrane would have the center of vibration at its geometrical center. In the tympanal membrane, however, the centers of vibration are not at the geometrical center, and their positions differ for different modes of vibration. The centers of all the modes of vibration of the entire membrane are located in the thick-membrane-end of the tympanum; but the center of the first mode is at the thin membrane (Fig. 9) whereas the centers of higher modes are in the thick membrane (Fig. 7). The centers of vibration of the thin-membrane system are located nearer the geometrical center of the tympanum (Fig. 7 and 8). Here again, the position of the center is not constant; at some frequencies it is at the geometrical center of the thin membrane (Fig. 8); at other frequencies it is at the area of attachment of the a- and b-cells, i.e. near the edge of the thin membrane (Fig. 7).

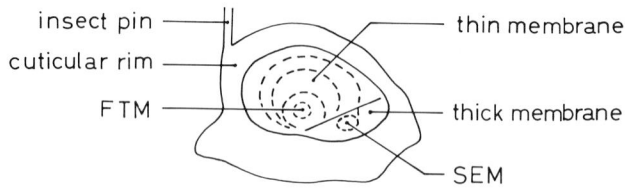

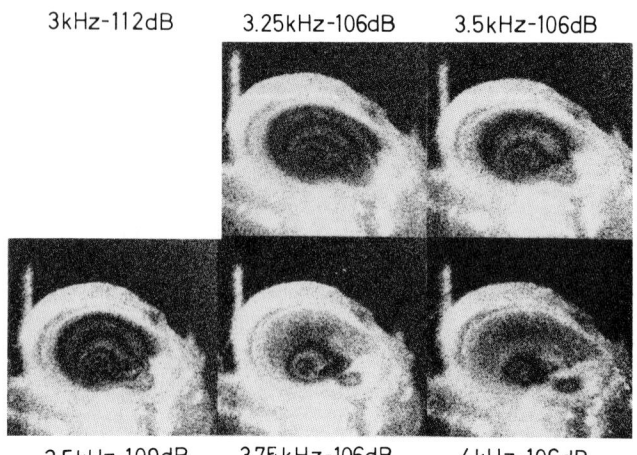

Fig. 7 Holographic pictures of the vibrations in the frequency range 3-4 kHz. Above: The orientation of the isolated ear, and the approximate positions of the centers of the fundamental mode of the thin membrane (FTM) and of the second mode of the entire membrane (SEM). Below: The vibration patterns; the dark and light lines on the pictures are loci of equal amplitudes of vibration. Note the concentration of the FTM vibration, when the frequency is varied from 3 to 3.75 kHz. (The 3 kHz vibration pattern has been drawn from a holographic picture of bad technical quality. This picture was from another preparation.

This may seem surprising, but because of the peculiar shape of the thin membrane (Fig. 2) the area of attachment of the a- and b-cells is both at the edge of the thin membrane and near to its center.

6.5 kHz-104dB   7kHz-104dB   7.5 kHz-104dB

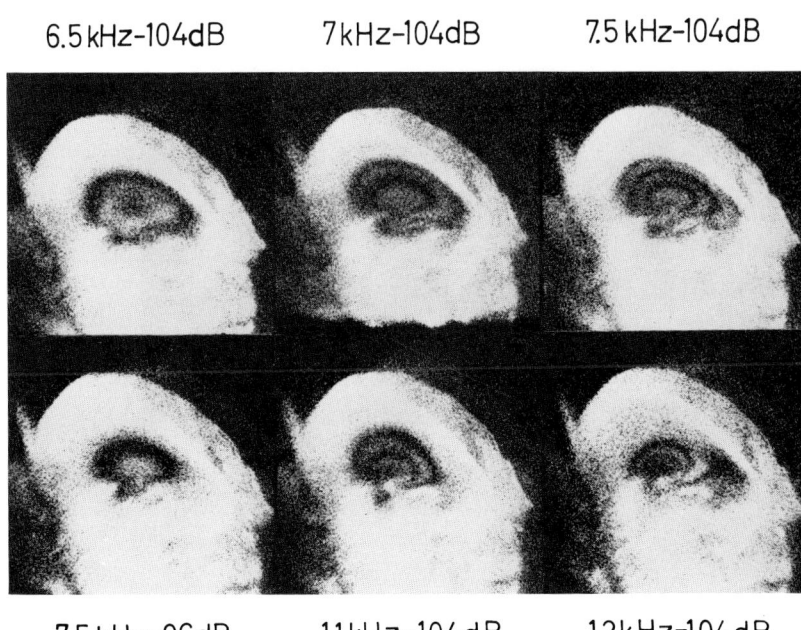

7.5 kHz-96dB   11kHz-104dB   12kHz-104dB

Fig. 8   Holographic pictures of the second
        and third mode of vibration of the
        thin-membrane system. The orienta-
        tion of the isolated ear is similar
        to Fig. 7. The three upper pictures
        show the increasing amplitude of
        vibration as the second resonance
        frequency (8 kHz) is approached.
        The pictures at 11 and 12 kHz show
        the concentration of the area of
        vigorous vibration as the third re-
        sonance frequency (13 kHz) is ap-
        proached.

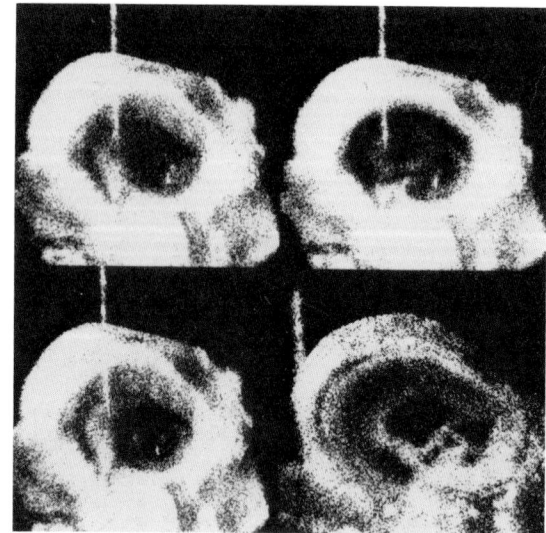

Fig. 9   Holographic pictures of vibration patterns in the isolated ear. Left: The fundamental mode of the entire-membrane system. Note that the center of vibration is in the thick-membrane corner of the tympanum. Right: Two unexpected patterns of vibration (see the discussion). In three of the pictures the insect pin is also seen on a part of the membrane. In fact, the pin was behind the membrane, and reflected light was transmitted through the membrane.

Measurements with the capacitance electrode confirm the difference in spatial position of the thin and entire membrane vibrations. The entire membrane system governs the phase and amplitude of the thick-membrane-end of the membrane (Fig. 2), whereas the values in the opposite end of the membrane are close to those expected for the thin membrane system. Between these "zones of influence" there is a "zone of interaction", where the behavior of the membrane is determined by both vibrations. Normally, the influence from the thin membrane system is the stronger, because the damping of this system is about three times less than that of the entire membrane system (see Michelsen, 1971 b).

A surprising feature of some of the tympanal vibrations is their spatial concentration. For example, the vibrations derived from the entire membrane system may bo rostricted to a very small area (SEM on Fig. 7). This is also true for some of the thin membrane vibrations, e.g. the fundamental mode at 3.75-4 kHz (FTM on Fig. 7) and the third mode at 12 kHz (Fig. 8). The patterns of vibration have been discussed in detail earlier (Michelsen, 1971b). It should be mentioned that at 5 and 9.5 kHz two unexpected vibrations have been observed (Fig. 9). Their nature is not clear, but they do not seem to affect the receptor cells very much.

6. The mechanism of frequency discrimination

The sensitivity of the a- and b-cells has a maximum at 3.74 and 3.46 kHz, respectively. In the frequency range 3-4 kHz a very dramatic change in the vibration pattern can be observed on the holograms (Fig. 7). At 3 kHz the fundamental mode of the thin-membrane system (FTM) is almost at the center of the tympanum, but as the frequency increases the FTM becomes more concentrated and moves towards the Müller organ (Fig. 7). At higher frequencies the center of the vibration again moves towards the center of the thin membrane.

The frequency selectivity of the a- and b-cells is in reasonable agreement with the observed vibrations. However, the differences between the two groups are not explained by the events shown on the holograms. Unfortunately, the capacitance electrode was too large to allow the fine details in the vibration of the adjoining attachment areas of the a- and b-cells to be resolved. A theory has been proposed to explain the differences between the groups (Michelsen, 1971b), but a final solution of the problem has to await experiments with more sensitive equipment. The secondary sensitivity maximum of the a-cells is probably caused by the second mode of the thin-membrane system, whereas that of the b-cells coincides with the unexpected vibration at 5 kHz.

The c-cells may have up to three frequencies of maximum sensitivity: 1.5 kHz, 2.5-3 kHz, and 8 kHz (see Fig. 3). The 8 kHz response is probably due to the second mode of the thin membrane. The response at 2.5-3 kHz does not correspond to any of the expected resonances. The experiments show that the response at 1.5 kHz is due to the fundamental mode of the entire-membrane system, and that the response at 2.5-3 kHz is caused by the interaction between the fundamental modes of the entire and thin part of the tympanum.

Different types of vibration have been found in different recordings, when the capacitance electrode is placed close to the folded body (the attachment area of the c-cells, see Fig. 2). They include an almost pure 1.8 kHz response (Fig. 10, I), a 3.4 kHz response (Fig. 10, III) and gradual series of intermediate types (Fig. 10, II). Their nature can be seen from the phase relationships (Fig. 10). The 1.8 kHz and

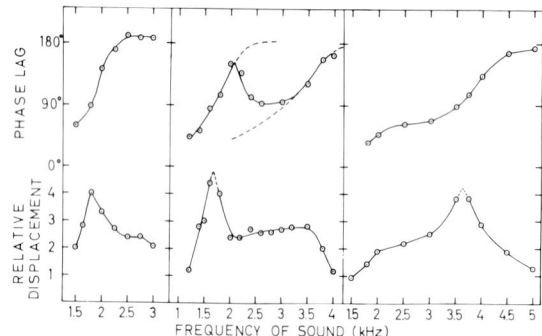

Fig. 10   Variation in amplitude and phase lag measured with the capacitance electrode placed close to the folded body (c-cells). I and III are extreme types which almost correspond to the fundamental modes of the entire and thin membrane, respectively. II is an intermediate type. Further explanation in the text.

3.4 kHz responses are almost equal to those expected for the fundamental modes of the entire- and thin-membrane systems, respectively. The phase lag is about 90°, when the amplitude of vibration is a maximum (cf. Fig. 5).

The response type II (Fig. 10), which is similar to the most common response curve of the c-cells, appears to be a compromise between the types I and III. This response type is very close to what can be expected for the "zone of interaction" between the "zones of influence" of the two fundamental modes: at

low frequencies (around 1.8 kHz) the variation of
phase and amplitude is governed by the fundamental
mode of the entire tympanum. Around 3.4 kHz the be
havior is mainly determined by the fundamental mode
of the thin membrane. Between these frequencies, a
dramatic change of phase is observed, corresponding
to a gradual shift in the relative "influence" of the
two vibrations. The reason that the 3.4 kHz vibration does not produce any peak in the amplitude of
type II may be that the fundamental mode of the thin
membrane in now interacting with the second mode of
the entire membrane (expected at 4.2 kHz).

The d-cells are specialized in responding to frequencies above 10 kHz (Fig. 3), and they appear to record
the third and fourth mode of vibration of the thin-
membrane system. The amplitude- and phase-relationships illustrated in Fig. 11, left, were recorded in

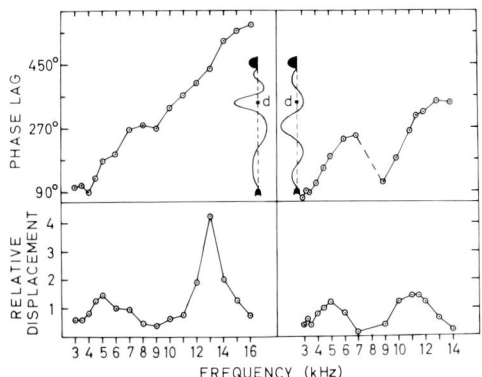

Fig. 11 Amplitude and phase measured with the capacitance electrode close to the pyriform
vesicle (d-cells). Left: the normal case;
the third mode (at 13 kHz) is so askew that
its center is at the d-cell area of attachment. Right: a more symmetrical vibration;
the pyriform vesicle is not at the center
of vibration. Note the decrease in phase at
the passing of the nodal circle.

most preparations when the capacitance electrode was
placed close to the attachment point of the d-cells
(see Fig. 2). The amplitude is a maximum at 13 kHz
(cf. Fig. 3 and 6). The amplitude is a minimum around

8 kHz. The reason for this behavior is that the area of attachment of the d-cells is close to the nodal circle of the second mode at resonance. This can be seen if the capacitance electrode is moved.

From Fig. 5 it is seen that in an ideal membrane the position of the node in the second mode should correspond to the part of the membrane between the two nodal circles in the third mode. The phase-relationships show that this is not true (Fig. 11, left). At 13 kHz the displacement is delayed about 450° with respect to the driving force, and not 270° as one would expect (see Fig. 5). This means that the d-cells must respond to the center of the third mode and not to the "bubble" between the two nodal circles. Thus, the third mode is very asymmetrical. This is also suggested by the holograms (Fig. 8).

The position of the d-cells is unique, since normally they avoid responding to the second mode by being near the nodal line at resonance, but at the same time they pick up the largest amplitude of the third mode by attaching to its center and not to the membrane between the nodal circles. In a few preparations, however, the third mode was not so askew (Fig. 11, right). In this case one can see a decrease in phase, indicating the passing of the inner nodal circle.

7. The role of the Müller organ

The findings described above indicate that the excitation of the receptor cells is roughly proportional to the vibration of their attachment area. The anatomy of the Müller organ is rather complicated, seemingly more so than necessary for the simple task of picking up the transverse vibrations of the attachment areas. The attachment parts of the tympanum have been referred to as "areas", but (except for the pyriform vesicle of the d-cells) they are certainly not simple thickenings of the cuticle (see Schwabe, 1906). The styliform body (b-cells) has the shape of an hour-glass, which is fastened to a plate at the membrane-end. The shape of the hollow, elevated process is often described as that of a cup, but in fact it bends at some distance from the tympanal membrane. Finally, the folded body is a surprisingly large and complicated, folded thickenings of the membrane. The possibility remains that the Müller organ is not just a passive observer of the tympanal vibrations, but that it plays an active role in the transduction process.

Two techniques have recently been used to investigate this possibility. Mechanical stimuli delivered from a "mini shaker" (Brüel & Kjær, type 4810) were applied through a glass rod to various parts of the ear. The exact magnitude and form of the stimulus was controlled by means of a "laser-Doppler-shift-vibratometer", which has been built as a prototype by DISA Elektronik, Copenhagen. This apparatus allows vibrations from areas with a diameter of 50 µm to be measured up to 100 kHz. The lower velocity limit is $10^{-5} - 10^{-4}$ m/sec and the lower amplitude limit is about 50 Å. This apparatus was also used to measure the vibration of the Müller organ in some of the experiments.

In some experiments, most of the tympanal membrane was cut away so that the behavior of the isolated Müller organ could be investigated. The preparation consisted only of the Müller organ surrounded by very little tympanal membrane. The vibrations were delivered with the stimulating rod placed perpendicularly to the outer surface of the Müller organ. This preparation had a threshold curve (Fig. 12), which followed a line of constant acceleration down to a displacement amplitude of about 6 Å (r.m.s.). The threshold acceleration was about 0.4 m/sec^2 (r.m.s.).

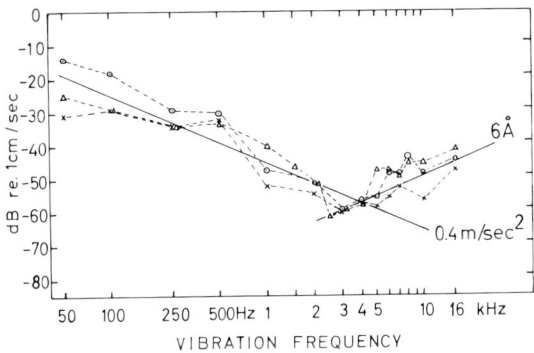

Fig. 12   The isolated Müller organ stimulated with mechanical vibration: threshold curves from three experiments.

The transduction mechanism responsible for this curious behavior is not known, but the transfer functions are almost linear. This is not the case when the tympanum is left intact (Fig. 13). The tympanum now

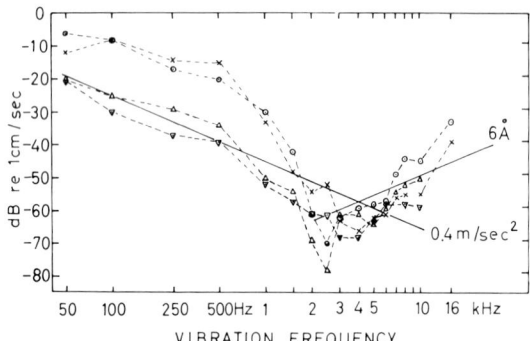

Fig. 13 The tympanal organ stimulated with mechanical vibration. For explanation, see the text.

plays a great role in determining the shape of the threshold curve. On Fig. 13 the two lower curves are from experiments in which the mechanical vibration was directed towards the Müller organ. These curves follow the line of constant acceleration up to 1 kHz, where the tympanal resonances start. The two upper curves are from experiments in which the vibration was directed towards the thin part of the tympanum (about half way between the edge and the d-cells). The lower sensitivity to low and high frequencies reflects the damping effect of the membrane impedance.

It was mentioned above ("expected vibrations") that a large number of irregular vibrations could be expected, if the membrane was not driven by an evenly distributed force. Preliminary laser measurements suggest that this is in fact the case. It is not really interesting to know the exact nature of these vibrations. The important thing is that vibrations in the membrane do influence the Müller organ, even when the mechanical vibrations are directed towards the Müller organ (and perpendicularly to the membrane). This would suggest that the Müller organ can pick up not only the vibrations perpendicular to the membrane, but also vibrations in the plane of the tympanum.

This idea is suggested, but not proven, by the experimental results just mentioned. Direct evidence for the existence of vibrations in the plane of the tympanum was obtained by directing the laser beam (of the Doppler-shift-vibratometer) towards the Müller organ as shown in Fig. 14. The ear was stimulated

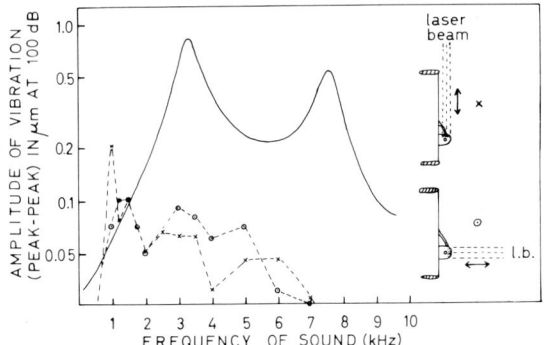

Fig. 14 The vibrations of the Müller organ parallel to and transverse to the membrane (broken lines). For comparison, the expected vibration of the center of the thin membrane is shown (solid line). Further explanation in the text.

with sound, so that irregular vibrations could be avoided. In the experiments marked with X, the vibrations of the Müller organ in the plane of the tympanum were measured. The circles give the vibrations in the direction perpendicular to the membrane. For comparison, the calculated (and experimentally verified) vibrations of the center of the thin membrane are given in solid line. It should be remembered that these vibrations co-exist with those of the entire membrane.

These pilot experiments show that the Müller organ performs vigorous vibrations in the frequency range 1-8 kHz. It is interesting that the d-group is the only group insensitive to this range and is the only group attaching to an attachment body of simple shape. Much more work is needed to clear up the exact nature of these vibrations; the laser beam should also be focused on the different parts of the Müller organ, so that it can be seen whether or not it moves as a unit.

8. Conclusions

The locust ear is able to discriminate sound frequencies. The physical basis of this ability is two sets of resonances, corresponding to the circularly symmetrical modes of the thin part and of the entire tympanum, respectively. The receptor cells attach to four different cuticular bodies. Their selectivity has several causes. The two sets of vibrations are located in different areas of the membrane, but their positions change with frequency. Furthermore, the vibrations are often spatially concentrated, and the two sets of vibrations can interact. The attachment areas of the receptor cells are a (or some) hundred µm apart, so they experience quite different vibrations in the direction perpendicular to the membrane. A group of receptors may also avoid responding to a certain vibration by attaching near one or more nodal lines.

The present working hypothesis on the function of the Müller organ is the following: It is sensitive not only to vibrations perpendicular to the membrane, but also to vibrations (variations in tensile strain) in the plane of the tympanum. This behavior is similar to that of a spider sitting at the border of its web, and it may turn out to be a sort of vectorial analysis. This idea explains why the Müller organ, situated near the border of the membrane, can detect vibrations far away on the membrane. It also explains most of the anatomical peculiarities of the Müller organ. However, the Müller organ is not a passive observer of the membrane vibrations. It goes into vigorous vibrations with both perpendicular and parallel orientation to the plane of the membrane. These vibrations may well turn out to play an important role in the function of the ear as a frequency analyzer.

Acknowledgements

The recent experiments reported were supported by grants from NATO and Statens naturvidenskabelige Forskningsraad. Mr. Buchhave, M. Sc. (DISA Elektronik) kindly placed the laser-vibratometer at my disposal and assisted in the experiments.

References

Gray, E.G. (1960). The fine structure of the insect ear. Phil. Trans. B 243, 75-94.

Michelsen, A. (1966). Pitch discrimination in the locust ear: observations on single sense cells. J. Insect Physiol. 12, 1119-1131.

Michelsen, A. (1971 a). The physiology of the locust ear. I. Frequency sensitivity of single cells in the isolated ear. Z. Vergl. Physiol. 71, 49-62.

Michelsen, A. (1971 b). The physiology of the locust ear. II. Frequency discrimination based upon resonances in the tympanum. Z. Vergl. Physiol. 71, 63-101.

Michelsen, A. (1971 c). The physiology of the locust ear. III. Acoustical properties of the intact ear. Z. Vergl. Physiol. 71, 102-128.

Popov, A.V. (1965). Electrophysiological studies on peripheral auditory neurons in the locust. J. Evol. Biochem. Physiol. 1, 239-250.

Schwabe, J. (1960). Beiträge zur Morphologie und Histologie der tympanalen Sinnesapparate der Orthopteren. Zoologica 20, 1-154.

DISCUSSION

DAVIS: I should like to look at this from the point of view of the nerve. I feel certain intuitively that setting up the nerve impulse in the ear you have studied is very much like exciting a pacinian corpuscle. There must be some dendritic termination that is sensitive to deformation. In order to get deformation, there must be a differential movement of some sort, corresponding to what in the mammalian ear is provided by the tectorial membrane and reticular lamina, the relative movement between them, and the bending of cilia. What do you know about the stiffness of your organ as a whole? Are the different parts attached quite firmly to one another like malleus and inclus in the middle ear? It is really differential movement between the points of attachment that you should examine. You have given a beautiful description of the vibration as a whole, but how does it produce deformation in the nerve terminals?

MICHELSEN: The vibration of the Müller-organ certainly suggests that we should look at relative movement of the receptor cells and not only at the absolute movement of their dendrites. From direct measurements of the stiffness we know that there is not much difference in the compliance of different parts of the membrane (see Michelsen, 1971a). However, the anatomy of three of the attachment bodies is very complex (Fig. 2). We do not know anything about their stiffness and their freedom of motion relative to each other. I hope that we can use the new laser vibrometer to make direct measurements of the freedom of motion, but this will be a rather difficult experiment to do.

GRIFFIN: How much effect does the removal of the whole structure from the insect's body have on the mechanical properties of the membrane? Have you made some comparisons with the mechanical situation when at least the thorax of the insect is still there?

MICHELSEN: The membrane is surrounded by a cuticular rim, which is very solid at most of the circumference of the tympanum, but fairly weak at the ventral-anterior corner. Thus, the mechanics of the membrane may change, when it is cut out. However, the resonance frequencies remain almost the same, so there does not appear to be any drastic change in the mechanics. The main difference between the isolated and intact ear is in the acoustical conditions, i.e. in the magnitude of the driving force and in the acoustic impedance of the membrane acoustics of the intact system are so complicated that we are forced to work on the isolated system, if we want to separate the acoustical and mechanical parameters of the system.

GRIFFIN: Could I elaborate that question a little bit? I should think these optical methods would let you check as to whether you were getting at least the main properties the same as in the intact insect.

MICHELSEN: Yes, we can do it now by means of the new laser vibrometer, and we certainly are going to do these experiments.

STEELE: The design of this system is interesting. It has been known for a long time that a stretched membrane would be very poor as the basilar membrane in the cochlea. In contrast a plate instead of a stretched membrane for this system would be undesirable, since the natural frequencies would be too dense. How did you determine that, is there tension in the membrane?

MICHELSEN: In this system there are two sets of resonances, so the natural frequencies are rather dense. I measured the compliance by driving a transducer against the membrane. On the basis of this measurement I calculated the effective tension.

STEELE: Yes, but this assumes that it does have tension. Did you establish that it is under tension?

MICHELSEN: If you cut a slit in the tympanum, the hole adopts the shape of a convex lens, so the membrane is under tension. It is physically speaking a "membrane" and not a plate, since free tympana are quite lose ("flabby").

STEELE: One more question, what is the relative mass between the body and the membrane?

MICHELSEN: The mass of the Müller organ (the "body") is about 35 micrograms and that of the thin membrane about 10 micrograms. The "effective mass" of the membrane varies somewhat with the acoustical conditions, because it is composed of a real mass and the reactive component of the radiation impedance.

SCHWARTZKOPPF: I was very much surprised to see how close some of the results we got in the second and third order neuron resemble your findings about changes of phase relations within the tympanic displacements. There is a Figure in a paper of Dr. Kalmring in which the oblique ascent of responses from low frequency to high equals the phase lag curve you gave. And there is another type of unit in Kalmring's paper in which the phase influences producing 2 maxima are represented by the behavior of single units in the ventral cord. I think there apparently is a very close relation.

MICHELSEN: The frequency sensitivity of the second of third order neurons reflects that of the primary receptor cells. However, the frequency analysis of the locust ear is based upon the occurrence of maxima of vibration amplitude, and not upon an exploration of the phase relationships. So, I do not think that your interpretation is correct.

Reference:

Kalmring, K. (1971). Akustische neuronen im unterschlundganglion der wanderheuschrecke Locusta migratoria. Z. Vergl. Physiol. 72, 95-110.

SUBJECT INDEX

A

Acetylcholine, released in olivocochlear nerve fibers, 396
Acoustico-lateralis system, *see* lateral line system
Acoustic trauma, 249-251
Adaptation, 334, 638, 653, 656, 660-662, 691, 800, *see also* temporary threshold shift
Adequate sound stimuli, 623-673
  segmentation in time, 625-631
  spectral characteristics of, 625-627
  time-dependent features of, 623-673
  time structure, 628
Aging, effect of in "region of best response" *see* death, effect of in basilar membrane response
Amplitude modulated sounds, coding of, 593-619
Anoxia, *see* cochlear microphonics, effects of oxygen shortage on
Anteroventral nucleus, 511-517
Antibiotics, cochleotoxic, 128, 242-252
Asymmetrical neurons, 704-707
  excitatory areas of, 704-707
  lateral inhibition of, 704
ATP-ase activity, 438-442, 444-445

B

Backward masking, 813-816
Basilar membrane
  location of maximum vibration amplitude along, 423
  morphology of, 125-183, 423-424
Basilar membrane motion, 336, 338, 340, 348-349, 352, 356-357, 361-366, 426, 434, 443, 520-531, *see also* phenomena, nonlinear review of

dc effects of, 101-104
nonlinear model for, 579
nonlinearities in, 523-527
Basilar membrane, observations of mechanical disturbances along, *see* fuzziness detection
Bats, *see also* feature extraction in auditory system of
  echolocation in, *see* echolocation
  frequency discrimination in, 702-703
Behavior, *see also* echolocation
  hunting behavior, bats, 668
  relation to auditory system, 624
Binaural hearing, cortical mechanisms in, *see* cortical mechanisms in binaural hearing
Binaural neural interaction, 779
Bioaccoustical pulse trains, 667-669
Biological sounds, *see* natural sounds
Body movement, effect of in neural recording, 753, 769
Bullfrog
  components of croak of, 721
  reception of croak of, 676, 723-724
Bushy cell, 480, 482-485

C

Calyx of held, 488-9, 491
Central auditory neurons, 696-699
  excitatory area of, 697-699
  functional organization of, 623-673
  impulse-count, function of, 699
  inhibitory areas of, 697-699
Central masking, 788-808
  binaural activity in, 792, 793, 800, 803
  calculated and empirical data, comparison of, 796-802
  decay, 790-791, 798-799, 807-808
  driven neural firing rate in, 793-796, 798-799, 803

935

SUBJECT INDEX

linearity in, 803-804
  manifestation of, defined, 788
  psychophysiological theory of, 792-796
  steady-state conditions, 788-791, 800-802
  theoretical tuning curves, 796-797
  transient conditions, 788-792, 799-802
Characteristic frequency, definition of, 563
Chopper pattern neurons, 461-466, 469-476, 505
Click, detection of, 829, 836-842, 846
Clicks
  as echolocation and orientation sounds in cetaceans, 853
  latency of responses to, 461-464
Cocaine, effect of, 315
Cochlea, physiology of, correlated to cochlear pathology, 251-253
Cochlear hair cells, pathology of, 235-256
  correlated to cochlear physiology, 251-253
  method for study of, 237
  morphology of, 236-256
Cochlear hydrodynamics, see hydrodynamics
Cochlear mechanics, three periods of research on, 119-121
Cochlear microphonics, 260-264, 279-288, 293, 305, 529, see cochlear potentials
  definitions of CM+ and CM−, 427
  dependence of temperature in, 424, 435-437, 441, 444-445
  effects of biochemicals on, 425, 437-440, 444-445
    cyanide poisoning, 425, 437-438, 444-445
    ouabain, 438-440, 444-445
  effects of oxygen shortage on, 427-437
    latency period, 430-431
    time course of, 429-435
Cochlear models, 11-44, 45, 69-81, 261, 527-530, 541
  as mechanisms to explain cochlear sharpening, 527, 541
  correlations with physiological data, 75-81
  displacement modes of organ of Corti, 70-72
  eddies, 82, 93
  phase integral solution, 73-75
  plate strip in infinite fluid, 72-73

Cochlear nerve fiber
  characteristic frequency of, 524
  two tone suppression in, 527, 541, 553
Cochlear nonlinearities, 11-41, 540, 542
Cochlear nucleus
  responses of, 455-478
  units, dynamic properties of, methods to investigate, 597-609
Cochlear potentials, 335-376, see also nonlinearity
  cochlear microphonics, 335-376, 423-452
  distortion processes, 356-363, 366
  effect of olivocochlear efferents, 377-421
  inner versus outer hair cells, 349-356, 365, 373, 375
  summating potential, 77, 84, 86, 92, 335-337, 346-348, 363-364, 375
  tuning curves (CM and SP) 336, 346-348
Cochlear receptor
  innervation of, see organ of Corti, innervation of
  morphology of, 185-234, 235-256, 273-306
Cochlear sharpening, see frequency sharpening
Combination tones, 527, 531, 565, 576, 582
Complex aural beats, 12, 24, 39-40
Complex periodic sound, responses to, 512-515
Complex sounds, 720-722, see also bioacoustical pulse trains
  hyper-complex neurons, 724
  neurons responding to only 722-725
Cortical fields, 750-752
Cortical mechanisms in binaural hearing, 758-763
Cues
  direction, 758
  distance, 758
Cyanide, see cochlear microphonics, effects of biochemicals on
Cytoarchitectonic approach in systematic analysis of auditory nuclei, 494

D

Dale's law, 496
Deafness, genetic inducement of, 237-241

Death, effect of
  in basilar membrane response, 105-111,
    see also listings under post-mortem
  on basilar membrane tuning, see post-
    mortem cochlear mechanics
Doppler shift, measurements in locust ear,
  927-929, 932-933
d-tubocurarine, effect of on cochlear
  potentials, 390-421

E

Echolocation, 678, 849-892
  adaptations of pulse repetition rate in,
    856-857
  discrimination between similar targets,
    875-876
  discriminative training, 876-879
  Doppler compensation, 868-870, 879,
    890
  in bats, 850-851, 855-879, 890-892
  in birds, 851
Echolocation
  in humans, 854-855
  in porpoises, 852, 856, 866
  in whales, 852, 856
  neurophysiological adaptations for, 866
  of flying insects, 857-860, 891
  off responses of CW bats, 870-871
  orientation sounds
    comparative morphology of, 860-866
    sensitivity reduction during emission
      of, 867-868
  phylogenetic range of, 850-855
  relationship to other sensory channels,
    855-856
  sensitivity and acuity in, 872-875
Eddies, cochlear, 11, 32-41, 45-47
  as result of basilar membrane motion, 47
Efferent crossed . . . nucleus, 773-784
  frequency function, 777-779
  intensity function, 777-779
  latency, 776
  pure tones applied, 775
Efferent inhibition of activity in primary
  auditory neurons, 394
Efferent system, 261-262, 377-421, see
  efferent fibers, action of

Eighth nerve, 265, 336, 356, 359, 361-362,
  366, 797-803, 807, 797-803, 825
  effect of removal of on basilar membrane
    tuning, 58 60
Elongate cell, 488
Endocochlear DC potential, (EP), 427,
  432-433, 439-442
Excitation, psychoacoustic, see temporal
  effects in psychoacoustic excitation

F

Fatigue, see temporary threshold shift
Feature extraction in auditory system of
  bats, 675-744
  assumptions for, 680-682
  "feature detectors," definition of, 681
Fish, see also lateral line system
  impulses from saccular neurons of, 676
  measurements from lateral line organs of,
    273-306
Flaxedil, 393
FM–specialized neurons, 707-714
  absence of excitatory area, 710
Forward masking, 813-818
Frequency analysis in locust ear, see locust
  ear
Frequency selectivity, 464-467, see also
  temporal effects in psychoacoustic
  excitation
Frequency selectivity of cochlea, 519-546
  broad frequency selectivity: relation to
    broad tuning curves, 519, 523, 527
  "extra filtering," 526
  mechanical and neural: comparisons of,
    519-527
  Mössbauer techniques in, 519-520
  neural and psychophysical, comparisons
    of, 542-545
  variations in, among species, 527
Frequency sharpening, evidence for "second
  filter," 527-535
  nature of second filter, 532-542
Frequency threshold curves 519-546, see
  also tuning curves
  acoustic grating stimulus in testing,
    535-545, 553
  gated tonal stimuli in determination of,
    520

pathological: similarity to basilar membrane response, 523
treated as a linear filter, 532-535
Fuzziness detection, 95-117

G

GABA, 392
Gentamicin, effect of, 293, see also corticotoxic antibiotics
Glossopharyngeal nerve, 323-325, 330
Glycin chloride, effect on cochlear potentials, 392

H

Hair cells, see also cochlear hair cells
development of, 294-298
in acoustico-lateralis system of fish, 893, 909
physiology of individual, 273-306
efferent fibers, action of, 287-294, 303-305
efferent synaptic transmission, 286-287
electrical excitability, 279-280
electrical properties and responses, 274-276
membrane potential and resistance, 276-278
receptor potential, 278-286, 290, 303
time constant, 278-279
Hearing, specialized, see specialized hearing in animals
Hemicholinicum effect on cochlear potentials, 391
Hydrodynamic principles (in cochlear mechanics), 11-47, 552
capillary waves, 14-18
gravity waves, 14-18
interface waves, 38-40
surface waves, 11, 14-21, 30-31
traveling waves, 11, 13, 20-31

I

Inferior colliculus, development of in echolocating bats, 890

Information bearing elements in animal sounds, 675-744
delivery of, 686-690
excitatory area, definition of, 690-691
in bullfrog's croak, 676
in echolocation, 678-680, 696, 702, 703, 725
in human speech sonograms, 676-678
in orientation sounds, 678-681, 702-703, 710-711, 718, 722
in saccular neurons of fish, 676
Inhibition, see also efferent system
Inhibition in cochlear nucleus, 487-489, 495
Inhibition in hair cells, 291-292, 303-304
Inhibition, lateral, 535-538
Inhibitory tones, dynamic properties of compared to excitatory tones, 609-615
Injury, effect of on cochlear response patterns, 108-110
Integration, see minimum integration time
Interface wares, see hydrodynamics
Intracochlear potentials, see cochlear potentials
Ionic receptive mechanism in acoustico-lateralis system, see lateral line system

K

Kanamycin, 64, 92, 268-269, 336-338, 349, 352-354, 362, 365, 374, 545, see also antibiotics, cochleotoxic
Kinocilium, 423, 426, 443
displacement of sensory hair cells toward, 12

L

Labyrinth organ of vertebrates, compared to lateral line system, 423-424, 426
Lagena, 423
Lasers, see fuzziness detection
Latency in response to clicks, see clicks
Lateral line organ, see also fish, measurements from lateral line organs of
Lateral-line system, 307-334, see also labyrinth organ chemical stimulation of, 309-330, 334

electrical stimulation of, 307, 316-317
mechanical stimulation of, 308-310, 317-319, 325
Locust ear
  anatomy of, 913
  best frequencies for, 917-918
  frequency discrimination of, 913-915, 930
  mechanism for frequency discrimination of, 923-926
  in vibrations, 915-923
  illustrated, 920-922
  mechanics of, 911-934
  Müller organ's role in, 926-930, 932-934
  vibration centers of, 919, 930

M

Masking, see central masking, monaural masking, backward masking, forward masking
  Huffman sequences used in studies of, 832
Menieres disease, 47, 267
Metabolism, dependence of inner ear potentials in lower vertebrates upon, see cochlear microphonics
Minimum integration time, 829-846
  as function of frequency, 832-835, 842
  critical masking interval in investigation of, 839-841, 842
  definition of, 830
  temporal modulation transfer function in investigation of, 835-839, 842
"Mistuned consonances," see complex aural beats
Monaural masking, 789, 791, 792, 793
Mössbauer effect, 49-67
  Doppler phenomenon, 49
Müller organ, 915, 926-930, 932-934

N

Natural sounds, features of, 624-629
  cue for distance, 629
  movement of sound source, 629
Neural analysis of amplitude modulated sounds, 725-731
  attenuation, 731, 744

Neural coding at higher levels, 623-784
Neural network models illustrated, 700, 706, 708
Neurons, classification of single in terms of responses to information-bearing elements, 682-685
  asymmetrical neurons, 683
  impulse-count function, 683
  in table, 684
  in terms of directional sensitivity or binaural interaction, 685
  in terms of recovery cycles, 685
  phasic units, 685
  symmetrical neurons, 683
  tonic units, 685
Neurons, patterns of single in auditory cortex of monkey, 745-772
  best frequencies, 746, 748, 758-759
  excitability of, 753
  gradient in responsiveness, 750
  response properties of, 752
  spike-count and SPL, 753-757
Noise modulated sounds, responses to, 602-609
Noise specialized neurons, 714-715
Nonlinear behavior of auditory nerve fibers, 512-517
Nonlinear phenomena, review of, 558-576
  combination click stimulation, 569-576
  single click stimulation, 565-582
  single tone stimulation, 558-564, 576-582
  two tone stimulation, 564-565, 579-582
Nonlinear response properties of single cochlear nerve fibers, 555-591
Nonlinearity, 53-62, 65-66, 337, 345, 356-357, 363-365
Nonlinearity, cochlear, 11-47
  amplitude-dependent, 39-41
  amplitude-independent, 39-41
Nonlinearity, essential, 529-531
Nonlinearity in hydrodynamics, 556
Nonlinearity, in sinusoidally amplitude modulated tones, 597-602

O

Octopus cell, 481, 484-487, 493-494
"Off" response, 489

Olivocochlear inhibition, *see* efferent
  systems
"On" pattern, 471, 478, 505
"On" response of octopus cell, 487, 494
Organ of Corti, 251, 260, 277-286, 423,
  438
  antibiotic injury of, 244-248
  genetic injury in, 237-241
  innervation of, 185-234
    afferent nerve supply of, 196-205,
      210, 215, 219, 221, 224
    efferent nerve supply of, 185-199,
      205, 224, 233
    inhibitory action of efferents on
      afferent nerve fibers, 224
    role of outer hair cell system in,
      223-225
    spiral ganglion cells, behavior of,
      206-214, 216-218, 220-221,
      224-225, 232
    types of nerve fibers participating in,
      186
  normal, morphology of, 125-183
    sensory cells, 126-132
      inner hair cells, 126-129
      outer hair cells, 127, 129-132
    supporting cells, 132-137
      Deiters' cells, 134-135
      Hensen cells, 135
      inner border cells, 133
      inner phalangeal cells, 134
      pillar cells, 134
Organon spirale, *see* organ of Corti
Orientation behavior, *see* echolocation
Orientation sounds, 678
Ototoxic antibiotics, *see* antibiotics,
  cochleotoxic
Ouabain, *see* cochlear microphonics, effects
  of biochemicals on
Oxygen shortage, effects on cochlear
  microphonics, *see* cochlear micro-
  phonics, effects of oxygen shortage on

P

Pacinian corpuscle, 259-260
Papilla basilaris, 423-424, 434, 442
  afferent nervous supply of, 424

"Pauser" pattern, 471-476, 505-506
Peripheral auditory neurons, 691-696
  adaptation in, 691
  excitatory area in, 691-694
  inhibitory area in, 691-694, 696
  post-stimulus time histograms of,
    691-696
  tuning curve of, 694
peripheral sensory mechanisms, *see* hair
  cells, physiology of individual
Phase-locked response, 511-515
Phonemes in animals, 723, *see also* sonograms
  sonograms
Pinna, role in human localization, 826-827
Pit organs, 309-310, 312, 321, 325
Pitch discrimination, 251-253
Post-mortem cochlear mechanics, 49-67
Potentials, in inner ear of lower vertebrates,
  see cochlear microphonics
Psychoacoustic characteristics, physiological
  correlates of, 787-808

R

Recruitment of loudness, 267-269
Reticular laminar flaw, 81-86
  nonlinearity, source of, 82-83
  viscous flaw between parallel plates,
    83-86

S

Saccular microphonic, 896-902, 909-910
Sensory behavior, *see* psychoacoustic
  characteristics
Short tone burst stimuli, responses to,
  467-475, 506
Signal detection theory, 877-878, 891
Signal transformation, 489
Sinusoidal amplitude modulated tones,
  responses to, 632-667
  optimal rates, 664-666, *see also*
    adaptation
Sinusoidal modulated tones, responses to,
  594-602
Sinusoidally modulated white noise bursts,
  responses to, 632-667

SUBJECT INDEX

Sleep, effect of on neuron discharge, 753, 771
Specialized hearing in animals, 849-934
Spiral ganglion cells, see organ of Corti, innervation of
Stellate cell, 480, 482-483, 488, see also octopus cell
Steven's power law, 792
Strychnine hydrochloride, effect of cochlear potentials, 390-421
Sub-tectorial membrane fluid motion, 69-93
Summating potential, 427, 429, 433-434, 436, 442-444, 452
 origin of, 40
Superior olivary complex, responses of, 455-478, 508
Superior temporal plane, tonotopic organization of, 745-752
Swimbladder, in hearing, 893-910
 acoustical properties of cod swimbladder, 902-906
 as displacement amplifier, 899
 in fish with bladder-ear connection, 894-895
 in fish without bladder-ear connection, 895-902
Synaptic organization in auditory nervous system, see auditory nervous system

T

Taste organ, 321, 323-325, 328
Tectorial membrane, 351, 362
Tegmentum vasculosum, 424-425, 433, 439, 441-442
Telephone principle, 913-914
Temperature, effect of on basilar membrane tuning, 56

Temporal effects in psycho-acoustic excitation, 809-827
 critical durations, 819-821, 826
 periodical change, 816-818
 quick change, 813-816
 slow changes, 811-813
 statistical change, 818-819
Temporal window, see minimum integration time
Temporary threshold shift, 262-263
Tetrodotoxin (TTX) effect of, 312-315
 on cochlear potentials, 390-421
Threshold duration shift following different stimuli, 638
Threshold shift, see temporary threshold shift
Trapezoidal body, 490-491
Triangularly modulated clicks, responses to, 632-667
 optimal rate, 664-666, see also adaptation
Two $f_1 - f_2$, see cochlear potentials and distortion processes
Two-tone inhibition (or suppression), 564, 580, 694
Tympanal organ in locust illustrated, 912-934

V

von Bekesy, George, biography, 3-9

W

Water response, 327-329
Weberian ossicles, 894-895
White noise, in measurement of temporal effects, 818-819